Handbook of
The Psychology of Aging

The Handbooks of Aging
Consisting of Three Volumes

Critical comprehensive reviews of
research knowledge, theories, concepts, and issues

Editor-in-Chief
James E. Birren

Handbook of the Biology of Aging
Edited by Edward J. Masoro and Steven N. Austad

Handbook of the Psychology of Aging
Edited by James E. Birren and K. Warner Schaie

Handbook of Aging and the Social Sciences
Edited by Robert H. Binstock and Linda K. George

Handbook of
The Psychology of Aging
Sixth Edition

Editors
James E. Birren and K. Warner Schaie

Associate Editors
Ronald P. Abeles, Margaret Gatz,
and Timothy A. Salthouse

AMSTERDAM • BOSTON • HEIDELBERG • LONDON
NEW YORK • OXFORD • PARIS • SAN DIEGO
SAN FRANCISCO • SINGAPORE • SYDNEY • TOKYO

ELSEVIER

Academic Press is an imprint of Elsevier

Cover photo credit: © *Corbis*

Elsevier Academic Press
30 Corporate Drive, Suite 400, Burlington, MA 01803, USA
525 B Street, Suite 1900, San Diego, California 92101-4495, USA
84 Theobald's Road, London WC1X 8RR, UK

This book is printed on acid-free paper. ∞

Library of Congress Cataloging-in-Publication Data
Handbook of the psychology of aging / editors, James E. Birren, K. Warner Schaie ;
associate editors, Ronald P. Abeles, Margaret Gatz, Timothy A. Salthouse.-- 6th ed.
     p. cm. -- (The handbooks of aging)
   Includes bibliographical references and indexes.
   ISBN 0-12-101264-6 (casebound : alk. paper) -- ISBN 0-12-101265-4 (pbk. : alk. paper)
1. Aging--Psychological aspects. I. Title: Psychology of aging. II. Birren, James E. III.
Schaie, K. Warner (Klaus Warner), 1928- IV. Abeles, Ronald P., 1944- V. Gatz,
Margaret. VI. Salthouse, Timothy A. VII. Series.
   BF724.55.A35H36 2005
   155.67--dc22

                                                2005025193

British Library Cataloguing-in-Publication Data
A catalogue record for this book is available from the British Library.

ISBN 13: 978-0-12-101264-9 (casebound)
ISBN 10: 0-12-101264-6 (casebound)

ISBN 13: 978-0-12-101265-6 (paperback)
ISBN 10: 0-12-101265-4 (paperback)

For all information on all Elsevier Academic Press publications
visit our Web site at www.books.elsevier.com

PRINTED IN THE UNITED STATES OF AMERICA
05 06 07 08 09 10   9 8 7 6 5 4 3 2 1

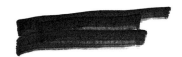

Contents

Part One
Concepts, Theory, and Methods in the Psychology of Aging

Part Two
Biological and Social Influences on Aging and Behavior

Part Three
Behavioral Processes and Aging

Part Four
Complex Behavioral Concepts and Processes in Aging

Contributors

Numbers in parentheses indicate the page number on which the author's contribution begins.

Ronald P. Abeles, National Institutes of Health, Office of Behavioral and Social Sciences Research, Bethesda, Maryland 20892–9205

Carolyn M. Aldwin (85), Department of Human Development & Family Sciences, Oregon State University Corvallis, Oregon 97330

James E. Birren (477), UCLA Center on Aging, Los Angeles, California 90095-6980

Gerard Brugman (445), University of Utrecht, De Uithof, Utrecht, The Netherlands

Laura Carstensen (343), Department of Psychology, Stanford University, Stanford, California 94305

Stanley J. Colcombe (57), Department of Psychology, Beckman Institute, University of Illinois at Urbana-Champaign, Champaign, Illinois 61820

Jennifer Dave (407), University of Southern California, Department of Psychology, Los Angeles, California 90089

Monica Fabiani (57), Department of Psychology, Beckman Institute, University of Illinois at Urbana-Champaign, Champaign, Illinois 61801

Geoff R. Fernie (425), Toronto Rehabilitation Institute, University Centre, Toronto, Ontario, Canada M5G 2A2

Margaret Gatz, Department of Psychology, University of Southern California, Los Angeles, California 90089-1061

Paul W. Griffin (363), Assistant Professor of Psychology Pace University Pleasantville, New York 10570

Alan Hartley (183), Scripps College, Claremont, California 91711

Thomas M. Hess (379), Department of Psychology, North Carolina State University, Raleigh, North Carolina 27695-7650

Scott M. Hofer (15), Department of Human Development and Family Studies, Pennsylvania State University, University Park, Pennsylvania 16802

William J. Hoyer (209), Department of Psychology, Syracuse University, Syracuse, New York 13244

Brian Kaskie (407), University of Iowa, Health Management and Policy, Iowa City, Iowa 52242

Bob G. Knight (407), Andrus Gerontology Center, University of Southern California, Los Angeles, California 90089-0191

Arthur F. Kramer (57), Department of Psychology, Beckman Institute, University of Illinois at Urbana-Champaign, Champaign, Illinois 61820

Neal Krause (499), Dept. of Hlth. Beh. and Hlth. Educ., The University of Michigan, Ann Arbor, Michigan 48109-2029

Shu-Chen Li (288), Center for Lifespan Psychology, Max Planck Institute for Human Development, D-14195 Berlin, Germany

Leah Light (261), Department of Psychology, Pitzer College, Claremont, California 91711

Ulman Lindenberger (289), Center for Lifespan Psychology, Max Planck Institute for Human Development, D-14195 Berlin, Germany

Jennifer Margrett (315), Department of Psychology, West Virginia University, Morgantown, West Virginia 26506-6040

Michael Marsiske (315), Department of Clinical and Health Psychology, University of Florida, Gainesville, Florida 32610-0165

Mara Mather (343), University of California, Santa Cruz, Department of Psychology, Santa Cruz, California 95064

Bonnie Meyer (233), Educational Psychology, Pennsylvania State University, University Park, Pennsylvania 16802

Joseph A. Mikels (343), Department of Psychology, Stanford University, Stanford, California 94305

Daniel K. Mroczek (363), Purdue University, Center on Aging & the Life Course, Department of Child Development & Family Studies West Lafayette, Indiana 47907-2055

Karl M. Newell (163), College of Health and Human Development, Pennsylvania State University, University Park, Pennsylvania 16802

Crystal L. Park (85), Department of Psychology, University of Connecticut, Storrs, Connecticut 06269-1020

Carlee K. Pollard (233), Educational and School Psychology and Special Education, Pennsylvania State University, University Park, Pennsylvania 16802

Michaela Riediger (288), Center for Lifespan Psychology, Max Planck Institute for Human Development, D-14195 Berlin Germany

Timothy A. Salthouse (3), Department of Psychology, University of Virginia, Charlottesville, Virginia 22904

K. Warner Schaie, Department of Human Development and Family Studies, Department of Psychology, and Gerontology Center, The Pennsylvania State University, State College, Pennsylvania 16801

Rick J. Scheidt (105), School of Family Studies & Human Services, Kansas State University, Manhattan, Kansas 66506

Frank Schieber (129), University of South Dakota, Heimstra Human Factors Laboratories, Vermillion, South Dakota 57069-2390

Johannes J. F. Schroots (477), 1000 GC Amsterdam, The Netherlands

Charles T. Scialfa (425), University of Calgary, Department of Psychology, Calgary, Alberta, Canada T2N 1N4

Gia Robinson Shurgot (407), Andrus Gerontology Center, University of Southern California, Los Angeles, California 90089-0191

Martin Sliwinski (15), Syracuse University, Department of Psychology, Syracuse, New York 13244

Jacob J. Sosnoff (163), University of Illinois at Urbana-Champaign, Urbana, Illinois 61801

Avron Spiro, III (85, 363), VA Boston Healthcare System and Boston University Schools of Public Health and Dental Medicine, Boston, Massachusetts 02130

Robert Thornton (261), Linguistics and Cognitive Science, Pomona College, Claremont, California 91711

David E. Vaillancourt (163), Department of Movement Sciences, University of Illinois at Chicago, College of Applied Health Sciences, Chicago, Illinois 60608

Paul Verhaeghen (209), Department of Psychology, Syracuse University, Syracuse, New York 13244

George Vogler (41), Pennsylvania State University, Center for Developmental and Health Genetics, University Park, Pennsylvania 16802

Paul G. Windley (105), University of Idaho-Moscow, Architecture Department, Moscow, Idaho 83844-2451

Foreword

This volume is one of a series of three handbooks on aging: *Handbook of the Biology of Aging, Handbook of the Psychology of Aging,* and *Handbook of Aging and the Social Sciences. The Handbooks of Aging* series, now in its sixth edition, reflects the exponential growth of research and publications in aging research, as well as the growing interest in the subject of aging. Stimulation of research on aging by government and private foundation sponsorship has been a major contributor to the growth of publications. There has also been an increase in the number of university and college courses related to aging. *The Handbooks of Aging* have helped to organize courses and seminars on aging by providing knowledge bases for instruction and for new steps in research.

The Handbooks are used by academic researchers, graduate students, and professionals, for access and interpretation of contemporary research literature about aging. They serve both as a reference and as organizational tool for integrating a wide body of research that is often cross disciplinary. *The Handbooks* not only provide updates about what is known about the many processes of aging, but also interpretations of findings by well informed and experienced scholars in many disciplines. Aging is a complex process of change involving influences of a biological, behavioral, social, and environmental nature.

Understanding aging is one of the major challenges facing science in the 21st century. Interest in research on aging has become a major focus in science and in the many professions that serve aging populations. Growth of interest in research findings about aging and their interpretation has been accelerated with the growth of populations of older persons in developed and developing countries. As more understanding has been gained about genetic factors that contribute to individual prospects for length of life and life limiting and disabling diseases, researchers have simultaneously become more aware of the environmental factors that modulate the expression of genetic predispositions. These *Handbooks* both reflect and encourage an ecological view of aging, in which aging is seen as a result of diverse forces interacting. These *Handbooks* can help to provide information to guide planning as nations face "age quakes" due to shifts in the size of their populations of young and older persons.

In addition to the rise in research publications about aging, there has been a dramatic change in the availability of scientific literature since the first editions of *The Handbooks of Aging* were published. There are now millions of references available on line. This increases the need for integration of information. *The Handbooks* help to encourage integration of information from across disciplines and methods of gathering data about aging.

With so much new information available, one of the editorial policies has been the selection of new chapter authors and subject matter in each successive edition. This allows *The Handbooks* to present new points of view, to keep current, and to explore new topics in which new research has emerged. The sixth edition is thus virtually wholly new, and is not simply an update of previous editions.

I want to thank the editors of the individual volumes for their cooperation, efforts, and wisdom in planning and reviewing the chapters. Without their intense efforts and experience *The Handbooks* would not be possible. I thank Edward J. Masoro and Steven N. Austad, editors of the *Handbook of the Biology of Aging*; the editors of the *Handbook of Aging and the Social Sciences*, Robert H. Binstock and Linda K. George, and their associate editors, Stephen J. Cutler, Jon Hendrick, and James H. Schultz; and my co-editor of the *Handbook of the Psychology of Aging*, K. Warner Schaie, and the associate editors, Ronald P. Abeles, Margaret Gatz, and Timothy A. Salthouse.

I also want to express my appreciation to Nikki Levy, Publisher at Elsevier, whose experience, long term interest, and cooperation have facilitated the publication of *The Handbooks* through their many editions.

James E. Birren

Preface

The *Handbook of the Psychology of Aging* provides a basic reference source on the behavioral processes of aging for researchers, graduate students, and professionals. It also provides perspectives for personnel from other disciplines.

This sixth edition of the *Handbook* reflects the growing volume of literature about adult development and aging. The research literature on the psychology of aging continues to expand rapidly reflecting both the rising interest of the scientific community but also the needs of a growing older population. The growth of the research literature provides opportunities to replace chronological age as a convenient index to behavior changes with variables that are inherently causal and have the potential for control or modification. Academic interests and public interests are contributing to the emergence of the psychology of aging as a major subject in universities and research institutions. Issues of the psychology of aging touch upon many features of daily life, from the workplace and family life to policy matters of retirement, health care, social security and pensions. People are living much longer and living more active lives than they did in the early days of the 20th century when child psychology emerged as a research and teaching specialty.

The psychology of aging is complex and many new questions are being raised about how behavior is organized and how it changes over the course of life. Increasingly, results of longitudinal studies are providing insights into the causal factors in behavior changes associated with adult development and aging. They are contributing to understanding the role of behavior changes in relation to biological, health, and social interactions. Parallel advances in methodology are making it possible to study in greater detail, patterns and sub-patterns of behavior over the life span.

Facing the rapid growth in literature, the editors have had to make choices about what new topics to include in the handbook. Growth in research activity is not uniform and notable increases may be seen in neuropsychology, cognitive psychology and behavioral genetics, in relation to aging. Some topics covered in earlier editions of the *Handbook* are not included in the present edition. For this reason readers are advised to consult earlier volumes both for data and for interpretations. The previous editions should be consulted for a perspective on the development of the subject matter of the psychology of aging.

The editors have deliberately tried to seek new authors of chapters on established and important topics as well as authors of chapters on new topics. Thus an important feature of this edition is new topics and new authors of well established topics.

The chapters are organized into four divisions: Part I Concepts, Theory, and Methods in the Psychology of Aging; Part II Biological and Social Influences on Aging and Behavior; Part III Behavioral Processes and Aging; and Part IV Complex Behavioral Concepts and Processes in Aging.

Changes in the draft manuscripts were recommended by the review process. The draft of each chapter was reviewed by two associate editors and one of the senior editors. The senior editors thank the associate editors, Ronald P. Abeles, Margaret Gatz, and Timothy A. Salthouse for their advice about the selection of topics, authors, and their reviews of the chapter drafts. Their careful reading of the manuscripts and their detailed editorial suggestions are gratefully acknowledged. The assistance of Jenifer Hoffman in the editorial process is also gratefully acknowledged.

James E. Birren
K. Warner Schaie

About the Editors

James E. Birren

is associate director of the Center on Aging at the University of California, Los Angeles, and serves as an adjunct professor in medicine, psychiatry, and biobehavioral sciences. Dr. Birren's previous positions include serving as chief of the section on aging of the National Institute of Mental Health, founding executive director and dean of the Ethel Percy Andrus Gerontology Center of the University of Southern California, founding executive director of the Anna and Harry Borun Center for Gerontological Research at UCLA, and president of the Gerontological Society of the American, The Western Gerontological Society, and the Division on Adult Development and Aging of the American Psychological Association. His awards include the Brookdale Award for Gerontological Research, and the Sandoz Prize for Gerontological Research, and the award for outstanding contribution to gerontology by the Canadian Association of Gerontology. Authors of over 250 scholarly publications, Dr. Birren's

research interests include the causes and consequences of slowed information processing in the older nervous system and the relation of age to decision-making processes. He has developed a program of guided autobiography for research purposes and the application to groups of older adults.

K. Warner Schaie

is the Evan Pugh Professor of Human Development and Psychology at the Pennsylvania State University. He also holds an appointment as Affiliate Professor of Psychiatry and Behavioral Science at the University of Washington. He received his Ph.D. in psychology from the University of Washington, an honorary Dr. phil. from the Friedrich-Schiller University of Jena, Germany, and an honorary Sc.D. from West Virginia University, He received the Kleemeier Award for Distinguished Research Contributions from the Gerontological Society of America, the MENSA lifetime career award, and the Distinguished

Scientific Contributions award from the American Psychological Association. He is author or editor of 45 books including the textbook Adult Development and Aging (with S. L. Willis) now in its 5th edition. He has directed the Seattle Longitudinal Study of cognitive aging since 1956 and is the author of more than 250 journal articles and chapters on the psychology of aging. His current research interest is the life course of adult intelligence, its antecedents and modifiability, the early detection of risk for dementia, as well as methodological issues in the developmental sciences.

Ronald P. Abeles

is the special assistant to the director of the Office of Behavioral and Social Sciences Research in the Office of the Director, National Institutes of Health (NIH). Previously, he was the associate director for behavioral and social Research at the National Institute on Aging, NIH. He is also the chair of the NIH Coordinating committee for Behavioral and Social Sciences Research. He was the president of the Division on Adult Development and Aging of the American Psychological Association (APA) and chair of the Section on Aging and the Life Course of the American Sociological Association. Dr. Abeles is a fellow of the APA, the American Psychological Society, the Society of Behavioral Medicine, and the Gerontological Society of America. He is a recipient of the NIH Director's Award and twice the recipient of the NIH Award of Merit for "leadership and contributions to the advancement of behavioral and social research on aging" and "for the exceptional leadership in advancing a program of research to understand and apply knowledge about the relationship between psychosocial factors and

health." He has edited books or published articles and chapters on aging and social psychology, health behaviors, quality of life, sense of control and the interface between social structure and behavior.

Margaret Gatz

is the professor of psychology, gerontology, and preventive medicine at the University of Southern California and foreign adjunct professor in medical epidemiology and biostatistics at the Karolinska Institute in Stockholm, Sweden. She is a fellow of the American Psychological Association, American Psychological Society, and Gerontological Society of America. She has served as chair of the Behavioral and Social Sciences Section of the Gerontological Society of America and as associate editor of Psychology and Aging. She has been recognized by the APA Division 20 Distinguished Research Achievement Award, APA Committee on Aging Award for the Advancement of Psychology and Aging, the Master Mentor Award of the Retirement Research Foundation and Division 20, the Distinguished Mentorship Award from the Gerontological Society BSS section, and the Apple of Knowledge for important contributions to development of research through the University College of Health Sciences, Jönköping, Sweden. Her research concerns mental health issues in older adults.

Timothy A. Salthouse

is the Brown-Forman Professor of Psychology at the University of Virginia. He is a fellow of the Gerontological Society of America, the American Association for the Advancement of Science, the American Psychological Society, and Divisions 3 and 20 of the American Psychological Association. He is a former president of Division 20 (Adult Development and Aging) of the American Psychological Association, and a past editor of the journal Psychology and Aging. He has received the Distinguished Research Contribution Award from Division 20 and the William James Fellow Award from the American Psychological Society. His primary research areas are age-related effects on cognitive functioning and the role of experience and knowledge in minimizing the consequences of those effects.

Part One

Concepts, Theory, and Methods in the Psychology of Aging

One

Theoretical Issues in the Psychology of Aging

Timothy A. Salthouse

Much of the research literature in many scientific disciplines can be categorized as primarily addressing empirical, methodological, or theoretical issues. Empirical articles attempt to provide tentative answers to specific questions, methodological articles tend to focus on how to ask answerable questions, and a major goal of theoretical articles is to specify which questions are the most important to ask. The current chapter is primarily concerned with theoretical issues relevant to contemporary research in the psychology of aging, and thus it is focused more on questions than on answers. However, at the outset it is important to acknowledge that no attempt was made to be comprehensive in the coverage of theoretical issues, nor to link the material to the literature in the philosophy of science. Furthermore, the goal was not to review contemporary theories in the field of aging, but rather to stimulate consideration of a number of issues that appear to be central to theoretical speculations in the psychology of aging. Indeed, a major thesis of this chapter is that there is currently a great deal of confusion about what should be considered a psychological theory of aging, at least in part because there is little consensus with respect to the critical questions that should be addressed in order to qualify as a theory of aging. Because the author is most familiar with research on age differences in cognitive functioning, most of the examples are drawn from that research domain, but the issues are assumed to be applicable to many different domains.

At least two well-recognized advantages of theories are that they organize a great deal of information in a parsimonious manner and they serve to guide future research. One of the primary ways in which theories influence the direction of research is by identifying major issues that ultimately must be addressed by a satisfactory theory. By specifying which questions are interesting and important and, by omission, which are not, theories serve to focus research.

The focusing-of-research function is essential because a nearly infinite number of questions could be asked in most research areas, and the vast majority of them could be justified by the claim that their answers are not yet known. However, not all questions are equally important or informative, and a major role of theories

Handbook of the Psychology of Aging
Copyright © 2006 by Academic Press.

Table 1.1
Major Theoretical Questions in the Psychology of Aging

Question	Issue	Elaboration
What?	In what psychological respects do people of different ages vary?	*What* refers to the phenomenon to be explained.
When?	At what ages do the changes occur?	*When* refers to the timing of the phenomenon.
Where?	Which hypothetical aspects, theoretical components, or neuroanatomical substrates are primarily involved in the phenomenon?	*Where* refers to conceptual or neuroanatomical localization.
Why?	What is responsible for the developmental changes?	*Why* refers to the causal determinants of the phenomenon.
How?	What are the mechanisms by which the developmental changes occur?	*How* refers to the manner by which the cause exerts its effect.

is to specify which research questions are central and which are peripheral or irrelevant.

I. A Taxonomy of Major Questions

It is helpful to begin by considering a taxonomy of major questions that ultimately must be addressed by a successful theory. In addition to providing a systematic basis for evaluating theories, the taxonomy may also be useful in understanding how theories differ from one another and why it is often not feasible to make direct comparisons among theories.

The taxonomy, which is summarized in Table 1.1, conceptualizes major issues in the psychology of aging in terms of questions concerning the what, when, where, why, and how of the phenomenon of age-related differences in some aspect of behavior. Each of the questions is important because a phenomenon could be considered to be well understood, and the theory would be considered to provide a compelling explanation of the phenomenon, if all of the questions had convincing answers.

The question of *what* is clearly relevant to distinctions among theories because the answer will affect the intended scope of the theory. For example, if the theory is primarily concerned with age differences in a limited aspect of behavior, then it would probably be considered relatively narrow in scope. In contrast, if the phenomenon is defined in general terms that encompass many different types of variables, then it would be viewed as fairly broad.

How a theory answers the question of what will also determine which aspects of the phenomenon are considered primary, and perhaps somewhat analogous to the central "disease," and which are considered secondary, and possibly more analogous to "symptoms" of the disease. For example, a variable that is interpreted as representing merely one of many possible manifestations of the phenomenon of primary interest might not be considered a high priority for theory-relevant research.

Because the answer to the question of what serves to specify the primary focus of a theory, this information needs to be considered before attempting to compare two or more theories. For example, if theories differ in their answers to the question of what, comparisons among them may not be meaningful because at a fundamental level they are not addressing the same phenomenon.

To illustrate, two theories may both be concerned with adult age differences in measures of speed, and hence from a certain perspective they might be considered similar. However, one of the theories might be primarily concerned with describing the relations among reaction time measures of speed in adults of different ages (Cerella, 1990), whereas another might attempt to explain the relations between a theoretical construct of processing speed and adult age differences in a variety of measures of cognitive functioning (Salthouse, 1996). Because in the former case the answer to the what question refers to the relation among reaction times in different age groups whereas in the latter case it refers to the role of speed in age-related differences in cognitive performance, the theories are not addressing the same phenomena, and consequently it may not make sense to attempt to make direct comparisons among them.

The question of *when* is relevant to the evaluation of theories because if the theory assumes that the phenomenon begins early in adulthood, then the theorist needs to consider what can be learned by studying age differences very late in life, whereas if the theory assumes that the phenomenon begins late in life, then the relevance of observations in early adulthood needs to be considered. In other words, if a theory's answer to the question of when is very late in life, then research on young adults may not be directly relevant to the theory, but if the phenomenon is assumed to begin early in life, then research restricted to older adults may be of limited value. Whether findings from research on adults from different age ranges are relevant to the theory will therefore be determined by the theory's conceptualization of the phenomenon. Many studies compare a sample of young college students with a sample of adults between 60 and 80 years of age, others restrict their focus to adults

above a certain age, such as 50 or 70, and a few studies compare adults across a wide range of 18 to 90 or older. However, depending on the theory's answer to the question of when, it may not be meaningful to treat each of these types of data as equally applicable to the theory because, for example, changes before age 60 may not be viewed as reflecting the same phenomenon or might not be postulated to involve the same mechanisms as changes that occur after age 80.

Most of the theoretical attempts to address the question of *where* have tried to localize age-related effects within some type of conceptual or neuroanatomical model of the behavioral variable of interest. To illustrate, at least five approaches to localization have been employed by researchers investigating influences associated with increased age on aspects of cognitive functioning. In each case a number of conceptually distinct "loci" for age-related influences have been postulated, and a primary goal of the research conducted within that perspective was to determine which of the possible loci have the greatest relations to age. For example, researchers working with correlation-based structural models have attempted to localize age-related influences within models of the organization of cognitive variables such as at the level of individual variables, the level of first-order factors, or the level of higher order factors. Researchers working with componential models have attempted to localize the influences within qualitatively different processing components that are postulated to contribute to performance on the task. Theorists who have proposed stage models attempt to localize age-related influences within components that are postulated to represent an ordered sequence between input and output, such as encoding, storage, and retrieval in the case of memory. Theorists working with computational models attempt to determine which specific parameters of one or more equations intended to describe relations between hypothetical processes and observed measures of performance are most susceptible to age-related effects. Finally, researchers working within a neuroscience perspective have attempted to localize age-related influences to particular areas of the brain that are active during the performance of relevant cognitive tasks.

Although the question of where, in the form of either conceptual or neuroanatomical localization, has been the focus of a great deal of aging-related research in the area of cognitive functioning, it actually may be the least important of the major theoretical questions. The reason is that while it is clearly useful to be more precise about the exact nature of the observed differences, it is still important to know why and how a given theoretical aspect or neuroanatomical region is affected and not others. In a sense, therefore, rather than functioning as an explanation, answers to the question of where can be considered to provide a more specific level of description of the phenomenon. This is not to say that there is no value in localization research, but rather that localization primarily serves to supply a more precise characterization of exactly what needs to be explained.

Perhaps the most intuitively obvious question regarding developmental phenomena is *why* they occur. A fundamental question for any developmental phenomenon is what are the precursors or determinants of the phenomenon? The question of why is often closely linked to the question of *how* because the latter focuses on the specific manner by which the postulated causes (i.e., the hypothesized answer to why) produce the phenomenon. A successful answer to the question of why should therefore be accompanied by a fairly thorough understanding of the basis for the developmental trends of interest, and a successful answer to the question of how should specify the mechanisms underlying any interventions or moderators that might be found to alter the rate of aging.

Theories can obviously differ in the level of analysis used in attempting to answer the questions of why and how. For example, the explanatory mechanisms could be very distal, perhaps involving characteristics of the social or cultural environment when the individuals were young, or they could be proximal and at the same conceptual level or measured at the same time as the to-be-explained phenomenon. The degree of reductionism incorporated into a theory largely reflects the preference of the theorist, but it is important to recognize that there may be some practical limits on reductionism if it is considered desirable to use the same level of description in characterizing the phenomenon and in specifying possible answers to the why and how questions. To illustrate, it may be very difficult in the context of a single theory to interpret age-related changes in relatively high-level concepts such as life goals or reasoning ability in terms of biochemical reactions at the synapses of individual neurons.

II. Criteria for Evaluating Explanations

Because the questions of why and how are fundamental with respect to evaluating theories of psychological aging, it is important to consider how the adequacy of their answers might be assessed. Five criteria that could be used to evaluate theoretical hypotheses addressing the why and how of age-related effects in behavior are outlined in Table 1.2. These are obviously not the only possible criteria that could be used to evaluate aging-related hypotheses, but when

Table 1.2
Proposed Criteria to Evaluate Theoretical Hypotheses in Aging

Criterion	Elaboration
Construct validity	Do the variables used to represent the critical construct reflect the hypothesized construct exclusively and exhaustively?
Age relation	Is the construct related to age in the expected direction?
Criterion relation	Is the construct related to the criterion in the expected direction?
Statistical mediation	Is the age relation on the criterion reduced after statistical control of the variation in the construct?
Effective intervention	Is the age relation on the criterion altered substantially when the level of the construct is manipulated in an experiment with random assignment?

considered together they appear to be relatively comprehensive. If all of the criteria were to be satisfied, one could probably be confident that the hypothesis provided plausible answers to the questions of the why and how of the phenomenon. Moreover, explicit recognition of the existence of multiple criteria may minimize the tendency for advocates of a particular theory to emphasize only one or two of the criteria, which could lead to distorted evaluations of the relative merits of different theories.

In much of the subsequent discussion the relations of age on some aspect of cognitive functioning will be used as the phenomenon of primary interest, and thus the theoretical hypothesis should specify a mechanism by which increased age is presumed to be associated with lower levels of cognitive functioning. Most of the hypotheses postulate that aging leads to a change in one or more critical constructs that are responsible for many, if not all, of the age-related differences in the relevant measure of cognitive functioning. Aging is typically not considered a causal factor itself, but rather is viewed as a dimension along which causal influences operate.

The first criterion is construct validity, which is essential to establish that the variable actually represents what it is intended to represent. It is widely recognized in many areas of psychology that few variables are "pure" in the sense that the variable has a one-to-one correspondence with a particular theoretical process or construct. Two analytical approaches have been used to deal with the problem that observed variables are imperfect indicators of the theoretical constructs of primary interest. One approach involves attempting to rule out extraneous influences and to isolate the critical construct by a combination of experimental design (e.g., multiple task conditions) and analysis (e.g., subtraction, process dissociation). The second approach consists of trying to converge on what the construct represents by obtaining multiple indicator variables of the construct from each research participant and focusing on what these variables have in common that is distinct from what is common among variables assumed to represent alternative constructs.

The two analytical methods derive from different traditions within psychology, and thus it is not surprising that researchers working from different perspectives vary in their preference for one procedure or the other. Regardless of the method used to investigate the meaning of the variables, however, establishment of construct validity is a critical criterion for theoretically relevant research because one must have confidence that the key constructs are assessed appropriately before hypotheses about their roles in aging-related phenomena can be meaningfully evaluated. Although this point may seem obvious, it is surprising how much research in the psychology of aging relies on theoretical constructs that have only face validity. For example, within the field of cognition there is apparently very little evidence of convergent/discriminant validity for such frequently mentioned constructs as processing resources, attentional capacity, inhibition, and executive functioning.

A causal hypothesis of the age relations in cognitive functioning is not plausible if the critical construct is not related both to age and to cognition, and thus the second and third criteria listed in Table 1.2 also need to be satisfied for a developmental explanation to be convincing. However, because a great many variables are related to age, the second criterion of a relation between age and the construct is not very diagnostic by itself. Furthermore, most cognitive variables are positively correlated with one another, and thus the third criterion of a relation between construct and cognition is also not very informative in isolation. Moreover, even if both the second and the third criteria are satisfied, one cannot necessarily infer a causal linkage among the three variables because, for example, the construct–cognition relation may be age specific. To illustrate, use of a strategy (construct) may only be effective in improving performance (cognition) among high-functioning young adults, or an increase in stimulus intensity (construct) may only be effective in improving performance (cognition) among older adults with sensory impairments. In both of these cases the construct is unlikely to be involved in the age-related differences in cognition, and this lack of involvement would be revealed by the fourth criterion, statistical mediation.

The rationale for the statistical mediation criterion is that if the critical construct contributes to the mediation of age–cognition relations, then the strength of the relation between age and cognition should be reduced if there was little or no variation in the level of the construct. Variation in the level of the construct could be reduced by equating people on the hypothesized mediator by selection or matching, but these methods typically result in small samples with low statistical power. A more effective procedure is to control the variation in the construct by means of statistical adjustment, which is why this criterion is known as statistical mediation.

Because many causal factors are likely to be operating simultaneously for most aspects of behavior, it is probably unrealistic to expect any candidate hypothesis to be the exclusive cause of aging-related phenomena such that statistical mediation accounted for all of the age-related effects. However, if there is not at least some attenuation of the age–cognition relations after restriction of the variation in the critical construct, then there would be little evidence that the construct is involved in the phenomenon under investigation.

Statistical mediation can be a powerful tool, but it should be distinguished from causal mediation because evidence of statistical mediation is sometimes interpreted erroneously as implying that the hypothesized mediator is *the* causal factor. For example, assume that a researcher hypothesizes that age-related declines in some aspect of health cause age-related declines in a particular type of cognitive functioning. If the researcher then finds substantial attenuation of the relation between age and cognition after statistical control of the variation in relevant measures of health, it may be tempting to infer that declining health is a major cause of age-related cognitive decline.

However, it is important to realize that an inference of this type is not valid, and in the field of logic it is known as the fallacy of affirming the consequent. The contrast of this invalid form of reasoning with a valid form, known in logic as *modus tollens*, can be illustrated by expressing both types of arguments in abstract terms, with p representing the hypothesis that age-related decreases in health contribute to age-related cognitive decline and q referring to a discovery of statistical mediation.

Fallacy of affirming the consequent
   If p then q
   q
   Therefore p

Modus tollens
   If p then q
   Not q
   Therefore not p

Note that although it may seem counterintuitive, a finding that the age-related effects in the relevant measure of cognition are reduced substantially after control of the variation in the hypothesized mediating construct of health does not imply that the hypothesis is confirmed. The reason is that many other possible factors could contribute to the attenuation of age–cognition relations after statistical control of a potential mediator such as health. In contrast, the valid form of the argument is directly informative about the plausibility of the hypothesis because a discovery of a *failure* to find substantial attenuation of the age-cognition relations after control of the variation in health (i.e., not q) would be inconsistent with the hypothesis (i.e., not p). Statistical mediation results can therefore provide evidence relevant to the validity of causal hypotheses, but primarily when the outcome fails to support the theoretical prediction. As the philosopher Karl Popper (Popper, 1959) and others have pointed out in

other contexts, however, tests such as statistical mediation can be viewed as opportunities to falsify a causal hypothesis, and thus confidence in a hypothesis should increase when it is successful at surviving serious attempts at falsification, in this case in the form of tests of statistical mediation.

Although the first through the fourth criteria listed in Table 1.2 are necessary, they are not sufficient to definitively establish the credibility of a developmental theory or hypothesis. All of these criteria must be satisfied for the hypothesis to be capable of explaining relations between age and cognition, but even if these conditions are met, the hypothesis and the critical construct still may not have a truly causal role in the phenomenon. Only the final criterion of effective intervention will yield unambiguous evidence that the hypothesized construct and its associated mechanism are sufficient to explain the age–cognition relations because if the construct is truly causal, then manipulation of the level of the construct should alter the age–cognition relation.

In light of the potential informativeness of interventions, it is not surprising that there has been considerable interest in various types of intervention research among researchers investigating aging. Both practical and theoretical benefits could be expected from successful interventions, but two issues need to be considered in the design and interpretation of intervention studies to ensure that the results are truly relevant to the theoretical speculations.

First, for pragmatic reasons of time and expense, most experimental interventions have focused on short-term outcomes, such as improvement in the level of a particular variable immediately after the intervention. If the intervention is judged to be successful based on comparisons involving the appropriate types of controls (e.g., random assignment to groups that are treated identically except for the critical intervention component), then the manipulated factor can be inferred to affect performance on that variable. In other words, if individuals are randomly assigned to treatment and control groups and the groups are found to differ significantly on the criterion variable after the intervention, then it is reasonable to conclude that the manipulated factor has a causal effect on the level of performance. Moreover, if the participants in the study vary in age, it may also be possible to reach conclusions about the effectiveness of the intervention across different periods of adulthood.

What is often not recognized, however, is that short-term interventions are not necessarily relevant to the effect of the manipulated factor on the relations between age and the target variable of interest. In order to determine whether the intervention has an impact on processes of aging, individuals in the treatment and control groups must be monitored for a long enough period to detect possible alterations in the relations between age and the target variable. Only if the relation between age and the variable is altered after the intervention could one validly infer that the intervention was relevant to the effects of age on the construct of interest, and this determination requires that the effects of the intervention be monitored for an extended period. The most informative contrast from an intervention designed to alter effects of aging is therefore not the difference between the treatment and the control group immediately after the intervention or even a contrast between these groups at various intervals after the beginning of the intervention. Instead it is a comparison of the slopes of the functions relating the target variable to age. Because slopes represent rate of change over time, they should be considered the key outcome variable in intervention research designed to modify rates of aging. Unfortunately, very few intervention studies have monitored individuals for decades, or even for years, after the intervention and apparently none have reported comparisons of intervention and control groups on measures of rates of age-related change. Short-term effects can be important for practical reasons, but they are not necessarily informative about the effects of an intervention on the rate of age-related change of the target variable. For example, a large immediate effect might dissipate rapidly and have no effect on the rate of aging or the immediate effect could be small but might accumulate over years or decades such that it led to a substantial modification of the relation between age and the relevant behavior.

Another important issue to consider in attempting to relate the outcomes of interventions to theories of psychological aging is the breadth of the intervention effects because the results may not be of much practical or theoretical interest if the effects are restricted to a very small set of highly similar variables. To illustrate, a researcher might find that with appropriate training a group of middle-aged adults is able to improve their memory for faces and that the benefits persist over an extended period such that these individuals experience a smaller age-related change in measures of face memory over the next 20 years than control individuals who did not receive the training. Although these would be very impressive results, they might nevertheless be of limited interest if there was no generalizability of the intervention benefit to memory for other types of information, such as names, stories, telephone numbers, and recipes.

Research findings with a very specific outcome could still have theoretical value, but only if the results of the intervention are comparable in scope to the phenomenon represented by the theory's answer to the question of what. In other words, if a theory characterizes the phenomenon as age-related influences on many aspects of cognitive functioning but the intervention is found to affect only a limited type of memory, then results of the intervention would likely only be relevant to a portion of the theory.

Although capable of providing some of the most convincing evidence relevant to theories of aging, the criterion of effective intervention obviously poses a major challenge. Not only are most interventions difficult to implement, but it is extremely expensive and time-consuming to monitor individuals for a long enough period after the introduction of an intervention to allow an evaluation of its effects on rates of aging, which is the outcome of primary interest for theories of aging.

III. Evaluating Criteria

Determination of the degree to which a given criterion in Table 1.2 is satisfied is likely to be somewhat subjective, although quantitative indices such as correlations and effect sizes can be used to assist in evaluating some of the criteria. However, the mere process of articulating criteria such as those in Table 1.2 may facilitate progress in theoretical development and understanding. For example, consideration of the criteria when thinking about one's theory may suggest the type of research that is needed to further explore the viability of theoretical hypotheses.

The classification scheme presented in Table 1.2 may also be useful in helping explain some of the differences in perspective among theorists who investigate psychological aging. Some theorists appear to have emphasized the first and third criteria and have tended to neglect the remaining criteria, whereas other theorists have emphasized the second and fourth criteria while ignoring the others. It is therefore not surprising that there is sometimes a lack of communication or conflict if the theorists do not share the same values, which in this case can be conceptualized as the perceived importance of the different criteria. However, to the extent that each criterion in Table 1.2 is relevant to the validity of the hypotheses, they should all be considered in evaluating the adequacy of theoretical explanations.

IV. Theoretical Progress

It is sometimes lamented that there has been relatively little progress in developing and evaluating theories of psychological aging (Bengston & Schaie, 1999). It is certainly true that no consensus has yet emerged as to the most convincing or comprehensive theory in any area of the psychology of aging. This final section of the chapter considers three conceptual and methodological factors that may have limited theoretical progress in the psychology of aging.

The first limiting factor is a failure on the part of many researchers to consider phenomena broader than what is assessed by single variables. Variables do not exist in isolation, and consequently misleading conclusions might be reached if researchers attempt to interpret age-related effects on a particular variable as though they existed in a vacuum. Although it is obviously easier to focus on one variable rather than on many, there is now considerable evidence that age-related effects on different cognitive (and likely noncognitive) variables do not occur independently. Furthermore, most theories are concerned with relations at the level of theoretical constructs, and it is very unlikely that any single variable exhaustively and exclusively represents a given theoretical construct in psychology. Failure to consider influences on the variable of interest in the context of age-related influences on other variables may therefore result in a distorted characterization of the nature of the phenomenon and could impede progress in the ultimate discovery of explanations.

A second issue relevant to theoretical progress concerns the importance of maintaining close linkages between the theory and potentially relevant empirical observations. In particular, the level of abstraction in the theoretical discussion should be appropriate to link the speculations to data in a testable manner. On the one hand, if the theoretical speculations are too broad and the concepts are too vague to have specific operationalizations or if they allow many potentially contradictory operationalizations, then the speculations may not be testable. The theoretical concepts could still serve as guiding assumptions, but they might better be viewed as a framework, or as a set of biases, rather than as a true scientific theory. On the other hand, if the theoretical speculations are highly specific, as they might be if they are based on formal computational models that incorporate many assumptions that are only weakly related to observable behavior, then they again may not be testable. Exercises of this type can be useful in indicating the sufficiency of a particular set of assumptions, but unless they can be established to be directly related to observable aspects of behavior, they may not be amenable to rigorous evaluation.

A third factor that may have limited theoretical progress in contemporary research on psychological aging is the frequent failure to relate one's results to earlier findings in order to ensure that there is cumulative progress. Researchers sometimes appear to act as though their results with a particular variable are completely novel and unrelated to all past research, when this is seldom, if ever, the case. Although the goal of research is the discovery of new information, unless linkages are established with prior results there is a risk that the information is not truly new, in which case no progress will be made. A major role of theory is to integrate information, which includes previously established information as well as information that is assumed to be new.

V. Conclusion

The major theses of this chapter were that a primary purpose of theories of psychological aging is to provide answers to major questions (cf. Table 1.1) and that at least five criteria (cf. Table 1.2) should be considered when evaluating the validity of answers to those questions. It was suggested that communication among theorists, and comparisons of theories, may have been hampered in the past because only a subset of questions and criteria have typically been considered in the description and evaluation of theories. Finally, the chapter concluded with three suggestions that might contribute to more rapid process in the development and evaluation of theories of psychological aging: (a) adopting a broader perspective than a focus on a single variable to ensure that the theory is addressing the "disease" and not merely the "symptoms"; (b) maintaining a close linkage between the level of theoretical discourse and the level of empirical observation to ensure that the theoretical speculations actually address, and are influenced by, empirical results; and (c) ensuring cumulative progress by placing new results in the context of already established results.

References

Bengston, V.L., & Schaie, K.W. (1999), *Handbook of theories of aging.* New York: Springer.

Cerella, J. (1990). Aging and information-processing rate. In J. E. Birren & K. W. Schaie (Eds.), *Handbook of the psychology of aging* (3rd ed.) (pp. 201–221.). San Diego: Academic Press.

Popper, K.R. (1959). *The logic of scientific discovery.* London: Hutchinson.

Salthouse, T. A. (1996). The processing-speed theory of adult age differences in cognition. *Psychological Review, 103,* 403–428.

Two

Design and Analysis of Longitudinal Studies on Aging

Scott M. Hofer and Martin J. Sliwinski

Developmental scientists seek to understand how and why cognition, emotion, personality, health, and many other psychological characteristics change in individuals as they age. For understanding aging, longitudinal studies provide many advantages relative to cross-sectional studies, as between-person age comparisons cannot provide a basis for disentangling changes due to aging from stable individual characteristics, average between-person trends, or population selection and mortality effects, for example. However, longitudinal studies also present unique and significant design and data analysis challenges that can limit their utility for advancing theory. The purpose of this chapter is to examine recent progress in longitudinal research for testing theories of aging and to draw attention to what we believe are important challenges facing developmental scientists involved in longitudinal aging research.

Such an examination cannot proceed without first establishing a frame of reference for evaluating approaches to longitudinal design and data analysis.

In the late 1970s, Baltes and Nesselroade (1979) offered five rationales of longitudinal research that provide a framework for advancing developmental and aging theory: (1) Direct identification of intraindividual change; (2) direct identification of interindividual differences in intraindividual change; (3) analysis of interrelationships of change; (4) analysis of causes of intraindividual change; and (5) analysis of causes of interindividual differences in intraindividual change. Although it is fair to assert that many practicing aging researchers are familiar with these rationales, it is equally fair to remark that this framework has not influenced longitudinal aging research to the extent that it should. These five rationales clarify an often neglected complexity of longitudinal research, namely the necessity of measuring and modeling change at two distinct levels of analysis: the intraindividual (or within-person; WP) and the interindividual (or between-person; BP). The primary thesis of this chapter is that aging researchers should pay more attention to developing theoretically informative models of intraindividual change before devoting effort toward analysis of individual differences in change.

Remarkable national and international efforts have produced over 40 major longitudinal studies of individuals 50 years of age and older (for review, see Schaie & Hofer, 2001), representing an enormous potential wealth of information on within-person changes with age. However, relatively little attention has been given to developing theoretically sophisticated models of intraindividual-level change. Additionally, the inferential and statistical issues that complicate the analysis of longitudinal aging data are often cited as limiting factors for the development of theories and models of aging based on "within-individual" longitudinal designs. Although longitudinal data are admittedly more complex than cross-sectional data, longitudinal data contain information necessary to directly address within-person change processes and related inferential issues of attrition and mortality selection that must be ignored in cross-sectional data because these processes are inaccessible. Such direct assessment of WP processes is necessary for understanding developmental and aging-related changes.

Nevertheless, many theories and models of aging are based solely on results from cross-sectional studies of individuals varying in age. Several competing accounts of cognitive aging (e.g., resource deficit theories, inhibition theory, common factor models, processing speed theory) attempt to identify and isolate cognitive processes, operations, and constructs that can account for observed cognitive age differences. Although the specifics of these theories differ, they all derive from a common finding in cross-sectional cognitive aging studies: that the effects of chronological age differences are not statistically independent, but are shared among different types of cognitive and noncognitive variables (e.g., Salthouse, 2005; Salthouse,

Hambrick, & McGuthry, 1998). A key challenge facing these theories, one that is largely unaddressed, is to describe and explain the formal characteristics of changes that occur *within* aging individuals. It is not sufficient for a theory to identify basic cognitive processes that differ as a function of chronological age. A sufficient theory of cognitive aging must also provide a model of *how* aging influences these cognitive processes. This process orientation is underdeveloped in current theories because most studies treat "aging" as a BP characteristic—as an age "difference." For example, a common assumption in cognitive aging research is that continuous and smooth population age trends observed in age-heterogeneous cross-sectional samples reflect continuous and smooth cognitive changes occurring within aging individuals. However, depending on the cause, cognitive loss with aging may not be continuous, but rather stochastic and discontinuous. Absent of disease, does aging produce a "graceful degradation" of cognitive function or is cognitive loss better characterized as a probabilistic transition between stages or plateaus of functioning? Such questions, with particular answers true of some people and perhaps not of others, must be addressed by the direct observation of intraindividual change in the context of longitudinal designs.

Several other issues motivate the emphasis on longitudinal study for understanding aging. First, cognitive change reflects developmental as well as pathological processes and involves external influences that interact with both of these processes within individuals (e.g., Nilsson et al., 2004). Second, evidence for the importance of the life span developmental perspective is provided in findings that early patterns of development are predictive of later changes (e.g., Hayward & Gorman, 2004). We expect that complex interactive effects are associated with multiple causal influences (e.g., comorbidity), with cumulative effects of risk factors, and perhaps with age-specific (delayed) causal action (e.g., Rutter, 1988; Seeman, Singer, Rowe, & McEwen, 2001). Third, population selection (i.e., mortality) is a natural population dynamic related to chronological age and is accessible only in longitudinal studies. Inferences regarding change and causal processes may be obscured if mortality and selection processes are not taken into account (e.g., Vaupel & Yashin, 1985).

I. Research Design and Inferential Scope

Developmental researchers can make use of a variety of research designs and analytic models to examine aging-related changes. These different designs and methods of analysis emphasize different aspects of population and individual change and are best viewed as complementary approaches but must be considered in regards to questions posed for answers to be most useful and interpretable.

What can be learned from cross-sectional and longitudinal designs can be summarized in terms of levels of analysis and inferential scope. Table 2.1 shows several levels of analysis based on multiple-cohort, BP, and WP approaches, all of which have recent examples in the area of aging research. For example, intercohort differences (Table 2.1) can be examined to evaluate whether different contexts have lasting effects on individuals reaching maturity (e.g., Alwin & McCammon, 2001). Population average trends show that fluid ability begins to decline at an earlier age and at a steeper rate than crystallized knowledge (e.g., McArdle et al., 2002). A number of theories and hypotheses derive from variance decomposition and factor models, which are based on between-person differences (e.g., Lindenberger & Baltes, 1997; Salthouse & Ferrar-Caja, 2003) with typical findings that age-related variance

Table 2.1
Levels of Analysis (from Populations to Individuals)[a]

1. Inter cohort differences
Aggregate effects of broad contextual differences in same age / different birth cohort groups
2. Average population trends
Aggregate between-person (or within-person) age trends
3. Between-person differences
Factor and regression decomposition models of age-related variance
4. Between-person differences in within-person rates of change
Unconditional and conditional (w/covariates) growth curve models
5. Interrelationships among within-person rates of change
Multivariate growth curve models
Bivariate dual change score models
6. Aggregate within-person variability
Correlations among SD within-person
7. Coupled within-person processes
Within-person correlation (analysis of detrended time-specific residuals)
Dynamic factor analysis

[a]Available timescales often decrease across levels of analysis. Adapted from Hofer (2004).

is largely shared among cognitive, sensory, psychomotor, and functional tasks and that common factor models account for the patterns of covariance (e.g., see Hofer, Berg, & Era, 2003). Christensen, Hofer et al. (2001) found no association of education on the rate of cognitive decline in four cognitive measures while controlling for health status and sex. Sliwinski, Hofer, and Hall (2003) found that associations among rates of change in memory, speed, and verbal fluency were attenuated after removing individuals with preclinical dementia. Strauss et al. (2002) found reliable correlations among within-person variability in cognitive and functional indicators (see also Siegler, 1994). Within-person correlations (i.e., coupling), based on the analysis of residuals (after removing intraindividual mean and trend), provide information regarding the correlation of within-time variation in functioning across variables (Almeida, 2005; Sliwinski et al., 2003a). While each level of analysis provides information regarding aging-related change, the inferences and interpretations possible from any single level of analysis have distinct and delimited ramifications for theories of aging (e.g., Hofer, Berg, & Era, 2003) and are dependent on time sampling as well as other design characteristics.

Different longitudinal study designs provide different types of information and opportunities for analyses regarding between-person differences and within-person change. For example, longitudinal designs permit cross-sectional analysis of between-person variation in age at the initial assessment in addition to longitudinal BP/WP analysis of change in mean trends, rates of change, and WP coupling. Sequential cohort studies permit comparisons across birth cohorts, cross-sectionally and longitudinally (Schaie, 1965). Other designs and analyses necessarily require that we

aggregate or ignore other important sources of change and variation (e.g., Schaie, 1973; Nesselroade, 1988). For example, the analysis of cohort differences often ignores within-individual and between-individual variability and emphasizes average effects. Analyses that focus on rates of change, such as the analysis of growth curves, emphasize variation in individual-level change as expressed as a deviation from the population average change function and often ignore information from individual variation in time-specific residuals. The emphasis on between-person age differences in age must usually ignore important population processes associated with attrition and mortality selection, as well as differences in historical contexts related to birth cohort, in making inference to a single population of aging individuals. In addition, analysis of cross-sectional age differences usually confounds average BP differences (mean BP age trend) and within-person change and variation (e.g., Hofer, Flaherty, & Hoffman, 2006). However, research that focuses on within-person variability and covariability requires that the higher order levels of between-person differences and within-person change be controlled as these can contribute to spurious associations. The central idea is that these levels of analysis are complementary and carry different information about aging-related changes.

The levels of analysis described earlier correspond roughly to different temporal, including historical (i.e., birth cohort), sampling frames. The interpretation, comparison, and generalizability of parameters derived from different temporal samplings must be carefully considered. The temporal characteristics of change and variation must be taken into account, as different sampling intervals will likely lead to different results requiring different interpretations for both within and between-person processes (Boker &

Nesselroade, 2002; Martin & Hofer, 2004). For example, correlations of change in two variables over time will likely be quite different for short temporal intervals (minutes, hours, days, or weeks) in contrast to change across many years, as is the case for many of the longitudinal studies on aging. Measurement interval is also critical for the prediction of outcome variables and establishing evidence for leading versus lagging indicators (Gollob & Reichardt, 1987). The measurement burst design described by Nesselroade (1991) is a compromise between single-case time-series and conventional longitudinal designs and permits the examination of WP processes (within measurement burst) and change in processes (across measurement bursts) over time.

A. Comparing Levels of Analysis: Within Person and Between Person.

Most studies whose results support general factor theories of cognitive aging, (i.e., the general slowing and common cause/dedifferentiation hypotheses) are cross-sectional and based on the analysis of individuals varying broadly in age. The assumption is that between-person differences provide an appropriate representation of within-person changes. Much of what we take as established empirical findings (e.g., the centrality of speed) is grounded in analyses that depend on these untested assumptions of *ergodicity* (Molenaar, 2004; Molenaar, Huizenga, & Nesselroade, 2003). Modeling health indicators is especially problematic in this regard because the within-person processes associated with health-related changes are likely to be highly selected in cross-sectional samples (i.e., resulting from nonparticipation of persons with greater declines in health) and are thus unlikely to be well understood by between-person comparisons even at the population level.

Evaluating and developing new theories using within-person designs are critical for scientific progress, as results from within-person and between-person analyses often do not agree (Molenaar et al., 2003; Sliwinski & Hofer, 1999; Zimprich, 2002a). For example, Sliwinski and Buschke (1999; 2004) showed that within-person declines in speed do not mediate within-person declines in memory function, although they observed the typical speed mediation effect at the between-person level of analyses. One reason for such differences across BP and WP approaches is that age-related mean differences are part of the estimates of association in cross-sectional studies. The high levels of association between age-dependent outcomes that are often reported from age-heterogeneous samples can result simply from average population age differences and not necessarily from associations between individual "rates of aging" (for derivation of cross-sectional covariances from linear change models (both fixed and random effects) see Hofer, Flaherty, & Hoffman, 2006; Hofer & Sliwinski, 2001; for extension to polynomial change models, see Zimprich, 2002b). The reliance on between-person information is a shortcoming that must be remedied for continued theoretical and methodological progress (Hofer & Sliwinski, 2001; Kraemer et al., 2000). Longitudinal studies of long-term change represent a necessary step in confirming or disconfirming theories and hypotheses of aging and permit the direct analysis of influences that may only be demonstrated as "tenable" by cross-sectional analysis of individual differences.

However, analyses of longitudinal data do not necessarily reflect strong emphasis on intraindividual modeling. The third rationale of Baltes and Nesselroade (1979) focuses on the examination of interrelationships in behavioral change. There are two ways in which this objective can be accomplished. Several longitudinal studies have examined the extent to which time-related changes on different cognitive variables are correlated. The focus of these analyses is on individual differences in estimates of intraindividual change and is therefore a between-person level analysis (on WP change outcomes). Although modeling between-person correlations among rates of cognitive change is theoretically informative, it is not the only way in which to formulate predictions regarding the interrelationships in change. An alternative approach involves modeling within-person associations among cognitive variables (e.g., Horn, 1972; Sliwinski et al., 2003b; Sliwinski & Buschke, 1999, 2004; MacDonald, Dixon, Cohen, & Hazlitt, 2004; MacDonald, Hultsch, & Dixon, 2003) to test predictions regarding the relationships among change on different cognitive variables. The distinction between these two approaches is most apparent when we articulate the type of question each can answer. The conventional between-person analysis of correlated rates of change can answer questions such as "Are individuals who are changing more (or less) rapidly on one variable also changing more (or less) rapidly on another?" The within-person analysis can address questions such as "Does performance on a set of variables rise and fall together over time?" The different time scales that these estimates refer to can be quite different—change over extended periods compared with short-term cross-occasion fluctuations—and so make these results complementary and require joint interpretation of quite different conceptualizations of change (as in Table 2.1). Sliwinski and Buschke (2004) suggested that in order to keep these two types of analyses clearly distinguished that we refer to the former

as *correlated* between-person change and the latter as *coupled* within-person change.

B. Interrelationships in Behavioral Change: Evidence for Correlated and Coupled Change in Longitudinal Studies on Aging

There is substantial evidence of "shared" age-related effects on cognitive variables from cross-sectional research (e.g., Baltes & Lindenberger, 1997; Salthouse, Hambrick, & McGuthry, 1998). There is also a growing body of evidence for associations in age-related cognitive change at two levels of analysis. The most common level focuses on correlated rates of change, which involves estimating a slope or change parameter for each individual and correlating these estimates across different variables (e.g., Anstey, Hofer, & Luszcz, 2003; Christensen et al., 2004; Ghisletta & Lindenberger, 2004; Hertzog, Dixon, Hultsch, & MacDonald, 2003; Hofer et al., 2002; Hultsch et al., 1992, Johansson et al., 2004; Mackinnon et al., 2003; Sliwinski et al., 2003a,b; Wilson et al., 2002; Zimprich & Martin, 2002). For example, Zimprich and Martin (2002) reported a correlation of .53 between rates of memory change and speed change. Wilson et al. (2002) showed that a single factor accounted for 62% of the variance among change slopes. Both of these results indicated weaker associations than might be expected, given cross-sectional findings (see Verhaeghen & Salthouse, 1997). One possibility for this discrepancy is that the follow-up period in most longitudinal studies is relatively short compared to the age range examined in cross-sectional studies. Another reason why common factor models work better in accounting for cross-sectional data than longitudinal data is that cross-sectional analyses of age-heterogeneous samples are confounded by average age-related trends and do not permit sensitive assessment of the myriad dynamic and progressive processes that can cause cognitive loss in old age (e.g., Hofer & Sliwinski, 2001; for review, see Hofer, Flaherty, & Hoffman, 2006).

However, even if the magnitude of correlated change was on par with expectations from cross-sectional research, this would not imply evidence of a common cause. Wilson et al. (2002) interpreted correlated rates of change as indicating the "accumulation of common age-related conditions that can affect multiple cognitive systems (p. 190)." Such age-related conditions could include both nonnormative influences (e.g., Alzheimer's or vascular disease) and normative age-graded influences (e.g., structural and functional brain changes). This insight suggests that even if age-related cognitive change were very highly correlated, this would reflect common age *effects*, and not necessarily a common *cause*. Sliwinski et al. (2003b) reported results consistent with this interpretation of correlated change by estimating correlations among measures of memory, speed, and verbal fluency, including only data obtained prior to the diagnosis for individuals with incident dementia. Between-person correlations among rates of change were moderate and consistent (.56–.61), but were attenuated (.34–.48) when individuals with preclinical dementia were removed. Individual differences in rates of change were close to zero when a disease process model (time-to-diagnosis) was applied to model change in individuals with dementia diagnosis. These results demonstrate how aggregation of heterogeneous groups of individuals (e.g., those with and without dementia) can lead to high correlations among rates of change and also demonstrate that these correlations can be near to zero in the case of a single significant cause of cognitive decline (i.e., dementia).

In contrast to correlations among rates of change, the other level at which interrelationship in behavioral change can be examined is the within-person or intraindividual level. Sliwinski and Buschke (1999, 2004) evaluated the processing speed hypothesis by examining how intraindividual change in speed could predict intraindividual change in other cognitive measures. In both of these studies, they demonstrated that speed and memory change were coupled within individuals. However, tests of mediation indicated that intraindividual changes in speed could not account for a substantial proportion of the within-person change in memory. MacDonald, Hultsch, Strauss, and Dixon (2003b) performed a similar analysis to examine whether within-person changes in the digit symbol substitution test could be predicted by changes in more basic measures of speed. Their findings indicated evidence of coupling, but also found that much of the within-person change in the digit symbol test was not accounted for by corresponding changes in processing speed. In another analysis, MacDonald, Hultsch, and Dixon (2003) found that wave-to-wave changes in trial-to-trial response time variability predicted corresponding cognitive changes within individuals. Sliwinski et al. (2003b) found that within-person correlations among memory, speed, and verbal fluency were notably higher in a group of individuals with preclinical dementia compared to their age peers without dementia.

Sophisticated models of intraindividual change tend to be time based in the sense that change is treated to be a function of time between measurement occasions, anchored at defined reference points (e.g., date of birth, date of the baseline test). However, theorists view age-related behavioral change to be a function of structural and functional brain changes, disease progression, changes in health, and changes in other cognitive and psychosocial functions. We view the growing emphasis on intraindividual modeling (Hultsch et al., 2000; Molenaar, Huizenga, & Nesselroade, 2003; Nesselroade, 2001; 2004) as a very promising step for research on aging. This approach takes full advantage of longitudinal data by bringing our analytic models in line with our theorizing through developing process-based models of intraindividual change.

Longitudinal "process-based" models will often involve centering on an event or state of a process of interest in order to compare individual change relative to a common organizing time structure. Alternative time structures in our longitudinal models are used to identify a more interpretative basis for individual change. In operationalizing the construct of "aging," we can use chronological age (time since birth, e.g., McArdle et al., 2004) or time specifications based on the occurrence of particular events or processes (i.e., morbidity, mortality; e.g., time prior/since diagnosis of dementia; e.g., Sliwinski, Hofer, & Hall, 2003). Other approaches treat time as an ordinal variable (study wave or attrition, e.g., Anstey et al., 2003; Hertzog et al., 2003). A key objective for any of these approaches is to measure change related to aging processes and distinguish these changes from changes due to processes, such as health changes, that are merely *associated* with age. This type of inference relates to the normative/nonnormative distinction. Normative processes and events are strongly age graded and occur in all or nearly all individuals, whereas nonnormative processes/events are individual specific or subsample specific (i.e., that the majority of individuals will not experience) and are not well predicted by chronological age (Baltes & Nesselroade, 1979). We have previously argued that the nearly exclusive use of chronological age as the time basis for modeling intraindividual change will result in overestimating the importance of normative age-graded influences and underemphasize the importance of non-normative influences that affect subsets of the population (Sliwinski, Hofer, & Hall, 2003a).

C. Evidence for Distinct Patterns of Change

Recent developments in growth mixture models (Muthén, 2001) may have particular relevance to aging studies, with several well-known studies providing evidence for differential growth patterns. Using individual response patterns in a longitudinal setting with repeated measurements to define trajectories, growth mixture models (a) identify homogeneous groups of individuals or trajectory classes, (b) assign each participant a probability of belonging to a particular trajectory class, and (c) use class membership information to estimate the influence of individual characteristics on trajectory shape. Other forms of cluster analysis have been used to identify patterns of individual differences and trajectories in gerontological studies (Aldwin, Spiro, Levenson, & Cupertino, 2001; Maxson, Berg, & McClearn, 1996, 1997; Smith & Baltes, 1997), but these are cross-sectional in design. Smith and Baltes (1997) applied cluster analysis to time one assessments of intellectual, personality, self-related, and social functioning in the Berlin aging study and identified nine distinct subgroups, with four subgroups exhibiting positive patterns of functioning that were associated with younger age status. Maxson et al. (1996) investigated the survival probabilities for five subgroups identified by cluster analysis in the Gothenburg, H-70 study with the finding that disability in any one domain (cognitive performance, physical health, functional capacity, subjective well-being, and social contacts) had a greater effect on subsequent functioning and mortality than the average level of performance across all areas.

II. Understanding Heterogeneity in Age-Related Processes

Although much of the previous research has been performed in the context of so-called healthy aging, there is sufficient evidence to indicate that changes in cognition and health are strongly related. However, theories of cognitive aging have not taken morbidity and population mortality selection sufficiently into account in the interpretation of results or theoretical propositions. Important next steps in cognitive aging research will emphasize the interplay between cognition and health from a multiple-process orientation. Such understanding of change in cognition with age requires the better identification of aging-related changes produced by disease processes (i.e., morbidity, comorbidity, mortality). Health can have both direct and indirect effects on cognitive decline. Direct effects of health on cognition are those related to pathological changes in the integrity of the neurological, cardiovascular, and cerebrovascular systems. The link between health and cognition may be indirect in that consequences of disease (frailty, level of arousal) impact the level of cognitive reserve, affecting older adults more because of their lower reserve thresholds. Broader changes, such as physical disablement and mental health functioning, that are related to health indicators, must also be considered as well as potential long-term cumulative effects of income, education, and health-care access.

Assuming that aging is a highly complex, dynamic, and multidimensional process, influences that cause changes in multiple outcomes (i.e., systems) are likely to differ across individuals, implying that there will be different patterns of biological and psychological aging (e.g., Shanahan & Hofer, 2005). This assumption is central to a science based on individual differences—that we can identify and intervene in processes that cause or result in individual differences in aging-related outcomes. Here we can distinguish between "common cause" and "common outcome" and consider that common causes might lead to different outcomes and that different causes can lead to common outcomes. For example, different aging-related and/or disease-related processes may influence multiple systems within an individual. Age-related environmental influences or health-related changes may be unique to each individual, although different causative "aging" influences may appear to have a common outcome in the population when analyses are based on the aggregate sample (e.g., Hofer et al., 2003; Sliwinski et al., 2003a). This heterogeneity and increasing disease risk with age are probably sources of the difficulty in differentiating aging-related changes from changes associated with disease processes. Additionally, changes in health may result from a complex interaction of life span influences, including formal education, occupational status, behavioral risk and health factors, and genetic risk factors for cardiovascular and other disease.

By definition, normative causes of cognitive loss occur in most individuals as they age (e.g., Bäckman et al., 2000). However, there is compelling evidence for the operation of processes that cause cognitive loss in a restricted (but not trivial) subset of aging individuals. The development of preclinical dementia (Haan et al., 1999; Hall et al., 2000; Rubin et al., 1998; Sliwinski et al., 2003b), the progression of subclinical cardiovascular disease (Haan et al., 1999), and respiratory dysfunction (Albert et al., 1995) have all been demonstrated to substantially impact rates of cognitive decline. Hassing et al. (2004a,b) reported significant changes in cognitive outcomes related to type 2 diabetes mellitus across a 6-year interval in a sample of octogenarians with evidence for increased risk of decline associated with comorbidity of diabetes and hypertension. These processes, although increasing in prevalence and severity with age, are not strongly correlated with chronological age in cross-sectional analyses. The identification of normative changes may thus depend on measuring nonnormative changes.

III. Methodological Issues in the Study of Aging-Related Change

Inferential and statistical issues that complicate the analysis of longitudinal aging data are often cited as limiting factors for the development of theories and models of aging based on within-individual designs. Directly pertinent to modeling change and deriving useful inferences are two major challenges that require resolution in repeated measures studies: population inference in the context of attrition and mortality and differential gains in performance related to retest effects. Differential survival and participant nonresponse are related to many or most aging-related outcomes, and learning or retest effects are almost inevitably observed with repeated cognitive assessments. However, similar issues are present in cross-sectional studies, but are intractable (e.g., population mortality is indistinguishable from sample selection) and have generally been overlooked. The mortality selection dynamic cannot be understood by single-occasion sampling of different age groups in which attrition has already occurred to different degrees and possibly for different reasons. Analyses of longitudinal data provide the opportunity to directly address attrition

and mortality selection, essential for understanding aging-related changes in health and cognitive outcomes. This section reviews two important inferential issues regarding individual change processes: population selection (i.e., attrition and mortality) and retest effects.

A. Inference and the Processes of Mortality and Attrition in Longitudinal Studies on Aging

While state-of-the-art techniques for analyzing incomplete data have been developed (e.g., Diggle & Kenward, 1994; Schafer & Graham, 2002) and are in relatively wide use, the application of these methods to longitudinal samples in late life remains problematic, both conceptually and computationally. These methods and their corresponding assumptions are based on the notion of a single, accessible population. However, in longitudinal aging studies, at each new wave of testing the sample becomes less representative of the population from which it originated and generalizations from the sample of continuing participants to the initial population become difficult to justify (Nesselroade, 1988; Vaupel & Yashin, 1985). Whereas some forms of nonparticipation can logically permit inference to a single population, such inference is impossible in the case of mortality because individuals have left the population of interest. Therefore, inferences regarding change must be defined as conditional on the probability of surviving or remaining in the study, in interaction with chronological age (Harel, 2003; Kurland & Heagerty, 2004, 2005). In addition, the incomplete data mechanism in studies of aging is not likely to be "missing at random" (i.e., that the probability of missing to be dependent on covariates or prior states), an important assumption of these methods because aging-related outcomes are known to be related to mortality and study nonparticipation (Cooney, Schaie, & Willis, 1988; Riegel, Reigel, & Meyer, 1967; Siegler & Botwinick, 1979; Streib, 1966).

Assuming initial representative sampling, in age-heterogeneous samples, with or without follow-up, inference to individual aging processes is not possible in the aggregate analysis because initial sample selection is confounded with population mortality. In the case of longitudinal follow-up, however, individual and population change processes can be evaluated and interpreted with inferences regarding aging-related changes made conditional on morbidity, mortality, and other attrition processes. Statistical approaches for dealing with mortality and ignorable nonresponse have been developed and permit conditional separation of aging-related changes from other decline processes (mortality, disease-related change). Conditional selection related to mortality in longitudinal studies is often dealt with statistically by either ignoring missing values in maximum likelihood analysis, creating a covariate representing mortality status, with a time-varying covariate representing years to death, or simply treating data as complete within blocks (e.g., Diehr & Patrick, 2003; Diehr et al., 2002; DuFouil, Brayne, & Clayton, 2004; Guo & Carlin, 2004; Johansson et al., 2004; Harel, 2003; Kurland & Heagerty, 2005). Inferences in such approaches are defined as conditional on the probability of surviving and/or remaining in the study and alleviate some concerns with current state-of-the-art approaches that provide inferences to a single population of aging individuals.

B. Retest Effects on Study of Intraindividual Change

Retest (i.e., practice, exposure, learning, reactivity) effects have been reported in a number of longitudinal studies on aging that focus on cognitive outcomes (e.g., Ferrer, Salthouse, Stewart, & Schwartz, 2004; Hultsch et al., 1998; Rabbitt, Diggle, Smith, Holland, & McInnes, 2001; Schaie, 1988, 1996). The issue is that estimates of longitudinal change may be attenuated due to gains occurring as a result of repeated testing, potentially persisting over long intervals (e.g., Schaie, 1996; Willis & Schaie, 1994). Complicating matters is the potential for improvement to occur differentially, related to ability level, age, or task difficulty and which may be due to any number of related influences, including warm-up effects, initial anxiety, and test-specific learning, such as learning content and strategies for improving performance. Differential retest gains such as these confound the identification of differential age-related changes (e.g., in older adults, retest may not be manifest as an increase in performance, but as an attenuated decrease in performance). For example, Zimprich et al. (2004), relating retest gains to long-term change, found that short-term practice gains in processing speed were positively associated with long-term (6-year) changes in processing speed in a sample of older adults.

Several procedures have been proposed for estimating, and ultimately controlling for, retest effects in the context of longitudinal studies on aging (e.g., Ferrer, Salthouse, Stewart, & Schwartz, 2004; McArdle, Ferrer-Caja, Hamagami, & Woodcock, 2002; Rabbitt et al., 2001). Design-based approaches have been reported, making use of either variable retest intervals (e.g., McArdle & Woodcock, 1997) or sequential sample comparison, in which individual samples would differ in terms of test exposure but not age or cohort (e.g., Schaie, 1973). The unique design of the Seattle longitudinal study, and other studies with sequential recruitment, permits retest effects to be evaluated by comparing individuals at the same age who were tested previously with individuals assessed for the first time. Parallel test forms and emphasis on sufficient pretesting have also been used to minimize retesting effects with mixed results.

A recent statistical approach relies on modeling the divergence of between-person age differences and within-person age changes and is based on a specification of the piecewise linear growth curve model (Ferrer et al., 2004; McArdle et al., 2002; Rabbitt et al., 2001). This model, similar in concept to what is gained from sequential sample comparison, permits the estimation of linear or step function changes in retest gains as distinct from "age" changes. Unfortunately, these statistical models rely on strong and often untested assumptions (no difference across birth cohorts; random selection related to attrition and mortality) and require that the initial sample be sufficiently heterogeneous in age to utilize the initial BP age-based heterogeneity in "untested" ability to "control" for test exposure. These models cannot be estimated if the age structure closely approximates the time-in-study intervals (e.g.,in the extreme case of an age-homogeneous longitudinal study) because test exposure is confounded with within-person change. Results of age-related change controlling for practice effects are highly congruent with results from the BP age differences alone.

There are additional conceptual difficulties in the consideration of whether retest or learning effects are a problem that requires a statistical solution. For example, what is the interpretation of the change function that remains after we correct for individual retest effects? At the individual level, is it reasonable to "correct" an individual's change slope to that which would have been obtained if repeated testing had not been performed? Learning is a fundamental feature of development in general and of repeated

testing. Fundamentally, the statistical correction of retest effects results in an unobservable construct of average within-person change in an untested individual, anchoring by between-person age differences as these represent the first assessment exposure.

Retest effects might best be considered as an outcome of interest, with evaluation focused on change in learning processes over time. Widely spaced occasions of measurement , typical of many longitudinal studies, may not be conducive to this perspective that requires intensive measurement bursts spaced over longer periods. Considering long-term change as conditional on previous testing experience makes inferences more complex with generalizability across studies with different characteristics potentially more difficult. However, treating retest or learning effects as outcomes may provide a more realistic framework for understanding change in constructs influenced by learning gains.

IV. Statistical Analysis of Longitudinal Studies of Aging

There are a number of excellent resources for the analysis of longitudinal data (e.g., Fitzmaurice, Laird, & Ware, 2004; Hertzog & Nesselroade, 2003; Singer & Willett, 2003; Snijders & Bosker, 1999). This section provides a brief description with key references for several of the most pertinent statistical models for longitudinal data analysis described in this chapter.

A. Random Coefficients (Latent Growth Curve) Models: Estimating Initial Status and Rate of Change in Cognitive and Other Outcomes

Conceptually, growth curve analysis involves estimating within-individual regressions of the outcome on the temporal metameter and on expected predictors of these individual regression parameters. The level 1 model summarizes individual level outcome data at three or more temporal occasions in terms of "true" initial level of performance (intercept), slope (improvement or rate of change), and error (residual) parameters. The level 2 model estimates fixed (i.e., average) and random (i.e., varying) intraindividual differences and can include predictors of individual/group differences in level 1 parameters (i.e., intercept, slope). Detailed descriptions of these methods (e.g., Snijder & Bosker, 1999; Verbeke & Molenberghs, 2000) and examples using structural equation modeling programs are available elsewhere (e.g., Ferrar & McArdle, 2003).

The univariate random coefficients model (Laird & Ware, 1982) is expressed as

$$y_{ij} = \beta_0 + \beta_1(time_{ij}) + U_{0i} + U_{1i}(time_{ij}) + R_{ij} \qquad (1)$$

where y_{ij} is the dependent variable (e.g., memory) measured at time j in person i, $time_{ij}$ is person i's time (or age) at wave j, β_0 is the average intercept, β_1 is the average slope, U_{0i} is the random intercept for person i, U_{1i} is the random slope for person i, and R_{ij} is the residual for person i at time j. The between-person variance components, $Var(U_{0i})$ and $Var(U_{1i})$, reflect individual differences in level and rate of change, respectively. The within-person variance component $Var(R_{ij})$ reflects the variability of each individual from their predicted values at each measurement time. Alternative specifications of time (age, time in study, time to event/diagnosis) are easily implemented in this model and can be evaluated in terms of comparability of within-person and between-person components (e.g.,

Miyazaki & Raudenbush, 2000; Sliwinski & Buschke, 1999). The power to detect change and correlates of change can be enhanced by increasing the number of occasions (Willett, 1989), by increasing the variability between occasions (Singer & Willet, 2003), or by increasing the reliability of the measurements either by modeling factor level constructs (e.g., Anstey et al., 2003; Hofer et al., 2002; McArdle, 1988) or by intensive measurement designs that make use of aggregate scores (i.e., reducing systematic and error variability by aggregating short-term assessments).

B. Multivariate Random Coefficients (Growth Curve) Analysis

Multivariate latent growth curve models permit direct assessment of correlated level and rates of change across variables. The structure of individual differences in change provides the basis for understanding the relative independence or interdependence of aging-related processes. Multivariate models can be estimated simultaneously (e.g., Johansson et al., 2004; Sliwinski, et al., 2003a) or as a two-stage process where the predicted intercepts and slopes are output for secondary analysis (e.g., Wilson et al., 2002). The degree to which the associations among rates of change are attenuated by covariates, representing individual differences in age, context, or health status, provides a basis for understanding the influence of particular individual characteristics on accounting for heterogeneity in common change processes.

The conventional random coefficients model [Equation (1)] can be extended to the multivariate case by introducing dummy variables to indicate each dependent variable. In the case of three outcome variables, three dummy variables would be integrated into the model to produce a multivariate random coefficients model. Formally, let the dependent variables be indexed by $h = 1, \ldots m$, let the dummy variables be indexed by $d = 1, \ldots s$, and let $d_h = 1$ if $s = m$, and $d_h = 0$ otherwise. The multivariate random coefficients aging model is written as

$$
\begin{aligned}
y_{hij} = & \sum_{s=1}^{m} \beta_{0s} d_{shij} + \sum_{s=1}^{m} \beta_{1s} d_{shij}(time_{ij}) \\
& + \sum_{s=1}^{m} U_{0si} d_{shij} + \sum_{s=1}^{m} U_{1si} d_{shij}(time_{ij}) \\
& + \sum_{s=1}^{m} R_{sij} d_{shij} \qquad (2)
\end{aligned}
$$

The bivariate dual change score model (BDCSM; McArdle & Hamagami, 2001; Ferrer & McArdle, 2004) uses an alternative specification of change extended to lead–lag associations among detrended difference scores (for examples, see Ghisletta & Lindenberger, 2004; McArdle et al., 2004), permitting both constant and proportional estimates of change.

C. Piecewise Cross-Time Analysis: Evaluation of Discontinuous Change across Age Periods

In the basic latent growth curve approach, curvilinear slope parameters are used to describe accelerating or decelerating changes in functioning across repeated measurements, and individual differences are parameterized as deviations from these slopes. In contrast, *piecewise growth curve models* permit the estimation of multiple slope factors for distinct periods of measurement, such as pre- and postretirement, as well as correlated rates of change across these distinct periods (e.g., Jones & Meredith, 2000). Alternate representations of multiple intercept and slope

models can be evaluated, such as an overall linear and quadratic slope for complete life span data, with a third slope representing transitional deviations over a particular time period. Statistical techniques are available for evaluating whether multiple slopes and intercepts are required and where the change points that link distinct slopes reside (e.g., Hall et al., 2000).

D. Within-Person Correlation Analysis (i.e., Coupling)

Models of correlated age slopes at the between-person level are typically based on linear individual trajectories over time, with the time-to-time dynamics considered as unmodeled error components. This ignores the pattern and coupling of cognitive change at the intraindividual (time-varying) level of analysis. Focused analysis of coupled change provides information regarding the relative amount of change exhibited by an individual during a given time period on one variable that is similar to the relative amount of change on other variables. This provides complementary evidence regarding the structure or commonality of within-person change processes.

The multivariate model (described earlier) produces covariance matrices for between-person variance components (i.e., random intercepts and random age slopes) denoted as $\Sigma = \text{cov}(U_j)$ and for within-person variance components denoted as $T = \text{cov}(R_{ij})$. Sliwinski et al. (2003a) used an unconditional multivariate model (i.e., omitting all predictor variables except age when a time in study basis vector is modeled) to decompose variance and covariances into their within-person and between-person components (see Snijders and Bosker, 1999, p. 203).

E. Growth Mixture Models: Identification of Subgroups of Individuals Exhibiting Particular Patterns of Change

The assumption motivating the use of growth mixture modeling (Muthén, 2001) is that the sample is composed of members from more than one population that each exhibit distinct patterns of change. Instead of conceptualizing individual differences in change over time as varying continuously about a single population slope, mixture models permit the identification of multiple population patterns of change that better account for individual-level patterns of change. Individuals probabilistically belong to discrete groups that are distinguished by qualitatively different growth trajectories and other characteristics.

F. Comparison of Measures over Time: Factorial Invariance

Factorial invariance (FI) is a foundational aspect of empirical research and essential for longitudinal evaluations that implicitly require the comparability of constructs (e.g., across occasions). Evidence for measurement invariance is obtained within a confirmatory factor analytic framework using structural equation modeling approaches for estimation. A logical hierarchy of constraints in factor invariance models begins with configural invariance (Horn, McArdle, & Mason, 1983), which requires only that the number of factors and pattern of salient factor loadings be equivalent across groups. Using this model as a baseline, Meredith's (1993; see also Hofer, Horn, & Eber, 1997; Meredith & Horn, 2001) hierarchy of increasingly stringent constraints on the factor model is fit to data: (1) *weak FI* (also known as "metric" invariance) involves equivalence of factor-variable regressions (i.e., factor loadings); (2) *strong FI* adds

constraints on manifest intercept (mean) terms and requires that one of the factor means be fixed to specify the metric of the latent variables; and (3) *strict FI* further constrains unique variances to be equivalent. Extending factorial invariance analyses to multiple occasions permits the rigorous evaluation of measurement comparability within a single sample across age periods.

G. Comparison of Results across Longitudinal Studies of Aging: Meta-analysis and Extensions

Comparison of results across studies is sometimes complex given the differences in study samples (e.g., cohort, culture, age range), design (e.g., age heterogeneous versus age homogeneous, number and span of repeated assessments), specificity and sensitivity of measures, methods of statistical analysis, and ways in which results are reported. A more rigorous approach for the scientific comparison of complex findings across longitudinal studies, permitting direct comparison of results, would be extremely valuable. Increased collaboration among investigators on longitudinal investigations with the aim of coordinating analyses and harmonizing measurements across studies would permit direct and immediate comparison of results.

Currently, evaluating the comparability of particular study results, often based on different variables and study characteristics, remains a challenge. Typical meta-analytic methods for comparing results are based on the effect size and variability of parameter estimates across studies and feature a parameter-by-parameter assessment. New developments in methods for combining evidence from studies with different measurements and other characteristics permit evaluation of theoretical hypotheses with the potential for reconciliation of cross-sample differences by sample-level and individual-level characteristics (e.g., Spiegelhalter & Best, 2003). In general, the advantages of simultaneous cross-study analysis and comparison are that it can (1) permit the inclusion of study and country-level variables to account for potential differences in results across studies; (2) provide increased sample sizes for the oldest ages and for particular health conditions (i.e., rare events); and (3) provide immediate evidence with regard to the replicability and generalizability of findings.

V. Summary

Longitudinal studies have direct implications for explanatory theories of development and aging. The evidence we have obtained thus far from long-term longitudinal and intensive short-term longitudinal studies indicates remarkable within-person variation in many types of processes, even those once considered as highly stable (e.g., personality; Mroczek & Spiro, 2003). Although we emphasize that aging and human development is fundamentally a within-person process and that this is where our research should focus, we understand the practical limitations that have led to the reliance on between-person age differences as a surrogate of within-person change. We have outlined many of the assumptions that are made by relying on BP information and that in many cases, these assumptions are untenable or untestable. From both theoretical and empirical perspectives, between-person differences are a complex function of initial individual differences and intraindividual change and covariation. The identification and understanding of these different sources of between-person differences and developmental and aging-related changes require the direct observation of within-person change.

There are many challenges for the design and analysis of strict within-person studies and large-sample longitudinal studies and these will differ according to purpose. The challenges of strict within-person studies include limits on inferences given the smaller range of contexts and characteristics available within any single individual. Certainly, the study of fixed or relatively stable person characteristics (i.e., genetic differences) necessitate a between-person design. In addition, the thorny issue of gains associated with repeated testing requires focus on the dynamic processes themselves rather than considering the counterfactual of what change would have occurred in the absence of repeated testing. In general, combination (WP, BP) studies are necessary for comprehensive understanding of within-person processes of aging—people differ in their responsivity to influences of all types, to the complex effects of aging. The strength of the many existing longitudinal studies is that they permit the simultaneous examination of within-person processes in the context of between-person variability, differences in change, and between-person moderation of within-person processes. Temporal sampling is important in this regard, and recent studies incorporating "process" variables using intensive burst measurements within the context of long-term longitudinal studies permit the direct study of change in intraindividual variability and intraindividual change.

The focus of this chapter is on ways to achieve an integrative understanding of aging-related changes. We must seek comprehensive, developmental theories that combine both between-person and within-person sources of information from results based on appropriate designs and tenable assumptions. Even so, we do not expect that these two general sources of variability will correspond. There is good evidence that between-person differences are important modifiers of within-person processes and that within-person processes are important components of subsequent between-person differences. It is also essential for our continued understanding of change that our interpretations of results and theoretical developments be sensitive to different temporal sampling spans as these will likely reflect different WP processes and influences.

There is a growing consensus that understanding processes as they transpire within individuals should serve as the foundation for developmental and aging science but also that we cannot discount the importance of between-person differences in within-person processes. The study of within-person change emphasizes the interplay among cognitive, emotional, and physiological characteristics in the development and changing contexts that occur over time and thus is sensitive to the temporal sampling of the design. Such understanding requires many different levels of analysis (e.g., birth cohort, average population change, correlated and coupled change) that are each complementary and necessary perspectives on the dynamics of aging. It is only within the context of longitudinal studies on aging that the critical comparison of both between-person differences and within-person change processes can be evaluated in the same sample of aging individuals. Furthermore, the longitudinal approach provides opportunities to identify processes of change other than the simple passage of time (i.e., chronological age) that account for population and individual-level change.

References

Albert, M. S., Jones, K., Savage, C. R., Berkman, L., Seeman, T., Blazer, D., & Rowe, J. W. (1995). Predictors of cognitive change in older persons: MacArthur studies of successful aging. *Psychology and Aging, 10*, 578–589.

Aldwin, C. M., Spiro, A., III, Levenson, M. R. & Cupertino, A. P. (2001). Longitudinal findings from the normative aging study. III. Personality, individual health trajectories, and mortality. *Psychology and Aging, 16*, 450–465.

Almeida, D.M. (2005). Resilience and vulnerability to daily stressors assessed via diary methods. *Current Directions in Psychological Science, 14*, 64–68.

Alwin, D. F., & McCammon, R. J. (2001). Aging, cohorts, and verbal ability. *Journals of Gerontology: Series B: Psychological Sciences & Social Sciences, 56*, S151–S161.

Anstey, K. J., Hofer, S. M., & Luszcz, M. A. (2003). A latent growth curve analysis of late life cognitive and sensory function over eight years: Evidence for specific and common factors underlying change. *Psychology and Aging, 18*, 714–726.

Bäckman, L., Ginovart, N., Dixon, R. A., Robins Wahlin, T. B., Wahlin, Å., Halldin, C., & Farde, L. (2000). Age-related cognitive deficits mediated by changes in the striatal dopamine system. *American Journal of Psychiatry, 157*, 635–637.

Baltes, P.B., & Lindenberger, U. (1997). Intellectual functioning in old and very old age: Cross-sectional results from the Berlin Aging Study. *Psychology and Aging, 12*, 410–432.

Baltes, P. B., & Nesselroade, J. R. (1979). History and rationale of longitudinal research. In J. R. Nesselroade & P. B. Baltes (Eds.), *Longitudinal research in the study of behavior and development*. New York: Academic Press.

Boker, S. M., & Nesselroade, J. R. (2002). A method for modeling the intrinsic dynamics of intraindividual variability: Recovering the parameters of simulated oscillators in multi-wave panel data. *Multivariate Behavioral Research, 37*, 127–160.

Christensen, H., Hofer, S. M., Mackinnon, A. J., Korten, A. E., Jorm, A. F., & Henderson, A. S. (2001). Age is no kinder to the better educated: Absence of an association established using latent growth techniques in a community sample. *Psychological Medicine, 31*, 15–27.

Christensen, H., Mackinnon, A., Jorm, A. F., Korten, A., Jacomb, P., Hofer, S. M., & Henderson, S. (2004). The Canberra longitudinal study: Design, aims, methodology, outcomes and recent empirical investigations. *Aging, Neuropsychology, & Cognition, 11*, 169–195.

Cooney, T. M., Schaie, K. W., & Willis, S. L. (1988). The relationship between prior functioning on cognitive and personality dimensions and subject attrition in longitudinal research. *Journal of Gerontology, 43*, 12–17.

Diehr, P., & Patrick, D. L. (2003). Trajectories of health for older adults over time: Accounting fully for death. *Ann Intern Med., 139*, 416–20.

Diehr, P., Williamson, J., Burke, G. L., & Psaty B. M. (2002). The aging and dying processes and the health of older adults. *Journal of Clinical Epidemiology, 55*, 269–78.

Diggle, P. J., & Kenward, M. G. (1994). Informative dropout in longitudinal data analysis (with discussion). *Applied Statistics, 43*, 49–94.

DuFouil, C., Brayne, C., & Clayton, D. (2004). Analysis of longitudinal studies with death and dropout: A case study. *Statistics in Medicine, 23*, 2215–2226.

Ferrer, E., & McArdle, J. J. (2003). Alternative structural models for multivariate longitudinal data analysis. *Structural Equation Modeling, 10*, 493–524.

Ferrer, E., & McArdle, J. J. (2004). An experimental analysis of dynamic hypotheses about cognitive abilities and achievement from childhood to early adulthood. *Developmental Psychology, 40*, 935–952.

Ferrer, E., Salthouse, T. A., Stewart, W. F., & Schwartz, B. S. (2004). Modeling age and retest processes in longitudinal studies of cognitive abilities. *Psychology and Aging, 19*, 243–259.

Fitzmaurice, G., Laird, N., & Ware, J. (2004). *Applied longitudinal analysis.* New York: Wiley.

Ghisletta, P., & Lindenberger, U. (2004). Static and dynamic longitudinal structural analyses of cognitive changes in old age. *Gerontology, 50*, 12–16.

Gollob, H. F., & Reichardt, C. S. (1987). Taking account of time lags in causal models. *Child Development, 58*, 80–92.

Guo, X., & Carlin, B. P. (2004). Separate and joint modeling of longitudinal and

event time data using standard computer packages. *The American Statistician, 58*, 16–24.

Haan, M. N., Shemanski, L., Jagust, W. J., Manolio, T. A., & Kuller, L. (1999). The role of APOE ε4 in modulating effects of other risk factors for cognitive decline in elderly persons. *Journal of the American Medical Association, 282*, 40–46.

Hall, C.B., Lipton, R.B., Sliwinski, M.J., & Stewart, W.F., (2000). A change point model for estimating onset of cognitive decline in preclinical Alzheimer's disease. *Statistics in Medicine, 19*, 1555–1566.

Harel, O. (2003). *Strategies for data analysis with two types of missing values.* Ph.D. dissertation. Department of Statistics, The Pennsylvania State University, University Park, PA.

Hassing, L. B., Grant, M. D., Hofer, S. M., Pedersen, N. L., Nilsson, S. E., Berg, S., McClearn, G. E., & Johansson, B. (2004a). Type 2 diabetes mellitus contributes to cognitive change in the oldest old: A longitudinal population-based study. *Journal of the International Neuropsychological Society, 4*, 599–607.

Hassing, L. B., Hofer, S. M., Nilsson, S. E., Berg, S., Pedersen, N. L., McClearn, G. E., & Johansson, B. (2004b). Comorbid type 2 diabetes mellitus and hypertension acerbates cognitive decline: Evidence from a longitudinal study. *Age and Ageing, 33*, 355–361.

Hayward, M.D., & Gorman, B.K. (2004). The long arm of childhood: The Influence of early-life social conditions on men's mortality. *Demography, 41*, 87–107.

Hertzog, C., Dixon, R. A., Hultsch, D. F., & MacDonald, S. W. S. (2003). Latent change models of adult cognition: Are changes in processing speed and working memory associated with changes in episodic memory? *Psychology and Aging, 18*, 755–769.

Hertzog, C., & Nesselroade, J. R. (2003). Assessing psychological change in adulthood: An overview of methodological issues. *Psychology and Aging, 18*, 639–657.

Hofer, S. M., Berg, S., & Era, P. (2003). Evaluating the interdependence of aging-related changes in visual and auditory acuity, balance, and cognitive functioning. *Psychology and Aging, 18*, 285–305.

Hofer, S. M., Christensen, H., MacKinnon, A. J., Korten, A. E., Jorm, A. F., Henderson, A. S. & Easteal, S. (2002). Change in cognitive functioning associated with apoE genotype in a community sample of older adults. *Psychology and Aging, 17*, 194–208.

Hofer, S. M., Horn, J. L., & Eber, H. W. (1997). A robust five-factor structure of the 16PF: Evidence from independent rotation and confirmatory factorial invariance procedures. *Personality and Individual Differences, 23*, 247–269.

Hofer, S. M., & Sliwinski, M. J. (2001). Understanding ageing: An evaluation of research designs for assessing the interdependence of ageing-related changes. *Gerontology, 47*, 341–352.

Hofer, S. M., Sliwinski, M. J., & Flaherty, B. P. (2002). Understanding aging: Further commentary on the limitations of cross-sectional designs for aging research. *Gerontology, 48*, 22–29.

Hogan, J. W., Roy, J., & Korkontzelou, C. (2004). Handling drop-out in longitudinal studies. *Statistics in Medicine, 23*, 1455–1497.

Horn, J. (1972). State, trait and change dimensions of intelligence. *British Journal of Educational Psychology, 42*, 159–185.

Horn, J. L., McArdle, J. J., & Mason, R. (1983). When is invariance not invariant: A practical scientist's look at the ethereal concept of factor invariance. *The Southern Psychologist, 1*, 179–188.

Hultsch, D. F., Hertzog, C., Dixon, R. A., & Small, B. J. (1998). *Memory changes in the aged*. New York: Cambridge University Press.

Hultsch, D. F., Hertzog, C., Small, B. J., McDonald-Miszczk, L., & Dixon, R. A. (1992). Short-term longitudinal change in cognitive performance in later life. *Psychology and Aging, 7*, 571–584.

Hultsch, D. F., MacDonald, S. W. S., Hunter, M. A., Levy-Bencheton, J., & Strauss, E. (2000). Intraindividual variability in cognitive performance in older adults: Comparison of adults with mild dementia, adults with arthritis, and healthy adults. *Neuropsychology, 14*, 588–598.

Johansson, B., Hofer, S. M., Allaire, J. C., Maldonado-Molina, M., Piccinin, A. M., Berg, S., Pedersen, N., & McClearn, G. E. (2004). Change in memory and cognitive functioning in the oldest-old: The effects of proximity to death in genetically related individuals over a six-year period. *Psychology and Aging, 19*, 145–156.

Jones, C. J., & Meredith, W. (2000). Developmental paths of psychological health from early adolescence to later adulthood. *Psychology and Aging, 15*, 351–360.

Kraemer, H. C., Yesavage, J. A., Taylor, J. L., & Kupfer, D. (2000). How can we learn about developmental processes from cross-sectional studies, or can we? *American Journal of Psychiatry, 157*, 163–171.

Kurland, B. F., & Heagerty, P. J. (2004) Marginalized transition models for longitudinal binary data with ignorable and non-ignorable drop-out. *Statistics in Medicine, 23*, 2673–2695.

Kurland, B. F., & Heagerty, P. J. (2005). Directly parameterized regression conditioning on being alive: Analysis of longitudinal data truncated by deaths. *Biostatistics, 6*, 241–258.

Laird, N., & Ware, J. (1982) Random-effects models for longitudinal data. *Biometrics, 38*, 963–974.

Lindenberger, U., & Baltes, P. B. (1994). Sensory functioning and intelligence in old age: A strong connection. *Psychology and Aging, 9*, 339–355.

Little, R. J. A. (1995). Modeling the dropout mechanism in repeated-measures studies. *Journal of the American Statistical Association, 90*, 1112–1121.

MacDonald, S. W. S., Dixon, R. A., Cohen, A., & Hazlitt, J. E. (2004). Biological age and 12-year cognitive change in older adults: Findings from the Victoria Longitudinal Study. *Gerontology, 50*, 64–81.

MacDonald, S. W. S., Hultsch, D. F., & Dixon, R. A. (2003). Performance variability is related to change in cognition: Evidence from the Victoria longitudinal study. *Psychology and Aging, 18*, 510–523.

MacDonald, S. W. S., Hultsch, D. F., Strauss, E., & Dixon, R. A. (2003). Age-related slowing of digit symbol substitution revisited: What do longitudinal age changes reflect? *Journals of Gerontology: Series B: Psychological Sciences and Social Sciences, 58*, P187–P194.

Mackinnon, A., Christensen, H., Hofer, S. M., Korten, A., & Jorm, A. F. (2003). Use it and still lose it? The association between activity and cognitive performance established using latent growth techniques in a community sample. *Aging, Neuropsychology, and Cognition, 10*, 215–229.

Martin, M., & Hofer, S. M. (2004). Intraindividual variability, change, and aging: Conceptual and analytical issues. *Gerontology, 50*, 7–11.

Maxson, P. J., Berg, S., & McClearn, G. (1996). Multidimensional patterns of aging in 70-year-olds: Survival differences. *Journal of Aging and Health, 8*, 320–333.

Maxson, P. J., Berg, S., & McClearn, G. (1997). Multidimensional patterns of aging: A cluster-analytic approach. *Experimental Aging Research, 23*, 13–31.

McArdle, J. J. (1988). Dynamic but structural equation modeling of repeated measures data. In J. R. Nesselroade & R. B. Cattell (Eds.). *The handbook of multivariate experimental psychology* (Vol. 2, pp. 561–564). New York: Plenum Press.

McArdle, J. J., Ferrer-Caja, E., Hamagami, F., & Woodcock, R. W. (2002). Comparative longitudinal structural analyses of the growth and decline of multiple intellectual abilities over the life span. *Developmental Psychology, 38*, 115–142.

McArdle, J. J., & Hamagami, F. (2001). Latent difference score structural models for linear dynamic analyses with incomplete longitudinal data. In L. M. Collins & A. G. Sayer (Eds.), *New methods for the analysis of change* (pp. 139–175). Washington, DC: American Psychological Association.

McArdle, J. J., Hamagami, F., Jones, K., Jolesz, F., Kikinis, R., Spiro, A., III, & Albert, M. S. (2004). Structural modeling of dynamic changes in memory and brain structure using longitudinal data from the normative aging study. *Journals of Gerontology: Series B: Psychological Sciences and Social Sciences, 59*, P294–P304.

McArdle, J. J., & Woodcock, R. W. (1997). Expanding test-retest designs to include developmental time-lag components. *Psychological Methods, 2*, 403–435.

Meredith, W. (1993). Measurement invariance, factor analysis and factorial invariance. *Psychometrika, 58*, 525–543.

Meredith, W., & Horn, J. L. (2001). The role of factorial invariance in modeling growth and change. In L.M. Collins & A.G. Sayer (Eds.), *New methods for the analysis of change* (pp. 204–240). Washington, DC: American Psychological Association.

Miyazaki, Y., & Raudenbush, S. W. (2000). Tests for linkage of multiple cohorts in an accelerated longitudinal design. *Psychological Methods, 5*, 44–63.

Molenaar, P. C. M. (2004). A manifesto on psychology as idiographic science: Bringing the person back into scientific psychology, this time forever. *Measurement: Interdisciplinary Research and Perspectives, 2, 201–218.*

Molenaar, P. C. M., Huizenga, H. M., & Nesselroade, J. R. (2003). The relationship between the structure of interindividual and intraindividual variability: A theoretical and empirical vindication of developmental systems theory. In U. M. Staudinger, Lindenberger (Eds), *Understanding human development: Dialogues with lifespan psychology (pp. 339–360).* Dordrecht, Netherlands: Kluwer Academic Publishers.

Mroczek, D. K., & Spiro, A., III (2003). Personality structure and process, variance between and within: Integration by means of a developmental framework. *Journals of Gerontology: Series B: Psychological Sciences and Social Sciences, 58*, 305–306.

Muthén, B. (2001). Latent variable mixture modeling. In G. A. Marcoulides & R. E. Schumacker (Eds.), *New developments and techniques in structural equation modeling* (pp. 1–33). Lawrence Erlbaum Associates.

Nesselroade, J. R. (1988). Sampling and generalizability: Adult development and aging research issues examined within the general methodological framework of selection. In K. W. Schaie, et al. (Eds.), *Methodological issues in aging research.* (pp. 13–42). New York: Springer.

Nesselroade, J. R. (1991). The warp and woof of the developmental fabric. In R. Downs, L. Liben, & D. S. Palermo (Eds.), *Visions of aesthetics, the environment, and development: The legacy of Joachim F. Wohwill* (pp. 213–240) Hillsdale, NJ: Erlbaum.

Nesselroade, J. R. (2001). Intraindividual variability in development within and between individuals. *European Psychologist, 6,* 187–193.

Nesselroade, J. R. (2004). Intraindividual variability and short-term change. *Gerontology, 50,* 44–47.

Nilsson, L., Adolfsson, R., Bäckman, L., de Frias, C. M., Molander, B., & Nyberg, L. (2004). Betula: A prospective cohort study on memory, health and aging. *Aging, Neuropsychology, and Cognition, 11,* 134–148.

Rabbitt, P. M. A. (1993). Does it all go together when it goes? The Nineteenth Bartlett Memorial Lecture. *Quarterly Journal of Experimental Psychology: Human Experimental Psychology, 46A,* 385–434.

Rabbitt, P., Diggle, P., Smith, D., Holland, F., & Innes, L. M. (2001). Identifying and separating the effects of practice and of cognitive ageing during a large longitudinal study of elderly community residents. *Neuropsychologia, 39,* 532–543.

Riegel, K. F., Riegel, R. M., & Meyer, G. (1967). A study of the drop-out rates in longitudinal research on aging and the prediction of death. *Journal of Personality and Social Psychology, 4,* 342–348.

Rubin, E. H., Storandt, M., Miller, J. P., Kinscherf, D. A., Grant, E. A., Morris, J. C., & Berg, L. (1998). A prospective study of cognitive function and onset of dementia in cognitively healthy elders. *Archives of Neurology, 55,* 395–401.

Rutter, M. (1988). *Studies of psychosocial risk: The power of longitudinal data.* Cambridge: Cambridge University Press.

Salthouse, T. A. (2005). From description to explanation in cognitive aging. In R. J. Sternberg & J. E. Pretz (Eds.), *Cognition and intelligence: Identifying the mechanisms of the mind* (pp. 288–305). Cambridge: Cambridge University Press.

Salthouse, T. A., & Ferrer-Caja, E. (2003). What needs to be explained to account for age-related effects on multiple cognitive variables? *Psychology and Aging, 18,* 91–110.

Salthouse, T. A., Hambrick, D. Z., & McGuthry, K. E. (1998). Shared age-related influences on cognitive and noncognitive variables. *Psychology and Aging, 13,* 486–500.

Schafer, J. L., & Graham, J. W. (2002). Missing data: Our view of the state of the art. *Psychological Methods, 7,* 147–177.

Schaie, K. W. (1965). A general model for the study of developmental problems. *Psychological Bulletin, 64,* 92–107.

Schaie, K. W. (1973). Developmental processes and aging. In C. Eisdorfer & M. P. Lawton, (Eds). *The psychology of adult development and aging (pp. 151–156).* Washington, DC: American Psychological Association.

Schaie, K. W. (1973). Methodological problems in descriptive developmental research on adulthood and aging. In J. R. Nesselroade, H. W. Reese, (Eds.), *Life-span developmental psychology: Methodological issues.* Oxford, England: Academic Press.

Schaie, K. W. (1988). Internal validity threats in studies of adult cognitive development. In M. L. Howe & C. J. Brainard (Eds.), *Cognitive development in adulthood: Progress in cognitive development research (pp. 241–272).* New York: Springer-Verlag.

Schaie, K. W. (1996). *Intellectual development in adulthood.* Cambridge, England: Cambridge University Press.

Schaie, K. W., & Hofer, S. M. (2001). Longitudinal studies of aging. In J. E. Birren & K. W. Schaie (Eds.), *Handbook of the psychology of aging* (pp. 53–77). San Diego: Academic Press.

Seeman, T. E., Singer, B., Rowe, J., & McEwen, B. (2001). Exploring a new concept of cumulative biological risk: Allostatic load and its health consequences: MacArthur Studies of Successful Aging. 98, 4770–4775. *Proceeding of the National Academy of Sciences.*

Shanahan, M. J., & Hofer, S. M. (2005). Social context in gene-environment interactions: Retrospect and prospect. *Journal of Gerontology: Behavioral and Social Sciences, 60B* (Special Issue I), 65–76.

Siegler, R.S. (1994). Cognitive variability: A key to understanding cognitive development. *Current Directions in Psychological Science, 3,* 4–5.

Siegler, I. C., & Botwinick, J. (1979). A long-term longitudinal study of intellectual ability of older adults: The matter of selective subject attrition. *Journal of Gerontology, 34,* 242–245.

Singer, J. D., & Willett, J. B. (2003). *Applied longitudinal data analysis: Modeling change and event occurrence.* London: Oxford University Press.

Sliwinski, M., & Buschke, H. (1999). Cross-sectional and longitudinal relationships among age, memory and processing speed. *Psychology and Aging, 14,* 18–33.

Sliwinski, M., & Buschke, H. (2004). Modeling intraindividual cognitive change in aging adults: Results from the Einstein aging studies. *Aging, Neuropsychology, and Cognition, 11,* 196–211.

Sliwinski, M. J., & Hofer, S. M. (1999). How strong is the evidence for mediational hypotheses of age-related memory loss? A commentary on Luszcz and Bryan. *Gerontology, 45,* 351–354.

Sliwinski, M. J., Hofer, S. M., & Hall, C. (2003a). Correlated and coupled cognitive change in older adults with and without clinical dementia. *Psychology and Aging, 18,* 672–683.

Sliwinski, M. J., Hofer, S. M., Hall, C., Bushke, H., & Lipton, R. B. (2003b). Modeling memory decline in older adults: The importance of preclinical dementia, attrition and chronological age. *Psychology and Aging, 18,* 658–671.

Sliwinski, M., Lipton, R.B., Buschke, H., & Stewart, W.F. (1996). The effect of preclinical dementia on estimates of normal cognitive function in aging. *Journal of Gerontology: Psychological Sciences, 51B,* P217–P225.

Smith, J., & Baltes, P. B. (1997). Profiles of psychological functioning in the old and oldest old. *Psychology and Aging, 12,* 458–472.

Snijders, T., & Bosker, R. (1999). *Multilevel analysis: An introduction to basic and advanced multilevel modeling.* Thousand Oaks, CA: Sage Publications.

Spiegelhalter, D. J., & Best, N. G. (2003) Bayesian approaches to multiple sources of evidence and uncertainty in complex cost-effectiveness modeling. *Statistics in Medicine, 22,* 3687–3709.

Strauss, E., MacDonald, S. W. S., Hunter, M., Moll, A., & Hultsch, D. F. (2002). Intraindividual variability in cognitive performance in three groups of older adults: Cross-domain links to physical status and self-perceived affect and beliefs. *Journal of the International Neuropsychological Society, 8,* 893–906.

Streib, G. F. (1966). Participants and drop-outs in a longitudinal study. *Journal of Gerontology, 21,* 200–209.

Vaupel, J. W., & Yashin, A. I. (1985). Heterogeneity's ruses: Some surprising effects of selection on population dynamics. *American Statistician, 39,* 176–185.

Verbeke, G., & Molenberghs, G. (2000). *Linear mixed models for longitudinal data.* New York: Springer-Verlag.

Verhaeghen, P., & Salthouse, T. A. (1997). Meta-analyses of age-cognition relations in adulthood: Estimates of linear and nonlinear age effects and structural models. *Psychological Bulletin, 122,* 231–249.

Willis, S.L. & Schaie, K.W. (1994). Cognitive training in the normal elderly. In F. Forette, Y. Christen, & F. Boller (Eds.), *Plasticité cérébrale et stimulation cognitive* (pp. 91–113). Paris: Foundational National De Gérontologie.

Willett, J. B. (1989). Some results on reliability for the longitudinal measurement of change: Implications for the design of studies of individual growth. *Educational and Psychological Measurement, 49,* 587–602.

Wilson, R. S., Beckett, L. A., Barnes, L. L., Schneider, J. A., Bach, J., Evans, D. A., & Bennett, D.A. (2002). Individual differences in rates of change in cognitive abilities of older persons. *Psychology and Aging, 17,* 179–193.

Zimprich, D. (2002a). Cross-sectionally and longitudinally balanced effects of processing speed on intellectual abilities. *Experimental Aging Research, 28,* 231–251.

Zimprich, D. (2002b). Cognitive development in old age: The significance of processing speed and sensory functioning for cognitive aging. Doctoral Dissertation, University of Hamburg.

Zimprich, D., Hofer, S. M., & Aartsen, M. J. (2004). Short-term versus long-term longitudinal changes in processing speed. *Gerontology, 50,* 17–21.

Zimprich, D., Martin, M. (2002). Can longitudinal changes in processing speed explain longitudinal age changes in fluid intelligence? *Psychology and Aging, 17,* 690–695.

Part Two

Biological and Social Influences on Aging and Behavior

Three

Behavior Genetics and Aging

George P. Vogler

Genetics as a field has undergone dramatic development during the time when the *Handbook of the Psychology of Aging* has been publishing chapters on behavior genetics and aging. There are two fundamentally different approaches used to study genetics and aging. The first is an approach that has been used since the early 20th century to quantify the extent of genetic influences based on statistical estimates of latent (unobserved) genetic influences using genetically informative samples such as twins. Methodological developments using this approach permit us to conduct genetically informative longitudinal analyses to characterize the nature of stability and change in age-related behavioral traits over time. The second approach is based on molecular genetic techniques to identify the effects of specific genes. This approach capitalizes on advances that have occurred primarily in the past two decades. It has been applied successfully to diseases that are influenced by one (or very few) major gene and is now being used to attempt to identify specific genetic factors for traits that are much more complex in their etiology, including multiple genes of small effect that are

functioning within a complex environment. Traits with this complex pattern of etiology include age-related behavioral traits such as cognitive function and decline. Technological developments in molecular genetics provide us with new opportunities to identify specific genes and to consider how they function in an interacting network of other genes, environmental influences, and developmental change over time as they influence complex traits. This chapter provides a brief discussion of the theoretical issues that underlie our conception of how genetics can have an impact on age-related behavior, followed by consideration of research approaches that are used in contemporary studies. Finally, recent research findings are surveyed briefly.

I. Theoretical Aspects of Genetics and Aging

Individual variability in age-related outcomes has long been recognized. These outcomes are diverse and include life span (both reduced through adverse events and extended through factors that confer exceptional longevity), health-related outcomes, and functional abilities, including cognitive function. This chapter focuses on the latter.

A. Mendelian Genetics and Major Genes

Mendelian genetics is based on the insightful recognition by Gregor Mendel in the 19th century that observed patterns of inheritance were consistent with a mechanism where there were pairs of elements at each gene, with one element inherited from each parent. The forms of these elements (alleles) acted jointly to produce the phenotype (a term used by geneticists to denote the observed trait) in an individual, but retained their distinct identity so that they could segregate independently for transmission to the next generation. The principles of Mendelian genetics have been especially useful in identifying the genetic etiology of major medical disorders that result from the strong effect of a single major gene on the phenotype. As of February 2005, there were 15,870 entries catalogued in Online Inheritance in Man (OMIM, 2005). However, it is likely that Mendelian major genes are relatively insignificant in their effects on aging and cognition and that a multifactorial model in which many genes function and interact with other genes and environmental influences is a more appropriate model.

B. Quantitative Genetics and Polygenic Traits

Traits that are of the most interest in behavioral genetics and aging do not generally have genetic influences that are due to the effects of single major genes. With the exception of some specific genetic factors related to forms of Alzheimer's disease, accounting for perhaps only 1–2% of all cases

(Plassman & Breitner, 1997), the cognitive and personality traits that are of interest in aging research are due to the effect of many genes, each of which has a small effect, rather than single major genes. Quantitative genetic theory, which was developed well before anything was known about the physical nature of the genetic material (e.g., Fisher, 1918), builds on the idea that complex traits are characterized by a continuous quantitative scale of measurement that arises from the aggregate influence of many small genes.

A widely applied research design is the classical twin study (see summary of research results using twin studies described later). This design permits assessment of the heritability of a phenotype and the shared genetic variance between multiple phenotypes. Twin studies are particularly useful in studies of aging because they do not require data from multiple generations, in contrast to other family designs for which parent–offspring data are needed and which are impractical to obtain in the study of age-related traits. Twin studies have been extremely useful in establishing with confidence the relative magnitude of genetic influences on behavioral outcomes that are relevant to aging.

One of the most important advances in the past decade has been the development of technologies and methodologies to identify the effect of specific genetic loci. In the context of the effect of a major Mendelian locus, identification of the effect of a major gene using linkage to DNA markers is straightforward. In the context of the effect of an individual locus embedded within the broader context of a multifactorial polygenic system, detection of the effect of any individual locus becomes more challenging, both because the effect of any one locus is expected to be small and because there are numerous other effects on the phenotype that tend to mask or modify the influence of any single locus. This presents a challenge both in the detection of loci for complex traits and in the interpretation in terms of confidence in the results when replication among multiple studies is often inconsistent.

C. Molecular Genetics

The ability to identify major genes exploded once the availability of DNA markers became widespread. A DNA marker is a type of DNA variability that is measurable at the molecular level and whose chromosomal location is known. Markers can be of several types, with the most frequently used involving variability in the length of a DNA fragment or substitution of one nucleotide in the DNA sequence for a different nucleotide. Because the location of a marker is known, if there is an association between variability in the DNA marker and in the trait of interest it implies that there is a gene that has an effect on the trait in the chromosomal region near the known location of the marker.

There have been several general approaches to the incorporation of molecular markers into the search for genes for complex traits. One approach is exploratory, where markers of known location selected that are distributed throughout the genome, and linkage approaches are taken to identify chromosomal regions that are likely to contain genes that are relevant for the trait under investigation. These approaches tend to point to very broad regions that contain many genes. The success of such approaches depends on whether the regions contain genes of known function that are likely candidate genes for further investigation. A second approach is more confirmatory in nature, where more intensive investigation of known candidate genes is undertaken. This approach depends on the appropriateness of the selected candidate genes, as genes that

are related to the trait but that are not investigated will be overlooked. However, the ability to identify polymorphisms (multiple forms of genes) within the functional or regulatory regions of known genes makes it possible to identify in detail the nature of the genetic polymorphism that affects the phenotype.

D. Genetics and Development

Because aging can be considered to be a developmental phenomenon, it is important to recognize that genetic influences can be dynamic rather than static. While the coding sequence and polymorphisms within the coding sequence are fixed, the genome is dynamic in terms of what genes are expressed at a particular time or in a particular tissue. Several approaches are beginning to be applied to understand the nature of the dynamics of genetic factors as they relate to aging.

One approach is to conduct linkage types of analyses using a panel of markers but looking for differences in the patterns of linkage across multiple ages. Using this approach, it is possible to detect changes in loci that are detected as having an influence on the phenotype at different ages. This approach presents a number of challenges. Significantly, because the effects of any particular locus on a complex phenotype such as cognitive performance are likely to be small, low statistical power to detect effects and the problem of false-positive results when conducting exploratory studies using a large number of markers make it difficult to interpret changes in the pattern of linkage results. What appears to be change over time could be the result of low power and a high rate of false-positive results. Thus, it important to replicate results before claiming evidence of change in linkage patterns over time.

A second approach involves a radically different technology that uses gene expression. If there are developmental effects, one important mechanism is differences in the expression of genes at different ages. Gene expression studies evaluate whether a gene is being actively transcribed into RNA under a particular set of conditions (e.g., a particular age). While this technology has a lot of promise in informing us about developmental change, there are challenges. Normally a large number of genes are evaluated—many thousands. In this situation, standard statistical procedures for determining whether there are significant differences in different age groups break down. How to deal with this issue is an area that is the focus of much investigation at present. A second issue is that in order to obtain a sample of tissue to assay RNA levels, invasive procedures are required. For behavioral phenotypes, this means that brain tissue is needed to assess neurotransmitter expression levels under different conditions. This limits the experimental design to animal studies for most applications of relevance to aging and behavior.

II. Research Approaches and Issues

A. Determining the Importance of Genetic Factors in Aging

1. Heritability and the Importance of Context

The key question that is addressed in studies of heritability is the importance of genetic factors in contributing to variability in a trait relative to nongenetic factors. This is done formally by quantifying the proportion of variance within a defined population that can be attributed to genetic factors. This concept, termed heritability, is a population parameter that is applicable to the particular population in its particular environment at a particular time. Even though genes are generally considered to be fixed at conception, their relative impact as assessed by heritability can be altered, sometimes dramatically, by changes in the composition of the population being investigated (e.g., one population might be genetically homogeneous for a trait, exhibiting very little genetic variability, whereas another population might have substantial genetic heterogeneity, resulting in greater relative genetic variability), by environmental changes within a population (if there is an environmental change resulting in greater environmental variability, the relative importance of genetic effects will be reduced even if there is no change in the absolute magnitude of genetic influences), or by differences within a population at different periods of development (genes that are actively transcribed at one period of development exhibit genetic variability whereas there will be no genetic variability for those genes if they are not actively transcribed at a different period of development).

It is also important to recognize that, as a population parameter, heritability does not apply directly to individuals. For example, a heritability of 0.4 means that 40% of the variance in a particular population is due to genetic effects. However, it does not mean that the phenotype of any individual in the population is 40% due to genes and 60% due to environmental factors.

Many studies have been done over the years to establish the heritability for a variety of traits. With the availability of increasingly sophisticated molecular genetic methods for identifying genes and characterizing their molecular basis of action, it is tempting to dismiss heritability studies as outdated. However, it is important to establish the relative importance of genetic factors prior to embarking on expensive molecular genetic studies. Furthermore, with dramatic changes in factors, such as demographics of the elderly, changes in medical care, and changes in options for long-term care, the context in which heritability estimates have been made has changed so that heritability estimates from older studies may no longer be accurate estimates of the current impact of genetic factors.

2. Twin Studies

The primary strategy for characterizing individual differences in age-related characteristics has been to use twin studies. While there have been several important twin studies of aging conducted in the United States, there has also been a remarkable wealth of information generated from twin studies conducted in Scandinavia. This reflects, in part, the superb population registry information that is available in Scandinavian countries, not possible in the United States, that permits ready identification of population cohorts of elderly twins and linkage to a wealth of health information.

The Swedish Twin Registry was established in the 1950s and has been expanded over the years with assessment of different cohorts to focus on common complex diseases with current screening of all twins born in 1958 or earlier (Lichtenstein et al., 2002). Included in the registry are approximately 70,000 twin pairs yielding more than 370 publications. The Swedish Adoption Twin Study of Aging (SATSA; Pedersen et al., 1991) was developed from the registry. The study has contributed substantially to twin study information on cardiovascular disease risk factors, allergy and respiratory symptoms, cancer risk, psychiatric disorders and substance use and abuse, and cognitive decline and dementia. The OCTO-Twin study was also derived from the registry. The Danish Twin Registry includes twin pairs born in Denmark between

1870 and 1930 (Hauge et al., 1968). It has been used to address a variety of research questions in aging, including investigation of genetic influences on general health and cognition (Christensen et al., 1999).

The National Heart, Lung and Blood Institute (NHLBI) twin study (e.g., Swan et al., 1990; Reed et al., 1993) is a study of white male veterans of World War II and the Korean war. While the original and primary focus of this study has been on cardiovascular risk factors (Feinleib et al., 1977), as the twins have become older a focus has emerged on the cognitive performance and its relationship to cardiovascular risk factors over the life span (e.g., Carmelli et al., 1998; Swan & Carmelli, 2002; Swan et al., 1990, 1992, 1998, 1999).

Another study of veterans, the Vietnam Era Twin Study (e.g., Goldberg et al., 1990a, 1990b), includes over 2000 male monozygotic twin pairs who both served on active military duty during 1965–1975. These twins have been evaluated on a variety of health and cognitive factors periodically throughout adulthood and continue to be followed longitudinally.

The Minnesota Twin Study of Adult Development and Aging covers a broad age range but consists of a modest subset of twins who have been investigated with respect to age-relevant issues. These include memory performance (Finkel & McGue, 1993) and functional age (Finkel, Whitfield, & McGue, 1995).

While there are clearly environmental influences such as schooling, occupation, and lifestyle habits that can influence health and cognitive functioning in adults (e.g., Cerhan et al., 1998), these have largely been emphasized in epidemiological studies that do not include a substantial genetic component. In contrast, genetically informative twin studies of aging have generally emphasized the quantitative genetic model and have not focused on specific aspects of the environment in the context of this model. An exciting challenge for contemporary researchers is to integrate more informative environmental assessments into innovative quantitative genetic designs.

B. Detecting the Effects of Specific Genetic Loci

Once it has been established that genetic factors are significant and remain significant as aging progresses, the challenge is to identify the specific loci that are involved. This can be accomplished using linkage analysis of pedigree data or affected sibling pairs, which are approaches that are frequently applied to relate genetic markers to qualitative traits such as the presence or absence of a diagnosis of dementia. These approaches can also be applied to the investigation of quantitative traits that have a continuous scale of measurement, such as cognitive performance measures. Genetic loci that affect such continuously varying measures are called quantitative trait loci (QTL). Other study designs, such as the analysis of siblings, are also useful for QTL analysis. Association studies use individuals selected from a population rather than relatives. Whereas linkage studies can identify loci that affect a trait over a fairly broad chromosomal region, association studies that do not include relatives can only detect loci that are the functional gene or that are very close to the functional gene.

1. Candidate Gene Approaches

If prior information is available that points to a particular known gene as likely to be involved in a trait or if the biological mechanism underlying a trait is well understood, then it is possible to focus on that locus, either through testing for linkage or association with DNA markers that are very close but that are not part of the functional gene or through searching for polymorphisms within the coding and regulatory regions of a known gene. With current technology, it is possible to search for single nucleotide polymorphisms (SNPs that are a change in a single nucleotide in a DNA sequence) within the exons (coding regions) and regulatory regions and to relate SNP variability to variability in the phenotype. This is most likely to succeed if the SNP results in a change in the amino acid sequence of the resulting gene product (nonsynonymous SNP), as there is redundancy in the genetic code such that there are many instances where change in a nucleotide does not change the amino acid that is encoded. However, even if the amino acid sequence is unchanged, it is possible for a SNP to have an effect on the gene product through change in the physical properties of the DNA strand that could impact the ability of a gene to be transcribed. An interesting example of this approach is the finding of a relationship between one of four SNPs in the Werner's syndrome gene for premature aging and cognitive function in elderly Danish twins (Bendixen et al., 2004). Interestingly, a rare allele at the SNP is suggested to have a beneficial effect on cognitive performance.

2. Exploratory Approaches

For complex traits for which the underlying genetic architecture is not clear, an exploratory analysis that examines a set of DNA markers distributed throughout the genome is more appropriate. This approach, if successful, will identify broad chromosomal regions that are likely to contain genes that influence the trait. Further detailed work is then required to narrow the region in order to ultimately identify the gene involved.

While genomic databases have become useful in providing information about genes in particular locations, it is usually the case that the number of genes in a region is very large. Approaches that look for associations between a marker and a trait at the population level provide a much finer resolution but would require a dramatically and impractically larger set of markers to saturate the genome. As the technology for SNP genotyping improves and becomes less expensive, this approach may become more feasible in the future.

C. Sampling: Challenges and Opportunities

1. The Effect of Selective Survival on Genetic Studies

A challenge in research on aging arises in the effect of selective survival. In the absence of life span data or information on individuals who are deceased or otherwise unavailable to be included in a study, researchers are limited to studying survivors, who may not be representative of the population from which they were drawn. The problem of selective survival is particularly acute in some genetically informative designs, such as a twin study, where selection for participation is often conditional on both members of a twin pair being available at the initiation of the study. A related issue in longitudinal studies is the drop-out rate. If the drop-out rate is affected by particular genetic or environmental factors that, for example, impact a particular disease, then the remaining participants will provide biased inference regarding those genetic or environmental factors. The deleterious effects of this kind of bias can be overcome to some extent by the use of imputation or weighting schemes that have been well developed by survey researchers.

2. Genetic studies of exceptional survivors

Exceptional survival (ES) can be defined arbitrarily as survival to 100 years of age. While this threshold is arbitrary, the use of centenarians provides a convenient reference point. Regardless of the precise definition of exceptional survival, such individuals have several characteristics that make them particularly useful in studying age-related factors in the absence of serious morbidity due to disease, cognitive decline, or functional disability. One characteristic of ES is maintenance of independent functioning late in life, such that morbidity is compressed in life, making centenarians a useful human model of disease-free or disease-delayed aging (Perls et al., 2002a, b). There appear to be three profiles of centenarians for age-associated diseases (hypertension, heart disease, diabetes, stroke, nonskin cancer, skin cancer, osteoporosis, thyroid condition, Parkinson's disease, chronic obstructive pulmonary disease, and cataracts): survivors who had a diagnosis of illness prior to age 80, delayers who did not have age-associated disease until after age 80, and escapers who reached age 100 without developing age-associated disease (Evert et al., 2003).

Because of selective mortality, individuals who have a genotype that contributes to earlier mortality will be more likely to be absent from a population of ES individuals. This results in changes in genotypic and allele frequencies in survivors in favor of protective alleles or absence of deleterious alleles. This phenomenon has been termed demographic selection (Vaupel et al., 1998). For example, the APOE ε4 allele frequency drops with a corresponding increase in the relative frequency of the ε2 allele (Schächter et al., 1994; Rebeck et al., 1994). A somewhat counterintuitive increase in homozygosity in centenarians is reported by Bonafè et al (2001). This finding could be due to either progressive loss of one allele during aging or progressive selection with age of homozygotes, potentially due to selection for homozygotes that are more effective at dealing with a variety of stressors (Franceschi et al., 2000). Demographic selection is important for enhancing the possibility of detecting genetic loci of significance to exceptional survival because the selection process provides a "cleaner" phenotype relative to younger nonsurvivors. Reduction of heterogeneity is an important step for enhancing the likelihood that relevant loci will be detected with a greater degree of statistical certainty.

D. Modeling Complexity

A challenge in the investigation of age-related behavioral traits is the complexity of the phenotypes. Those related to the maintenance or decline of cognitive function with age are likely to be multifactorial in their etiology, including a role for many genes (a polygenic system). The quantitative genetic perspective discussed previously assumes such a multifactorial system. Linkage and association approaches, in contrast, are designed primarily to detect the effect of a single locus, sometimes in the context of a handful of other loci. A challenge is in the development of models that accurately describe the situation that occurs in polygenic systems as we move from modeling influences on the phenotype as abstract components of variance to the identification of individual factors, both genetic and environmental. One of the most well-integrated approach is the multipoint linkage analysis of quantitative trait loci embedded within a more general variance component method, as implemented in the computer package SOLAR (Almasy & Blangero, 1998). To date, this approach has not been applied to cognitive outcomes but has been

applied to cardiovascular outcomes in the Framingham Heart Study (Diego et al., 2003). Results indicated a genotype by age interaction for fasting glucose and systolic blood pressure for the polygenic component of variance and a quantitative trait locus by age interaction for a linkage signal on chromosome 17 for systolic blood pressure.

Just as our understanding of genetic influences on complex traits is improving as it becomes possible to incorporate information on specific genetic loci into models, it is important to develop tools that also incorporate measurable aspects of relevant environmental influences. One of the most significant measures that affects a variety of health and functional outcomes and that most likely includes environmental aspects is socioeconomic status (SES). The relationship between SES and morbidity and mortality is well established (reviewed by Preston & Taubman, 1994).

While incorporation of measured aspects of the genotype and environment into variance component models is an important step in accurately characterizing the relationships among factors that affect age-related phenotypes, it is increasingly clear that the true nature of these relationships is more complex than a standard regression or covariance-based model is designed to accommodate. It is likely that the relationships among causal factors include linear effects, nonlinear effects, interactions among factors, feedback loops, redundant pathways, dynamic change over time, and so on (Heller & McClearn, 1995). While some of these issues can be modeled with appropriate data, few studies have the sample size, study design, or massively repeated measure data that would be required. To take advantage of the statistical power that is realized in moving from latent variable models to measured genotype and environment for estimating more complex nonlinear effects, it will be necessary to reconceptualize the study design that is required. Careful consideration needs to be given to the sample size and the frequency and type of longitudinal assessment so that it will be possible to understand more fully how genetic factors act in the broader context of other genes and environmental factors rather than in isolation.

III. Research Findings

A. The Stability of Heritability for Cognitive Functioning in Aging

One perspective on the stability of genetic influences in old age predicts that, as environmental insults accumulate over time and as physiological systems begin to break down with age, the importance of genetic effects relative to environmental effects would diminish with advancing age. In contrast to this expectation, the heritability for cognitive functioning appears to be relatively stable over time, perhaps with some decline in heritability in older cohorts. Finkel et al. (1998) found in the Swedish Adoption/ Twin Study of Aging (SATSA) that heritability for cognitive abilities remain stable over two 3-year intervals for younger individuals when the SATSA sample was divided into younger and older cohorts, but that there may be decreases in heritability for general cognitive performance over time in the older cohort. Using a latent growth curve model, Reynolds, Finkel, Gatz, and Pedersen (2002) found that genetic influences were generally more important for the cognitive ability level, whereas environmental or stochastic processes were more important in the rate of change. A similar pattern was observed in the Longitudinal Study of Aging Danish Twins (McGue & Christensen, 2002). There was increasing influence of genetics on functional abilities with age (Christensen et al., 2000),

and high heritability for level but not for rate of change of cognitive functioning in twins 70 years and older assessed up to four times over 8 years (McGue & Christensen, 2002), with little influence of age, gender, or social contact on heritability (McGue & Christensen, 2001). While there appears to be some evidence of a decline in heritability from longitudinal studies, genetic influences remain substantial even in very old twins, as demonstrated in octogenarian Swedish twins (McClearn et al., 1997) and Danish twins aged 75 and older (McGue & Christensen, 2001). Becuase change in cognitive ability is predicted by proximity to death, as well as chronological age (Johansson et al., 2004), it is possible that differences within twin pairs on mortality-related factors contribute to the modest reduction in heritability in the oldest old.

B. Comorbidity of Cognitive Functioning with Genetically Influenced Health Outcomes

Given the relationship described earlier between mortality and changes in the pattern of genetic influences on cognition, it is noteworthy that there is substantial evidence showing relationships between a variety of health outcomes and cognitive performance. A substantial amount of work has been done in this area using information from the Framingham Heart Study. Cognitive performance has been demonstrated to be negatively related to poor serum cholesterol levels (Elias et al., 2005), midlife stroke risk profile (Seshadri et al., 2004) and 10-year stroke risk (Elias et al., 2004), blood pressure (Elias et al., 1998, Elias et al., 2004), obesity in men (Elias et al., 2003), and type II diabetes (Elias et al., 1997). Moderate alcohol consumption, in contrast, resulted in superior cognitive performance. Each of these health conditions has a genetic component. It would be of value to investigate the extent to which the covariance between these conditions and cognitive functioning reflects genetic factors for the health conditions. This covariance could contribute to changes in the genetic structure of influences on cognitive ability in the elderly as these health conditions become more acute, thus potentially altering the apparent genetic architecture of cognitive function with age due to the increasing impact of correlated health conditions.

C. Genetic Factors in Dementia

Substantial work has been done on genetic factors in dementia, and it is not possible to do a thorough review in this chapter. However, there are several noteworthy general conclusions regarding genetics and dementia. The genetic factors that have been identified are different for familial or early onset Alzheimer's disease in contrast to late onset dementia. Three genes have been identified for familial or early onset Alzheimer's disease: the amyloid precursor protein gene, presenilin 1, and presenilin 2 (for reviews, see Schott, Fox, & Rossur, 2002; Rademakers, Curtis, & Van Broecthoven, 2003; Zekanowski et al., 2004). Genetic influences on late onset dementia, in contrast, are less clear. There is one clear genetic risk factor that has substantial support in the literature. This is the $\varepsilon 4$ allele of the apolipoprotein E (APOE) gene (Corder, Saunders et al., 1993; for reviews, see Ashford & Mortimer, 2002; Raber, Huang, & Ashford, 2004), which appears to account for a substantial portion of the risk of developing late onset dementia. There is some evidence that this effect is not observed across all ethnic groups. Some studies suggest that the frequency of Alzheimer's disease is independent of the APOE genotype in African Americans (e.g.,

Tang et al., 1998) and the relationship is less pronounced in white Hispanics (Harwood et al., 2004). There also is evidence from a large meta-analysis of 5930 Alzherimer disease patients and 8607 controls of a sex difference in the relationship of APOE and risk of developing dementia (Farrer et al., 1997). A very large number of reports of linkage analysis are published each year, but the results are inconsistent and challenging to interpret. Kamboh (2004) summarized recent genome-wide linkage or linkage-disequilibrium studies for late onset Alzheimer's disease and found compelling evidence for linkage to regions on chromosomes 6, 9, 10, and 12. Bertram and Tanzi (2004) summarized 90 studies reported in 2003 and identified three loci on chromosomes 6, 10, and 11 that were positive in three or more independent studies. There are beginning to be replicated reports of other genes involved in Alzheimer's disease, such as CYP46A1 contributing to variability in β-amyloid metabolism (Johansson et al., 2004) and ABCA1 on chromosome 9, which is involved in cholesterol metabolism (Katzov et al., 2004). Despite substantial progress and massive efforts to understand the genetic factors in Alzheimer's disease, much work remains to be done before a full understanding of the genetics of dementia is realized.

IV. New Tools and New Perspectives

A. The Information Explosion from the Genome Sequence Projects

The widespread availability of databases that contain information regarding positions of genes, their function, sequence, and sequence variability is an enormously useful tool for identifying genes that influence complex traits. It is routine to go from the identification of regions of chromosomes using linkage or association approaches to look for potential candidate genes and to obtain information regarding sequence variations that can help identify the functional polymorphisms that result in variability in complex traits. As the information in these databases is expanded and refined, it will be increasingly useful.

B. Gene Expression Studies

The identification of polymorphisms that affect behavioral traits in aging is related to variability in the genetic constitution of individuals that is fixed. Gene expression, however, can vary within individuals as a function of a variety of factors, including development and aging, tissue, and exposure to environmental agents. It is noteworthy that loci detected for age-related traits are not necessarily constant from age group to age group. Variability in what loci are relevant as a function of age is likely due to differences in gene expression at different ages. Because gene expression studies generally examine the expression of thousands of genes at a time, it is a methodological challenge to disentangle true expression differences as a function of age from spurious differences that arise as a result of chance. An interesting area for future research is to determine if phenotypic differences that are a function of polymorphisms at a locus are due to differences in the level at which the gene is expressed.

A limitation of gene expression studies is that they require tissue samples to determine the level of RNA production in a particular tissue under a particular set of circumstances. Because the genes that are of most interest for cognition and dementia involve factors such as neurotransmitters in specific brain regions, it is impossible to conduct expression studies in humans. This is one area where animal models such as mouse models are critical

for expression studies of age-related cognitive phenotypes to be feasible.

C. Integrative Models

This chapter has identified a number of areas that have the potential to extend our understanding of genetic influences on age-related behavioral traits, particularly maintenance or deterioration of cognitive function, beyond the traditional quantitative genetic models that decompose the phenotypic variance into latent genetic and environmental components or linkage and association studies that are used to identify specific genes through candidate gene or genome-wide linkage approaches without consideration of other important contexts. While substantial progress has been made in understanding genetic factors on aging and cognition, it is timely to consider extension of standard models to more fully integrate the information that is becoming available from multiple domains in order to characterize these influences and their interrelationships in a manner that is more consistent with what actually occurs.

These extensions include models that incorporate individual risk factors explicitly. These include measures of environmental assessment. Further research is needed to identify those relevant aspects of the environment that are appropriate candidates for inclusion in a model. Similarly, individual genetic risk factors can be incorporated as linkage and candidate gene approaches identify measurable specific genetic factors. Current methods are limited in terms of statistical power for the detection of interactions, both epistatic interactions among genetic factors and gene–environment interactions. With appropriate sampling, the incorporation of specific measurable genetic and environmental factors will enhance our ability to identify these interactions, which are increasingly recognized as important in studies of other organisms.

Models that truly recognize that multiple genetic and environmental influences function as a complex system will ultimately be the most accurate characterization of how cognitive function is maintained in aging. At present, progress in developing realistic complex system models in this area has been limited. It is likely that the data requirements are more substantial than most current studies can provide. One area that is potentially ripe for a complex systems approach is in gene expression, where data are available on thousands of loci and characterization of the relationships among these loci will be technically difficult. Despite the challenges, development of a systems approach and the investment of resources to obtain the appropriate data for a complex systems model are challenges worth meeting as we strive to characterize the nature of genetic and environmental influences on behavioral outcomes in aging completely and accurately.

V. Conclusions

There is substantial evidence in the literature that genetic influences remain important and substantially stable with aging, although there may be changes in the genetic architecture in the oldest old, particularly as mortality is approached. Identification of specific genetic influences has progressed for Alzheimer's disease, but progress in identifying specific alleles that affect general cognitive ability or cognitive decline has been limited. Continued effort is required to identify both specific genetic factors and specific environmental factors that are significant in change and stability in cognitive outcomes in aging. As these factors are identified, new opportunities will arise to model them explicitly,

including interactions among factors and, ultimately, to develop a complex systems model that provides a good approximation of the true mechanisms that affect cognitive functioning in aging.

Maintenance of cognitive function is one of the most significant factors related to aging. We are on the verge of dramatic new opportunities to understand fully the nature of genetic and environmental factors on this process. Ultimately, the identification of specific, measurable genetic and environmental risk factors has the potential to lead to individualized interventions designed to optimize the maintenance of cognitive function through old age. While the relationships among these risk factors are complex and present a challenge to disentangle, it is a challenge worth facing given the demographic factors leading to an increasing elderly population surviving to increasingly older ages.

References

Almasy, L., & Blangero, J. (1998). Multipoint quantitative-trait linkage analysis in general pedigrees. *American Journal of Human Genetics, 62,* 1198–1211.

Ashford, J. W., & Mortimer, J. A. (2002). Non-familial Alzheimer's disease is mainly due to genetic factors. *Journal of Alzheimer's Disease, 4,* 169–177.

Bendixen, M. H., Nexo, B. A., Bohr, V. A., Frederiksen, H., McGue, M., Kolvraa, S., & Christensen, K. (2004). A polymorphic marker in the first intron of the Werner gene associates with cognitive function in aged Danish twins. *Experimental Gerontology, 39,* 1101–1107.

Bertram, L., & Tanzi, R. E. (2004). Alzheimer's disease: One disorder, too many genes? *Human Molecular Genetics, 13 Spec. No. 1,* R135–R141.

Bonafè, M., Cardelli, M., Marchegiani, F., Cavallone, L., Giovagnetti, S., Olivieri, F., Lisa, R., Pieri, C., & Franceschi, C. (2001). Increase of homozygosity in centenarians revealed by a new inter-*Alu* PCR technique. *Experimental Gerontology, 36,* 1063–1073.

Carmelli, D., Swan, G. E., Reed, T., Miller, B., Wolf, P. A., Jarvik, G. P., & Schellenberg, G. D. (1998). Midlife cardiovascular risk factors, APOE, and cognitive decline in elderly male twins. *Neurology, 50,* 1580–1585.

Cerhan, J. R., Folsom, A. R., Mortimer, J. A., Shahar, E., Knopman, D. S., McGovern, P. G., Hays, M. A., Crum, L. D., & Heiss, G. (1998). Correlates of cognitive function in middle-aged adults. Atherosclerosis Risk in Communities (ARIC) Study Investigators. *Gerontology, 44,* 95–105.

Christensen, K., Holm, N.V., McGue, M., Corder, L., & Vaupel, J. W. (1999). A Danish population-based twin study on general health in the elderly. *Journal of Ageing and Health, 11,* 49–64.

Christensen, K., McGue, M., Yashin, A., Iachine, I., Holm, N. V., & Vaupel, J. W. (2000). Genetic and environmental influences on functional abilities in Danish twins aged 75 years or older. *Journal of Gerontology: Medical Sciences, 55A,* M446–M452.

Corder, E. H., Saunders, A. M., Strittmatter, W. J., Schmechel, D. E., Gaskell, P. C., Small, G. W. et al (1993). Gene dose of apolipoprotein E type 4 allele and the risk of Alzheimer's disease in late onset families. *Science, 261,* 921–923.

Diego, V. P., Almasy, L., Dyer, T. D., Soler, J. M. P., & Blangero, J. (2003). Strategy and model building in the fourth dimension: A null model for genotype x age interaction as a Guaussian stationary stochastic process. *BiomedCentral Genetics, 4 Suppl. 1,* S34–S38.

Elias, M. F., Elias, P. K., Sullivan, L. M., Wolf, P. A., & D'Agostino, R. B. (2003). Lower cognitive function in the presence of obesity and hypertension: The Framingham heart study. *International Journal of Obesity and Related Metabolic Disorders, 27,* 260–268.

Elias, M. F., Robbins, M. A., Elias, P. K., & Streeten, D. H. (1998). A longitudinal study of blood pressure in relation to performance on the Wechsler Adult Intelligence Scale. *Health Psychology, 17,* 486–493.

Elias, M. F., Sullivan, L. M., D'Agostino, R. B., Elias, P. K., Beiser, A., Au, R., Seshadri, S., DeCarli, C., & Wolf, P. A. (2004). Framingham stroke risk profile and lowered cognitive performance: *Stroke, 35,* 404–409.

Elias, P. K., Elias, M. F., D'Agostino, R. B., Cupples, L. A., Wilson, P. W., Silbershatz, H., & Wolf, P. A. (1997). NIDDM and blood pressure as risk factors for poor cognitive performance: The Framingham Study. *Diabetes Care, 20,* 1388–1395.

Elias, P. K., Elias, M. F., D'Agostino, R. B., Silbershatz, H., & Wolf, P. A. (1999). Alcohol consumption and cognitive performance in the Framingham Heart Study. *American Journal of Epidemiology, 150,* 580–589.

Elias, P. K., Elias, M. F., D'Agostino, R. B., Sullivan, L. M., & Wolf, P. A. (2005). Serum cholesterol and cognitive performance in the Framingham heart study. *Psychosomatic Medicine, 67,* 24–30.

Elias, P. K., Elias, M. F., Robbins, M. A., & Budge, M. M. (2004). Blood pressure-related cognitive decline: Does age make a difference? *Hypertension, 44,* 631–636.

Evert, J., Lawler, E., Bogan, H., & Perls, T. (2003). Morbidity profiles of centenarians: Survivors, delayers, and escapers. *Journal of Gerontology: A. Biological Science and Medical Science, 58,* 232–237.

Farrer, L. A., Cupples L. A., Haines, J. L., Hyman, B., Kukull, W. A., Mayeux, R., Myers, R. H., Pericak-Vance, M. A., Risch, N., & van Duijn, C. M. (1977). Effects of age, sex, and ethnicity on the association between apolipoprotein E genotype and Alzheimer disease: A meta-analysis. *Journal of the American Medical Association, 278,* 1349–1356.

Feinleib, M., Garrison, R. J., Fasitz, R. R., Christian, J. C., Hrubec, Z., Borhani, N. O., Kannel, W. B., Rosenman, R., Schwartz, J. T., & Wagner, J. O. (1977). The NHLBI Twin Study of cardiovascular risk factors: Methodology and summary of results. *American Journal of Epidemiology, 106,* 284–295.

Finkel, D., & McGue, M. (1993). The origins of individual differences in memory among the elderly: A behavior genetic analysis. *Psychology and Aging, 8,* 527–537.

Finkel, D., Whitfield, K., & McGue, M. (1995). Genetic and environmental influences on functional age: A twin study. *Journal of Gerontology: Psychological Science, 50,* P104–P113.

Finkel, D., Pedersen, N. L., Plomin, R., & McClearn, G. E. (1998). Longitudinal and cross-sectional twin data on cognitive abilities in adulthood: the Swedish Adoption/Twin Study of Aging. *Developmental Psychology, 34,* 1400–1413.

Fisher, R. A. (1918). The correlation between relatives on the supposition of Mendelian inheritance. *Transactions of the Royal Society of Edinburgh, 52,* 399–453.

Franceschi, C., Valensin, S., Bonafè, M., Paolisso, P., Yashin, A., & De Benedictis, G. (2000). The network and the modeling theories of aging. *Experimental Gerontology, 35,* 869–896.

Goldberg, J., Eisen, S. A., True, W. R., & Henderson, W. G. (1990a). A twin study of the effects of the Vietnam conflict on alcohol drinking patterns. *American Journal of Public Health, 80,* 570–574.

Goldberg, J., True, W. R., Eisen, S. A., & Henderson, W. G. (1990b). A twin study of the effects of the Vietnam War on post-traumatic stress disorder. *Journal of the American Medical Association, 263,* 1227–1232.

Harwood, D. G., Barker, W. W., Ownby, R. L., St George-Hyslop, P., Mullan, M., & Duara, R. (2004). Apolipoprotein E polymorphism and age of onset for Alzheimer's disease in a bi-ethnic sample. *International Psychogeriatrics, 16,* 317–326.

Hauge, M., Harvald, B., Fischer, M., et al. (1968). The Danish Twin Register. *Acta Geneticae Medicae et Gemellologiae, 2,* 315–331.

Heller, D. A., & McClearn, G. E. (1995). Alcohol, aging, and genetics. In T. Beresford & E. Gomberg (Eds.), *Alcohol and aging* (pp. 99–114), New York: Oxford University Press.

Johansson, A, Katzov, H., Zetterberg, H., Feuk, L., Johansson, B., Bogdanovic, N., Andreasen, N., Lenhard, B., Brookes, A. J., Pedersen, N. L., Blennow, K., & Prince, J. A. (2004). Variants of CYP46A1 may interact with age and APOE to influence CSF Abeta42 levels in Alzheimer's disease. *Human Genetics, 114,* 581–587.

Johansson, B., Hofer, S. M., Allaire, J. C., Maldonado-Molina, M. M., Piccinin, A. M., Berg, S., Pedersen, N. L., & McClearn, G. E. (2004). Change in cognitive capabilities in the oldest old: The effects of proximity to death in genetically related individuals over a 6-year period. *Psychological Aging, 19,* 145–156.

Kamboh, M. I. (2004). Molecular genetics of late-onset Alzheimer's disease. *Annals of Human Genetics, 68,* 381–404.

Katzov, H., Chalmers, K., Palmgren, J., Andreasen, N., Johansson, B., Cairns, N. J., Gatz, M., Wilcock, G. K., Love, S., Pedersen, N. L., Brookes, A. J., Blennow, K., Kehoe, P. G., & Prince, J. A. (2004). Genetic variants of ABCA1 modify Alzheimer disease risk and quantitative traits related to beta-amyloid metabolism. *Human Mutation, 23,* 358–367.

Lichtenstein, P., DeFaire, U., Floderus, B., Svartengren, M., Svedberg, P., & Pedersen, N. L. (2002). The Swedish Twin Registry: A unique resource for clinical, epidemiological and genetic studies. *Journal of Internal Medicine, 252,* 184–205.

McClearn, G. E., Johansson, B., Berg, S., Pedersen, N. L., Ahern, F., Petrill, S. A., & Plomin, R. (1997). Substantial genetic influence on cognitive abilities in twins 80 or more years old. *Science, 276,* 1560–1563.

McGue, M., & Christensen, K. (2001). The heritability of cognitive functioning in very old adults: Evidence from Danish twins aged 75 years and older. *Psychology and Aging, 16,* 272–280.

McGue, M., & Christensen, K. (2002). The heritability of level and rate-of-change in cognitive functioning in Danish twins aged 70 years and older. *Experimental Aging Research, 28,* 435–451.

Online Mendelian Inheritance in Man, (OMIM) (2005). McKusick-Nathans Institute for Genetic Medicine, Johns Hopkins University (Baltimore, MD) and National Center for Biotechnology Information, National Library of Medicine (Bethesda, MD). World Wide Web URL: http://www.ncbi.nlm.nih.gov/omim.

Pedersen, N. L., McClearn, G. E., Plomin, R., Nesselroade, J. R., Berg, S., & DeFaire, U. (1991). The Swedish Adoption Twin Study of Aging: An update. *Acta Geneticae Medicae et Gemellologiae, 40,* 7–20.

Perls, T., Kunkel, L. M., & Puca, A. A. (2002a). The genetics of exceptional human longevity. *Journal of the American Geriatrics Society, 50,* 359–368.

Perls, T., Levenson, R., Regan, M., & Puca, A. (2002b). What does it take to live to 100? *Mechanisms of Ageing and Development, 123*, 231–242.

Plassman, B. L., & Breitner, J. C. (1997). The genetics of dementia in late life. *Psychiatric Clinics of North America, 20*, 59–76.

Preston, S. H., & Taubman, P. (1994). Socioeconomic differences in adult mortality and health status. In L. G. Martin & S. H. Preston (Eds), *Demography of aging.* Washington, DC: National Academy Press.

Raber, J., Huang, Y., & Ashford, J. W. (2004). ApoE genotype accounts for the vast majority of AD risk and AD pathology. *Neurobiology of Aging, 25*, 641–650.

Rademakers, R., Cruts, M., & Van Broeckhoven, C. (2003). Genetics of early-onset Alzheimer dementia. *Scientific World Journal, 3*, 497–519.

Rebeck, G. W., Perls, T. T., West, H. L., Sodhi, P., Lipsitz, L. A., & Hyman, B. T. (1994). Reduced apolipoprotein epsilon 4 allele frequency in the oldest old: Alzheimer's patients and cognitively normal individuals. *Neurology, 44*, 1513–1516.

Reed, T., Carmelli, D., Christian, J. C., Selby, J. V., & Fabsitz, R. R. (1993). The NHLBI male veteran twin study data. *Genetic Epidemiology, 10*, 513–517.

Reynolds, C. A., Finkel, D., Gatz, M., & Pedersen, N. L. (2002). Sources of influence on rate of cognitive change over time in Swedish twins: An application of latent growth models. *Experimental Aging Research, 28*, 407–433.

Schächter, F. (1998). Causes, effects, and constraints in the genetics of human longevity. *American Journal of Human Genetics, 62*, 1008–1014.

Schächter, F., Faure-Delanef, L., Guenot, F., Rouger, H., Froguel, P., Lesueur-Gnot, L., & Cohen, D. (1994). Genetic associations with human longevity at the APOE and ACI loci. *Nature Genetics, 6*, 29–32.

Schott, J. M., Fox, N. C., & Rossor, M. N. (2002). Genetics of the dementias. *Journal of Neurology, Neurosurgery and Psychiatry, 73*, 1127–1132.

Seshadri, S., Wolf, P. A., Beiser, A., Elias, M. F., Au, R. Kase, C. S., D'Agostino, R. B., & DeCarli, C. (2004). Stroke risk profile, brain volume, and cognitive function: The Framingham Offspring Study. *Neurology, 63*, 1591–1599.

Swan, G. E., & Carmelli, D. (2002). Evidence for genetic mediation of executive control: A study of aging male twins. *Journal of Gerontology: Psychological Sciences, 57B*, P133–P143.

Swan, G. E., Carmelli, D., Reed, T., Harshfield, G. A., Fabsitz, R. R., & Eslinger, P. J. (1990). Heritability of cognitive performance in aging twins: The National Heart, Lung, and Blood Institute Twin Study. *Archives of Neurology, 47*, 259–262.

Swan, G. E., DeCarli, C., Miller, B. L., Reed, T., Wolf, P. A., Jack, L. M., & Carmelli, D. (1998). Association of midlife blood pressure to late-life cognitive decline and brain morphology. *Neurology, 51*, 986–993.

Swan, G. E., LaRue, A., Carmelli, D., Reed, T., & Fabsitz, R. R. (1992). Decline in cognitive performance in aging twins: Heritability and biobehavioral predictors from the National Heart, Lung, and Blood Institute Twin Study. *Archives of Neurology, 49*, 476–481.

Swan, G. E., Reed, T., Jack, L. M., Miller, B. L., Markee, T., Wolf, P. A., DeCarli, C., & Carmelli, D. (1999). Differential genetic influence for components of memory in aging adult twins. *Archives of Neurology, 56*, 1127–1132.

Tang, M. X., Stern, Y., Marder, K., Bell, K., Gurland, B., Lantigua, R., Andrews, H., Feng, L., Tycko, B., & Mayeux, R. (1998). The APOE-epsilon 4 allele and the risk of Alzheimer disease among African Americans, whites, and Hispanics. *Journal of the American Medical Association, 279*, 751–755.

Vaupel, J. W., Carey, J. R., Christensen, K., Johnson, T. E., Yashin, A. I., Holm, N. V., Iachine, I. A., Kannisto, V., Khazaeli, A. A., Liedo, P., Longo, V. D., Zeng, Y., Manton, K. G., & Curtsinger, J. W. (1998). Biodemographic trajectories of longevity. *Science, 280*, 855–860.

Zekanowski, C., Religa, D., Graff, G., Filipek, S., & Kuznicki, J. (2004). Genetic aspects of Alzheimer's disease. *Acta Neurobiologiae Experimentalis, 64*, 19–31.

Four

Contributions of Cognitive Neuroscience to the Understanding of Behavior and Aging

Arthur F. Kramer, Monica Fabiani, and Stanley J. Colcombe

I. Introduction

The field of cognitive neuroscience in general and more specifically the application of neuroscientific methods and theories to the study of cognitive aging have blossomed in the past decade, largely as the result of the development of functional magnetic resonance imaging (fMRI) techniques. However, it is important to note that the use of neuroimaging techniques to study brain and cognitive differences and changes during the adult life span has been ongoing for the past several decades through the application of electrophysiological techniques, including the recording of electroencephalographic activity (EEG) and event-related brain potentials (ERPs; for a review, see Fabiani & Wee, 2001). Clearly, much has been learned about age-related differences and changes in cognitive function and differences in the timing of mental processes from this earlier research. However, electrophysiological techniques do not lend themselves to the unambiguous localization of the sources of brain activity that

support the multitude of perceptual, cognitive, and action-based processes of interest to researchers who study aging. Hence new techniques were needed to augment scalp-recorded bioelectric recording methods in order to start mapping the way in which neural circuits relate to cognitive processes and the manner in which both brain and mind change across the adult life span.

As described later, over the past decade converging neuroscientific operations have be used to examine both the timing of mental processes [e.g., ERPs, event-related optical signals [EROS], and the localization of cortical processors [e.g., MRI, fMRI, positron emission tomography (PET), EROS, near-infrared (NIRS)] that support cognition and performance. For the most part the collection of these multiple measures has taken place in parallel experiments and then been related during analyses of data. Indeed, the patterns of activation indexed by PET and fMRI recordings have been used as a starting point for the localization of sources of scalp-recorded ERPs (e.g., Di Russo et al., 2003). The simultaneous collection of neuroimaging measures that provide different perspectives on the relationship between brain and mind, e.g., the joint recording of ERPs or optical signals and fMRI, is also developing at a rapid pace and will likely be an important focus during the next decade (e.g., Toronov et al., 2003).

Given the brief nature of the articles in the *Handbook of the Psychology of Aging*, the scope of this chapter is necessarily restricted. For example, although both normal aging and the examination of age-related pathologies are of considerable interest we will, for the most part, confine our discussion to nonpathological aging. We will also restrict our discussion of the application of cognitive neuroscience methodologies to the study of a subset of illustrative cognitive processes of interest to aging researchers, namely attention and memory. The organization of the chapter takes the following format. We begin with a brief discussion of a number of methodologies that have been utilized in the study of the cognitive neuroscience of aging. Next we provide a brief description and discussion of the patterns of age-related differences and changes (in the limited subset of studies that have examined changes over time in brain and cognition within individuals) in brain activation that have been observed and the functional significance of these changes in terms of cognition and performance. We then describe how the cognitive neuroscience approach, i.e., examination of the relationship between measures of brain function and cognition, has enhanced our understanding of age-related differences and changes in attentional and memory processes. Finally, we provide some speculations on the future of the cognitive neuroscience of aging by describing a few promising areas of investigation.

However, before moving on to the central topics of this chapter, we briefly provide the context in which the cognitive neuroscience of aging has been studied. In human cognitive aging research there have been a variety of different theoretical explanations proffered to account for decreases in fluid or process-based abilities across the adult life span. Fluid or process-based abilities are largely independent of experience and instead depend on the speed of processing, reasoning, and memory encoding and retrieval. These processes show substantial declines in both cross-sectional and longitudinal studies during the course of normal aging (Park et al., 2003; Schaie, 2002). However, it has generally been observed that knowledge-based or crystallized abilities (i.e., the extent to which a person has absorbed the contents of culture), such as verbal knowledge and comprehension, continue to be maintained or improve over the life span (Baltes, Staudinger & Lindenberger, 1999).

In the cognitive aging literature, explanations for age-related declines in process-based or fluid abilities fall into two broad classes of theories. General or common cause explanations suggest that a common factor may be responsible for age-related declines (Park, 2000). Common factor models have suggested that a number of different factors, including speed of processing, working memory, inhibition, or diminished sensory functions, may be responsible for cognitive decline observed across a variety of different tasks. For example, Salthouse (1996) argued that processing speed serves as a common factor in age-related cognitive decline. Assuming a model of information processing in which different operations (e.g., perception, decision making, response selection and execution) are performed in a serial fashion, he suggested that the time to perform later operations is reduced when a large proportion of the available time is occupied by the execution of earlier operations. Thus, slowed processing that occurs during the normal course of aging has a cascading effect on information processing. Furthermore, it is assumed that slowed processing can also result in loss of the output of earlier operations, as a result of decay, before these outputs can be integrated with the output of later processing operations. Thus, in this way slowed processing also leads to decrements in working memory. Similar arguments have been made for the primacy and centrality of processes such as working memory (Craik & Byrd, 1982), inhibition of extraneous and task-irrelevant information in the environment and in memory (Hasher & Zacks, 1988), deficits in sensory and motor function (Lindenberger & Baltes, 1997), and attentional or processing resources (Hartley, 1992). Indeed, a variety of studies have shown that such processes, especially processing speed, can often account for a large proportion of age-related variance across a wide assortment of tasks and environments.

An alternative to common factor models of cognitive aging are proposals that age-related cognitive decline is multifaceted with different processes changing across the adult life span at different rates. Support for these specific factor models has been provided by studies that have either equated younger and older adults' performance on some facets of a task and observed changes in other facets of a task, or statistically controlled for general age-related changes and still observed changes in other aspects of performance (Schmiedek & Li, 2004). The results of these studies, however, do not preclude the possibility that both relatively general and more process-specific factors will contribute to cognitive changes in cognition across the adult life span. Indeed, general and specific cognitive changes may be reflected differentially in age-related changes in different aspects of human brain structure and function. This issue are discussed further later.

II. Approaches to the Study of Cognitive Neuroscience

This section briefly describes techniques that have been used in the examination of human brain structure and function. We also illustrate how these techniques have been used to examine some specific questions concerning changes in brain and cognition across the adult life span.

A. Assessing Brain Structure

The *in vivo* assessment of age-related differences in brain structures using MRI-based methods has taken many forms and is perhaps the fastest growing branch of human neuroimaging. This section presents a brief overview of the general approaches currently employed before turning to findings gleaned from these methods in subsequent sections. This overview is limited to noninvasive methods, which have largely developed over the past decade and have allowed investigators to examine issues that could previously only be addressed postmortem.

A gross measure of brain atrophy with age is sometimes computed by measuring the volume of the gray and white matters of the brain, relative to some standard. For example, Smith and colleagues (2002) proposed the use of a normalized brain volume metric, where brain images are segmented into gray and white tissue maps. The maps are then registered into a standard spatial template, and the volumes of the gray and white matters are corrected for spatial scaling, thus yielding an estimate of the relative amount of gray and white matter for each subject, constrained to a common space. This measure can provide a surprisingly accurate cross-sectional estimate of brain atrophy, although it cannot provide information about any regional differences in shrinkage.

Diffusion tensor imaging (DTI) is an MRI technique that provides a mechanism to indirectly assess microstructures of the brain, particularly the white matter tracts, by estimating nonrandomness in the diffusion of water through axonal fibers (Basser et al., 1994; Pierpaoli & Basser, 1996). In DTI, one employs a series of brain scans that are differentially sensitive to the diffusion of water in different directions, thus allowing the researcher to track the pattern of water diffusion in the brain. From these scans the researcher can derive several useful measures. One of the principal outcomes involves *anisotropy*, the degree of nonrandom diffusion of the water, at every point measured in the brain. When the myelin sheaths that surround axonal fibers in the white matter deteriorate, water may diffuse through these tissues in a more random fashion. Thus, by assessing the randomness of water diffusion through myelinated axonal fibers, the researcher can assess the integrity of these structures. Additionally, the researcher can use the information about the principal direction of the water's diffusion through the white matter to trace the path of the myelinated axons, which can be useful in assessing the structural connectivity between different brain regions. However, although this technique can tell us a great deal about the integrity of the myelin sheaths surrounding axons and the rough paths they follow in the brain, the usefulness of DTI in assessing brain structures is generally limited to the white matter and can tell us very little about the volume or integrity of the gray matter cell bodies or their dendrites.

Another approach used to assess differences in brain structure involves manually tracing predefined regions of the gray (e.g., hippocampus) or white (e.g., corpus callosum) matters on a high-resolution MRI scan (e.g., Raz, 2000). This hand-tracing approach allows the researcher to measure regionally specific individual differences in brain volume and is often thought of as the "gold standard" neuroimaging volumetric technique. Hand tracing the volume of specific brain regions can be very useful in determining the relationship between regional volumetric losses and changes in the cognitive processes thought to be supported by these regions, as addressed later. However, this approach requires a high degree of anatomical knowledge and training and can be very time-consuming, which precludes hand tracing every potentially relevant region of the brain. Thus, researchers using hand-tracing methods must limit the number of brain regions they measure and, in the case of very large regions (e.g., the dorsolateral prefrontal cortex), often must sample only a portion of the region of interest.

Another approach gaining in popularity is voxel-based morphometry (VBM; e.g., Ashburner & Friston, 2000), in which high-resolution MRI brain scans are coregistered into a common spatial coordinate system and then semiautomatically segmented into three-dimensional maps of gray matter, white matter, and cerebrospinal fluid (CSF). The researcher can then interrogate each point in the gray, white, and CSF maps for systematic variation with some other variable of interest (e.g., age, cognitive performance). The semiautomatic nature of the technique allows a high degree of replicability, is much faster than hand-tracing techniques, and the researcher can evaluate structural variation throughout the brain, unconstrained by a priori regions of interest. For better or worse, the researcher does not necessarily need a great degree of anatomical training to employ this method. Although VBM has shown good concordance with hand-tracing studies in well-defined regions (e.g., the hippocampus; Good et al., 2002), its fidelity with hand-tracing outcomes in more structurally heterogeneous regions of the brain (e.g., the frontal cortex) has been questioned (e.g., Tisserand et al., 2002). Finally, it should be noted that it is unclear what changes at the cellular level (e.g., myelin loss, cell body shrinkage, cell loss, reductions in dentritic interconnections) underlie changes in volume assessed by VBM. Thus, although useful in describing gross changes in regional brain volumes, VBM may lack adequate statistical power to detect subtle changes in highly heterogeneous regions of the brain (Colcombe et al., 2005; Gunning-Dixon & Raz, 2003). Additionally, it is important to note that neither VBM nor the other neuroimaging techniques reviewed earlier can provide the sort of specificity in the underlying cellular changes that are available with the traditional histological methods applied to nonhuman animals.

B. Electrical Recording of Brain Activity

Electrophysiological measures of brain function include EEG (Davidson, Jackson, & Larson, 2000), ERPs (Fabiani, Gratton, & Coles, 2000), and magnetoencephalography (MEG; Hari, Levanen, & Raij, 2000). These techniques measure the electrical (EEG, ERPs) or magnetic (MEG) fields generated by populations of neurons that are simultaneously active. In the case of EEG the focus is typically on spontaneously generated rhythms and their modification in the presence of intervening events or processes [event-related desynchronization or (ERD), Babiloni et al., 2004], whereas ERPs (and MEG) are typically analyzed as time-locked responses to internal or external events.

Not all neuronal activity is recordable from the surface of the scalp. Much of the electrical activity that can be recorded at a distance is assumed to originate from the dendritic trees of large pyramidal neurons rather than from other cell populations and is postsynaptic (graded) in nature. Further, only activity originating in structures with open-field configurations (i.e., where the dendrites of the neurons are aligned to form a dipole) can be measured from the scalp surface (Allison, Wood, & McCarthy, 1986; Nunez, 1981). For EEG and ERPs, this translates into a bias toward activity occurring in gyri. For MEG, because of the orientation of magnetic fields with respect to their corresponding electric fields and because of the characteristics of the recording apparatus, this leads to a bias toward sources oriented tangentially with respect to the surface of the scalp, and therefore to a bias for activity occurring inside sulci.

These electrophysiological methods are well established and are considered the gold standard for temporal resolution because they index neuronal activity directly, rather than indirectly, as fMRI and PET. However, because electrical activity summates over space and time, it is very difficult to reconstruct the exact origin of scalp-recorded potentials. Therefore, the spatial resolution of these methods is limited and can only be modeled through complex algorithms (for a brief review, see Fabiani et al., 2000). MEG yields a better spatial resolution than EEG or ERPs because magnetic fields decay more quickly with distance than electric fields and because they are less influenced by intermediate layers of tissue (scalp, skull, etc.). This allows for a more precise modeling of the activity of neural generators, especially when only a few generators can be assumed to be concurrently active.

Taken together, these methods have provided very useful insights into the aging brain, especially with respect to the timing of spontaneous physiological activities (i.e., their basic rhythms) and of brain cognitive processes. However, it is important to note that with aging several anatomical and physiological changes may occur that will affect the propagation of electrical and magnetic signals to the scalp. As reviewed in other sections of this chapter, age-related changes in brain anatomy include a reduction of gray and white matter and a consequent increase in cerebrospinal fluid. In addition to the volumetric reduction of brain tissues, the skulls of aging adults are usually more calcified than those of young adults, and there may also be loss of subcutaneous fat. These characteristics should be kept in mind when results obtained with different methods and age groups are compared. For example, experimental designs that include within-group comparisons and that make use of statistical procedures to avoid misattribution of variance (McCarthy & Wood, 1985) may be more powerful for highlighting age-related differences in cognitive processes. Later in this chapter we review some of the main results obtained with these methods in the study of cognitive aging.

C. Optical Imaging Techniques

Optical methods are one of the most recent developments in brain imaging (for reviews, see Villringer & Chance 1997; Gratton & Fabiani, 1998, 2001a, b) used in cognitive neuroscience research. These methods, as applied to the study of the human brain, are noninvasive and are based on the measurement of changes in the parameters of near-infrared (NIR; 690- to 1000-nm wavelengths) light as it diffuses through active compared to inactive brain tissue. Light propagation in tissue can be best described as a diffusion process, which is influenced by two main parameters: scattering and absorption. Measurements can be taken at the scalp by placing several light sources (optic

fibers coupled with laser diodes) and detectors (fiber-optic bundles coupled with photo-multiplier tubes) in appropriate montages.

With time-resolved instrumentation (Gratton et al., 1997), two types of data can be collected: (a) data indexing neuronal activity (EROS; Gratton & Fabiani, 1998, 2001a, b) and (b) data reflecting hemodynamic activity (NIRS; e.g., Villringer & Chance 1997; Choi et al., 2004), such as absolute and relative changes in the concentration of oxy- and deoxyhemoglobin in the tissue.

EROS data possess a good combination of spatial and temporal resolution. In fact, because they index neuronal activity, their temporal resolution is of the order of milliseconds, and compares well with that of ERP data (Gratton et al., 1997, 2001; Rinne et al., 1999; DeSoto et al., 2001). They also possess a subcentimeter spatial resolution in that, unlike electrical activity, scattering changes are localized with a point-spread function of less than 15 mm (Gratton & Fabiani, 2003).

Hemodynamic (NIRS) data, similar to BOLD fMRI data, are limited in their temporal resolution by the intrinsic characteristics of hemodynamic effects, which typically lag neuronal activity of a few seconds. Their spatial resolution varies. With animal models and appropriate methods the resolution can be of the order of micrometer, and can be used to describe, among others, columnar (e.g., Malonek & Grinvald, 1996) and barrel (Masino & Frostig, 1996) organization *in vivo* and with great precision. In humans, the spatial resolution is subcentimeters and depends in part on the coregistration methods used (Whalen et al., in preparation).

The main limitation of these methods (when used noninvasively) is their lack of penetration — a few centimeters within the tissue (Gratton et al., 2000) — which makes it very difficult to image structures that are deep into the brain and/or surrounded by white matter (which is highly reflective). However, notwithstanding these limitations, these methods could be very useful for the study of aging, especially with respect to examining changes in connectivity between brain areas and also changes in the relationship between neuronal and hemodynamic signals that may occur during aging. These types of data are reviewed briefly later.

D. Positron Emission Tomography and Functional Magnetic Resonance Imaging

The field of cognitive neuroscience has benefited tremendously from the utilization of relatively noninvasive *in vivo* neuroimaging techniques. This section reviews two of the more widely used techniques: positron emission tomography and functional magnetic resonance imaging. Although a thorough overview of the methods is far beyond the scope of this chapter, we hope to give the reader a basic familiarity with some of the underlying mechanisms, assumptions and limitations of each technique.

Both PET and fMRI utilize biophysiological correlates of neural activity to infer the involvement of cortical regions in a given cognitive task. In the case of PET, participants are injected with molecules that carry a positron-emitting isotope (e.g., ^{15}C, ^{11}C), which then are carried into the brain where they aggregate in metabolically active areas. As the unstable isotopes decay, they emit a positron, which, after traveling a few millimeters on average, eventually collides with an electron. Both particles are destroyed, resulting in the emission of γ rays, which are then detected by an array of γ ray sensors surrounding the head of the participant. Because the γ rays are emitted in a predictable pattern (180° apart), the site of the collision between the emitted positron and the electron can be localized spatially, allowing the researcher to identify the concentrations of positron-emitting isotopes in the brain and thus infer the relative level of activity of each region of the brain (Phelps et al., 1986). This process evolves rather slowly, on the order of ~45 s (Volkow, Wang, Fowler & Hitzemann, 1997), and therefore typically allows investigators to get a global assessment of the regions involved in a task with no temporal specificity.

fMRI is a technique that takes advantage of the fact that oxygenated blood has a different magnetic resonance signal than deoxygenated blood, or the surrounding tissues. This process evolves more quickly than that of PET. As neurons fire, they initially deplete the local oxygenated blood pool. After a short interval (1–2 s), the local cerebrovasculature responds to this oxygen depletion by increasing the flow of oxygenated blood into the region for a short time (3–5 s) before returning oxygenated blood levels back to normal (12–16 s). Researchers using fMRI can then track the change in the resonance signal throughout the brain and correlate these changes with the onset of a given cognitive task, which allows one to identify cortical regions that are involved with task performance (for a review, see Frackowiak et al., 2003).

One of the clear advantages of PET is the ability to translate detected signals into biologically meaningful units (e.g., glucose metabolization or regional cerebral blood flow; e.g., Brickman et al., 2003). In contrast, the signal changes detected by fMRI methods vary along arbitrary units that do not translate directly into an absolute metric of biological function. Another advantage of PET is the ability for researchers to design isotope-tagged molecules that bind to specific biologically relevant elements, such as dopamine receptors. This allows one to map out not only brain function, but also other potentially important individual differences in brain chemistry. Perhaps the most obvious disadvantage of PET is that the participants must be injected with a radioactive substance, whereas fMRI uses the native contrast of naturally occurring biological processes to infer function. fMRI also has the advantage of improved temporal resolution, which allows the researchers to resolve inferred neural activity from rapidly presented stimuli (e.g., Burock et al., 1998) or even self-paced events (e.g., Maccotta, Zacks, & Buckner, 2001) on a trial-by-trial basis. This allows the researcher to separate and compare, for example, correct trials from error trials (Hester, Fassbender, & Garavan, 2004), remembered vs. forgotten trials (Morcom et al., 2003), or intermixed trials of varying difficulty (Olson et al., 2004). In contrast, given the slow evolution of the signal changes, PET studies must utilize blocked designs, where the participant responds to repeated trials of a given type (e.g., Cabeza, Anderson, Houle, Mangels, & Nyberg, 2000). This precludes the use of more standard cognitive experimental designs, where trials of each type are often intermixed and balanced for order of presentation. Additionally, it is not possible to resolve neural activity to individual trials (e.g., errors), and neural activity from all trials within the block becomes averaged together. Further, compared to electrophysiological and optical methods, both fMRI and PET cannot resolve activity within a trial because of the intrinsically slow course of hemodynamic and metabolic phenomena that follow neuronal activity. Nonetheless, PET and fMRI studies have contributed greatly to our understanding of cortical function and the age-related changes in these functions. Finally, although fMRI appears to be emerging as the tool of choice for many cognitive neuroscientists, it is clear that both techniques will continue to provide insights into cognitive neurosciences into the foreseeable future.

E. Transcranial Magnetic Stimulation

Another technique that has proven increasingly useful in the study of the neuronal underpinnings of perception, cognition, and action is referred to as transcranial magnetic stimulation (TMS). TMS has also been used to study and treat disorders such as depression and schizophrenia (Robertson et al., 2003). TMS involves the application of a brief magnetic pulse to the scalp. This pulse induces localized electromagnetic fields, which alter the electrical field in the brain below the stimulator. TMS has been produced through a number of different coil designs, the most popular of which is a figure eight that induces an electrical field underneath the intersection of the two loops of the coil. TMS can be delivered as a single pulse or as a repeated series of pulses, which temporally extend the impact of the stimulation on the brain tissue below the coil. TMS is considered a safe and minimally invasive method and has been used in hundreds of studies with both patients and normal volunteers ranging from children to older adults (Sulekha & Hoston, 2002). However, it is important to note that, prior to the establishment of safety guidelines, repeated pulse TMS was observed to induce seizures in a small number of healthy volunteers.

TMS has been used to study the chronometry of mental processes as well as the connectivity among different brain regions that support a variety of perceptual, cognitive, and motor functions. TMS works by interrupting processing in the tissue below the coil — in essence causing a temporally and spatially localized virtual lesion that is both reversible and transient. For example, Grosbas and Paus (2002) examined whether the frontal eye fields, which serve an important role in the control of voluntary saccades, are also involved in the control of covert attention. Single pulse TMS was presented either before or after the onset of a target to which subjects were to respond. An increased reaction time (RT) cost was found for the invalidly cued trials, but only when the TMS pulse was delivered over the right FEF. These results were interpreted in terms of dominance of the right hemisphere for attentional control. Other studies have begun to utilize TMS jointly with fMRI, EEG, or ERP recordings to capitalize on the relative strengths of each technique. For example, Rushworth et al. (2002) examined the role of the presupplementary motor area (pre-SMA)—a frontal region previously observed to be active in task-switching paradigms—in switching between tasks and responses. They found that the application of repeated TMS over the pre-SMA disrupted switching between different responses as indexed by fMRI, but only when the TMS was applied just prior to the switch.

Although TMS has not yet been widely used in the study of brain and cognitive changes that occur during the course of normal aging, a number of studies have demonstrated that TMS may be safely used with older adults, and other studies have begun to examine how best to accommodate TMS parameters to changes in cortical morphology that are associated with aging (Kozel et al., 2000). Therefore, we anticipate that the next version of the handbook will likely include a detailed discussion of how TMS has been used to examine age-related changes in cognition as well as the use of TMS in the treatment of age-related neurological disorders.

III. Patterns of Age-Related Differences in Brain Structure and Function

This section briefly describes and discusses some general results concerning changes in brain structure and function across the adult life span.

A. Structural Differences

The human brain tends to show reductions in volume starting around the age of 30. However, much as in the cognitive literature reviewed earlier, these losses are not at all uniform. Correlations between age and cortical volume have been reported to be the largest for prefrontal regions, somewhat smaller for temporal and parietal areas, and small and often nonsignificant for sensory and motor cortices (e.g., Head et al., 2002; Raz, 2000). In general, the disproportionate changes in brain structure across the adult life span parallel findings of age-specific changes in executive control and a subset of memory processes that are supported in large part by prefrontal, parietal, and temporal regions of the brain (Robbins et al., 1998; Schretlen et al., 2000). Similar findings from DTI have shown that the integrity of white matter microstructures of the brain decline with age (Mosley et al., 2002); again, these losses are significantly greater in the frontal regions of the cortex (Head et al., 2004). The close match between the regional declines in brain structure and the cognitive processes that they ostensibly subserve suggests that volumetric losses in these regions of the brain underlie at least some part of the cognitive declines seen in aging humans.

Indeed, several studies have formally evaluated the idea that declines in specific cortical regions result in deterioration of the cognitive processes subserved by these regions. For example, hand-traced estimates of prefrontal gray matter volume in cross-sectional samples significantly predict age-correlated reductions in performance on frontally mediated executive tasks such as the Wisconsin card sorting test (Gunnin-Dixon & Raz, 2003) and verbal working memory (Head, et al., 2002). Another set of studies linked the hippocampal volume of older adults to their long-term memory performance (across several weeks), even when accounting for the effects of age on memory (Walhvod et al., 2004). Similarly, O'Sullivan et al. (2001), in a DTI study of white matter integrity, found that deterioration in the frontal white matter tracts, which allow the frontal hemispheres to communicate, significantly predicted poorer performance on the trails B task, which is considered a classic neuropsychological test of frontal lobe function. Finally, Colcombe and colleagues (2005) examined the relationship between differences in brain structure and function in older adults who performed a variant of the flanker task, which is also considered an assessment of executive function. They found, similar to O'Sullivan et al. (2001), that older adults who were better able to inhibit incongruent stimuli in a flanker task also had greater volume in the frontal white matter tracts, as measured by VBM. Additionally, older adults who showed reduced frontal white matter volume also showed significantly greater contralateral frontal lobe recruitment (i.e., the extent to which these areas are activated) during task performance, thus demonstrating that changes in brain structure can impact both cognitive performance and patterns of cortical recruitment.

Perhaps more impressively, several studies have linked longitudinal changes in brain structure to declines in cognition. That is, not only do individual differences in current brain structure impact cognitive performance in aged individuals, but the change in these structures across time also predicts cognitive decline. For example, Rusinek and colleagues (2003) assessed changes in regional brain structures and cognitive performance across a 6-year period. They found that older adults who showed evidence of cognitive decline also

showed significant atrophy in the medial temporal lobe. In another study, Rodrigue and Raz (2004) tested older adults at two time points separated by 5 years. They found that declines in the hand-traced volume of the entorhinal cortex were significantly related to declines in memory performance across the 5-year period. In combination, these results highlight the idea that changes in the integrity of the gray matter regions that subserve local cortical processing, in the mylenated axonal fibers that allow effective communication between different cortical processors, and in the patterns of cortical recruitment all may have a critical role in describing the changes in cognitive performance of aging adults.

B. Functional Differences

1. Patterns of Age-Related Difference in PET and fMRI Activation

As described in Section I, studies that have examined the relationship between changes in perception, cognition, and action across the adult life span have asked whether such changes are specific or general in nature. Although the great majority of neuroimaging studies that have examined age-related differences have done so within the context of a limited number of paradigms and therefore cannot explore intraindividual performance or brain activation patterns across selective aspects of cognition as in the cognitive aging literature (e.g., Salthouse, 1996), some general data patterns have been observed across studies. For example, it has often been reported that older adults show lower levels of activation than younger adults in a wide variety of tasks and brain regions (Logan et al., 2002; Stebbins et al., 2002; Madden et al., 1996). Two different interpretations have been offered for such data. One is that aging is associated with an irreversible loss of neural resources. As described earlier, there are clearly a number of structural and functional changes that occur in the brain across the adult life span (Morrison & Hof, 1997; Raz, 2000). Another interpretation is that resources are available but inadequately recruited. Support for this hypothesis has been provided by Logan et al. (2002), who found that underrecruitment of prefrontal regions could be reduced when old adults were instructed to use semantic association strategies during word encoding. Activation in the prefrontal cortex was reduced for older as compared to younger adults when word memorization depended on self-initiated encoding strategies. However, age-related underrecruitment was reduced substantially when old and younger adults were encouraged to use specific encoding strategies. Such results suggest that, at least under some conditions, reduced age-related cortical activation is reversible with instructions and training (see additional discussion of this issue in Section V,B).

Another common finding is that older adults also show nonselective recruitment of brain regions. That is, relative to younger adults performing the same task, older adults often show the recruitment of different brain areas in addition to those activated in the younger adults. One variant of nonselectivity that has been observed is the activation of different but nonhomologous brain regions in young and old adults. For example, in a study of focused and divided attention Madden et al. (1997) observed that older adults showed weaker activity than young adults in the occipital cortex while also showing stronger activation than young adults in the prefrontal cortex. These data were interpreted as evidence for strategic differences in the processing of task-relevant stimuli. In a study of face encoding and retrieval, Grady and colleagues (2002) found that activity in hippocampal and orbitofrontal regions for younger adults was correlated positively with recognition memory for faces. However, for older adults, recognition performance was predicted by positive correlations in the right prefrontal and parietal regions. These data, when viewed in the context of the extant memory literature, appear to suggest a general compensatory role for the temporoparietal and prefrontal regions across different memory tasks for older adults.

A second variety of nonselective recruitment, the bilateral activation of homologous brain regions, has been codified into a model of neurocognitive aging by Cabeza (2002). The model, referred to as hemispheric asymmetry reduction in older adults (HAROLD), suggests that cortical activity under similar circumstances tends to be less lateralized in older than in younger adults. Bilateral activation for older adults has been demonstrated in a number of different paradigms, including episodic encoding (Rosen et al., 2002), episodic retrieval (Cabeza et al., 2002), working memory (Reuter-Lorenz et al., 2000), and face matching (Grady et al., 2000). For example, in a classic study by Reuter-Lorenz et al. (2000), PET data were recorded as older and younger adults performed verbal and spatial working memory tasks. In the frontal lobes, activation was predominately left lateralized for verbal and right lateralized for spatial working memory for the younger adults. However, older adults showed a pattern of bilateral activation for both types of memory tasks.

An important question with regard to this asymmetry is whether the additional activity observed for the older adults is compensatory or a marker of cortical decline (i.e., a failure to recruit specialized neural processors). At present, this is an open question, with a number of studies reporting that older adults who perform better on a task show bilateral recruitment of homologous areas, whereas older adults who perform more poorly show unilateral activation (Cabeza et al., 2002; Rosen et al., 2002; Reuter-Lorenz et al., 2000). However, other studies have either failed to find a relationship between laterality and performance (Logan et al., 2002; Madden et al., 2002) or reported unilateral prefrontal activation for better-performing old adults and bilateral activation for poorer-performing older adults (Colcombe et al., 2005; Nielson et al., 2002).

Thus far, studies like those described earlier that have associated patterns of brain activation of old and young adults with performance quality have done so through comparisons between individuals. Clearly, it is important in the future to examine the relationship between patterns of cortical recruitment and performance quality *within* subjects. Ideally, examination of this relationship should take place in studies with graded cognitive challenges, as well as in intervention studies whose goal is to enhance cognition and brain function of older adults. Evaluation of the generality of asymmetry reduction across different perceptual, cognitive, and motor processes is also an important goal for the future.

The HAROLD model discussed earlier presents one framework in which to conceptualize age-related changes in the brain circuits that underlie cognition and performance. However, there are also several other frameworks that are important to note. Reuter-Lorenz and Mikels (2005) have proposed the compensation related utilization of neural circuits (CRUNCH) model to account for age-related differences in brain function and cognition. The CRUNCH model suggests that, with declining neural efficiency, additional neural circuitry is required at lower levels of task demands. Compensation can take several forms, including

bilateral recruitment of homologous brain regions or recruitment of different brain regions for older as compared to younger adults. Because, according to CRUNCH, older adults should reach their resource limits sooner than younger adults, the model predicts (1) poorer performance for older than for younger adults on more complex tasks and (2) underrecruitment for old relative to younger adults as tasks become more difficult. Older adults should show a smaller change than younger adults in PET or fMRI activation as tasks become more difficult. These predictions are generally consistent with extant data. For example, DiGirolamo et al. (2001) found that older adults displayed a larger increase in activation in the dorsolateral prefrontal cortex (DLPFC) and anterior cingulate than younger adults when comparing a fixation control condition to the performance of numerical judgment tasks. However, younger adults showed much larger increases in activation in these brain regions when the individual numeric comparison tasks were contrasted with a task-switching condition in which subjects were required to frequently switch between different numeric judgment tasks. Older adults also showed larger performance costs when comparing single task and switching conditions. Of course, the CRUNCH hypothesis requires additional validation with a variety of different tasks and subject populations to determine the generality of the proposal.

A somewhat similar proposal has been made in the form of the cognitive reserve (CR) hypothesis. CR has been defined as the ability of individuals to cope with advancing brain pathology through either at set of acquired skills or inherent abilities. Operationally, CR has often been defined in terms of level of education, IQ, occupational status, or other lifestyle factors (Habeck et al., 2003; Stern et al., 2003; Scarmeas et al., 2003).

The concept of CR was initially introduced in an attempt to explain the imperfect coupling between the degree of brain pathology and cognition. Studies found that a substantial number of individuals who, upon histological examination, were found to have Alzheimer's disease were without behavioral symptoms during life (Ince, 2001). This behavioral sparing appears to be moderated by high levels of education or IQ (Snowdon et al., 2000).

Several neuroimaging studies have been conducted to examine the neuro-underpinnings of CR. For example, Scarmeas et al. (2003) examined the relationship between regionally specific measures of the difference in PET activation between nonverbal memory conditions that differed in task difficulty and a measure of CR (which was derived from measures of reading, IQ, and years of formal education). Different negative and positive correlations between CR and regionally specific PET activation were found for older and younger adults (see also Habeck et al., 2003; Stern et al., 2003). That is, the brain regions that showed the most substantial change as a function of task difficulty were different for old and young adults. These data, although preliminary, may suggest that different neural networks subserve difficulty-based compensation in young and old adults.

Proposals such as HAROLD, CRUNCH, and CR might be taken to suggest that relatively general compensatory strategies can be adopted to offset age-related declines in cognition (although future studies may suggest that effective compensatory strategies are much more process specific). However, one might ask whether there is any empirical evidence for general cognitive decline, as suggested by the cognitive aging literature (Salthouse, 1996). Indeed, a study by Cabeza et al. (2004; see also Grady et al., 2003) investigated this issue

by requiring subjects to perform three different tasks — working memory, visual attention, and episodic retrieval — and then examined the common and task-specific age-related differences across tasks. Evidence for both general and process-specific age differences were observed. For example, across all three tasks older adults showed weaker occipital activity and stronger frontal and parietal activity than younger adults. Such data may support the sensory deficit hypothesis of cognitive aging, with the frontoparietal circuit being employed to compensate for sensory deficits. Other age-related differences in activation patterns varied across tasks. Although additional research is clearly needed, these initial data appear to suggest, like the cognitive aging literature, both general and specific changes in brain function across the adult life span. Knowledge of the relationship between different types of age-related decline, which is general or specific, may be quite useful in targeting intervention strategies to reduce or possibly reverse age-related decline in perception, cognition, and action.

2. Patterns of Change in the Timing of Brain Events

As mentioned earlier, electrophysiological and fast optical measures, unlike hemodynamic measures, yield data with very good temporal resolution and therefore allow for an examination of age-related changes in the temporal patterns of brain responses. This section provides a brief and therefore necessarily selective review of the main types of data obtained in this domain.

Alterations in the EEG of older adults have been reported for many years and are characterized by changes in the frequency of the α rhythm and by slowing and some abnormalities in other aspects of the recordings (for a review, see Woodruff-Pak, 1997). These effects are hypothesized to be due to diminished arousal to the cortex from the reticular formation.

In the case of ERP data, age-related phenomena can be classified as (a) changes in the latency of a specific ERP component, signifying a delay in the processing that the component is assumed to index; (b) changes in the amplitude of a specific ERP component, signifying a decrease in the strength or intensity of the processing; (c) changes in the distribution of effects across electrodes (scalp distribution), which is taken to index a change in the neuronal generators contributing to the effects, and therefore in the strategies or set of processes used for performing a task; and (d) changes in the pattern of habituation of responses over time and/or with stimulus repetition, which can signal a change in the temporal dynamics of processes and their interaction.

It is important to note that ERP effects in latency, amplitude, and, to some extent, scalp distribution can interact and are potentially confusable. For example, when latency variability increases across trials, as is often the case in aging, the average amplitude of these trials may be apparently decreased (because of lack of synchronization of the effects over time) even in the absence of diminished amplitude on single trials. By the same token, if some ERP responses are delayed and not others, their overlap may change, leading to an apparent change in the distribution of effects over the scalp.

Notwithstanding these caveats, ERP data provide a window on the relative occurrence of cognitive processes in aging compared to young adulthood. Given the crucial role of slowing in many theories of aging, they allow for the testing of hypotheses concerning the occurrence of delays and bottlenecks within the processing system (for a review, see Fabiani & Wee, 2001). For example, several age-related changes in the P300 ERP component have been reported, including increased latency and decreased amplitude (Ford & Pfefferbaum, 1991; Polich, 1991, 1996; Polich, Howard, & Starr, 1983; see also Fjell & Walhovd, 2004), suggesting the existence of a delay in encoding and decision processes.

A number of studies suggest that older adults may be slower (or unable) to cease processing stimuli that are irrelevant and/or repeated compared to young adults who quickly stop responding to these same stimuli. For example, early sensory ERP components, such as the auditory N100 (peak latency: 100 ms after stimulus onset), are maintained in older adults with sound repetition (Alain & Woods, 1999; Golob et al., 2001; Fabiani et al., in press), even when the repeated tones are irrelevant and should be ignored. Similarly, the mismatch negativity component of the ERP (latency: approximately 200 ms after stimulus onset), which is calculated as the *difference* between the response to unattended deviant and standard stimuli, appears to be reduced with aging, likely because the response to the standard (repeated) stimuli is *increased* (Low et al., 2001). These data suggest that older adults have difficulty filtering out stimuli that should no longer be processed and is well in line with aging theories stressing the decreased efficiency of inhibitory processes (Hasher & Zacks, 1988).

These effects, possibly indicating lack of or reduced inhibitory suppression of brain responses that should be no longer be needed, are also evident later in the information processing chain. The P3a or novelty P3 (latency: approximately 300 ms after stimulus onset) is elicited by unexpected or novel stimuli that typically also elicit an orienting response. Note that in the typical paradigms in which a novelty P3 is elicited, novel stimuli do not require a response and should be ignored.

The novelty P3 is reduced greatly in patients with dorsolateral prefrontal lesions, suggesting a possible frontal origin (Knight, 1984). Because aging is accompanied by a shrinkage of frontal brain tissue and by problems that mimic some of the effects obtained in frontal patients (West, 1996; Moscovitch and Winocur, 1992), a number of studies have examined the patterns of novelty P3 responses in aging (Friedman & Simpson, 1994; Fabiani & Friedman, 1995; Fabiani, Friedman, & Cheng, 1998; Friedman, Simpson, & Hamberger, 1993). As a whole, these studies indicate that orienting-like novelty P3 responses are more persistent in older adults than in young adults. For example, Friedman and Simpson (1994) found that when novel stimuli were repeated, this response was maintained over a longer time in older than younger adults. Similarly, Fabiani and Friedman (1995) found that novelty-like responses were also elicited by target (repeated) stimuli in young adults, but only for the first few repetitions, after which these responses subsided. In contrast, in older adults, these same responses were maintained over many blocks of trials, suggesting an inability to suppress processes that were no longer relevant. Finally, Fabiani et al. (1998) found that the extent to which this frontal novelty P3 component was maintained when it was no longer necessary was highly correlated with neuropsychological tests of frontal function.

These ERP results suggest that reduced inhibitory processes at different levels of the system play important roles in shaping the cognitive changes occurring in normal aging. They are also in line with observations, made in a number of fMRI studies, of increased and/or more diffuse activity in older than younger adults (e.g., Cabeza et al., 2002; Reuter-Lorenz et al., 2000). Similar to fMRI data, these ERP data are open to different interpretations

as to their function—whether compensatory or signaling processing failures—although much of the evidence reviewed earlier would suggest the latter.

In order to better understand the nature of these differential patterns of activities across age groups and their roles in the information processing flow, it is potentially very useful to examine the order and type of activation of different brain areas. This is difficult to do with both ERP and fMRI recordings because these two methods trade off spatial and temporal resolution. In a optical imaging study, Gratton et al., (2005) illustrated the utility of a multimodal approach affording specificity in both domains. In this study, younger and older adults were engaged in a cued spatial Stroop task in which the words "above" and "below" were presented above and below fixation. A cue preceding each trial indicated to the subject whether to respond based on the meaning or position of the upcoming stimulus. The focus of the study was on the activity elicited by the cue, with the hypothesis that on trials in which task switching was required, old task rules should be suppressed and new task rules activated. Results showed an asymmetry in frontal lobe activation in young adults, with switches to verbal (meaning) rules activating primarily the left DLPC, and switches to position (spatial) rules activating the homologous area in the right hemisphere. As expected based on fMRI data in similar paradigms, older adults showed bilateral activation of DLPFC during switches. However, activation of the incorrect cortex was *delayed* with respect to that of the appropriate one. We hypothesized that the reason for the bilateral activity in older adults was a reduction or delay in the inhibitory control exerted by active areas in the "correct" hemisphere over those in the "incorrect" hemisphere. We further assumed that the size of the anterior third of the corpus callosum (CC) would mediate these inhibitory effects. Results confirmed these hypotheses. In subjects with large CCs (mostly young adults), there was evidence of negative lagged cross-correlations between the two DLPFC cortices, suggesting that activity in the appropriate hemisphere would lead to activity of the opposite sign (inhibition) of the incorrect hemisphere with some (150 ms or so) delay. Further, these negative cross-correlations were also associated with small behavioral switch costs in RT. However, in subjects with small CCs (mostly older adults), these inhibitory processes were absent or delayed, thus presumably leading to bilateral activation and the larger switch costs in RT observed in this group. This study, as the only one of this type, is mostly illustrative of an approach that could potentially greatly improve our understanding of the mechanisms underlying cognitive processes in aging.

IV. Application of Cognitive Neuroscience to the Study of Attention and Memory

This section briefly describes and discusses recent research that has employed a cognitive neuroscience approach to the study of memory and attention across the adult life span.

A. Attention

Interest in attentional processes has been increasing from both a psychophysical and a neuroscience perspective in recent years. Several issues have served as a major focus of this interest. One such focus has been on the understanding of the mechanisms that underlie the control of attention as well as the expression of attention. In general, this research has suggested that attentional control is mediated, in large part, by a frontoparietal network, whereas the expression of

attention is reflected in regions of cortex responsible for the processing of specific attributes of stimuli, such as spatial location, color, shape, and motion, (Pessoa et al., 2003). With respect to visual spatial attention, Corbetta and Shulman (2002) have argued that there are two separate but interacting networks. A dorsal frontoparietal system subserves the generation of attentional sets that provide top–down guidance for attentional control, whereas a right lateralized ventral system is thought to be responsible for the detection of unexpected events in a stimulus-driven manner.

Age-related changes in the mechanisms of attentional control have been examined in the context of visual search paradigms (for a more extensive review of this topic, see Madden et al., 2005). For example, Madden and colleagues (1997, 2002) have examined age-related differences in feature search, which requires a combination of bottom–up and top–down control, with a conjunction search, which entails primarily a top–down search. In general, in the conjunction search condition, older adults showed less of an increase in ventral pathway activation and more of an increase in frontal activation (i.e., as compared to the feature search condition; Madden et al., 1997) than younger adults. These results may indicate an attempt to compensate for insufficient processing in the ventral pathway with increased activation of top–down control mechanisms in the frontal cortex. Consistent with the CRUNCH and CR models, older adults also showed a higher level of ventral activation than younger adults in the feature search condition (Madden et al., 2002). Indeed, this high level of activation in the "easy" search condition may be responsible for the difficulty that older adults had in increasing activation in the ventral pathway in the more difficult conjunction search condition.

Another important area of investigation of attentional processes has been the influence of aging on the control of interference or inhibition. In this regard, Milham et al. (2002) examined age-related differences in brain activation in the Stroop paradigm. In this paradigm, subjects are instructed to respond to the color of ink in which a word is presented and ignore the word. However, this is difficult to do when the word is incongruent with the ink color (e.g., the word red presented in blue ink). Milham et al. (2002) found that younger adults showed more activation in the DLPFC—a brain region that aids in the maintenance of attentional sets—than older adults. This was true regardless of whether the word and ink color were compatible or incompatible. Older adults also showed more activation of the anterior cingulate cortex, an area that assists in the monitoring for potential response conflict, at lower levels of conflict (i.e., in the compatible condition) than younger adults. These data suggest that as a result of difficulty in maintaining a strong attentional set, older adults may need to activate conflict monitoring algorithms at lower levels of task difficulty (see also Nielson et al., 2002; West, 2004). As discussed earlier (see Colcombe et al., 2005), failures to inhibit task-irrelevant stimuli or stimulus characteristics may be due, in part, to age-related differences in white matter integrity.

Given the relative scarcity of neuroscientific studies on age-related changes in attentional processes, further research will be necessary to fully understand how aging influences attentional control and its instantiation in the brain. For example, while we know quite a bit about behavioral changes over the adult life span in the ability to switch priorities among concurrently performed tasks, little neuroscience research has been conducted to augment behavioral studies in developing integrative theories of multitask processing (for an exception, see DiGirolamo et al., 2001).

B. Memory

Cognitive memory research since the mid-1970s has clearly shown evidence suggesting the existence of multiple memory systems by means of behavioral dissociations of results in different conditions and/or groups (e.g., Tulving, 1987; Tulving & Schacter, 1990). Since the mid-1980s, cognitive neuroscience—through both functional and lesion animal and human studies—has augmented this view by showing that these different memory systems are likely supported by separable brain substrates (e.g., Squire, 2004). Further, and of central interest for this book, aging appears to differentially affect these substrates so that memory impairments observed with age further corroborate the multisystem view (e.g., Hay & Jacoby, 1999).

Although the precise mapping between brain substrates and dissociable cognitive constructs is still debated and incomplete, much has been learned about its essential elements. This section focuses on three particular aspects of memory that are central to aging research: (1) age-related dissociations between declarative and nondeclarative memory, such as those between recollection and priming; (2) the role of left and right prefrontal areas in recollection and familiarity phenomena, including source memory; and (3) the role of the prefrontal cortex in working memory function.

Both ERP (e.g., Friedman, 2000) and fMRI (e.g., Lustig & Buckner, 2004) research indicate that repetition priming effects are preserved in aging, as shown by (a) comparable RT advantages across age groups; (b) similar reductions in N400 and increase in P300 for ERP data (but see Joyce at al., 1998); and (c) similar reductions across groups in prefrontal activity, correlated with repetition-related response time reductions.

In tasks involving effortful retrieval and/or source judgments, older adults often show increased or more diffuse frontal activity compared to young adults in both fMRI (e.g., Cabeza et al., 2002; Morcom et al., 2003) and ERP (e.g., Li et al., 2004; but see Friedman 2000) studies.

Working memory studies have been reviewed in other sections of this chapter. As a summary, these studies suggest that older adults require activation of more areas, often bilaterally, to perform dual tasks or tasks imposing a heavy load on working memory (e.g., Reuter-Lorentz et al., 2000; Smith et al., 2001).

V. Summary and Future Directions

This chapter has reviewed some of the contributions that the cognitive neuroscience approach has produced so far in the area of aging. These include the existence of functional difference between younger and older adults both in the timing and sequence of brain processes and in the brain areas that are recruited during the performance of specific tasks. These age-related effects are likely to reflect differential strategic processes in task performance, as well as in anatomical and physiological changes in the brain substrate.

A large number of questions are still open to debate and will benefit from further research, including the functional significance of the additional recruitment often observed in older adults, and its underlying mechanisms, and brain-imaging-based approaches to the study of inhibitory processes. Also, within a network view of brain function (as compared to a localization-biased perspective), it will be important to explore the relationship between areas that are involved in memory, attentional, and other processes.

The remainder of this section briefly describes a couple of promising areas of research on aging and neurocognitive function.

A. Multi-modal Imaging

A multimodal imaging approach can be extremely beneficial to research on the cognitive neuroscience of aging. As reviewed in earlier sections of this chapter, the different brain imaging methods currently available provide data that are often complementary rather than redundant, with functional data further augmented by anatomical information. The combination of methods, although more theoretically and practically complex than the unimodal approach, can allow for the understanding of the relationship between different brain phenomena, such as blood flow and neuronal activity (Fabiani et al., 2004; Fabiani & Gratton, 2005). Because aging occurs on a background of overall changing physiology, and often in the presence of incipient or ongoing disease, a thorough understanding of age-related cognitive phenomena can benefit from an integrated approach (for a similar discussion, see Kutas & Federmeier, 1998).

B. Intervention Research

In addition to describing age-related declines in neurocognitive performance, strong and growing interest exists in identifying mechanisms that might be of use in offsetting or even reversing some of these declines. Although several decades of research have investigated the cognitive impact training interventions in older adults (Kramer et al., 2004), there exist relatively few neuroimaging studies that have examined the impact of training on neural recruitment or brain structure in aged individuals. However, we argue that controlled longitudinal assessments of cognitive and fitness training will prove a fertile future direction in the cognitive neuroscience of aging.

For example, Nyberg and colleagues (2003) trained younger and older adults to use the method of loci mnemonic strategy, where one learns to associate words that are to be memorized with a particular spatial location. Patterns of brain activation were then assessed both pre and posttraining using PET. They found that although both younger and older adults were able to learn the locations and understand that they were to associate the words with the locations, younger adults were better able to utilize the strategy than older adults. In fact, only half of the older adults showed any benefit from the training. This suggests that older adults have difficulty not in learning the strategy, but rather in successfully implementing the strategy to improve memory performance. In neuroimaging data, they found that younger adults showed an increase in dorsal frontal regions of the brain that are associated with mental imagery and integration of information in working memory, but that older adults showed no such difference. This, Nyberg and colleagues (2003) suggest, may reflect a deficit in the reserve capacity of older adults. That is, they may lack the additional neurocognitive resources to successfully implement the new strategy. However, both young and those older adults who showed an improvement in memory performance after method of loci training showed increased activity in the occipitoparietal and retreosplenial regions of the brain. These regions have been associated with spatial imagery and route-based learning, respectively. Thus, although not all older adults were able to benefit from the training, those who did showed similar changes in neural activation patterns to the younger adults in the

posterior regions of the brain. It seems that it is indeed possible to both engender improvements in memory performance and changes in neural recruitment in some older adults through cognitive training interventions, and that age-related limitations in the ability to benefit from cognitive training may result from reductions in frontal reserve capacity.

Older adults can, in fact, benefit from cognitive training, as seen earlier. In some cases, older adults can achieve greater gains from formal cognitive training interventions than their younger counterparts (Kramer et al., 1999; Scialfa et al, 2000). However, with few exceptions (e.g., Kramer et al., 1999), the benefits of cognitive training do not extend beyond the specific cognitive skill that was trained (Kramer et al., 2004). However, cardiovascular fitness training has shown great promise as a general moderator of cognition. Aerobically trained older adults show improvements in both simple and highly complex cognitive tasks, although the improvements are greatest in the more complex "executive" tasks thought to be mediated by the frontal and parietal lobes (Colcombe & Kramer, 2003). In one study, Colcombe and colleagues (2004) randomly assigned older adults to participate in either a cardiovascular exercise group or a control group for a 6-month period. These participants performed a version of the flanker task in which they were asked to identify the orientation of a central arrow cue that was surrounded by either congruent (e.g., "<<<<<") or incongruent (e.g., ">><>>") flanking items, while scanned in an fMRI protocol. They found that older adults who participated in the cardiovascular fitness training protocol were better able to ignore the misleading flanking items, but the control older adults were not. Importantly, exercising older adults showed increased neural activity in the frontal and parietal regions of the brain thought to be involved in directed attentional control and a reduction in the dorsal region of the anterior cingulate cortex, which is thought to be sensitive to behavioral conflict, or the need for increased cognitive control. Nonhuman animal data suggest that these effects may be engendered by exercise-induced increases in key neurochemicals such as brain-derived neurotrophic factor and insulin-like growth factor-1, which are known to increase neuronal survival, the growth of new interconnections between neurons, and the growth of new capillaries (see Cotman & Berchtold, 2002; Carro et al., 2001). The end result of exercise training then is a brain that is more plastic and adaptive to change and more able to survive the vagaries of the aging process.

Finally, Colcombe and colleagues (submitted) used VBM to assess longitudinal changes in the brain structure of older adults who were randomly assigned to participate in either a 6-month cardiovascular fitness training program or a nonexercise control group. They found that older adults who participated in the exercise group showed a significant increase in gray matter volume in regions of the frontal and superior temporal lobe compared to controls. Also, exercising older adults showed a significant increase in the volume of the anterior white matter tracts that allow the frontal lobes of the brain to communicate. These results suggest that even relatively short exercise interventions can begin to restore some of the losses in brain volume associated with normal aging. However, it should be noted that limitations of the VBM technique do not allow one to infer precisely what mechanism results in these changes (e.g., increase in cell body size, increased dendritic connections, increased capillary bed volume, increased glial size or number).

More research is needed to clearly flesh these issues out.

Acknowledgments

This research was supported by grants from the National Institute on Aging to Arthur Kramer and Stanley Colcombe (RO1 AG25032 and RO1 AG25667) and to Monica Fabiani (RO1 AG21887). Reprint requests should be sent to Arthur F. Kramer, University of Illinois, Beckman Institute, 405 N. Mathews Ave., Urbana, IL 61801 or via e-mail to akramer@cyrus.psych.uiuc.edu.

References

Alain, C., & Woods, D. L. (1999). Age-related changes in processing auditory stimuli during visual attention: Evidence for deficits in inhibitory control and sensory memory. *Psychology and Aging*, *14*, 507–519.

Allison, T., Wood, C. C., & McCarthy, G. (1986). The central nervous system. In M. G. H. Coles, S. W. Porges, & E. Donchin (Eds.), *Psychophysiology: Systems, processes, and applications* (pp. 5–25). New York: Guilford.

Ashburner, J., & Friston, K. J. (2000). Voxel-based morphometry: The methods. *Neuroimage. 11*, 805–821.

Babiloni, C., Babiloni, F., Carducci, F., Cappa, S.F., Cincotti, F., Del Percio, C., Miniussi, C., Vito Moretti, D., Rossi, S., Sosta, K., & Rossini, P.M. (2004). Human cortical rhythms during visual delayed choice reaction time tasks. A high-resolution EEG study on normal aging. *Behavioral Brain Research*, *153(1)*, 261–271.

Baltes, P. B., Staudinger, U. M., & Lindenberger, U. (1999). Lifespan psychology: Theory and application to intellectual functioning. *Annual Review of Psychology, 50*, 471–507.

Basser, P.J., Mattiello, J., & Le Bihan, D. (1994). Estimation of the effective self-diffusion tensor from the NMR spin echo. *Journal of Magnetic Resonance, 103(3)*, 247–254.

Brickman, A. M., Buchsbaum, M. S., Shihabuddin, L., Hazlett, E. A., Borod, J. C., & Mohs, R. C. (2003). Striatal size, glucose metabolic rate, and verbal learning in normal aging. *Cognitive Brain Research* *17(1)*, 106–116.

Burock, M. A., Buckner, R. L., Woldorff, M. G., Rosen, B. R., & Dale, A. M. (1998). Randomized event-related experimental designs allow for extremely rapid presentation rates using functional MRI. *Neuroreport 9(16)*: 3735–3739.

Cabeza, R. (2002). Hemispheric asymmetry reduction in old adults: The HAROLD model. *Psychology and Aging, 17*, 85–100.

Cabeza, R., Daselaar, S.M., Dolcos, F., Prince, S.E., Budde, M., & Nyberg, L. (2004). Task-independent and task-specific age effects on brain activity during working memory, visual attention and episodic retrieval. *Cerebral Cortex, 14*, 364–375.

Cabeza, R., Anderson, N. D., Houle, S., Mangels, J. A., & Nyberg, L. Age-related differences in neural activity during item and temporal-order memory retrieval: A positron emission tomography study. *Journal of Cognitive Neuroscience. Vol 12(1)*, 2000, 197–206.

Cabeza, R., Anderson, N. D., Locantore, J. K., & McIntosh, A. (2002). Aging gracefully: Compensatory brain activity in high performing older adults. *Neuroimage, 17*, 1394–1402.

Carro, E., Trejo, L. J., Busiguina, S., & Torres, Aleman, I. (2001). Circulating insulin-like growth factor 1 mediates the protective effects of physical exercise against brain insults of different etiology and anatomy. *Journal of Neuroscience, 21*, 5678–5684.

Choi, J., Wolf, M., Toronov, V., Wolf, U., Polzonetti, C., Hueber, D., Safonova, L.P., Gupta, R., Michalos, A., Mantulin, W., & Gratton, E. (2004). Noninvasive determination of the optical properties of adult brain: Near-infrared spectroscopy approach. *Journal of Biomedical Optics, 9(1)*, 221–229.

Colcombe, S., & Kramer, A.F. (2003). Fitness effects on the cognitive function of older adults: A meta-analytic study. *Psychological Science, 14*, 125–130.

Colcombe, S.J., Erickson, K.I., Raz, N., Webb, A.G., Cohen, N.J., McAuley, E., & Kramer, A.F. (2003). Aerobic fitness reduces brain tissue loss in aging humans. *Journal of Gerontology: Medical Sciences, 58*, 176–180.

Colcombe, S.J., Kramer, A.F., Erickson, K.I., & Scalf, P. (2005). The implications of cortical recruitment and brain morphology for individual differences in cognitive performance in aging humans. *Psychology and Aging*.

Colcombe, S.J., Kramer, A.F., Erickson, K.I., Scalf, P., McAuley, E., Cohen, N.J., Webb, A., Jerome, G.J., Marquez, D.X., & Elavsky, S. (2004). Cardiovascular fitness, cortical plasticity, and aging. *Proceedings of the National Academy of Sciences, 101*, 3316–3321.

Corbetta, M., & Shulman, G.L. (2002). Control of goal-directed and stimulus-driven control of attention in the brain. *Nature Reviews of Neuroscience, 3*, 201–215.

Cotman, C. W., & Berchtold, N. C. (2002). Exercise: A behavioral intervention to enhance brain health and plasticity. *Trends in Neuroscience, 25*, 295–301.

Craik, F.I. M., & Byrd, M. (1982). Aging and cognitive deficits: The role of attentional resources. In F.I. M. Craik & S. Trehub (Eds.), *Aging and cognitive processes* (pp. 191–211). New York: Plenum.

Davidson, R. J., Jackson, D.C., & Larson, C. L. (2000). Human electroencephalography. In J. Cacioppo, L. Tassinary, & G. Berntson (Eds.), *Handbook of psychophysiology* (pp. 53–84). New York: Cambridge University Press.

DeSoto, M. C., Fabiani, M., Geary, D. C., & Gratton, G. (2001). When in doubt, do it both ways: Brain evidence of the simultaneous activation of conflicting responses in a spatial Stroop task. *Journal of Cognitive Neuroscience, 13(4)*, 523–536.

DiGirolamo, G.J., Kramer, A.F., Barad, V., Cepeda, N., Weissman, D.H., Wszalek, T.M., Cohen, N.J., Banich, M., Webb, A. & Beloposky, A. (2001). General and task-specific frontal lobe recruitment in older adults during executive processes: A fMRI investigation of task switching. *Neuroreport, 12(9)*, 2065–2072.

Di Russo, F., Martinex, A., & Hillyard, S.A. (2003). Source analysis of event-related cortical activity during visuo-spatial attention. *Cerebral Cortex, 2003*, 486–499.

Fabiani, M., Brumback, C., Gordon, B., Pearson, M., Lee, Y., Kramer, A., McAuley E., & Gratton, G. (2004). Effects of cardio-pulmonary fitness on neurovascular coupling in visual cortex in younger and older adults. *Psychophysiology, 41*, S19.

Fabiani, M., & Friedman, D. (1995). Changes in brain activity patterns in aging: The novelty oddball. *Psychophysiology, 32*, 579–594.

Fabiani, M., Friedman, D., & Cheng, J. C. (1998). Individual differences in P3 scalp distribution in older adults, and their relationship to frontal lobe function. *Psychophysiology, 35*, 698–708.

Fabiani, M., & Gratton, G. (2005). Electro-physiological and optical measures of cognitive aging. In R. Cabeza, L. Nyberg, & D. Park (Eds.). *Cognitive neuroscience of aging: Linking cognitive and cerebral aging.* Oxford University Press.

Fabiani, M., Gratton, G., & Coles, M. G. H. (2000). Event–related brain potentials: Methods, theory and applications. In J. Cacioppo, L. Tassinary, & G. Berntson (Eds.), *Handbook of psychophysiology* (pp. 53–84). New York: Cambridge University Press.

Fabiani, M., Low, K. A., Wee, E., Sable, J. J., & Gratton, G. (in press). Reduced suppression or labile memory? Mechanisms of inefficient filtering of irrelevant information in older adults. *Journal of Cognitive Neuroscience.*

Fabiani, M., & Wee, E. (2001). Age-related changes in working memory function: A Review. In C. Nelson & M. Luciana (Eds.), *Handbook of developmental cognitive neuroscience* (pp. 473–488). Cambridge, MA: MIT Press.

Fjell, A.M., & Walhovd, K.B. (2004). Life-span changes in P3a. *Psychophysiology, 41(4)*, 575–583.

Ford, J. M., & Pfefferbaum, A. (1991). Event-related potentials and eyeblink responses in automatic and controlled processing: Effects of age. *Electroencephalography and Clinical Neurophysiology, 78*, 361–377.

Frackowiak, R.S.J., Friston, K.J., Frith, C., Dolan, R., Price, P., Zeki, S., Ashburner, J., & Penny, W.D. (2003). *Human brain function.* New York: Academic Press.

Friedman D. (2000). Event-related brain potential investigations of memory and aging. *Biological Psychology, 54(1-3)*, 175–206.

Freidman, D., & Fabiani, M. (1995). Memory and aging: An event-related brain potential perspective. In A. P. Allen & T.R. Bashore (Eds.), *Age differences in word and language processing. Advances in psychology* vol. 110, pp. 345–389. Amsterdam, Netherlands: North-Holland/Elsevier Science Publishers.

Friedman, D., & Simpson, G.V. (1994). ERP amplitude and scalp distribution to target and novel events: Effects of temporal order in young, middle-aged and older adults. *Cognitive Brain Research, 2(1)*, 49–63.

Friedman, D., Simpson, G., & Hamberger, M. (1993). Age-related changes in scal p topography to novel and target stimuli. *Psychophysiology, 30*, 383–396.

Golob, E. J., Miranda, G. G., Johnson, J. K., & Starr, A. (2001). Sensory cortical interactions in aging, mild cognitive impairment, and Alzheimer's disease. *Neurobiology of Aging, 22*, 755–763.

Good, C.D., Scahill, R.I., Fox, N.C., Ashburner, J., Friston, K.J., Chan, D., Crum, W.R., Rosson, M.N., & Frackowiak, R.S.J. (2002). Automatic differentiation of anatomical patterns in the human brain: Validation with stidues of degenerative dementias. *Neuroimage, 17*, 29–46.

Grady, C.L., Bernstein, L.J., Beig, S., & Siegenthaler, A.L. (2002). The effects of encoding task on age-related differences in the functional neuroanatomy of face memory. *Psychology and Aging, 17*, 7–23.

Grady, C.L., McIntosh, A.R., Beig, S., Keightley, cM.L., Burian, H., & Black, S. (2003). Evidence from functional neuroimaging of a compensatory prefrontal network in Alzheimer's disease. *The Journal of Neuroscience, 23*, 986–993.

Grady, C.L., McIntosh, A.R., Horwitz, B., & Rapoport, S.I. (2000). Age-related changes in the neural correlates of degreaded and nondegraded face processing. *Cognitive Neuropsychology, 217*, 165–186.

Gratton, E., Fantini, S., Franceschini, M. A., Gratton, G., & Fabiani, M. (1997). Measurements of scattering and absorption changes in muscle and brain. *Philosophical*

Transactions of the Royal Society of London: Biological Sciences, 352, 727–735.

Gratton, G., & Fabiani, M. (1998). Dynamic brain imaging: Event-related optical signal (EROS) measures of the time course and localization of cognitive-related activity. *Psychonomic Bulletin & Review, 5,* 535–563.

Gratton, G., & Fabiani, M. (2001). Shedding light on brain function: The event-related optical signal. *Trends in Cognitive Science, 5(8),* 357–363.

Gratton, G., & Fabiani, M. (2001). The event-related optical signal: A new tool for studying brain function. *International Journal of Psychophysiology, 42,* 109–121.

Gratton, G., & Fabiani, M. (2003). The event related optical signal (EROS) in visual cortex: Replicability, consistency, localization and resolution. *Psychophysiology, 40(4),* 561–571.

Gratton, G., Fabiani, M., Corballis, P. M., Hood, D. C., Goodman-Wood, M. R., Hirsch, J., Kim, K., Friedman, D., & Gratton, E. (1997). Fast and localized event-related optical signals (EROS) in the human occipital cortex: Comparisons with the visual evoked potential and fMRI. *NeuroImage, 6,* 168–180.

Gratton, G., Rykhlevskaia, E., Wee, E., Leaver, E., & Fabiani, M. (2005). White matter matters: Corpus callosum size is related to inter-hemispheric functional connectivity and task-switching effects in aging. Submitted for publication.

Gratton, G., Sarno, A. J., Maclin, E., Corballis, P. M., & Fabiani, M. (2000). Toward non-invasive 3-D imaging of the time course of cortical activity: Investigation of the depth of the event-related optical signal (EROS). *NeuroImage, 11,* 491–504.

Grosbras, M.-H., & Paus, T. Transcranial magnetic stimulation of the human frontal eye field facilitates visual awareness. [References]. *European Journal of Neuroscience. Vol 18(11)* 2003, 3121–3126.

Gunning-Dixon, FM., & Raz, N. (2003). Neuroanatomical correlates of selected executive functions in middle-aged and older adults: A prospective MRI study. *Neuropsychologia. 41(14),* 1929–1941.

Habeck, C., Hilton, H.J., Zarahn, E., Flynn, J., Moeller, J., & Stern, Y. (2003). Relation of cognitive reserve and task performance to expression of regional covariance networks in an event-related study of non-verbal memory. *Neuroimage, 20,* 1723–1733.

Hari, R., Levanen, S., & Raij, T. (2000). Timing of human cortical functions during cognition: Role of MEG. *Trends in Cognitive Science, 4(12),* 455–462.

Hartley, A.A. (1992). Attention. In F. Craik & T. Salthouse (Eds.), *The handbook of aging and cognition* (pp 3–49). Hillsdale, NJ: Erlbaum.

Hasher, L., & Zacks, R. (1988). Working memory, comprehension and aging: A review and a new view. In G. K. Bower (Ed.), *The psychology of learning and motivation* (pp. 192–225). New York: Academic Press.

Hay, J.F., & Jacoby, L.L. (1999). Separating habit and recollection in young and older adults: Effects of elaborative processing and distinctiveness. *Psychology and Aging, 14(1),* 122–134.

Head, D., Buckner, RL., Shimony, J. S., Williams, L. E., Akbudak, E., Conturo, T. E., McAvoy, M., Morris, J. C., & Snyder, A. Z. (2004). Differential vulnerability of anterior white matter in nondemented aging with minimal acceleration in dementia of the Alzheimer type: Evidence from diffusion tensor imaging. *Cerebral Cortex, 14(4),* 410–423.

Head, D., Raz, N., Gunning-Dixon, F., Williamson, A., & Acker, J. D. (2002). Age-related differences in the course of cognitive skill acquisition: The role of regional cortical shrinkage and cognitive resources. *Psychology and Aging, 17,* 72–84.

Hester, R., Fassbender, C., & Garavan, H. (2004). Individual differences in error processing: A review and reanalysis of three event-related fMRI studies using the Go/NoGo task. *Cerebral Cortex. 14(9),* 986–994.

Ince, P. (2001). Pathological correlates of late-onset dementia in a multi-center community-based population in England and Wales. *Lancet, 357,* 169–175.

Joyce, C.A., Paller, K.A., McIsaac, H.K., & Kutas, M. (1998). Memory changes with normal aging: behavioral and electrophysiological measures. *Psychophysiology, 35(6),* 669–678.

Knight, R. T. (1984). Decreased response to novel stimuli after prefrontal lesions in man. *Electroencephalography and Clinical Neurophysiology, 59*, 9–20.

Kozel, F.A., Nahas, Z., deBrux, C., Molly, M., Lorberbaum, J.P., Bohning, D., Risch, S.C., & George, M.S. (2000). How coil cortex distance relates to age, motor threshold, and antidepressant response to repetitive transcranial magnetic stimulation. *Journal of Neuropsychiatry & Clinical Neurosciences, 12*, 376–384.

Kramer, A. F., Bherer, L., Colcombe, S. J., Dong, W., & Greenough, W. T. (2004). Environmental influences on cognitive and brain plasticity during aging. *Journals of Gerontology Series A: Biological Sciences & Medical Sciences. 59(9)*, 940–957.

Kramer, A.F., Larish, J., Weber, T., & Bardell, L. (1999). Training for executive control: Task coordination strategies and aging. In D. Gopher & A. Koriat (Eds.), *Attention and performance XVII*. Cambridge, MA: MIT Press.

Kutas, M., & Federmeier, K.D. (1998). Minding the body. *Psychophysiology, 35(2)*, 135–150.

Li, J., Morcom, A.M., & Rugg, M.D. (2004). The effects of age on the neural correlates of successful episodic retrieval: An ERP study. *Cognitive and Affective Behavioral Neuroscience, 4(3)*, 279–293.

Lindenberger, U., & Baltes, P. B. (1997). Intellectual functioning in old and very old age: Cross-sectional results from the Berlin Aging Study. *Psychology & Aging, 12(3)*, 410–432.

Logan, J. M., Sanders, A. L., Snyder, A. Z., Morris, J. C. & Buckner, R. L. (2002). Under-recruitment and non-selective recruitment: Dissociable neural mechanisms associated with cognitive decline in older adults. *Neuron, 33*, 827–840.

Low, K. A., Wee, E., Sable, J. J., Gratton, G., & Fabiani, M. (2001). Effects of interstimulus delay on the mismatch negativity in young and older adults. *Psychophysiology, 38*, S62.

Lustig, C., & Buckner, R.L. (2004). Preserved neural correlates of priming in old age and dementia. *Neuron, 42(5)*, 865–875.

Maccotta, L., Zacks, J. M., & Buckner, R. L. (2001). Rapid self-paced event-related functional MRI: Feasibility and implications of stimulus-versus response-locked timing. *Neuroimage, 14(5)*, 1105–1121.

Madden, D.J., Turkington, T.G., Coleman, R.E., Provenzale, J.M., DeGrado, T.R., & Hoffman, J.M. (1996). Adult age differences in regional cerebral blood flow during visual word identification: Evidence from PET. *Neuroimage, 3*, 127–142.

Madden, D.J., Turkington, T.G., Provenzale, J.M., Denny, L.L., Lamgley, L.K., Kawk, T.C., & Coleman, R.E. (2002). Aging and attentional guidance during visual search. *Psychology and Aging, 17*, 24–43.

Madden, D.J., Turkington, T.G., Provenzale, J.M., Hawk, T.C., Hoffman, J.M., & Coleman, R.E. (1997). Selective and divided visual attention: Age-related changes in regional cererbral blood flow measure by H$_2$^{15}O PET. *Human Brain Mapping, 5*, 389–409.

Madden, D.J., Whiting, W.L., & Huettel, S.A. (2005). Age-related changes in neural activity during visual perception and attention. In R. Cabeza, L. Nyberg & D.C. Park (Eds.), *Cognitive neuroscience of aging: Linking cognitive and cerebral aging*. New York: Oxford University Press.

Malonek, D., & Grinvald, A. (1996). Interactions between electrical activity and cortical microcirculation revealed by imaging spectroscopy: Implications for functional brain mapping. *Science, 272(5261)*, 551–554.

Masino, S.A., & Frostig, R.D. (1996). Quantitative long-term imaging of the functional representation of a whisker in rat barrel cortex. *Proceedings of the National Academy of Sciences, USA, 93(10)*, 4942–4947.

McCarthy, G., & Wood, C. C. (1985). Scalp distribution of event related potentials: An ambiguity associated with analysis of variance models. *Electroencephalography and Clinical Neurophysiology, 62*, 203–208.

Milham, M.P., Erickson, K.I., Banich, M.B., Kramer, A.F., Webb, A., Wszalek, T., & Cohen, N.J. (2002). Attentional control in the aging brain: Insights from an fMRI study of the Stroop task. *Brain and Cognition, 49*, 277–296.

Morcom, A.M., Good, C.D., Frackowiak, R.S., & Rugg, M.D. (2003). Age effects on the neural correlates of successful memory encoding. *Brain, 126(Pt 1)*, 213–229.

Morrison, J.H., & Hof, P.R. (1997). Life and death of neurons in the aging brain. *Science, 278*, 412–419.

Moscovitch, M., & Winocur, G. (1992). The neuropsychology of memory and aging. In F. I. M. Craik & T. A. Salthouse (Eds.), *The handbook of aging and cognition* (pp. 315–372). Hillsdale, NJ: Erlbaum.

Mosley, M, Bammer, R. I., & Illes, J. (2002). Diffusion-tensor imaging of cognitive performance. *Brain and Cognition, 50*, 396–413.

Nielson, K.A., Langencker, S.A., & Garvan, H.P. (2002). Differences in the functional neuroanatomy of inhibitory control across the adult lifespan. *Psychology and Aging, 17*, 56–71.

Nunez, P. L. (1981). *Electric fields of the brain: The neurophysics of EEG.* London: Oxford University Press.

Nyberg, L., Sandblom, J., Jones, S., Neely, A. S., Petersson, K. M., Ingvar, M., & Backman, L. (2003). Neural correlates of training-related memory improvement in adulthood and aging. *Proceedings of the National Academy of Sciences of the United States of America. 100(23)*, 13728–13733.

Olson, I. R., Zhang, J. X., Mitchell, K. J., Johnson, M. K., Bloise, S. M., & Higgins, J. A. (2004). Preserved spatial memory over brief intervals in older adults. *Psychology and Aging, 19(2)*, 310–317.

O'Sullivan, M., Jones, D. K., Summers, P. E., Morris, R. G., Williams, S. C. R., & Markus, H. S. (2001). Evidence for cortical "disconnection" as a mechanism of age-related cognitive decline. *Neurology, 57*, 632–638

Park, D. C. (2000). The basic mechanisms accounting for age-related decline in cognitive function. In D. C. Park & N. Schwartz (Eds.), *Cognitive aging: A primer.* Philadelphia, PA: Psychology Press.

Park, D.C., Lautenschlager, G., Hedden, T. Davidson, N.S., Smith, A.D. & Smith, P.K. (2003). Models of visuospatial and verbal memory across the adult lifespan. *Psychology and Aging, 17*, 299–320.

Pessoa, L., Kastner, S., & Ungerleider, L.G. (2003). Neuroimaging studies of attention: From modulation of sensory processing to top-down control. *The Journal of Neuroscience, 23*, 3990–3998.

Phelps, M. E., Mazziotta, J. C., & Schelbert, H. (1986). *Positron emission tomography and autoradiography: Principles and applications for the brain and heart.* New York: Raven.

Pierpaoli, C., & Basser, P. J. (1996). Toward a quantitative assessment of diffusion anisotropy. *Magnetic Resonance in Medicine, 36(6)*, 893–906.

Polich, J. (1991). P300 in the evaluation of aging and dementia. In C. H. M. Brunia, G. Mulder, & M. N. Verbaten (Eds.) *Event-related potential research* (EEG Suppl. 42, pp. 304–323). Amsterdam, The Netherlands: Elsevier.

Polich, J. (1996). Meta-analysis of P300 normative aging studies. *Psychophysiology, 33(4)*, 334–353.

Polich, J., Howard, L., & Starr, A. (1983). P300 latency correlates with digit span. *Psychophysiology, 20*, 665–669, 1983.

Raz, N. (2000). Aging of the brain and its impact on cognitive performance: Integration of structural and functional findings. In F. I. M. Craik & T. A. Salthouse (Eds.), *The handbook of aging and cognition,* (2nd edition, p. 1–90). Mahwah, NJ: Lawrence Erlbaum.

Reuter-Lorenz, P. A., & Mikels, J.A. (2005). The aging mind and brain: Implications of enduring plasticity for behavioral and cultural change. In P. Baltes, P.A. Reuter-Lorenz, & F. Roesler (Eds.), *Lifespan development and the brain: The perspective of biocultural co-constructivism.* London: Cambridge University Press.

Reuter-Lorenz, P. A., Jonides, J., Smith, E. E., Hartley, A., Miller, A., Marshuetz, C., & Koeppe, R. A. (2000). Age differences in the frontal lateralization of verbal and spatial working memory revealed by PET. *Journal of Cognitive Neuroscience, 12*, 174–187.

Rinne, T., Gratton, G., Fabiani, M., Cowan, N., Maclin, E., Stinard, A., Sinkkonen, J., Alho, K., & Näätänen, R. (1999). Scalp-recorded optical signals make sound processing from the auditory cortex visible. *NeuroImage, 10*, 620–624.

Robbins, T. W., James, M., Owen, A. M., Shaakian, B. J., Lawrence, A. D., McInnes, L., & Rabbit, P. M. A. (1998). A study of performance from tests from the CANTAB battery sensitive to frontal lobe dysfunction in a large sample of normal volunteers: Implications for theories of executive functioning and cognitive aging. *Journal of the International Neuropsychological Society, 4*, 474–490.

Robertson, E.M., Theoret, H., & Pascual-Leone, A. (2003). Studies in cognition: The problems solved and created by transcranial magnetic stimulation. *Journal of Cognitive Neuroscience, 15*, 948–960.

Rodrigue, K. M., & Raz, N. (2004). Shrinkage of the entorhinal cortex over five years predicts memory performance in healthy adults. *Journal of Neuroscience. 24(4)*, 956–963.

Rosen, A., Prull, M., O'Hara, R., Race, E., Desmond, J., Glover, G., Yesavage, J., & Gabrieli, J. (2002). Variable effects of aging on frontal lobe contributions to memory. *Neuroreport, 13*, 2425–2428.

Rushworth, M.F.S., Hadland, K.A., Paus, T., & Sipila, P.K. (2002). Role of the human medial frontal cortex in task switching: A combined fMRI and TMS study. *Journal of Neurophysiology, 87*, 2577–2592.

Rusinek, H., De Santi, S., Frid, D., Tsui, W. H., Tarshish, C. Y., Convit, A., & de Leon, M. J. (2003). Regional brain atrophy rate predicts future cognitive decline: 6-year longitudinal MR imaging study of normal aging. *Radiology, 229(3)*, 691–696.

Safonova, L.P., Michalos, A., Wolf, U., Wolf, M., Hueber, D.M., Choi, J.H., Gupta, R., Polzonetti, C., Mantulin, W.W., & Gratton, E. (2004). Age-correlated changes in cerebral hemodynamics assessed by near-infrared spectroscopy. *Arch. Gerontol. Geriatr. 39(3)*, 207–225.

Salthouse, T. A. (1996). Processing-speed theory of adult age differences in cognition. *Psychological Review, 103*, 403–428.

Scarmeas, N., Zarahn, E., Anderson, K.E., Hilton, J., Flynn, J., Van Heertum, R.L., Sackeim, H.A., & Stern, Y. (2003). Cognitive reserve modulates functional brain responses during memory tasks: A PET study in healthy young and elderly subjects. *Neuroimage, 19*, 1215–1227.

Schaie, K.W. (2002). The impact of longitudinal studies on understanding development from young adulthood to old age.

In W.W. Hartup & R.K. Soldereisen (Eds.), *Growing points in developmental science* (pp. 307–328). Philadelphia, PA: Psychology Press.

Scialfa, C. T., Jenkins, L., Hamaluk, E., & Skaloud, P. (2000). Aging and the development of automaticity in conjunction search. *Journal of Gerontology: Psychological Sciences, 55(B)*, 7–46.

Schretlen, D., Pearlson, G. D., Anthony, J. C., Aylward, E. H., Augustine, A. M., Davis, A., & Barta, P. (2000). Elucidating the contributions of processing speed, executive ability, and frontal lobe volume to normal age-related differences in fluid intelligence. *Journal of the International Neuropsychological Society, 6*, 52–61.

Schmiedek, F., & Li, S.C. (2004). Toward an alternative representation for disentangling age-associated differences in general and specific cognitive abilities. *Psychology and Aging, 19*, 40–56.

Smith, E.E., Geva, A., Jonides, J., Miller, A., Reuter-Lorenz, P., & Koeppe, R.A. (2001). The neural basis of task-switching in working memory: Effects of performance and aging. *Proceedings of the National Academy of Sciences, 98(4)*, 2095–2100.

Smith, S.M., Zhang, Y., Jenkinson, M., Chen, J., Matthews, P.M., Federico, A., & De Stefano, N. (2002). Accurate, robust and automated longitudinal and cross-sectional brain change analysis. *NeuroImage, 17(1):*479–489.

Snowdon, D.A., Greiner, L.H., & Markesbery, W.R. (2000). Linguistic ability in early life and the neuropathology of Alzheimer's disease and cerebrovascular disease: Findings from the nun study. *Annual New York Academy of Sciences, 903*, 34–38.

Squire, L.R. (2004). Memory systems of the brain: A brief history and current perspective. *Neurobiology of Learning and Memory, 82(3)*, 171–177.

Stebbins, G.T., Carrillo, M.C. Desmond, J.E., Turner, D., Bennett, D., Wilson, R., Glover, G., & Gabrieli, J. (2002). Aging effects on memory encoding in the frontal lobes. *Psychology and Aging, 17*, 44–55.

Stern, Y., Zarahn, E., Hilton, H.J., Flynn, J., DeLaPaz, R., & Rakitin, B. (2003). Exploring the neural basis of cognitive reserve. *Journal of Clinical and Experimental Neuropsychology, 25*, 691–701.

Sulekha, A., & Hotson, J. (2002). Transcranial magnetic stimulation: Neurophysiological applications and safety. *Brain & Cognition, 50*, 366–386.

Tisserand, D. J., Pruessner, J. C., Arigita, E. J. S., van Boxtel, M. P. J., Evans, A. C, Jolles, J., & Uylings, H. B. M. (2002). Regional frontal cortical volumes decrease differentially in aging: An MRI study to compare volumetric approaches and voxel-based morphometry. *Neuroimage, 17(2)*, 657–669.

Toronov, V., Walker, S., Gupta, R., Choi, J.H., Gratton, E., Hueber, D., & Webb, A. (2003). The roles of changes in deoxyhemoglobin concentration and regional cerebral blood volume in the fMRI BOLD signal. *Neuroimage, 19(4)*, 1521–1521.

Tulving, E. (1987). Multiple memory systems and consciousness. *Human Neurobiology, 6(2)*, 67–80.

Tulving, E., & Schacter, D.L. (1990). Priming and human memory systems. *Science, 247(4940)*, 301–306.

Villringer, A., & Chance, B. (1997). Non-invasive optical spectroscopy and imaging of human brain function. *Trends in Neuroscience, 20(10)*, 435–442.

Volkow, N. D., Wang, G.-J., Fowler, J. S., Hitzemann, R. et al. Gender differences in cerebellar metabolism: Test-retest reproducibility. *American Journal of Psychiatry. Vol 154(1)* 1997, 119–121.

Walhovd, K. B., Fjell, A. M., Reinvang, I., Lundervold, A., Fischl, B., Quinn, B. T., & Dale, A. M. (2004). Size does matter in the long run: Hippocampal and cortical volume predict recall across weeks. *Neurology, 63(7)*, 193–1197.

West, R. L. (1996). An application of prefrontal cortex function theory to cognitive aging. *Psychological Bulletin, 120(2)*, 272–92.

West, R. L. (2004). The effects of aging on controlled attention and conflict processing in the Stroop task. *Journal of Cognitive Neuroscience, 16*, 103–113.

Woodruff-Pak, D. S. (1997). *The neuropsychology of aging* (Vol. 352). Cambridge, MA: Blackwell.

Five

Health, Behavior, and Optimal Aging: A Life Span Developmental Perspective

Carolyn M. Aldwin, Avron Spiro III, and Crystal L. Park

One of the most striking changes in the aging paradigm since the mid-1960s is the recognition of both individual differences and plasticity in the aging process. Some individuals become severely disabled in midlife, whereas others are running marathons in their seventies and even eighties (albeit rarely). Some of these individual differences are due to the plasticity of biological aging, i.e., the rate at which we age is modified by health behavior habits and by psychosocial factors such as personality processes and social context.

The purpose of this chapter is to review the behavioral and psychosocial factors that influence the rate from a life span developmental perspective. Some factors are aging accelerators, i.e., they appear to hasten decline in specific organ systems and/or more general physiological processes. These include health behavior habits, such as smoking and obesity, and personological factors, such as hostility, depression, and anxiety. Other factors, less well understood, appear to decelerate the rate of aging or to promote healthy aging, including exercise, diets low in saturated fats and high in antioxidants,

and, perhaps, psychosocial factors such as social support (see Carstensen, Mikels, and Mather, Chapter 15), sense of control, and emotional balance. We then propose a preliminary model of optimal aging, which may reflect a life span developmental perspective more closely than other theories of successful aging.

I. A Life Span Developmental Perspective: Toward Optimal Aging

While a life span perspective has long been accepted in adult development and aging, this approach is just starting to gain favor in epidemiology (Kuh & Ben-Shlomo, 2004). A life span perspective on health was proposed by Spiro (2001), which is characterized by several axioms. First, *health is a life-long process*. It has genetic origins; it develops during infancy, childhood, and adulthood as a result of gene–environment interactions, as well as elements of volition, and undergoes continuous change across the life span. Health during later life is an outcome of factors that play out across the life span (Power & Parsons, 2003).

Second, *health is characterized by multidimensionality*. In 1948, the World Health Organization defined health as "a state of complete physical, mental and social well-being and not merely the absence of disease or infirmity" (from http://www.who.int/about/definition/en/, accessed January 19, 2005). Although debate continues on the precise definition of health (and its counterparts, disease and illness), it is generally recognized to include several dimensions and to encompass multiple levels of analysis. This has implications for understanding optimal aging. If health is multidimensional, and some sort of decline in physical health is inevitable in late life, how can individuals optimize psychosocial well-being despite physical loss? While some hold that the different aspects of health become more tightly entwined in later life, there is also evidence of growing independence, especially in very late life. For example, physical pain may have less impact on psychological health among the very old (Frytak et al., 2001). Third, the obvious corollary is that the *study of health is inherently multidisciplinary*. Enhanced understanding of health is possible only as a result of multidisciplinary collaboration.

Fourth, *there are always gains and losses in development*. This principle of multidirectionality suggests a focus on positive as well as negative outcomes. However, most theories of successful aging focus on the prevention of loss (e.g., Rowe & Kahn, 1997) rather than what may be gained in optimal aging. While wisdom is an obvious component of optimal aging, it is difficult to show that wisdom increases with age (see Brugman, Chapter 20). However, how individuals cope with physical and social losses may be an essential component to the development of wisdom in later life (Levenson, Aldwin, & Cupertino, 2001).

Fifth, *health occurs in and is constrained by its sociohistorical context*. The influence of social context, in general, and socioeconomic status (SES), in particular (e.g., Adler & Snibbe, 2003), is increasingly recognized as an important influence on health and disease. In general, those with lower SES have reduced life expectancy, worse health behaviors, more restrictions on activities, worse well-being, and less access to health care. However, the influence of context on health should also be considered historically as well as socially, as the settings in which humans have lived have changed much over the past 500 years. The gains in longevity are greater since 1900 than in the whole previous span of human history.

A life span developmental approach will be used to examine factors that affect the rate of biological aging. These factors may also promote optimal aging, not only in terms of decelerating the rate of aging, but also promoting healthy adaptation in the face of losses in late life. First, however, we briefly review the current health status of older adults, including changes in life expectancy, morbidity, and mortality, as well as the behavioral or lifestyle factors widely acknowledged to affect the development of disease and thus the rate of aging.

II. Changing Health and Behavior of Older Adults

A. Improving Health of Older Adults

There has been a remarkable change in the life expectancy of people throughout the world. Life expectancy in 1900 was about 47 years, whereas today it is 74 for men and a remarkable 79 years for women (CDC, 2004). Figure 5.1a shows the change in age-adjusted mortality rates from 1965 to 2002 in the United States, during which time the overall rate (per

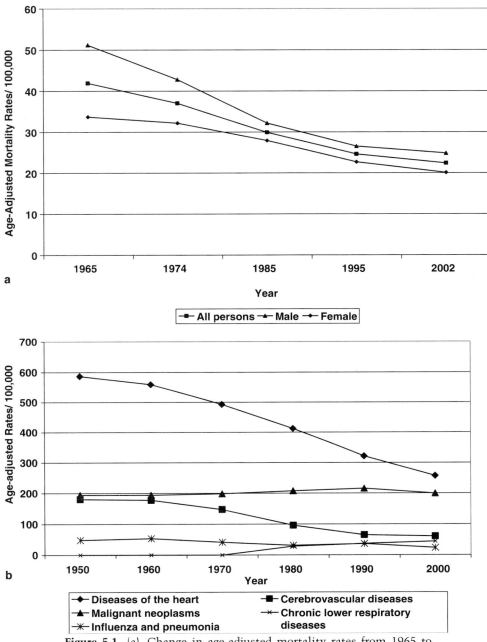

Figure 5.1 (a). Change in age-adjusted mortality rates from 1965 to 2002. Based on data from the Centers for Disease Control (2004). Health, United States, 2004, retrieved December 14, 2004 from http://www.cdc.gov/nchs/hus.htm. (b). Change in disease-specific mortality from 1950 to 2000. Based on data from the Centers for Disease Control (2004). Health, United States, 2004, retrieved December 14, 2004 from http://www.cdc.gov/nchs/hus.htm.

100,000 people) was halved, from slightly over 50 to about 25. The traditional gender gap in mortality rates had narrowed during this time period, although women still enjoy lower mortality rates than men.

This demographic shift is worldwide, with the net result of older populations in most of the countries of the world. This shift is not restricted to developed countries. In 2030, there will be twice as many older adults in developing countries as in Europe and North America (Kinsella & Velkoff, 2001). The economic consequences of this demographic shift, especially in the developing world, may be very severe; thus it is critical to examine ways to promote optimal aging.

Much of this change in life expectancy is due to a decrease in infant mortality and in infectious diseases. By the latter part of the 20th century, the distribution of age at death had changed, dramatically, with most deaths occurring late in life. While some of this increase in survival can be attributed to better medical practices, much of it is a reflection of better public health practices in sanitation, drinking water, nutrition, and food safety, as well as changes in health behavior habits. Consequently, there has been a shift in the cause of death, from acute to chronic illnesses. Figure 5.1b demonstrates secular trends in causes of death since the mid-1950s, based on data gathered by the CDC (2004). Since 1950, the rate of deaths due to heart disease has been more than halved, even as the rate of smoking has dropped in a similar pattern. Heart disease continues to be the leading cause of death, despite its dramatic decline, and deaths due to cardiovascular diseases such as stroke have also declined. Mortality from chronic obstructive pulmonary disease (COPD) increased slightly and now surpasses deaths from influenza and pneumonia. Cancer deaths have remained fairly stable and, for some groups, surpass heart disease (Greenlee et al., 2000).

B. Role of Health Behavior Habits

Mokdad and colleagues (2004) estimate that the leading causes of death in the United States are smoking, poor diet and physical activity, and alcohol consumption — *not* pathogens.

1. Smoking

The rate of cigarette smoking decreases with age; individuals over the age of 65 have the lowest rate of smoking in any adult group (10% or less, as opposed to a third of young adults). The exception to this is found among African-American males. Nearly 20% of African-American males over the age of 65 smoke, but the rate of smoking among young males aged 18–24 is only 22.8%, as opposed to 34.5% of white males overall (CDC, 2004). To some extent this decline in smoking rates with age is a function of aging and cohort effects, but it also reflects survival rates.

The health benefits of smoking cessation are well known. These have been summarized by the Surgeon General (1990; http://profiles.nlm.nih.gov/NN/B/B/C/T/_/nnbbct.pdf). Depending on the illness, most people receive immediate benefits of smoking cessation. Although the effect is stronger for younger adults, even older people may benefit from smoking cessation. For individuals without preexisting disease, risks are reduced to the levels of nonsmokers usually within 5 to 15 years. For individuals with established disease, quitting smoking may reduce the rate of decline. Most people quit smoking on their own, and a variety of aids exist, including nicotine patches, acupuncture, and hypnosis, as well as antidepressants. Individuals with a history of depression are more likely to be heavy smokers and have a difficult time with smoking cessation, and antidepressants such as buproprion may be helpful (Wilhelm et al., 2004). In general, health education programs are helpful in smoking cessation, with multimodal treatments most successful (Fiore, 2000). While the assumption is that older smokers are particularly resistant to smoking cessation programs, Fair (2003) found them to be as effective in older people as in younger ones and that nicotine patches are preferable to nicotine gum (especially for those with dentures).

2. Diet and Physical Activity

This dramatic decrease in smoking behavior, however, may be offset by a startling increase in obesity over the same time period. Figure 5.2 shows changes in obesity from the early 1960s to 2002, separately by sex, drawing on data from the CDC (2004). Being overweight was defined as having a body mass index (BMI) of 25 or greater, whereas obesity was defined as having a BMI of 30 or above. In 1960, about half of young men

had healthy weights and only 10% were obese, regardless of age. For those aged 30 and older, about 40% had healthy weights. By 2000, however, nearly 25% of men in their fifties and sixties were obese, and less than one-fifth of the men in their forties, fifties, and sixties had healthy weights.

The change in women was even more dramatic. In the 1960s, clear age differences in BMI were evident. About 70% of young women in their twenties had healthy weights and only 10% were obese, but only about 30% of women in their sixties had healthy weights and 20% were obese. In 2000, however, there were very few age differences in BMI; between 20 and 30% of women at all ages were obese. Only 35% of young women had healthy weights compared to 20% among women in their fifties and sixties.

Obesity is also a well-known risk factor for a variety of chronic illnesses in late

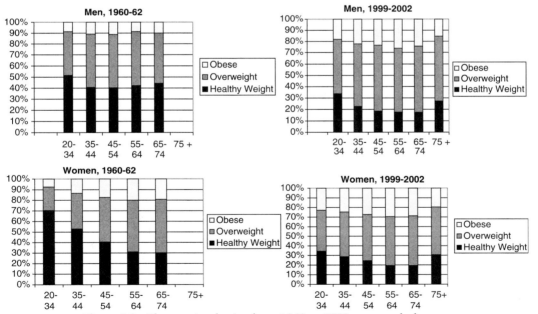

Figure 5.2 Changes in obesity from 1960 to 2002, separately by sex. Based on data from the Centers for Disease Control (2004). Health, United States, 2004, retrieved December 14, 2004 from http://www.cdc.gov/nchs/hus.htm.

life, including cardiovascular disease, diabetes, arthritis, blindness, and amputation (for physiological pathways, see Aldwin & Gilmer, 2004). Glucose intolerance usually precedes the onset of diabetes and is defined by the inability to adequately process glucose, leading to higher blood sugar levels. This in turn damages the ability of the pancreas to respond adequately with insulin, continuing the cycle. Diabetes accelerates the aging of both the sensory and the cardiovascular systems greatly and may affect mobility as well.

Diet, exercise, and weight loss can reverse glucose intolerance and can also help with early diabetes. Oral hypoglycemics are also a way to regulate glucose levels in the blood. In severe cases, insulin may be necessary to replace failing β cells in the pancreas. Adequate metabolic control is absolutely essential to prevent or at least delay the onset of the adverse effects of diabetes. While drugs such as metformin can help regulate blood glucose levels, Knowler et al. (2002) found that lifestyle interventions (e.g., intensive individual counseling promoting weight loss and exercise) decreased or delayed the onset of diabetes by over 50%, compared to about 38% with metformin alone.

Older adults are also at risk for undernutrition, especially if they are isolated, chronically ill, disabled (physically or cognitively), depressed, and/or have food insecurity due to inadequate financial resources. Diets low in calcium, protein, fluids, and calories lead to undernutrition, which can impair immune functioning, create electrolyte imbalances, leading to kidney or heart failure, and result in cognitive impairment. Institutionalized older adults in particular are at high risk for undernutrition (Palmer, 1997). Weight loss in later life is a serious risk factor for mortality (Tully & Snowdon, 1995). There is a J-shaped curve between weight and mortality: both under- and very overweight people have the highest mortality rates, whereas those who are slightly overweight have the lowest rates (Durazo-Arvizu et al., 1997). Thus, obesity is clearly an aging accelerator, but adequate fat reserves may be protective, especially in later life.

Both aerobic and anaerobic exercise can slow down the rate of aging, and not only by regulating weight. Exercise in late life can improve muscle strength, flexibility, walking, and standing balance (Keysor & Jette, 2001). Aerobic exercise improves cardiovascular function, strengthens the heart muscle, and lowers both low-density and total cholesterol levels, but increases high-density cholesterol levels. Although cardiac output decreases with age, older adults who are physically fit can increase their cardiac output 50% more than those who are not in good physical condition (Guyton & Hall, 1996). Aerobic exercise is also protective of pulmonary function and can increase vital capacity and VO_2 max, even in frail 85-year-old women (Puggaard et al., 2000).

While exercise can initially increase inflammatory processes, over time, it improves immune function. Moderate exercise enhances the production of antioxidants (Evans, 2000), although very strenuous exercise or exercise in very frail older adults may impair immune function (Bruunsgard & Pedersen, 2000). Nonetheless, long-term exercise programs appear to enhance immunity, and those with better pulmonary function have fewer respiratory infections in later life (Kostka et al., 2000). Further, even in late life, anaerobic or weight-bearing exercise can enhance muscle strength, slow down the rate of calcium loss from the bone, and improve balance, all of which may decrease the rate of falls and maintain functional capacity (Taaffe et al., 1996). Although there is less evidence regarding the impact of exercise on emotional, social, or physical disability in late life (Keysor & Jette, 2001), one study found that exposure to positive stereotypes of aging significantly increased gait speed and quality (Hausdorff, Levy, & Wei, 1999). More research is needed to study exercise, functional health, and disability in later life.

3. Alcohol Consumption

Currently, only 56% of Americans report alcohol use (CDC, 2004). Multiethnic individuals have the highest rate of drinking (62.1%), followed by whites (60.2%), Native Americans (48.6%), Blacks (40.3%), Hispanics (38.1%), and Asians (35.3%). Individuals 75 years and older, regardless of ethnicity, have the lowest rate of any demographic age group (30.4%), and nearly 80% of elders who do drink report being light drinkers.

While it is commonly believed that alcohol consumption decreases with age, Levenson, Aldwin, and Spiro (1998), using sequential data on men in the VA Normative Aging Study from 1972 to 1991, showed a more complex picture, with significant cohort, period, and age effects. In general, older cohorts of men consumed less, but all age groups increased consumption in the 1970s. While fewer older men drink, often due to problems with interactions with medications, those who maintained their drinking status often consumed nearly as much as they had when they were younger. A study of a different sample, however, did find decreases in alcohol consumption among elders who continued to drink (Moos et al., 2004). Levenson and colleagues (1998) found high rates of problem drinking among the youngest cohort, the baby boomers, who, in general, drank more than the older cohorts. Lemke and Moos (2003) showed that older men do at least as well in alcohol cessation programs as younger men. However, Johnson (1996) cautioned that old–old women may be at high risk for abusing alcohol and psychotropic medications to attempt to control pain and sleep problems.

III. Psychosocial Factors Affecting the Rate of Aging

This section considers three broad types of psychosocial factors that may affect the rate of aging: personality, religiousness/spirituality, and stress and coping processes.

A. Personality

There is now convincing evidence that personality, defined broadly to include traits, beliefs, affect, and attitudes, affects health, especially cardiovascular health (Aldwin et al., 2004; DeVellis & Devellis, 2001; Krantz & McCeney, 2001; Smith & Spiro, 2002). In particular, hostility (the toxic component in type A behavior), anxiety, and depressive symptoms are risk factors for cardiovascular disease, and thus can be considered aging accelerators. Although there is some evidence for the impact of these factors on immune function (Kiecolt-Gleser et al., 2002), evidence for the relationship between personality and cancer is much more controversial (McGee et al., 1994). Some exciting new developments focus on personality processes that can be protective factors, such as emotional stability, sense of control, and optimism.

1. Hostility

In 1978, the review panel on coronary-prone behavior and coronary heart disease presented striking evidence showing that hostility was comparable to smoking as a risk factor for cardiovascular disease. A meta-analysis showed that the risk level varies as a function of how hostility is measured, with interview measures stronger than self-report measures

(Miller et al., 1996). Nonetheless, individuals high in hostility have higher rates of both cardiovascular morbidity and mortality than less hostile individuals. The effect is stronger for men than for women, and may be stronger for middle-aged than older adults (Williams, 2000).

There are a number of pathways through which hostility can lead to cardiovascular disease. While some of this effect is mediated through poorer health behavior habits (e.g., smoking and higher BMIs), individuals high in hostility also have higher cardiovascular reactivity, especially to social stressors (Krantz & McCeney, 2002). Under stressors such as criticism, they respond with higher blood pressure and increases in serum lipid levels, especially low-density lipoproteins (LDLs) and triglycerides (Niaura et al., 2000). Thus, individuals who are high in hostility increase their risk of cardiovascular morbidity and mortality not only through their health behavior habits, but also through their physiological responses to stress.

2. Anxiety and neuroticism

Neuroticism appears to predict mortality independently of hostility (Surtees et al., 2003) and may be especially important in later life (Wilson et al., 2004). The relationship between neuroticism and mortality is not always consistent, however, and Friedman (2000) suggests that neuroticism may be problematic primarily under conditions of environmental stress.

Anxiety is related to both higher risks for CHD (Tennant & McLean, 2001) and sudden cardiac death (Kawachi et al., 1994). Eaker, Pinsky, and Castelli (1992) found that high-anxious women who did not work outside the home were eight and a half times more likely to die of sudden death than nonanxious women.

There are several possible pathways through which high anxiety can lead to

sudden death. Tennant and McLean (2001) reviewed evidence showing that under high anxiety, individuals release large amounts of catecholamines, which increase blood pressure and heart rate dramatically, resulting in ischemic problems, leading to myocardial infarctions (MIs), especially in those with underlying heart disease. Hyperventilation and emotional distress can also induce vasospasm and release platelets, which can cut off blood flow to the heart muscles, also resulting in MIs. Gorman and Sloan (2000) also reviewed evidence that individuals with high anxiety have poorer heart rate regulation, resulting in greater vulnerability to sudden releases of catecholamines, which can also result in overreaction to stressors.

3. Depression

Depressive symptoms can also result in higher levels of cardiovascular morbidity and mortality (Tennant & McLean, 2001), especially in men (Sesso et al., 1998). However, depressive symptoms in late life tend to be very unstable, and the effects on mortality may be relatively short-lived (Blazer et al., 2001). As individuals recover from depressive episodes, their mortality risk decreases. However, the effect may be strongest among those with preexisting cardiovascular disease (Lésperance et al., 2002).

Again, there appear to be multiple pathways through which depressive symptoms can affect health, including poorer health behavior habits, such as smoking and higher BMIs (Hayward, 1995), atherogenesis (Appels et al., 2000), arrhythmias (Ladwig, Kieser, & Konigh, 1991), and decreased heart rate variability (i.e., poorer regulation of the heart rate) (Light, Kathandopani, & Allen, 1998). A common symptom of depression is loss of appetite, and Pulska and colleagues (2000) found that depressive symptoms were related to mortality primarily among those elders who developed anorexia, as weight loss is a substantive risk for mortality in older adults.

4. Protective factors

Evidence for personality processes as protective factors is weaker, but nonetheless intriguing; more work is badly needed. Control is perhaps the most researched construct. In early experiments, individuals given control experienced less physiological arousal under stress than individuals with no control (Frankenhauser, 1978). Some studies have reported protective effects of control on morbidity and mortality, although the effects are not consistent across studies (DeVellis & DeVellis, 2001). Krause and Shaw (2000) suggested that some of the inconsistency in the literature reflects the difference between general control vs. situation- or role-specific control. In their study, global control did not predict mortality, but feelings of control in the most important social role did predict longevity.

Similarly, the effects of optimism on physical health have also been inconsistent. Some studies suggest that optimism is related to better self-reported health (Peterson, 1988), less cardiovascular disease (Kubzansky et al., 2001), better immune functioning (Kohout et al., 2002), and lower mortality (Giltay et al., 2004). However, optimism is often related to worse immune function, depending on the type of stressor and coping strategies (Segerstrom, 2001; Segerstrom, Castañeda, & Spencer, 2003), and is unrelated to survival in cancer patients (Schofield et al., 2004). Other studies have found little association with optimism and longevity (Schulz et al., 1996), and the findings for related constructs are similarly contradictory. For example, cheerfulness predicts premature mortality (Martin et al., 2002), whereas having a positive self-image predicts longevity (Levy et al., 2002).

The reasons for these inconsistencies are as yet unclear. In their review, Aldwin et al. (2004) suggested that optimism may be positively associated with better health outcomes in the absence of stressors or under acute stress, but is associated with poorer outcomes for persons under severe or chronic stress. Segerstrom et al. (2003) contrasted this model, which they termed the "affective" model, with the "persistence" model, which holds that optimists may have poorer immune function under stress because they persist at some physiological cost, but that they benefit in the long term. However, their chronic stressor was an examination, which is generally considered an acute stressor and has questionable relevance for elders compared to a chronic illness, for example. Distinguishing optimism from denial must also be better addressed.

Other personality factors may be important for health in late life. Ouellette and DiPlacido (2001) reviewed the relevance for health of hardiness and a sense of coherence (Antonovsky, 1987). The outcomes of most of the studies were either psychological or self-reported symptoms rather than morbidity or mortality, but results suggest that both constructs are related to better health. However, a sense of coherence may be an independent protective factor against premature mortality (Surtees et al., 2003).

Two newer constructs may hold particular promise for protecting health in later life, emotional stability and mindfulness. Spiro and colleagues (1995) found that emotional stability was inversely associated with the development of hypertension and that it was a much stronger predictor of hypertension in this sample than hostility. Aldwin and co-workers (2001) found that men who were high in emotional stability showed very little increase in self-reported symptoms from midlife to late life, suggesting that emotional stability may be a key component of successful aging. Indeed, to the extent that emotional lability such as anxiety, depressive symptoms, and hostility are risk factors because of cascade effects via changes in catecholamines, blood pressure, and cardiovascular reactivity in general, then it would make sense that emotional stability would be protective against such cascades.

Along similar lines, Langer (1989) proposed that mindfulness may be a health protective factor, especially in later life. Mindfulness is defined as the process of becoming aware of the environment and one's reactions to it, as well as one's internal states, which presumably allow a person to exercise better control. Alexander and colleagues (1989) conducted a study of the effectiveness of different types of interventions on 81 older adults residing in various institutional settings. They randomly assigned these individuals to one of four conditions: meditation, mindfulness training, relaxation, and a control group. The first two groups showed significant increases not only in mental health, but also in cardiovascular and cognitive function. After 3 years, all members of the meditation group and 87% of the mindfulness groups were still alive, compared to only about two-thirds of the control group. This accords with the growing evidence of the beneficial effect of meditation practice on cardiovascular health (Seeman, Dubin, & Seeman, 2003). More work is needed in older samples, especially given that older adults are the most likely users of complementary and alternative medicine, including prayer (Barnes et al., 2004).

B. Stress and Coping

Older adults are more vulnerable to physical stressors for a number of reasons (Aldwin & Gilmer, 2004). Age-related changes in the ability to regulate body temperature render elders more vulnerable to both heat and cold stress, as witnessed by recent mass fatalities of older adults during heat waves in both Europe and the United States. In later life, immune systems typically do not respond as well to new challenges as in younger years (Lutgendorf & Costanzo, 2003). As noted earlier, age-related decreases in heart rate regulation and disease-related changes in cardiovascular function may result in greater physiological strain on the heart in later life. At the cellular level, age-related decline in the ability to respond to stress is considered to be a major source of cellular senescence.

However, it is less clear whether older adults are more vulnerable to psychosocial stressors. Studies of common stressors in late life, such as caregiving, show that the immune systems of older adults are more vulnerable to stress, especially among those who are also depressed (Kiecolt-Glaser et al., 2002; Vitaliano, 1995). Other studies have shown that older adults are less vulnerable than middle-aged adults to some types of stressors. For example, Johnson and co-workers (2000) showed that spousal bereavement was associated with higher risks of mortality among middle-aged rather than older adults and that these effects could not be attributed solely to dyadic congruence in health behavior habits.

Further, in most studies of population trauma, such as the September 11 attacks, older adults typically appraised these as less stressful than younger adults (Park, Aldwin, Snyder, & Fenster, 2005). Similarly, older adults tend to report fewer problems, especially hassles (Aldwin & Levenson, 2001), which is counterintuitive, given the increased problems with chronic illness and disability in later life. However, they are more likely to report certain types of problems, such as bereavement and ill health of significant others. Aldwin et al. (1996) speculated that this decline in reported stress reflects the fact that there may be a shift from acute to chronic stress in later life, i.e., younger adults are more likely to experience stress related to rolechanges such as marriage, parenthood, and divorce, as well as losing a job. Older adults are more likely to be coping with health problems, which are usually chronic in nature and thus form part of the "background" of daily existence and only become "problems" when there is a flare-up or an acute episode. However, this ability to distance oneself from stress, in part by taking a broader perspective, may be a protective mechanism to avoid feeling distressed.

Hamarat et al. (2001) found that stress is a stronger predictor of life satisfaction in younger adults, whereas coping resources are better predictors of well-being in middle and later adulthood. Whether and how coping strategies change with age is a matter of some debate. Aldwin et al. (1996) found that older adults were just as effective copers as were adults in midlife (barring major cognitive impairments), as did Whitty (2003). However, older adults tend to use fewer coping strategies, which can be interpreted as supporting Baltes' (1997) theory of energy conservation in later life (see also Hobfoll, 2001).

In a qualitative study of the old–old in San Francisco, Johnson and Barer (1993) found that older adults maintained themselves in the community despite significant levels of disability by using a variety of management strategies and distancing techniques. They made extensive use of assistive devices, such as canes and walkers, and often arranged the furniture in their homes to allow them to brace themselves against falls while walking. To navigate the environment, they would spend much time in anticipatory coping, such as plotting out routes to avoid making left-hand turns. They also relied heavily on routinization of daily activities to decrease potential problems and

stress. In a quantitative investigation, Rothermund and Brandstadter (2003) argued that compensatory strategies, which include problem-focused attempts to correct for deficiencies, increase up until about age 70 and then accommodative strategies (acceptance) become primary.

In Johnson and Barer's (1993) study, older adults used a variety of emotion-focused strategies to deal with their health problems, such as positive comparisons. Even the most disabled of their respondents could point to someone who was either more disabled or had a different (and presumably) worse impairment. They dissociated their identities from their failing bodies and also made extensive use of denial and minimization. As one highly impaired woman said, "What can I say, I've had bypass surgery, I now have shingles, I'm isolated and lonely, I'm losing my strength and my confidence in myself. But glory to God, I'm feeling well" (Johnson & Barer, 1993, p. 75).

However, too much reliance on avoidant coping is a predictor of alcohol abuse in later life (Moos et al., 2004), but it is important to differentiate between avoidant coping and other types of emotion-focused coping (Stanton et al., 2000). Carstensen and colleagues (Chapter 15) argued that the social selectivity processes seen in later life can also be extended to coping in that individuals may focus more on regulating their emotional responses. Older adults may use dyadic coping strategies when dealing with memory problems (Dixon,1999), and Lawrence and Schigelone (2002) suggested that older adults living in communal situations may use more reciprocal assistance as a way of compensating for declines in individual resources.

However, there are relatively few studies of coping strategies and biomedical health outcomes among older adults.

While Vitaliano, Russo, and Niaura (1995) did find that avoidant coping was associated with higher cholesterol levels among caregivers, Yancura (2004) found that positive coping strategies were associated with higher high-density lipoprotein (HDL) levels in the NAS men. The physiological impact of stress and immune functioning among the elderly has been most studied in the context of caregiving, especially caregiving for Alzheimer's patients, showing that caregiving stress not only suppresses immune functioning during the process, but that the immune suppression lasts for up to a year (Kiecolt-Glaser et al., 2002; Patterson & Grant, 2003).

The relationships among age, coping, and immune function can be complex. Stowell, Kiecolt-Glaser, and Glaser (2001) found an interaction between active and avoidant coping and stress levels on immune cell proliferative responses. Under high stress, active coping was associated with higher proliferative levels, but under low stress, avoidant coping was associated with better immune performance, bolstering the argument given earlier that older adults are physiologically better off seeking to avoid stressors when possible. Some intriguing data by Vaillant (2002) also suggest that the use of "mature" defenses may also be associated with better longevity in later life. However, much work is still needed to fully understanding the pathways between coping and health, especially in later life (Aldwin & Park, 2004).

C. Religiousness and Spirituality

Religiousness and spirituality appear to be another factor for the health of the elderly that exerts complex effects (see Krause Chapter 22). Religiousness is highly prevalent in the United States and exerts a strong influence on both the social institutions and the personal lives of most Americans (Koenig, 2000). Nationwide polls demonstrate Americans' strongly held beliefs and widely held practices. For example, Gallup polls show that 96% of Americans believe in God or a universal spirit, 90% pray, 85% say religion is very or fairly important to them, and 41% attend religious services weekly or more often (Gallup Organization, 2004).

It has been suggested that religious and spiritual resources may become more salient and more closely linked to health in the elderly as health problems increase and other resources diminish. Although religious attendance falls off in later life due to health and mobility problems, levels of religiousness are typically higher in older people than in younger people (e.g., Pargament, 1997). For example, 73% of adults aged 65 and older say religion is very important to them compared to only 48% of 18 to 29 year olds (Gallup Organization, 2004).

The higher levels of religiousness of older individuals reflect a number of developmental influences. Clearly cohort effects are involved (Koenig, Kvale, & Ferrel, 1988), but there is also evidence that people become more religious or spiritual as they age (see Krause Chapter 22). To the extent that religiousness has salutary direct or indirect effects on health, the higher levels of religiousness observed among the elderly may also reflect survival effects. However, longitudinal data on multiple cohorts suggest that, regardless of cohort, people typically become more religious or spiritual as they age (Argue, Johnson, & White, 1999; Wink & Dillon, 2002), although not everyone experiences such increases (Ingersoll-Dayton, Krause, & Morgan, 2002).

In recent years, researchers have documented links between various dimensions of religiousness and lower rates of cancer, heart disease, alcoholism, and mental illness, as well as lower blood pressure, higher health-related quality of life, and higher levels of health behaviors (see George et al., 2002). The strongest findings, emerging from a number of large-scale epidemiological studies, are that more frequent attendance at religious services is related to lower mortality rates (Thoresen & Harris, 2002). Even when controlling for a variety of potential covariates, such as baseline health, social support, and health behaviors, attendance remains strongly and prospectively related to lower mortality (Oman et al., 2002). Religious attendance is associated with lower rates of a variety of illnesss, including alcoholism, cardiovascular disease, hypertension, and myocardial infarction (Miller & Thoresen, 2003).

The few studies that have examined links between other dimensions of religion and health have yielded mixed findings. In some studies, religious coping with illness was related to better recovery, but a number of other studies yielded null findings (see Powell et al., 2003). Many of these studies are difficult to interpret given the various ways in which both religion and health outcomes have been defined and the problems of such small, selective samples. In addition, it is clear that not all aspects of religion are helpful. Several studies have found aspects of religion that adversely affect mortality in elderly ill patients. One prospective cohort study of elderly inpatients found that experiencing religious struggle in the hospital (e.g., feeling punished or abandoned by God) increased mortality rates by 19–28% at the 2-year follow-up, even after adjusting for a variety of demographic, mental health, and physical health variables (Pargament et al., 2001).

While few studies have specifically examined the issue of religion and health in the context of aging, many studies of religion have been conducted with primarily older individuals. For example, results of a study of open-heart surgery patients (primarily older adults) found that perceiving strength and comfort from religion was related to a decreased risk of dying, controlling for age, previous history of cardiac surgery, and impairment in presurgery activities of daily living (Oxman, Freeman, & Manheimer, 1995). Some have suggested that religion may be particularly important in the lives and health of older individuals (e.g., Thorson, 2000) because of the higher levels of both religiousness and health problems that occur at later ages. To date, this remains an open question (for a review, see Park, 2005).

IV. What Is Optimal Aging?

From a life span developmental viewpoint, Rowe and Kahn (1997) appropriately defined healthy aging in terms of multiple dimensions: as absence of disease and good physical function, intact cognition, and an active engagement with life. Their model is hierarchical in that good physical health is considered to be primary to good cognitive and maintenance of activities of daily living (ADLs), which are, in turn, necessary for high levels of social integration and "productive" behavior. Using a similar definition, Vaillant (2002) examined lifelong predictors of successful aging. While he found no direct link between early childhood adversity and longevity in this smaller sample, he did find an indirect effect: stressful childhood environments affected mental health in midlife, which in turn was related to successful aging.

However, there may be problems with these hierarchical definitions of successful aging. Using Rowe and Kahn's (1997) criteria, Strawbridge et al. (2002) identified those who could be said to exhibit successful aging and their less successful compatriots in the Alameda County Population Study. They also asked individuals to indicate whether they felt themselves to be aging successfully and found considerable discrepancies between investigator-rated vs. self-rated success. For example, a third of individuals who had chronic physical illnesses rated themselves as aging successfully, whereas a third of those who were aging successfully by "objective" criteria did not consider themselves successful. Lawton (1999) argued that these definitions of successful aging rely too heavily on maintenance of typical functioning in midlife and ignore what may be qualitative shifts in late life in the valuation of life and its meaning. From a life span developmental perspective, what is missing from these definitions of successful aging is that losses are often balanced by gains. Standard definitions of successful aging fail to address what is gained in late life.

Using data from the Nun Study, Snowdon (2001) found that his "successful agers" were characterized by positive psychological characteristics, despite sometimes being profoundly physically disabled. These characteristics included happiness, intellectual curiosity, gratitude, deep spirituality, and a strong sense of community. Note that a sense of community may not require very active social integration, but would recognize that there may be social selectivity in late life (see Chapter 15), requiring a different allocation of social resources.

While not all elders become more religious, Vaillant (2002) found a deepening sense of spirituality, which he described as almost zen-like. Tornstam (1997) also observed that a certain amount of disengagement and quiet contemplation of life reflects a process of gerotranscendence (as opposed to disengagement), leading to alienation (Levenson et al., 2005). Gerotranscendence involves a decreasing reliance on external definitions of the self, a

deepening spirituality, and a greater sense of intergenerational continuity. From a life span developmental perspective, what is gained in late life as a counterbalance to losses may be wisdom. Baltes and Staudinger (2000) found little increase or even decreases in wisdom in late life, which may reflect a definition that focuses on social competence. Alternative views of wisdom that focus on characterological change (Wink & Dillon, 2000) or self-transcendence (Levenson et al., 2005) may be more likely to increase in late life—at least in some individuals.

Levenson et al. (2001) argued that the self-transcendence aspect of wisdom develops from coping with loss, which may force detachment from previous sources of identity. For example, the loss of social roles through retirement or bereavement or the loss of youthful good looks or physical capacity may force change in one's identity. A developmental process may result as individuals struggle to understand who they are without these external props. As in Tornstam's model, the self is no longer defined in terms of externals, and thus may become freer of external constraints and able to focus more on life's fundamentals. Empirically, Levenson et al. (2005) found correlations of self-transcendence with emotional stability and spirituality, which this review has suggested are associated with better health in later life.

From a life span developmental perspective, a definition of successful aging that focuses on only one model may be too limited. Baltes (1996) suggested that the term "optimal aging" may be more appropriate than "successful aging," in that individuals may choose to optimize different facets of their lives, depending on their current goal structures (Brandstadter & Rothermund, 2003). Optimal aging allows one to maximize whatever health one has by having the good judgment to avoid agents that accelerate the aging process and promoting those that retard it. Nonetheless, a certain level of detachment and wisdom may be necessary to learn to accept whatever level of illness and disability one has, thereby preserving mental health and as much social functioning as possible within the confines of disability. Thus, a life span developmental perspective affords a somewhat different image of optimal aging and suggests new ways of investigating this phenomenon, which focus on individual differences and plasticity in the aging process.

Acknowledgments

Preparation of this chapter was supported in part by grants from the National Institute on Aging (AG18436, to Daniel Mroczek; Avron Spiro, subcontract PI) and by a Veterans Affairs Merit Review from the Clinical Sciences Research and Development Program (to Avron Spiro). Correspondence should be addressed to Carolyn M. Aldwin, Chair, Deptartment of Human Development and Family Sciences, Oregon State University, 324 Milam Hall, Corvallis, OR 97331. Carolyn.Aldwin@oregonstate.edu.

References

Adler, N. E., & Snibbe, A. C. (2003). The role of psychosocial processes in explaining the gradient between SES and health. *Current Directions in Psychological Science, 12,* 119–123.

Aldwin, C. M. (1999). *Stress, coping, and development: An integrative approach.* New York: Guilford.

Aldwin, C. M., & Gilmer, D. F. (Eds.) (2004). *Health, illness, and optimal aging: Biological and psychosocial perspectives.* Thousand Oaks, CA: Sage.

Aldwin, C. M., & Levenson, M. R. (2001). Stress, coping, and health at mid-life: A developmental perspective. In M. E. Lachman (Ed.), *The handbook of midlife development* (pp. 188–214). New York: Wiley.

Aldwin, C. M., Levenson, M. R., & Gilmer, D. F. (2004). Interface between mental and physical health. In C. M., Aldwin, & D. F. Gilmer (Eds.), *Health, illness, and optimal aging: Biological and psychosocial perspectives* (pp. 227–253). Thousand Oaks, CA: Sage.

Aldwin, C. M., & Park, C. L. (2004). Coping and physical health: An overview. *Psychology and Health: Special Issue, Coping and Physical Health, 19,* 277–282.

Aldwin, C. M., Sutton, K. J., Chiara, G., & Spiro, A., III (1996). Age differences in stress, coping, and appraisal: Findings from the Normative Aging Study. *Journals of Gerontology: Psychological Sciences, 51B,* P179.

Aldwin, C. M., Spiro, A., III, Levenson, M. R., & Cupertino, A. P. (2001). Longitudinal findings from the Normative Aging Study. III. Personality, individual health trajectories, and mortality. *Psychology and Aging, 16,* 450–465.

Aldwin, C. M., & Yancura, L. A. (2004). Coping and health: A comparison of the stress and trauma literatures. In P. P. Schnurr & B. L. Green (Eds.), *Physical health consequences of exposure to extreme stress* (pp. 99–126). Washington, DC: American Psychological Association.

Alexander, C. N., Langer, E. J., Newman, R. I., Chandler, H. M., & Davies, J. (1989). Transcendental meditation, mindfulness, and longevity: An experimental study with the elderly. *Journal of Personality & Social Psychology, 57,* 950–964.

Antonovsky, A. (1987). *Unravelling the mystery of health: How people manage stress and stay well.* San Francisco: Jossey-Bass.

Appels, A., Bar, F. W., Bar. J., Bruggeman, C., & de Baets, M. (2000). Inflammation, depressive symptomatology, and coronary artery disease. *Psychosomatic Medicine, 62,* 601–605.

Argue, A., Johnson, D. R., & White, L. K. 1999). Age and religiosity: Evidence from a three-wave panel analysis. *Journal for the Scientific Study of Religion, 38,* 423–435.

Baltes, M. M. (1996). *The many faces of dependency in old age*. New York: Cambridge University Press.

Baltes, P. B. (1987). Theoretical propositions of life-span developmental psychology: On the dynamics between growth and decline. *Developmental Psychology, 24,* 611–626.

Baltes, P. B., & Baltes, M. M. (Eds.) (1990). *Successful aging: Perspectives from the behavioral sciences*. Cambridge, England: Cambridge University Press.

Baltes, P. B., & Staudinger, U. (2000). Wisdom: A metaheuristic (pragmatic) to orchestrate mind and virtue towards excellence. *American Psychologist, 55,* 122–136.

Barnes, P. M., Powell-Grinerm E., McFann, K., & Nahin, R. L. (2004). Complementary and alternative medicine use among adults: United States, 2002. *Advance Data from Vital and Health Statistics, No. 343,* Centers for Disease Control. http://www.cdc.gov/nchs/data/ad/ad343.pdf.

Blazer, D. G., Hybels, C. F., & Pieper, C. F. (2001). The association of depression and mortality in elderly persons: A case for multiple, independent pathways. *Journals of Gerontology: Medical Sciences, 65A,* M505–M509.

Bruunsgaard, H., & Pedersen, B. K. (2000). Special feature for the Olympics: Effects of exercise on the immune system: Effects of exercise on the immune system in the elderly population. *Immunology & Cell Biology, 78,* 523–531.

Centers for Disease Control (2004). *Health, United States, 2004*. National Center for Health Statistics, http://www.cdc.gov/nchs/hus.htm.

DeVellis, B. M., & DeVellis, R. F. (2001). Self-efficacy and health. In A. Baum, T. A. Revenson, & J. E. Singer (Eds.), *Handbook of health psychology* (pp. 235–248). Mahwayh, NJ: Lawrence Erlbaum Associates.

Dixon, R. A. (1999). Exploring cognition in interactive situations: The aging of $N+1$ minds. In T. M. Hess & F. Blanchard-Fields (Eds.), *Social cognition and aging* (pp. 267–290). San Diego, CA: Academic Press.

Durazo-Arvizu, R., Cooper, R., Luke, A., Prewitt, T., Liao, Y., & McGee, D. (1997). Relative weight and mortality in U.S.

blacks and whites: Findings from representative national population samples. *Annals of Epidemiology, 7,* 383–395.

Eaker, E. D., Pinsky, J., & Castelli, W. P. (1992). Myocardial infarction and coronary death among women: Psychosocial predictors from a 20-year follow-up of women in the Framingham Study. *American Journal of Epidemiology, 135,* 854–864.

Evans, R. I. (2001). Social influences in etiology and prevention of smoking and other health threatening behaviors in children and adolescents. In A. Baum, T. A. Revenson, & J. E. Singer (Eds.), *Handbook of health psychology* (pp. 459–468). Mahwah, NJ: Lawrence Erlbaum Associates.

Fair, J. M. (2003). Cardiovascular risk factor modification: is it effective in older adults? *Journal of Cardiovascular Nursing, 18,* 161–168.

Fiore, M. (2000). A clinical practice guideline for treating tobacco use and dependence: A US Public Health Service Report. *Journal of the American Medical Association, 283,* 3244–3254.

Frankenhaeuser, M. (1978). *Coping with job stress: A psychobiological approach*. Stockholm, Sweden: University of Stockholm.

Friedman, H. S. (2000). Long-term relations of personality and health: Dynamism, mechanisms, tropisms. *Journal of Personality, 68,* 1089–1107.

Frytak, J. R., Kane, R. A., Finch, M. D., Kane, R. L., & Maude-Griffin, R. (2001). Outcome trajectories for assisted living and nursing facility residents in Oregon. *Health Services Research, 36,* 91–111.

George, L., Ellison, C., & Larson, D. (2002). Explaining the relationships between religious involvement and health. *Psychological Inquiry, 13,*190–200.

Giltay, E. J., Geleijnse, J. M., Zitman, F. G., Hoekstra, T., & Schouten, E. G. (2004). Dispositional optimism and all-cause and cardiovascular mortality in a prospective cohort of elderly Dutch men and women. *Archives of General Psychiatry, 61,* 1126–1135

Gorman, J. M., & Sloan, R. P. (2000). Heart rate variability in depression and anxiety disorders. *American Heart Journal, 140*(4 Suppl. 4), 77–83.

Greenlee, R. T., Murray, T., Bolden, S., & Wingo, P. A. (2000). *Cancer statistics, 2000. CA, A Cancer Journal for Clinicians, 50,* 7–33.

Guyton, A. C., & Hall, J. E. (1996). *Textbook of medical physiology* (9th ed.). Philadelphia: Saunders.

Hamarat, E., Thompson, D., Zabrucky, K. M., Steele, D., Matheny, K. B., & Aysan, F. (2001). Perceived stress and coping resources availability as predictors of life satisfaction in young, middle-aged, and older adults. *Experimental Aging Research, 27,* 181–196.

Hausdorff, J. M., Levy, B. R., & Wei, J. Y. (1999). The power of ageism on physical function of older persons: reversibility of age-related gait changes. *Journal of the American Geriatrics Society, 47,* 1346–1349.

Hayward, C. (1995). Psychiatric illness and cardiovascular disease risk. *Epidemiological Review, 17,* 129–138.

Hobfoll, S. E. (2001). The influence of culture, community, and the nested-self in the stress process: Advancing conservation of resources theory. *Applied Psychology: An International Review, 50,* 337–370.

Ingersoll-Dayton, B., Krause, N., & Morgan, D. (2002). Religious trajectories and transitions over the life course. *International Journal of Aging and Human Development, 55,* 51–70.

Johnson, C., & Barer, B. M. (1993). Coping and a sense of control among the oldest old. *Journal of Aging Studies, 7,* 67–80.

Johnson, J. E. (1996). Sleep problems and self-care in very old rural women. *Geriatric Nursing, 17,* 72–74.

Johnson, N. J., Backlund, E., Sorlie, P. D., & Loveless, C. A. (2000). Marital status and mortality: The National Longitudinal Mortality Study. *Annals of Epidemiology, 10,* 224–238.

Kawachi, I., Sparrow, D., Vokonas, P. S., & Weiss, S. T. (1994). Symptoms of anxiety and risk of coronary heart disease: The Normative Aging Study. *Circulation, 90,* 2225–2229.

Keysor, J. J., & Jette, A. M. (2001). Have we oversold the benefit of late-life exercise? *Journals of Gerontology A: Biological Sciences & Medical Sciences, 56,* M412–M423.

Kiecolt-Glaser, J. R., McGuire, L., Robles, T. F., & Glaser, R. (2002). Psychoneuroimmunology: Psychological influences on immune function and health. *Journal of Consulting and Clinical Psychology, 70,* 537–547.

Kinsella, K., & Velkoff, V. A. (2001). *An aging world: 2001* (U. S. Census Bureau, Series P95-01-1). Washington, DC: Government Printing Office.

Knowler, W. C., Barrett-Connor, E,. Fowler, S. E, Hamman, R. F., Lachin, J. M., Walker, E. A., & Nathan, D. M. (2002). Reduction in the incidence of type 2 diabetes with lifestyle intervention or metformin. *New England Journal of Medicine, 346,* 393–403.

Koenig, H. G. (2000). Religion, well-being, and health in the elderly: The scientific evidence for an association. In J. A. Thorson (Ed.), *Perspectives on spiritual well-being and aging* (pp. 84–97). Springfield, IL: Charles C. Thomas.

Koenig, H. G., Kvale, J. N., & Ferrel, C. (1988). Religion and well-being in later life. *The Gerontologist, 28,* 18–28.

Kohut, M. L., Cooper, M. M., Nickolaus, M. S., Russell, D.R., Cunnick, J. E. (2002). Exercise and psychosocial factors modulate immunity to influenza vaccine in elderly individuals. *Journals of Gerontology: Series A: Biological Sciences & Medical Sciences, 57A,* M557–M562.

Kostka, T., Berthouze, S. E., Lacour, J., & Bonnefoy, M. (2000). The symptomatology of upper respiratory tract infections and exercise in elderly people. *Medicine and Science in Sports and Exercise, 32,* 46–51.

Krantz, D. S., & McCeney, M. K. (2002). Effects of psychological and social factors on organic disease: A critical assessment of research on coronary heart disease. *Annual Review of Psychology, 53,* 341–369.

Krause, N., & Shaw, B. A. (2000). Role-specific feelings of control and mortality. *Psychology of Aging, 15,* 617–26.

Kubzansky, L. D., Sparrow, D., Vokonas, P., & Kawachi, I. (2001). Is the glass half empty or half full? A prospective study of optimism and coronary heart disease in the Normative Aging Study. *Psychosomatic Medicine, 63,* 910–916.

Kuh, D., & Ben-Shlomo, Y. (Eds.) (2004). *A life course approach to chronic disease epidemiology* (2nd ed.). New York: Oxford University Press.

Ladwig, K. H., Kieser, M., & Konigh, J. (1991). Affective diseases and survival after acute myocardial infarction. *European Health Journal, 12,* 959–964.

Langer, E. J. (1989). *Mindfulness.* Reading, MA: Addison-Wesley.

Lawrence, A. R., & Schigelone, A. R. S. (2002). Reciprocity beyond dyadic relationships: Aging-related communal coping. *Research on Aging Special, Community context and aging, 24*(6), 684–704.

Lawton, M. P. (1999). Quality of life in chronic illness. *Gerontology, 45,* 181–183.

Lemke, S., & Moos, R. H. (2003). Treatment and outcomes of older patients with alcohol use disorders in community residential programs. *Journal of Studies on Alcohol, 64,* 219–226.

Lésperance, F., Frasure-Smith, N., Talajic, M., & Bourassa, M. G. (2002). Five-year risk of cardiac mortality in relation to initial severity and one-year changes in depression symptoms after myocardial infarction. *Circulation, 105,* 1049–1053.

Levenson, M. R., Aldwin, C. M., & Cupertino, A. P. (2001). Transcending the self: Towards a liberative model of adult development. In A. L. Neri (Ed), *Maturidade & Velhice: Um enfoque multidisciplinar* (pp. 99–116). Sao Paulo, BR: Papirus.

Levenson, M. R., Aldwin, C. M., & Spiro, A., III (1998). Age, cohort and period effects on alcohol consumption and problem drinking: Findings from the Normative Aging Study. *Journal of Studies on Alcohol, 59,* 712–722.

Levenson, M. R., Jennings, P. A., Aldwin, C. M., & Shiraishi, R. W. (2005). Self-transcendence, conceptualization and measurement. *International Journal of Aging & Human Development, 60,* 127–143.

Light, K. C., Kothandapani, R. V., & Allen, M. T. (1998). Enhanced cardiovascular and catecholamine responses in women with depressive symptoms. *International Journal of Psychophysiology, 28,*157–166.

Lutgendorf, S. K., & Costanzo, E. S. (2003). Psychoneuroimmunology and health psychology: An integrative model. *Brain, Behavior & Immunity, 17(4),* 225–232.

Martin, G. A. (1997). The genetics of aging. *Hospital Practice, 32,* 47–55.

Martin, L. R., Friedman, H. S., & Tucker, J. S. (2002). A life course perspective on childhood cheerfulness and its relation to mortality risk. *Personality & Social Psychology Bulletin, 28,* 1155–1165.

McGee, R., Williams, S., & Elwood, M. (1994). Depression and the development of cancer: A meta-analysis. *Social Science & Medicine, 38,* 187–192.

Miller, W. R., & Thoresen, C. E. (2003). Spirituality, religion, and health: An emerging research field. *American Psychologist, 58,* 24–35.

Miller, T. D., Smith, T. W., Turner, C. W., Guijarro, M. L., & Hallet, A. J. (1996). A meta-analytic review of research on hostility and physical health. *Psychological Bulletin, 119,* 322–348.

Mokdad, A. H., Markes, J. S., Stroup, D. F., & Gerlerding, J. L. (2004). Actual cases of death in the United States, 2000. *Journal of the American Medical Assn., 291,* 1238–1245.

Moos, R. H., Schutte, K., Brennan, P., & Moos, B. S. (2004). Ten-year patterns of alcohol consumption and drinking problems among older women and men. *Addiction, 99,* 829–838.

Niaura, R., Banks, S. M., Ward, K. D., Stoney, C. M., Spiro, A., III, Aldwin, C. M., Landsberg, M.D., & Weiss, S. T. (2000). Hostility and the metabolic syndrome in older males: The Normative Aging Study. *Psychosomatic Medicine, 62,* 7–16.

Oman, D., Kurata, J. H., Strawbridge, W. J., & Cohen, R. D. (2002). Religious attendance and cause of death over 31 years. *International Journal of Psychiatry in Medicine, 32,* 69–89.

Ouellette, S. C., & DiPlacido, J. (2001). Personality's role in the protection and enhancement of health: Where the research has been, where it is stuck, how it might move. In A. Baum, T. A. Revenson, & J. E. Singer (Eds.), *Handbook of health psychology* (pp. 175–194). New York: Guilford.

Oxman, T. E., Freeman, D. H., Jr., & Manheimer, E. D. (1995). Lack of social participation or religious strength and comfort as risk factors for death after cardiac surgery in the elderly. *Psychosomatic Medicine, 57,* 5–15.

Palmer, R. M. (1997). Acute hospital care. In C. K. Cassel, H. J. Cohen, E. B. Larosn, D. E.

Meier, N. M. Resnick, L. A. Rubvenstein, & L. B. Sorensen (Eds.), *Geriatric Medicine* (3rd ed., pp. 119–129). New York: Springer-Verlag.

Pargament, K. I. (1997). *The psychology of religion and coping: Theory, research, practice*. New York: Guilford.

Pargament, K. I., Koenig, H. G., & Tarakeshwar, N. (2001). Religious struggle as a predictor of mortality among medically ill elderly patients: A 2-year longitudinal study. *Archives of Internal Medicine, 61*, 1881–1885.

Park, C. L. (in press). Religious and spiritual issues in health and aging. In C. M. Aldwin, C. L. Park, & A. Spiro (Eds.), *Handbook of health psychology and aging*. New York: Guilford.

Park, C. L., Aldwin, C. M., Snyder, L., & Fenster, J. R. (2005). Coping with September 11: Uncontrollable stress, PTSD, and post-traumatic growth. Submitted for publication.

Patterson, T. L., & Grant, I. (2003). Interventions for caregiving in dementia: Physical outcomes. *Current Opinion in Psychiatry, 16*, 629–633.

Peterson, C. (1988). Explanatory style as a risk factor for illness. *Cognitive Therapy and Research, 12*, 117–130.

Powell, L. H., Shahabi, L., & Thoresen, C. E. (2003). Religion and spirituality: Linkages to physical health. *American Psychologist, 58*, 36–52.

Power, C., & Parsons, T. (2003). Overweight and obesity from a life course perspective. In D. Kuh & R. Hardy (Eds.), *A life course approach to women's health* (pp. 304–28). New York: Oxford University Press.

Puggaard, L., Larsen, J. B., Stovring, H., & Jeune, B. (2000). Maximal oxygen uptake, muscle strength and walking speed in 85-year-old women: Effects of increased physical activity. *Aging (Milano), 12*, 180–189.

Pulska, T., Pahkala, K., Laippala, P., & Kivelä, S.-L. (2000). Depressive symptoms predicting six-year mortality in depressed elderly Finns. *International Journal of Geriatric Psychiatry, 15*, 940–946.

Review Panel on Coronary-Prone Behavior and Coronary Heart Disease (1978). Coronary-prone behavior and coronary heart disease: A critical review. *Circulation, 65*, 1199–1215.

Rothermund, K., & Brandstädter, J. (2003). Coping with deficits and losses in later life: From compensatory action to accommodation. *Psychology & Aging, 18*(4), 896–905.

Rowe, J. W., & Kahn, R. L. (1997). Successful aging. *The Gerontologist, 37*, 433–440.

Schofield, P., Ball, D. Smith, J. G., Borland, R., O'Brien, P., Davis, S., Olver, I., Ryan, G., & Joseph, D. (2004). Optimism and survival in lung carcinoma patients. *Cancer, 100*, 1276–1282.

Schulz, R., Bookwala, J., Knapp, J. E., Scheier, M., & Williamson, G. M. (1996). Pessimism, age, and cancer mortality. *Psychology & Aging, 11*, 304–309.

Seeman, T. E., Dubin, L. F., & Seeman, M. (2003). Religiosity/spirituality and health: A critical review of the evidence for biological pathways. *American Psychologist, 58*, 53–63.

Segerstrom, S. C. (2001). Optimism, goal conflict, and stressor-related immune change. *Journal of Behavioral Medicine, 24*(5), 441–467.

Segerstrom, S. C., Castañeda, J. O., & Spencer, T. E. (2003). Optimism effects on cellular immunity: Testing the affective and persistence models. *Personality & Individual Differences, 35*(7), 1615–1624.

Sesso, H. D., Kawachi, I., Vokonas, P. S., & Sparrow, D. (1998). Depression and the risk of coronary heart disease in the Normative Aging Study. *American Journal of Cardiology, 82*, 851–856.

Smith, T. W., & Spiro, A. III. (2002). Personality, health, and aging: Prolegomenon for the next generation. *Journal of Research in Personality, 36*, 363–394. [Erratum, p. 661]

Snowdon, D. A. (2001). *Aging with grace: What the Nun Study teaches us about leading longer, healthier, and more meaningful lives*. New York: Bantam.

Spiro, A., III (2001). Health in midlife: Toward a life span view. In M. E. Lachman (Ed.), *Handbook of midlife development* (pp. 156–187). New York: Wiley.

Spiro, A., III, Aldwin, C. M., Ward, K. D., & Mroczek, D. K. (1995). Personality and the incidence of hypertension among older men: Longitudinal findings from the Normative Aging Study. *Health Psychology,* *14,* 563–569.

Stanton, A. L., Kirk, S. B., Cameron, C. L., & Danoff-Burg, S. (2000). Coping through emotional approach: Scale construction and validation. *Journal of Personality &* *Social Psychology, 78(6),* 1150–1169.

Stowell, J. R., Kiecolt-Glaser, J. K., & Glaser, R. (2001). Perceived stress and cellular immunity: When coping counts. *Journal of* *Behavioral Medicine, 24(4),* 323–339.

Strawbridge, W. J., Wallhagen, M. I., & Cohen, R. D. (2002). Successful aging and well-being: Self-report compared with Rowe and Kahn. *Gerontologist, 42,* 727–733.

Surgeon General (1990), *Health benefits of* *quitting smoking.* USDHHS, CDC. http://profiles.nlm.nih.gov/NN/B/B/C/T/_/nnbbct.pdf.

Surgeon General (2004). *The health conse-* *quences of smoking.* USDHHS, CDC. http://www.cdc.gov/tobacco/sgr/sgr_2004/pdf/).

Surtees, P., Wainwright, N., Luben, R., Khaw, K. T., & Day, N. (2003). Sense of coherence and mortality in men and women in the EPIC-Norfolk United Kingdom prospective cohort study. *American Journal of Epi-* *demiology, 158,* 1202–1209.

Taaffe, D. R., Pruitt, L., Pyka, G., Guido, D., & Marcus, R. (1996). Comparative effects of high- and low-intensity resistance training on thigh muscle strength, fiber area, and tissue composition in elderly women. *Clin-* *ical Physiology, 16,* 381–392.

Tennant, C., & McLean, L. (2001). The impact of emotions on coronary heart disease risk. *Journal of Cardiovascular Risk, 8,* 175–183.

The Gallup Organization. http://www.gallup.com/poll/focus/sr040302.asp

Thoreson, C. E., & Harris, A. H. S. (2002). Spirituality and health: What's the evidence and what's needed? *Annals of Behavioral* *Medicine, 24,* 3–13.

Thorson, J. A. (Ed.) (2000). *Perspectives on* *spiritual well-being and aging.* Springfield, IL: Charles C. Thomas.

Tornstam, L. (1997). Gerotranscendence: The contemplative dimension of aging. *Journal* *of Aging Studies, 11,* 143–154.

Tully, C. L., & Snowdon, D. A. (1995). Weight change and physical function in older women: Findings from the Nun Study. *Journal of the American Geriatric Society,* *43,* 1394–1397.

Vaillant, G. E. (2002). *Aging well: Surprising* *guideposts to a happier life.* Boston: Little, Brown.

Vitaliano, P. P., Russo, J., & Niaura, R. (1995). Plasma lipids and their relationships with psychosocial factors in older adults. *Journals of Gerontology: Series B: Psycho-* *logical Sciences & Social Sciences, 50(1),* P18–P24.

Whitty, M. T. (2003). Coping and defending: Age differences in maturity of defense mechanisms and coping strategies. *Aging* *& Mental Health, 7(2),* 123–132.

Williams, R. B. (2000). Psychological factors, health, and disease: The impact of aging and the life cycle. In S. B. Manuck, R. Jennings, B. S. Rabin, & A. Baum (Eds.), *Behavior, health, and aging* (pp. 135–151). Mahwah, NJ: Lawrence Erlbaum.

Wilhelm, K., Arnold, K., Nyven, H., & Richmond, R. (2004). Grey lungs and blue moods: Smoking cessation in the context of lifetime depression history. *Australian and New Zealand Journal of* *Psychiatry, 38,* 896–905.

World Health Organization (1948). The constitution of the World Health Organization. *WHO Chronicle, 1,* 21.

Wink, P., & Dillon, M. (2002). Spiritual development across the adult life course: Findings from a longitudinal study. *Journal* *of Adult Development, 9,* 79–94.

Yancura, L. A. (2004). How does coping get into the body? An examination of stress, coping, affect, and the metabolic syndrome in a sample of older men. Unpublished doctoral dissertation, University of California, Davis.

Six

Environmental Gerontology: Progress in the Post-Lawton Era

Rick J. Scheidt and Paul G. Windley

I. Introduction

A 75-year-old Swedish woman decides to cancel a local shopping trip after considering the problems posed for her by heavy traffic, poor sidewalks, and a user-unfriendly bus. An elderly married couple deals with the stresses involved in a move from their lifelong Los Angeles home to an assisted-living community located several miles away. Several relatively healthy Kansas elders with deep attachments to their homes and to their small rural town struggle to age in place in the face of seriously dwindling community supports and the steady deterioration of the town's physical and service infrastructure.

Such later-life scenarios are numerous, illustrating the increased demands often placed on elders by shifts in their personal resources and changes in their near and far environments. Environmental gerontology (also known as the study of *environment–aging* relations) is a loose confederation of disciplines (e.g., psychologists, sociologists, allied health professionals, architects, community planners,

social policy makers) devoted to understanding the behavioral and psychological implications of *encounters between elders and their environments*. The common hope is that this understanding may aid in the development of preventative and ameliorative interventions targeting both individual and environmental factors to affect a better "fit" between individuals and their environments, thus enhancing their quality of life.

The purpose of this chapter is to provide an update on issues of theory, method, and application in environmental gerontology occurring since Wahl's comprehensive evaluation in the last (5th) edition of this *handbook*. In that assessment, Wahl (2001) offered a mixed evaluation of progress in the science and application of environmental gerontology. More recently, several leaders in the field have engaged in productive introspection regarding its strengths and shortcomings. This is partially attributable to a "stock-taking" period initiated shortly before and following the death in 2001 of M. Powell Lawton, a multidimensional researcher

Handbook of the Psychology of Aging

and highly influential leader in the field (Scheidt & Windley, 2003). This internal evaluation of the field continued with the 2003 publication of a set of papers in *The Gerontologist* by leading experts who addressed gaps in the science and application of environmental gerontology. Their assessments, like that of Wahl, combined concern with cautious optimism. Illustrative concerns included the lack of uniformity of theory and methodology (Kendig, 2003); the lack of "sound theories," as well as conceptual and operational definitions to guide measurement, particularly in home environments (Gitlin, 2003a, p. 73); the need for greater psychometric integrity in environmentally related measures and for greater relevance of theoretical applications to both research and application (Wahl & Weisman, 2003); and the need for theoretical models and constructs that can accommodate temporal contexts as well as environmental activities to a greater extent (Golant, 2003). These are not minor concerns, of course, and address core components of any discipline that hopes to conduct healthy science.

To the benefit of the field, the most exciting and innovative progress in environmental gerontology is being modeled by those voicing the strongest concerns about these existing gaps in the field. Much of this recent work is strikingly international and European, focusing on the *home* environment, although the neighborhood environment is receiving increased attention as well. It includes strong theoretical and measurement contributions of university-based teams of occupational therapists such as Laura Gitlin (Thomas Jefferson University) and Suzanne Iwarsson and colleagues (Lund University), the interdisciplinary research team at the Center on Aging at Heidelberg University, including Hans-Werner Wahl, Frank Oswald, and Heidrun Mollenkopf; and the work of

the behavioral ecologists at the University of Wisconsin at Milwaukee, led by Gerald Weisman and students. We review these contributions. Due to space limitations, we exclude research in other important domains (e.g., technology). Comprehensive, in-depth reviews are contained in Wahl, Scheidt, & Windley (2004), devoted entirely to topics within environmental gerontology.

II. The Status of Theory

The most axiomatic statement in environmental psychology is Lewin's ecological equation, $B = f(P, E)$: Behavior is dependent on the qualities and dynamic interaction of both persons and environments. Lawton (1982) modified the equation to include $(P \times E)$, recognizing that subjective interpretations of environments affect how people behave. A handful of early theoretical (now classic) frameworks, developed around this axiom, drove policy and practice in environmental gerontology during the 1960s and 1970s, but this influence dissipated from the 1980s to the present time. In addition, little formal "middle-range" theorizing has occurred since the early 1980s (Lawton, 1998). Research and practice have largely been fueled by looser assumptions derived from these older grand-scale frameworks or from more specific models tailored to highly particularized contexts. The absence of well-articulated theory useful for stimulating empirical research and practice continues to occupy discussion. This section briefly evaluates the continuing influence of one classic framework, reviews and evaluates the development of a new theoretical perspective, and discusses theoretical work that attempts to sort out the meaning of critical concepts used in environment–aging research today.

A. A Classic Theory Revisited: Lawton and Nahemow's Competence-Press Model

In his 2001 review, Wahl warned of the inevitable limited shelf life of classical theories for addressing issues of relevance to current environmental gerontology (e.g., failing to deal adequately with individual differences in environment–aging relations). Over the past three decades, the founding theories have attained iconic status due to utility, as well as to the absence of fresher theoretical applications (Scheidt & Windley, 1998).

The most interesting thinking evolving from the recent period of theoretical introspection involves Lawton and Nahemow's competence-press model (1973), also referred to as the general ecological model (Scheidt & Norris-Baker, 2004). Simply, this classic model, which has evolved considerably from its initial formulation, holds that behavioral outcomes occur and vary as a function of personal competence and environmental press (Figure 6.1). *Environmental press* is environmental demands or contexts that normally would elicit some response among people. The impact upon the individual of these demands is mediated by *competence*, or one's "intrinsic performance potential, the maximal expectable performance in biological, sensorimotor, perceptual, and cognitive domains" (Lawton, 1998, p. 2). Outcomes resulting from these $P \times E$ encounters are represented in external (behavioral competence) or internal (psychological well-being) terms. As the model depicts, compared to more competent individuals, those with lower competence are apt to experience a wider range of environmental demands as aversive (termed the "environmental docility hypothesis"), making them more likely to be controlled by the environment. Alternatively, alongside perceived demands, those with

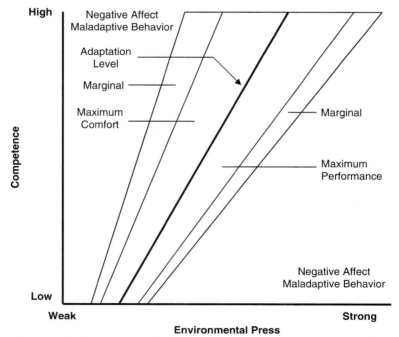

Figure 6.1 Lawton and Nahemow's competence-press model. Adapted from: Lawton and Nahemow (1973, p. 661). Reprinted with permission.

higher levels of competence are able to generate more resources and opportunities in environments, affording them greater control of the environment (Lawton, 1998).

The competence-press model remains the most influential model for research and practice assumptions in the field today. Illustratively, it forms the core of most accessibility research in occupational therapy and occupational science (Iwarsson & Stahl, 2003) and finds fresh praise for its application in new theory (Wahl & Lang, 2004). Nonetheless, Scheidt and Norris-Baker (2004) argue that the iconic status of the model has allowed it to serve functions that far outstrip tests of its empirical validity. Both Lawton and Nahemow acknowledged that tests of the basic assumptions of the model and its hypotheses are sparse, producing "mixed" results that contribute little to measurement. Because it has stood at the heart of environmental theorizing for so long, environmental gerontologists, including Lawton himself, used assessments of the empirical health of the model to draw conclusions about the state of health of theorizing in environmental gerontology as a whole. Over the past three decades, researchers have returned to the model again and again, adding to and changing taxonomic elements of each of its major environmental, individual, and outcome components in an attempt to revivify its empirical promise. Scheidt and Norris-Baker wonder whether these expectations

form the heart of a "rescue wish" for those seeking fresh perspectives in environmental gerontology and whether the continuing unparalleled preoccupation with the general ecological model may have actually constricted theory development by drawing energy and attention away from new theoretical pursuits (2004, pp. 48 and 49).

The heuristic strength of the competence-press model is well represented in two recent theoretical extensions.

Cvitkovich and Wister (2002) tested the general hypothesis that, compared to predictions afforded by the competence-press model, a greater amount of variation in psychological well-being (based on Lawton's valuation of life scale) can be predicted if individuals of varying competence are allowed to rate the degree that *multiple* environmental domains are able to meet their needs (termed P-E fit) and to *prioritize* these in terms of their importance for immediate life satisfaction. Environmental domains included housing and neighborhood resources, social support, and formal service support. This weighted *multilevel person–environment model* was supported among frail and nonfrail Vancouver older adults, with 31 and 30% improvement explained in well-being compared to the original competence-press model. Their revised model may be of aid in mapping changes in well-being tied to person–environment transactions across the life course, given that both competencies, as well as values placed on environmental resources and demands, change across adulthood.

Geboy and Diaz Moore (2005) extended the competence-press model to the organizational level of analysis, reconfiguring its basic constructs from an individual to a macro-level sphere. The *occupational competence-press model* (OCPM) employs five domains of organizational competence (structure, functions, knowledge, resource use, and interrelationships) derived from the organizational research literature. Environmental press is elaborated at the organizational level, emanating from both external and internal sources, as organizations are affected by the demands of internal microsystems as well as the larger external macrosystems. Organizational outcomes include efficacy in meeting goal-oriented outcomes at both individual and organizational levels. Hypothetical, potential applications of the OCPM are illustrated *for long-term care settings*, offering

...a way of looking at the complex interplay between organization, staff, physical setting, and the needs of a population of long-term care residents while allowing the accommodation of the needs of the individual resident to remain the focus point upon which resolution should be based (Geboy & Diaz Moore, 2004, p. 20).

The authors credit the "parsimony and accommodation" of the original competence-press model in the development of the OCPM (p. 20). The model has not been translated into measurement terms.

Both of these extensions address key theoretical gaps in environment–aging relations, accommodating *individual differences*, the *temporal* (life course) perspective, and domains of *environmental scale* and *complexity*.

B. New Theoretical and Conceptual Applications

Three types of theoretical applications typify new conceptual contributions to environmental gerontology. At the broadest level are efforts offering *conceptual guidance* regarding ways to advance the status of theory building in the field. Gitlin (2003a) cited promising efforts to insert environmental factors into existing theoretical models, including the international classification of functioning, disability, and health (ICF), as well as the research initiative Resources for Enhancing Alzheimer's Caregiver Health (REACH). The latter allows for assessment of and possible intervention with social and physical environmental stressors impacting caregiver stress (Gitlin & Gwyther, 2003). Golant (2003) argued persuasively that theories must include the influence of the temporal perspective on environments to a much greater extent. He also decried the absence of environmental behaviors and activities of older persons in contemporary theories. In a novel study reversing this trend, Diaz

Moore (2005) linked normative expectations and intentions for behavior to specific places within a dementia day care center. Ratings of affect (pleasure-to-anxiety ratios) of four groups of elderly residents at different competence levels varied as a function of the control demands of setting specific *"place rules"* or consistent, often implicit, associations between intentions and locations that may make regulatory demands on people in those locations (e.g., "staff may disturb client activities in any of the music room group's spaces"). Most relevant here, place rules constitute the "environmental press" in the competence-press model framing the study.

A second level of theoretical activity involves *development of more formal theoretical perspectives*. The most promising contribution here is Wahl and Lang's (2004) social–physical places over time (S.P.O.T) perspective. Based on Lang's (2003) goal-resource-congruence model of proactive social relationships across the life span, this meta-theoretical perspective gives primacy to *both* physical *and* social environments as individuals adapt to declines in personal competency and experience a sense of fore-shortened future. As they move from midlife through the later years, adults are predicted to display an adaptive dynamic within these environments, seeking and benefiting from an increased sense of belonging while exhibiting decreasing action potential. The evaluation of S.P.O.T. dynamics occurs against three criteria or themes drawn from person–environment fit models: stimulation and activation, safety and familiarity, and continuity and preservation of meaning. The latter two themes become increasingly important in old age. Adaptive responses to shifts in these themes are viewed as proactive. Greater refinement of these contextual criteria, the elaboration of additional criteria, and development of empirical measures suited to social and physical environments can allow S.P.O.T. to move us toward a developmentally informed, differential theory of environmental adaptation in the later years.

The third level of theoretically linked activity relates to the critical but relatively less dramatic task of clarifying the meaning of core concepts captured by various measures used in environment–aging studies. This work on *construct validity* strives to improve links between theory and measurement in environmental gerontology (Wahl & Weisman, 2003), often within existing theoretical models. Failure to clarify precisely what constructs are being measured, where one term begins and another ends, and how well they are represented in measures has led to well-deserved criticism in the past.

In recent years, however, exemplary work has been conducted by the Lund University occupational science team in the context of health and participation in everyday environments (Iwarsson & Stahl, 2003). The Lund team has done careful conceptual and empirical modeling to clarify person–environment constructs for both research and practice

purposes. The newly developed person–environment–activity (P-E-A) model (Figure 6.2) provides the most appropriate example of how "proper concepts are needed to form good theory, but good theory is needed to arrive at the proper concepts" (Iwarsson & Stahl, 2003, p. 63). Environmental "accessibility" has been theoretically conceived as "person–environment fit," representing both personal (functional capacity to perform) and environmental (barrier) components. Further, specific task-related behaviors constitute "activity." Subjective appraisals of efficacy and satisfaction with task-related activities define "usability." The components and the relations of this newly formulated P-E-A model have been carefully defined and differentiated in studies of physical accessibility of urban public buses for older users in Kristianstad, Sweden (Carlsson, 2002).

III. The Method Toolkit: Progress In Measurement

Successfully assessing predictors and outcomes of person–environment

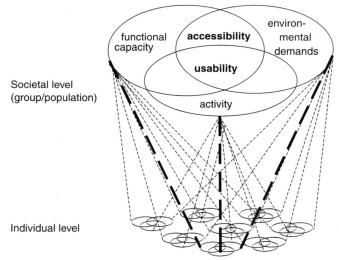

Figure 6.2 Person–environment–activity model of positioning of the concepts of accessibility and usability at individual and societal levels. Copyright G. Carlsson, 2002. Reprinted with permission.

transactions requires the marriage of both theory and measurement. Since 2000, the *home environment* has been the most frequently assessed target, with very recent efforts expanding to outdoor environments and public places (Iwarsson et al., 2004). The increased focus on the home environment is credited to rising public concern for health and care issues (Kendig, 2003), the strong preferences of elders themselves to remain in community-based home settings, particularly private homes, the increased interest of occupational therapists and allied health professionals in the reparative functions of home environments, and persisting data on time use and activity patterns showing that older people spent most of their time inside their homes. However, as Gitlin noted (2003b), measurement efforts have been hampered by factors such as the sheer complexity of the home setting and the lack of theoretically derived measurement approaches.

Although not plentiful in total number, newer measurement instruments reflect improved attention to psychometric properties, providing fundamental empirical support for reliability and validity. This is not typical of past assessment efforts (Wahl & Weisman, 2003). We briefly highlight three instruments that exemplify thoughtful and careful psychometric science. Each is derived from theoretical literature on person–environment relations. Two of these instruments—*the task management strategy index* (Gitlin et al., 2002) and *the housing-related control beliefs questionnaire* (Oswald et al., 2003)—are relative newcomers. Both focus on behavioral or psychological control and have solid "pilot study" status, but require further exploration, particularly in regard to predictive validity. The third, *the housing enabler* (Iwarsson, 2004), is designed to assess housing accessibility. It has had more extensive use and, although widely used

in Europe, is just beginning to receive the attention it deserves among researchers in the United States.

The *task management strategy index* (Gitlin et al., 2002) targets everyday behavioral strategies used by caregivers to cope with physical dependency and agitation in individuals with Alzheimer's disease and related disorders. With conceptual origins in the competence-press model, this self-report scale asks caregivers to endorse the frequency of use in the home of 19 *behavioral control* strategies (including environmental interventions) designed to compensate for functional losses at moderate to severe stages of dementia. Analyses of data drawn from two cross-sectional samples of Philadelphia family caregivers (including 255 from the REACH project) revealed evidence for solid construct validity and high internal consistency reliability. Gitlin et al. (2002) suggested that the current TMSI may be useful for identifying starting points for skill-oriented and educational interventions. Importantly, caregivers may learn that on many occasions it may be easier to affect changes in behavior by adjusting supporting environments as opposed to targeting directly elders with dementia.

The housing-related control beliefs questionnaire (Oswald et al., 2003) was developed on the premise that the proactive attitudes (Lawton, 1989) that elders show in dealing with environmental press in the home environment can be partially captured through assessments of psychological control orientations (internal control, external control: powerful others, and external control: chance). Items (23 in final scale) drawn from housing literature, as well as from studies on the functions of residential environments, were shaped to represent each control domain. Psychometric data drawn from two German samples—the largest $(N = 485)$ including participants of the Interdisciplinary Longitudinal Study on

Adult Development (ILSE)—were quite promising. The scale exhibits satisfactory internal consistency, retest reliability, and initial construct validity and generally confirmed predictions with socio structural variables (e.g., age and gender), objective and subjective environment-related variables (e.g., ownership, housing satisfaction), and general control beliefs (e.g., contributes unique variance) (Oswald et al., 2003). The scale has been put to work as an important component of the ENABLE-AGE project discussed later.

Based originally on the postoccupancy work of Steinfeld et al. (1979), the *housing enabler* is a novel system that affords "a *predictive, objective*, and *norm-based* assessment and analysis of accessibility problems in the physical home environment" from individual or population perspectives (Iwarsson, 2004b, p. 95). The instrument generates a total accessibility score based on combined interview and observational assessments of individual functional capacity and physical environmental barriers. Accessibility is defined in transactional terms, capturing specific P-E dynamics, making the enabler unique among measures. Careful exploration of the properties and uses of the enabler has been a major focus of the Lund team and inter rater reliability and content validity have been established. Illustrative here, Fange and Iwarsson (2003) explored the discriminant validity of *accessibility* and *usability* among a varied sample of 131 older Swedish urban residents. This subjective usability construct was assessed with the *usability in my home instrument* (UIMH), a P-E transactional measure assessing personal and social attributes, usability of sections of the housing environment, and housing supports and constraints on activity. At the most general level, accessibility and usability were found to be different, but related, concepts and the presumption that usability comprises an activity component were supported.

The housing enabler has been actively applied, stimulating research on accessibility on urban public transport (Carlsson, 2002) and adapted as an outcome measure to assess interventions targeting environmental barriers in public facilities (Iwarsson et al., 2004). Ongoing research with the enabler widens its use to outdoor environmental and public buildings at the local community level (Iwarsson, 2004) and housing adaptations useful for planning at the municipal level (Iwarsson, 2004). From its primary base in Sweden, the housing enabler traveled successfully to Europe. It was used in the ENABLE-AGE project, an innovative multinational, multidisciplinary, and multimethod European study conducted between 2001 and 2004. Environmental gerontologists from Sweden, Germany, United Kingdom, Hungary, and Latvia are exploring the influence of objective and subjective aspects of the home environment on "healthy aging," defined by behavioral (activity of daily living dependence), cognitive (life satisfaction), emotional (depression), and social participation domains (Iwarsson, 2004).

First results from the three-stage ENABLE-AGE Project (Oswald & Iwarrson, 2003) compared very old community dwelling samples from Sweden ($n = 397$) and Germany ($n = 450$). Although complex, results indicate that P-E fit measures of accessibility (ENABLER) and usability (UIMH) relate modestly but significantly to age and subjective health across both cultures. The advantages afforded by these P-E fit measures are illustrated nicely. The "stand-alone" measure of environmental barriers contributed very little to the understanding of healthy aging, although (ENABLER-defined) accessibility was related to aging in place, decreasing with increasing age and declines in subjective health. Further, aging in place is related to subjective housing aspects as well, including usability, place attachment, and housing-related control beliefs. Future analyses will examine differences across national samples, across subgroup variations among participants, and explore direct and indirect effects of predictors using latent variable modeling. ENABLE-AGE also produced qualitative analyses of adaptive transactions in the home environment and identified micro- and macroscale factors that affected social and community participation in very old age. Much data from the overall project remain to be published at this writing.

IV. Reflective Application: The Case For the Action Research Paradigm

The axiomatic focus on P-E fit and the intrinsic mission-oriented focus on quality of life issues put environmental gerontology at the heart of discussions of intervention, including ways to affect better data transfer to applied programs. As the previous brief review illustrates, there is a conscious effort to tighten the link between theory and measurement; further, the outcome domains often include affective and functional performance variables with immediate face validity. This more positivist flow of the research process—from theory to measurement to application—has come under increasing criticism by those seeking alternative ways of thinking about social science research in general (Flyvbjerg, 2001) and environmental gerontology specifically (Windley & Weisman, 2004). These alternative views range from matters of epistemology to issues of methodology and application. Space limits fuller discussion of these issues. However, in the context of the present review of reflective science in environmental gerontology, it seems appropriate to reflect on the contributions

of an alternative approach—the "action research paradigm"—linking research knowledge and application (Windley & Weisman, 2004).

At the philosophical and methodological core of action research are three basic principles outlined by Bradbury and Reason (2001): (1) action research should be done *with* people rather than *on* or *for* people; (2) understanding detailed contextual factors (e.g., case studies) is as important as understanding the general picture; and (3) and action research should produce knowledge that helps people understand and solve problems. With these basic principles in mind, we first review what action research is in the context of environmental gerontology. We explain why action research is a promising approach to a more complete understanding of environment and aging relationships. We then provide examples of action research in environmental gerontology and conclude with a discussion of how action research can advance the field of environmental gerontology in the future.

A. Action Research and Environmental Gerontology

Action research emerged from early efforts of Kurt Lewin (1946) to explore ways to analyze and act on social problems. Lewin argued that research in the social sciences should be integrated with concerns for application. Susman and Evered (1978) stated that the essential process of action research begins with a diagnostic phase of problem identification. A planning phase follows designed to identify alternative courses of action for solving the problem. In the next phase a course of action is taken followed by an evaluation phase that studies the consequences of the action. The final phase identifies findings that can be used to solve the problem. While small variations in procedures occur, action research is a cyclical, multistep process composed of a circle of planning, action, and fact finding about the results of a specific action (Lewin, 1947). Action research is collaborative knowledge building that involves clients, practitioners, consultants, and researchers whose collective aim is to produce practical knowledge useful to the everyday lives of people (Senge & Scharmer, 2001).

The argument for action research within an environmental context has been stressed since the early 1980s. For example, Sommer (1977) argued that action research is highly appropriate within an environmental context because it stresses the application of knowledge to important social, planning, and policy-related problems. In a similar vein, Weisman (1983) showed that although the application of action research in the field of environment and behavior studies generally has been characterized by "fits and starts," it shows promise as a vehicle for research application in architecture through the process of facility programming. More recently, action research has been effective in solving problems across a wide array of social, educational, and physical settings as reported by Reason and Bradbury (2001).

Environmental gerontology can benefit from action research through the tighter integration of theory and practice. That is, environmental design practitioners as well as health professionals seek to improve the quality of life of older people through environmental intervention informed by theory. However, there is a gap between theory and practice that must be narrowed before intervention can be more effective (Windley & Weisman, 1977). Windley and Weisman (2004) argued that the action research model is the most effective way to improve research application in environmental gerontology because it generates knowledge that is setting specific and problem

focused, unlike other research strategies that aim to develop generalizations and theory without concern for application. Specifically, Weisman (2003) showed how an action research perspective can provide information that leads to more therapeutic settings for people with dementia. An example of action research related to more general housing for older people is the work of Wisner, Stea, and Kruks (1997).

Thus, the primary purpose of action research in environmental gerontology is to improve the quality of life of older people through collaborative knowledge building that informs design and environmental modification of the social and physical living arrangements.

B. How Can Action Research Contribute to Environmental Gerontology?

The benefits of action research for a wide variety of fields have been amply demonstrated by several writers (e.g., Winter & Munn-Giddings, 2001; Reason & Bradbury, 2001) and are not reviewed here. In brief, the main benefits reported by these authors include (1) a more enriched understanding of phenomena by the potential involvement of all stakeholders as active participants in the research process, (2) the generation of information with high contextual validity in a form more suitable for application, and (3) an alternative research strategy that addresses the weaknesses of positivist-oriented research. However, the specific benefits for any given field depend on the needs of that discipline — its current knowledge base, theory status, and modes of practice.

We argue that action research contributes to the field of environmental gerontology in the following ways. First, Parmalee and Lawton (1990) noted that in the 1980s environmental gerontology as a field was stagnant due primarily to limited theoretical development and lack of integration of theory and practice. Progress in theory development and application since this time has been modest at best (Scheidt & Windley, 1998). Classic theories have come under increasing scrutiny. As noted, Scheidt and Norris-Baker (2004) believe that the long-standing functions of the classic competence-press model for future research should be reconsidered carefully, especially confusions between its epistemic and nonepistemic functions. They encourage the use of new approaches that focus on temporality and process within real-world, problem-specific contexts.

Second, action research capitalizes on the power of the case study to produce context specific information for application. In the spirit of what Stake (1994) called the "epistemology of the particular," environmental gerontology stands to benefit significantly from specific case studies that show potential causal relationships between environment and aging in various contexts. Flyvbjerg (2001) argued that in case study research, the "primacy of context" is essential to more enlightened practice because practice has always been based on context-dependent judgment. This is especially important in settings where it is difficult to obtain data from older people, such as in facilities for individuals with dementia. To effectively apply research in such settings, it is often necessary to triangulate data from various sources, such as from residents, family, and staff familiar with a specific setting. Because action research involves all stakeholders in the research process, triangulation is more likely to occur and can lead to more effective applications in a specific setting. However, Flyvbjerg (2001) noted that case studies also have broad implications:

The minutiae, practices, and concrete cases which lie at the heart of phronetic (applied) research are seen in their proper contexts; both the small, local context, which gives phenomena their immediate meaning, and the larger, international and global context in which phenomena can be appreciated for their general and conceptual significance (p. 138).

Thus, to the extent action research uses case study methodology, context-specific information will lead to more effective local problem solving. At the same time, the accumulation of specific case studies will add to our general understanding of phenomena in environmental gerontology — a "theories-in-use" perspective proposed by Argyris and Schon (1991).

Third, action research can bring needed change to traditional approaches in designing and managing facilities for older people. Schwarz (1997) has called for a new approach to nursing home design. His insightful critique shows how the medical model creates an institutional character in both design and management of nursing homes and does not promote the well-being of older residents. While providing efficiency in design and operation, nursing homes hinder individual autonomy. Such facilities need to develop more appropriate configurations and processes that increase life quality for those with chronic illness. Regnier (2002) has offered alternative ways of conceptualizing both housing and long-term care through the promotion of assisted living settings for older people. Located between congregate housing and long-term care, the assisted living concept aims to provide services to older people in residential settings that optimize the physical and psychological independence of older people. However, change is difficult. A significant barrier to change and improvement in traditional facilities is the strength and momentum of convention and regulation. Weisman (2003) demonstrated that many facilities for older people are embedded in tradition and have become "place types" or "frozen in place." Action research can bring about a "thaw" in such facility types and create circumstances where change can occur by applying four principles as outlined by Weisman: (1) adopt iterative group decision making where consensus is built through cycles of discussion and debate, (2) frame problems to be solved with a systemic approach that includes multiple perspectives from different levels of social aggregation, (3) consider general and local knowledge simultaneously when defining problems and evaluating actions, and (4) include training of researchers and other stakeholders as part of a action–research–training triangle. This training is aimed at preparing individuals to be agents of change.

C. Examples of Action Research in Environmental Gerontology

Most existing examples of action research across a broad spectrum of disciplines and scales of environment are anecdotal. There are few published examples in the field of environmental gerontology. This is partially due to problems of theory and practice integration discussed earlier as well as the overall newness of the field. Two case studies are described briefly to show the benefits of action research in environmental gerontology.

1. Brewster Village

Alden and Weisman (2003) described the replacement of a 100-year-old asylum located in Appleton, Wisconsin, with a 205 resident state-of-the-art long-term care facility for individuals with mental disability. Following the principles of action research described earlier by Weisman (2003), a team of individuals representing four different organizations (a county health center, architects office, a construction company, and a research institute at the University of Wisconsin) guided the development of the new facility over a 5-year period. A series of sight visits to other facilities and focus groups involving all stakeholders resulted in the development of project goals. These goals reflected a departure from traditional ways of conceiving of long-term care for older people, such as the provision of private rooms and decentralized dining facilities. Because these changes from tradition affected the entire system, a redefinition of staff duties was necessary to accommodate decentralized dining and other functions of the facility. Biweekly meetings were held among stakeholders throughout a 7-month period of schematic design to determine how the facility could meet project goals. During these meetings, general knowledge about the needs of long-term care was adapted to local circumstances and yielded six principles designed to create a noninstitutional environment: regulate sensory and social stimulation; create clusters of 13 to 14 residents; provide spaces for social interaction; facilitate spatial and social orientation; and create secure outdoor spaces (Figure 6.3). During this process, care was taken to educate staff and other participants in how to read architectural drawings and to envision how spaces in the facility would function. Once the facility was completed, project staff and researchers conducted a postoccupancy evaluation to assess whether the project met its goals (Alden & Weisman, 2003). Following the move to Brewster Village, quantitative measures showed positive change or no change for residents along 11 dimensions ranging from activity assessments and functioning to mood and anxiety measures. The only negative change was for a measure of communication/hearing. Staff experienced positive changes to working conditions and emotional climate, while families enjoyed the more home-like atmosphere and the visible improvement in quality of life among residents. Because action research is iterative, it is expected that subsequent environmental and operational changes

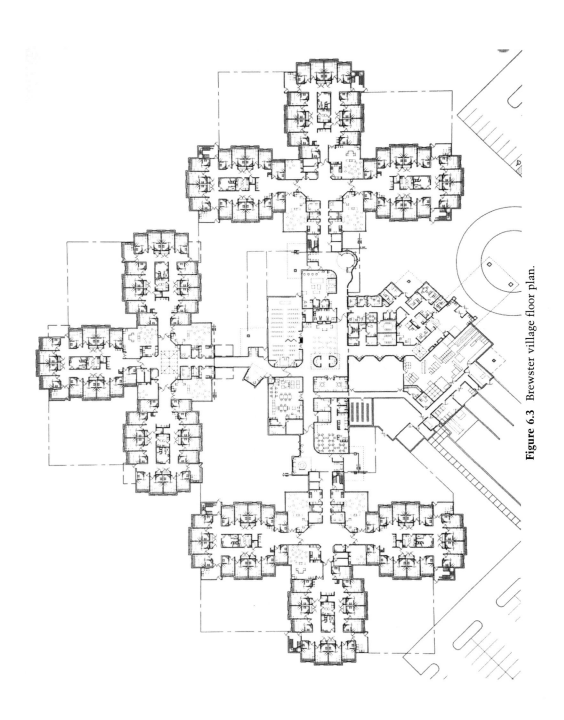

Figure 6.3 Brewster village floor plan.

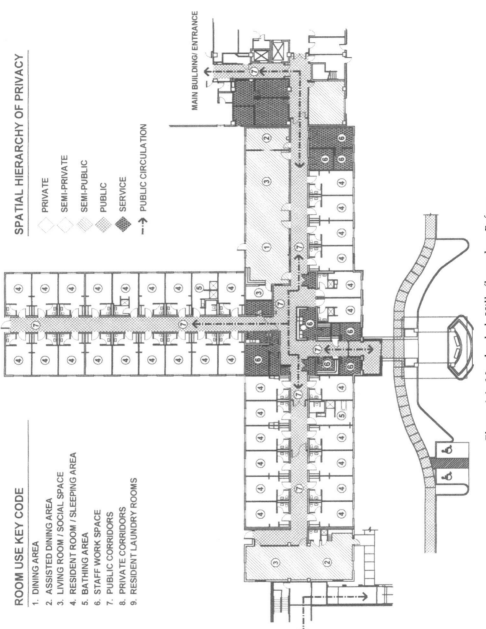

Figure 6.4 Meadowlark Hills floor plan: Before.

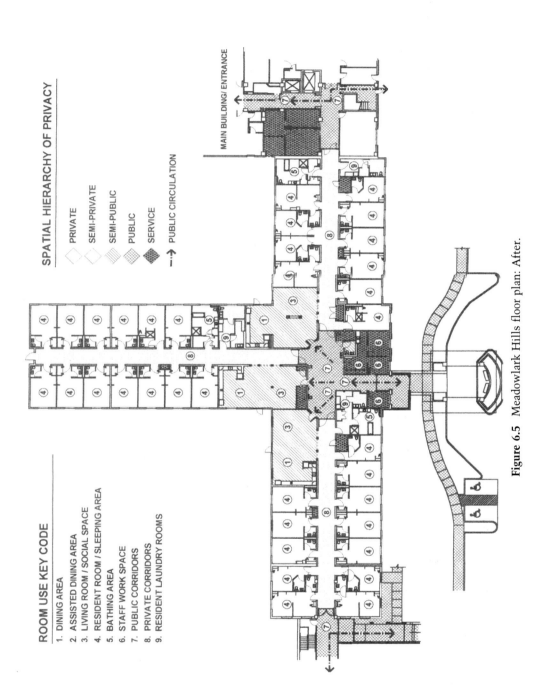

ROOM USE KEY CODE

1. DINING AREA
2. ASSISTED DINING AREA
3. LIVING ROOM / SOCIAL SPACE
4. RESIDENT ROOM / SLEEPING AREA
5. BATHING AREA
6. STAFF WORK SPACE
7. PUBLIC CORRIDORS
8. PRIVATE CORRIDORS
9. RESIDENT LAUNDRY ROOMS

SPATIAL HIERARCHY OF PRIVACY

◇ PRIVATE
◇ SEMI-PRIVATE
◈ SEMI-PUBLIC
◈ PUBLIC
◈ SERVICE
--→ PUBLIC CIRCULATION

MAIN BUILDING / ENTRANCE

Figure 6.5 Meadowlark Hills floor plan: After.

to the facility will be made following the evaluation. Alden and Weisman (2003) provide anecdotal evidence that tradition has been unfrozen in Brewster Village:

> those individuals who would have been described 100 years ago as "inmates of the poorhouse," and 50 years ago as "patients" in a medical-model nursing home, today view themselves as "villagers," active participants in their residential community (p. 27).

2. Meadowlark Hills

Based in the culture change movement within traditional long-term care, Kaup (2003) and colleagues conducted a postoccupancy evaluation of a traditional nursing home that was modified to improve the quality of life of residents and staff by making physical and organizational changes to the facility. In consultation with staff and residents, researchers documented resident and staff behavior within the facility before physical changes were made. Several problems were identified, including a lack of spatial hierarchy within the facility. For example, public areas and corridors were located adjacent to private rooms and bathing areas buffered only by doors between these spaces. The facility also lacked sufficient transitional or semi-private spaces between public and private areas. Thus, large numbers of residents congregated within small parlors or TV-watching areas, resulting in limited cohesiveness among residents. Following the facility assessment process involving all stakeholders, two goals guided the remodel: increase the residents' ability to identify with a family unit by grouping resident rooms into small household clusters and enhance resident autonomy and control by establishing the full range of spatial hierarchy within the facility. Physical changes to the facility included personalizing resident room entries by providing transitional porches; providing

transitional hallways between private and semiprivate areas of living units, thus avoiding the public domain; and arranging furniture within the semipublic spaces (dining and entertainment areas) that were more residential in character (Figures 6.4 and 6.5 — *before* and *after* floor plans). These modifications required changes in staff training and organizational policies to allow residents to benefit from the increased autonomy provided by the new facility. Ongoing evaluations will lead to further changes that promise to improve the quality of life of Meadowlark Hills residents.

V. Conclusion and Future Directions

While research on several empirical fronts continues to progress steadily, much recent progress in theory, method, and application domains has occurred in direct response to strong self-criticism of the field launched by several of its major leaders. To their credit and to the benefit of the field, those launching these criticisms have modeled the best aspects of the science in each of these realms. Much of this effort is characterized by "back to the basics" research practice, involving careful, systematic evaluation of key constructs. To date, most of this activity has focused on predictor constructs in both person and environment domains. Future work might examine more carefully the theoretical and measurement meanings captured by constructs assessing behavioral and affective outcomes, where research has been more uneven in this respect. For example, there is far less construct-related research on dimensions of subjective well-being than on psychological control among community-based populations (Pinquart & Burmedi, 2004).

Appraisal of the value of fundamental classic guiding models and development of fresh meta-theoretical perspectives characterize theoretical application. These efforts deal directly with missing gaps in theory, particularly related to temporality across the adult life span and to environmental scale and complexity. Compared to 5 years ago, there are more measures developed according to standard psychometric principles that offer evidence of fundamental construct validity for objective and subjective environmental constructs and of basic reliability and criterion-related validity. This small but important reformation has clearly benefited the field, particularly the focused study of home environments. Occupational health professionals who insist on close linkages between person–environment fit constructs and health-related interventions have had an enormous influence on this activity.

The complex question *of whether, where, and how* culture affects residential adaptations and healthy aging over time remains largely unaddressed. The multinational ENABLE-AGE project is historically unique in environmental gerontology. In addition to rich data on resident and residential predictors of healthy aging, it may be of value to those who seek to examine cultural similarities and differences in these cross-national housing contexts. Contextual paradigms linking culture to age-related changes in health (Scheidt, 2001) may prove useful to future research in this area.

The major momentum for much of the more reflective science in environmental gerontology is generated by the research teams at Lund, Heidelberg, Milwaukee, and Philadelphia (i.e., Thomas Jefferson University), including their important international collaborations. Can this momentum be maintained? Each site is defined by a "critical mass" of researchers and each continues to train competent students. It is difficult to predict, as resources and commitments so frequently shift, whether the efforts of these particular centers might be sustained over the coming years. However, judging from the productive research of second- and third-generation researchers coming from these and other sites, we are optimistic about a sustained future for environmental gerontology (Scheidt & Windley, 2003).

Like other disciplines within behavioral science, environmental gerontologists continue to grapple with the extrapolation of data to the realm of practice, i.e., affecting more efficient linkage between the meaning of statistical "effect sizes" and interventions designed to improve quality of life. We have argued that the action research paradigm is a most promising future direction for spawning innovative research-to-practice links. First, to aid transition to a more action-oriented research approach, we suggest that current research findings amenable to design application should be produced in a form easily understood by practitioners. Windley and Weisman (2004) described techniques for translating research information into guidelines for design application, such as pattern language and performance specifications. However, application does not necessarily follow from this translation process unless there is a plan for information dissemination. We propose the adoption of guidelines similar to those developed by Rogers (1995) for the dissemination of information to medical practitioners. In his view, successful application includes informing potential practitioners of innovative knowledge and assuring their decisional control regarding its programmatic use, evaluation, and possible continued adoption or discontinuance. Professional associations within environmental gerontology and related fields, and government and private research agencies, should take steps to encourage a more action research approach by promoting dialogue between researchers and practitioners, funding action research projects, and assuring avenues for publication and dissemination of action research findings.

Second, action research would benefit environmental gerontology with studies that focus on "place" rather than the traditional emphasis placed on the individual as the unit of analysis (Windley & Weisman, 2004). By "place" we mean the psychological, social, and architectural attributes of settings that contribute to how a place is experienced by individuals and groups. Shifting the focus of analysis from individuals to places has major implications for construct and measurement validity. Bradbury and Reason (2001) proposed five choice points that can broaden the *bandwidth of validity* for any given project: (1) foster maximal participation in the research group (2) ensure that the research is a benefit to participants (3) frame the project in people's experience and use investigative methods sensitive to context (4) target research questions of fundamental importance to participants, and (5) assure that the investigation can continue by leaving institutionalized infrastructures in place following an initial investigation.

Finally, a further development of environmental gerontology can occur by urging researchers and practitioners to conduct action research. For example, Windley and Weisman (2004) encouraged design and planning students and educators to focus on projects involving real clients. Students who have experience working with communities on real projects appreciate multiple points of view, serve effectively as facilitators of designer–client collaboration, and are adept at handling information generated through research—all of which are important in action research.

Finally, action research requires collaboration between researchers and practitioners, which is often resisted due to different epistemological orientations to knowledge (Schon, 1983). However, some land-grant universities, as part of their institutional missions, generate knowledge in cooperation with local communities to solve problems at a local level. The well-known land-grant model requires that researchers and all stakeholders engage in a continuous dialogue (van Beinum, 1998).

Translating existing information into application guidelines, focusing on place rather than the individual, and educating researchers and practitioners in the conduct of action research will enable this integration and accomplish Brulin's (2001) promise that action research will enlarge our concept of knowledge beyond what natural science can provide.

References

Alden, A., & Weisman, G. (2003). Inmates to villagers: The creation of Brewster Place. *Design*, March 22–27.

Argyris, C., & Schon, D. (1991). Participatory action research and action science compared. In W. Whyte (Ed*.), Participatory action research* (pp. 85–96). Newbury Park, CA: Sage Publications.

Bradbury, H., & Reason, P. (2001). Broadening the bandwidth of validity: Issues and choice-points for improving the quality of action research. In P. Reason & H. Bradbury (Eds.), *Handbook of action research: Participative inquiry and practice* (pp. 448–456). Newbury Park, CA: Sage Publications.

Brulin, G. (2001). The third task of universities or how to get universities to serve their communities. In P. Reason & H. Bradbury (Eds.), *Handbook of action research: Participative inquiry and practice* (pp. 440–445). Newbury Park, CA: Sage.

Carlsson, G. (2002). *Catching the bus in old age: Methodological aspects of accessibility assessments in public transport*. (From the Department of Clinical Neuroscience, Division of Occupational Therapy and the Department of Technology and Society, Division of Traffic Planning, Lund University). Lund, Sweden: Studentlitteratur.

Cvitkovich, Y., & Wister, A. (2002). Bringing in the life course: A modification to Lawton's ecological model of aging.

Hallym International Journal of Aging, 4(1), 15–29.

Diaz Moore, K. (2005). Utilizing place rules and affect to understand environmental fit. *Environment and Behavior.*

Fange, A., & Iwarsson, S. (2003). Accessibility and usability in housing: Construct validity and implications for research and practice. Paper presented as a part of a symposium entitled Psychological Dimensions of Aging in place: Processes and outcomes, November, 2003, Gerontological Society of America.

Flyvbjerg, B. (2001). *Making social science matter*. Cambridge, UK: Cambridge Press.

Geboy, L. D., & Diaz Moore, K. (2005). Considering organizational competence: A theoretical extension of Lawton and Nahemow's competence-press model. In H. Chaudhury & A. Mahmood (Eds.), *Proceedings of the environmental design research association*: (Vol. 1). Edmond, OK: EDRA.

Gitlin, L. (2003a). M. Powell Lawton's vision of the role of the environment in aging processes and outcomes: A glance backward to move us forward. In K. W. Schaie, H.W. Wahl, H. Mollenkopf, & F. Oswald (Eds.), *Aging independently: Living arrangements and mobility* (pp. 62–76). New York: Springer.

Gitlin, L. (2003b). Conducting research on home environments: Lessons learned and new directions. *The Gerontologist, 43(5)*, 628–637.

Gitlin, L., & Gwyther, L. (2003). In-home interventions: Helping caregivers where they live. In D. Coon, D. Gallagher-Thompson, & L. Thompson (Eds.), *Innovative interventions to reduce caregiver distress: A clinical guide* (pp. 139–160). New York: Springer.

Gitlin, L., Winter, L., Dennis, M., Corcoran, M., Schinfeld, S., & Hauck, W. (2002). Strategies used by families to simplify tasks for individuals with Alzheimer's disease and related disorders: Psychometric analysis of the Task Management Strategy Index (TMSI). *The Gerontologist, 42(1)*, 61–69.

Golant, S. M. (2003). Conceptualizing time and behavior in environmental gerontology: A pair of old issues deserving new thought. *The Gerontologist, 43(5)*, 638–648.

Iwarsson, S. (2004). Assessing the fit between older people and their physical environments: An occupational therapy research perspective. In H.W. Wahl, R. Scheidt, & P. Windley (Eds.), *Aging in context: Socio-physical environments. Annual review of gerontology and geriatrics* (Vol. 23, pp. 85–109). New York: Springer.

Iwarsson, S., Fange, A., Horbrandt, P., Carlsson, G., Jarbe, I., & Wijk, U. (2004). Occupational therapy targeting physical environmental barriers in buildings with public facilities. *British Journal of Occupational Therapy, 67(1)*, 29–38.

Iwarsson, S., & Stahl, A. (2003). Accessibility, usability, and universal design: Positioning and definition of concepts describing person–environment relationships. *Disability and Rehabilitation, 25(2)*, 57–66.

Kaup, M. L. (2003). Reshaping behaviors in nursing homes by reshaping nursing home architecture: A case study in the investigation of change. *Proceedings of the Environmental Design Research Association, 34*, 98–104.

Kendig, H. (2003). Directions in environmental gerontology: A multidisciplinary field. *The Gerontologist, 43(5)*, 611–615.

Lang, F.R. (2003). Social motivation across the lifespan: Developmental perspectives on the regulation of personal relationships and networks. In F. R. Lang & K. L. Fingerman (Eds.), *Growing together: personal relationships across the life span* (pp. 341–367). New York: Cambridge University Press.

Lawton, M.P. (1982). Competence, environmental press, and the adaptation of older people. In M.P. Lawton, P.G. Windley, & T.O. Byerts (Eds.), *Aging and the environment: Theoretical approaches* (pp. 33–59). New York: Springer.

Lawton, M.P. (1989). Environmental proactivity in older people. In V. L. Bengtson & K. W. Schaie (Eds.), *The course of later life* (pp. 15–23). New York: Springer.

Lawton, M.P. (1998). Environment and aging: Theory revisited. In R. J. Scheidt & P.G. Windley (Eds.), *Environment and aging theory: A focus on housing* (pp. 1–32). Westport, CT: Greenwood Press.

Lawton, M.P., & Nahemow, L. (1973). Ecology and the aging process. In C. Eisdorfer

& M. P. Lawton (Eds.), *Psychology of adult development and aging* (pp. 619–674). Washington, DC: American Psychological Association.

Lewin, K. (1946). Action research and minority problems. *Journal of Social Issues, 2*, 34–36.

Lewin, K. (1947). Frontiers in group dynamics. *Human Relations, 1*, 2–38. Reprinted in G.W. Levin, *Resolving social conflict in field theory in social science.* Washington DC: American Psychological Association.

Oswald, F., & Iwarsson, S. (2003). Aging in place and healthy aging in very old age: First results from the ENABLE-AGE project. Paper presented as part of a symposium entitled *Psychological Dimensions of Aging in Place: Processes and Outcomes*, November, 2003, Gerontological Society of America.

Oswald, F., Wahl, H.W., Martin, M., & Mollenkopf, H. (2003). Toward measuring proactivity in person–environment transactions in late adulthood: The housing-related control beliefs questionnaire. In R. Scheidt & P. G. Windley (Eds.), *Physical environments and aging: Critical contributions of M. Powell Lawton to theory and practice* (pp. 135–152). New York: The Haworth Press.

Parmalee, P., & Lawton, M.P. (1990). The design of special environments for the aged. In J. Birren & W. Schaie (Eds.), *Handbook of the psychology of aging* (pp. 464–488). San Diego, CA: Academic Press.

Pinquart, M., & Burmedi, D. (2004). Correlates of residential satisfaction in adulthood and old age: A meta-analysis. In H.W. Wahl, R. J. Scheidt, & P.G. Windley (Eds.), *Aging in context: Socio-physical environments: Annual review of gerontology and geriatrics* (Vol. 23, pp. 195–222.). New York: Springer.

Reason, P., & Bradbury, H. (Eds.). (2001) *Handbook of action research: Participative inquiry and practice.* Newbury, CA: Sage Publications.

Regnier, V. (2002). *Design for assisted living: Guidelines for housing the physically and mentally frail.* New York: Wiley.

Rogers, E. (1995). Lessons for guidelines from the diffusion of innovation. *Journal on Quality Improvement, 21/7*, 324–328.

Scheidt, R. (2001). Individual-cultural transactions: Implications for the mental health of rural elders. *Journal of Applied Gerontology, 20 (2)*, 195–213.

Scheidt, R.J., & Norris-Baker, C. (2004). The general ecological model revisited: Evolution, current status, and continuing challenges. In H.W. Wahl, R. J. Scheidt, & P.G. Windley (Eds.), *Aging in context: Socio-physical environments: Annual review of Gerontology and Geriatrics* (Vol. 23, pp. 34–58). New York: Springer.

Scheidt, R.J., & Windley, P.G. (Eds.) (1998). *Environment and aging theory: A focus on housing.* Westport, CT: Greenwood Press.

Scheidt, R. J., & Windley, P.G. (Eds.) (2003). *Physical environments and aging: Critical contributions of M. Powell Lawton to theory and practice.* New York: The Haworth Press.

Schon, D. (1983). *The reflective practitioner: How professionals think in action.* New York: Basic Books.

Schwarz, B. (1997). Nursing home design: A misguided architectural model. *Journal of Architectural and Planning Research, 14(4)*, 343–357.

Senge, P., & Scharmer, O. (2001). Community action research: Learning as a community of practitioners, consultants, and researchers. In P. Reason & H. Bradbury (Eds.), *Handbook of action research: Participative inquiry and practice* (pp. 238–249). Newbury, CA: Sage Publications.

Sommer, R. (1977). Action Research. In D. Stokols (Ed.), *Perspectives on environment and behavior: Theory, research and application* (p. 301). New York: Plenum.

Stake, R. (1994). Case studies. In N. Denzin & Y. Lincoln (Eds.), *Handbook of qualitative research* (pp. 236–247). Thousand Oaks, CA: Sage Publications.

Steinfeld, E., Schroeder, S., Duncan, J., Faste, R., Chollet, D., Bishop, M., et al. (1979). *Access to the build environments: A review of the literature.* Washington, DC: U.S. Government Printing Office.

Susman, G., & Evered, R. (1978). An assessment of the scientific merits of action research. *Administration Scientific Quarterly, 23*, 582–603.

van Beinum, H. (1998). On the practice of action research. *Concepts and Transformations, 3(12)*, 1–29.

Wahl, H. W. (2001). Environmental influences on aging and behavior. In J. E. Birren & K. W. Schaie (Eds.), *Handbook of the psychology of aging* (5th ed., pp. 215–237). New York: Academic Press.

Wahl, H. W., & Lang, F. R. (2004). Aging in context across the adult life course: Integrating physical and social environmental research perspectives. In H. W. Wahl, R. Scheidt, & P. Windley (Eds.), *Aging in context: Socio-physical environments* (Vol. 23, pp. 1–33). New York: Springer.

Wahl, H. W., Scheidt, R. J., & Windley, P.G. (2004). *Aging in context: Socio-physical environments: Annual review of gerontology and geriatrics* (Vol. 23). New York: Springer.

Wahl, H. W., & Weisman, G. (2003). Environmental gerontology at the beginning of the new millenium: Reflections on its historical, empirical, and theoretical development. *The Gerontologist, 43(5)*, 616–627.

Weisman, G. (1983). Environmental programming and action research. *Environment and Behavior, 15(3)*, 381–408.

Weisman, G. (2003). Creating places for people with dementia: An action research perspective. In K. Schaie, H.-W. Wahl, H. Mollenkopf, & F. Oswald (Eds.), *Aging independently: Living arrangements and mobility* (pp. 162–173). New York: Springer.

Windley, P., & Weisman, G. (1977). Social science and environmental design. *Journal of Architectural Education, 31(1)*, 16–19.

Windley, P. G., & Weisman, G. (2004). Environmental gerontology research and practice: The challenge of application. In H. W. Wahl, R. J. Scheidt, & P. G. Windley (Eds.), *Aging in context: Socio-physical environments: Annual review of Gerontology and Geriatrics* (Vol. 23, pp. 334–365). New York: Springer.

Winter, R., & Munn-Giddings, C. (2001). *A handbook for action research in health and social care*. London: Routledge.

Wisner, B., Stea, D., & Kruks, S. (1997). Participatory and action research methods. In E. Zube & G. Moore (Eds.), *Advances in environment, behavior, and design* (Vol. 4, pp. 271–295). New York: Plenum.

Part Three

Behavioral Processes and Aging

Seven

Vision and Aging

Frank Schieber

I. Introduction

Our ability to cope effectively with the environment begins with our capacity to process sensory input. Indeed, our senses have been carefully crafted by the forces of nature to effortlessly extract critical information from the world around us. Unfortunately, advancing adult aging brings with it systematic reductions in the efficiency of our sensory systems. This lost efficiency of low-level, automatic processing capacity often necessitates effortful, high-level compensatory processes that may tax already limited cognitive resources. Hence, sensory aging is of potentially great interest at all levels of psychological analysis (Schieber, 2003). The purpose of this chapter is to provide a contemporary overview of one aspect of sensory aging, namely age-related changes in vision and low-level visual information processing. This focus on vision does not discount the critical role played by the other major sensory systems, but instead is constrained by the author's breadth of expertise. This overview is by no means exhaustive. In fact, it merely samples important domains of investigative inquiry with a focus on basic aspects of vision and aging that have received significant attention in the research literature during the past decade. Several excellent reviews of the sensory aging literature prior to the contemporary period are available for readers in need of a more comprehensive and historical introduction to the topic (recommended readings include Corso, 1981; Kline & Scialfa, 1997; Fozard & Gordon-Salant, 2001).

II. Structural Changes in the Visual System

Any comprehensive review of vision and aging must begin with a consideration of the myriad age-related changes that occur in the eye, retina, and ascending visual pathways in the nervous system. Careful attention to this topic is also important because of continuing, but unresolved, efforts to attribute various aspects of visual aging to optical versus neurological mechanisms.

A. Optical Changes

1. Cornea

Light first enters the eye through the cornea (see Figure 7.1). The cornea is the major refractive element of the eye, accounting for approximately two-thirds of the power required to focus incoming light onto the retina (Geldard, 1972). Small changes in the curvature of the cornea result in remarkable changes in the quality of the retinal image. The curvature of the cornea tends to increase beyond 50 years of age. Most of this change is restricted to the horizontal meridian (Baldwin & Mills, 1981; Fledelius, 1988). Hence, corneal astigmatisms that emerge in later life tend to occur along the horizontal meridian — just the opposite of the pattern observed in younger adults with refractive error (Morgan, 1993). Changes in the internal microstructure of the cornea (rather than its anterior surface) result in age-related increases in the intraocular scattering of light in persons over 60 years of age. However, the magnitude of this effect

is small compared to the amount of increased scatter introduced by the senescent lens (Guirao, Redondo, & Artal, 2000; Artal et al., 2002).

2. Iris and Pupil

The amount of light that enters the eye is regulated by the pupillary aperture in the pigmented iris muscle. Through dilation and constriction the pupil of the typical young adult is capable of regulating retinal illumination over a 16:1 range (Geldard, 1972). However, as one grows older the average diameter of the pupil for a given value of illumination tends to become smaller — a condition referred to as *pupillary miosis*. Age differences in pupil diameter are greatest under low-illumination conditions (Winn et al., 1994). For example, in dim light the expected diameter of the pupil falls from an average of 7–8 mm at age 20 to approximately 4 mm by 80 years of age (Loewenfeld, 1979). Effective pupil size may be reduced further by *ptosis* — a common condition among older persons

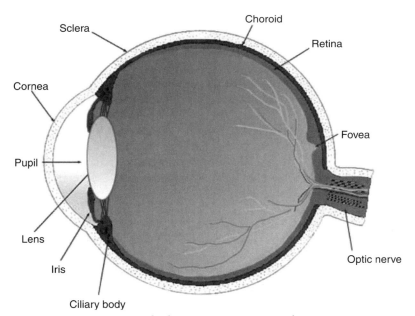

Figure 7.1 The human eye. Source: Webvision.

in which lost elasticity of the eye lid causes it to "droop" into the pupillary aperture (Theodore, 1975).

3. Lens

Light passing through the pupil next encounters the crystalline lens of the eye. In response to contractile forces exerted by the ciliary muscles, the lens can alter its shape, thereby changing its focusing power. This process, called accommodation, enables the lens to dynamically increase its focusing power as required for doing work at near viewing conditions. In young children, the maximum amplitude of accommodation enables the lens to add approximately 20 diopters of focusing power to the eye, thus enabling them to focus upon objects as close as 5 cm away. However, the maximum amplitude of accommodation decreases in a linear fashion from childhood onward. By the midforties, the average person has lost so much accommodative power that they can no longer adequately focus upon objects within arm's length (Hofstetter, 1965) — a normal age-related insufficiency of accommodation known as presbyopia. By the sixth decade of life, the amplitude of accommodation has been reduced to zero (Donders, 1864) and the need for reading glasses and/or bifocal lenses to perform near work becomes the norm. Presbyopia probably results from lost elasticity of the lens due to its continued growth across the life span rather than due to insufficiency in the ciliary muscles (Atchison, 1995).

The lens also becomes less transparent with increasing adult age (Weale, 1963). This increase in the optical density of the lens appears to be especially pronounced for short wavelength (i.e., blue) light (Said & Weale, 1959; Coren & Girgus, 1972). In addition to having increased optical density, the senescent lens also significantly increases the amount of off-axis light scatter within the eye (Mellerio, 1971; Whitaker, Steen, & Elliott, 1993; Guirao et al., 1999). Another optical aberration occurring within the aging lens is the accumulation of metabolic by-products that fluoresce when stimulated by 345- (ultraviolet) and 420 (visible violet) -nm light energy (Satchi, 1973).

4. Retinal Illumination and Contrast

The combined effects of diminished pupil diameter and increased lens opacity yield a 0.5 log unit (threefold) reduction in retinal illuminance between 20 and 60 years of age (Weale, 1963). It has been estimated that lens opacity accounts for a 0.2 log unit reduction in retinal illuminance, whereas pupillary miosis accounts for the remainder of the age-related loss in light reaching the retina (Elliott, Whitaker, & MacVeigh, 1990). The contrast of the retinal image also declines with advancing age due to increased intraocular scatter (van den Berg, 1995), as well as a generalized reduction in the modulation transfer function of the eye (Artal et al., 2003). Optical analysis suggests that much of this age-related reduction in the contrast of the image formed on the retina would be mitigated by reducing the resting size of the pupil (e.g., Guirao et al., 1999). Indeed, a study by Sloane, Owsley, and Alvarez (1988) suggests that the pupillary miosis commonly observed in older adults may represent a trade-off of the visual system between the demands of retinal illuminance and retinal contrast. Pupillary miosis does not represent an atrophic change in the iris, but rather a dynamic process acting to optimize retinal contrast and overall visual performance.

B. Sensorineural Changes

The most well-studied neural substrate of vision and aging is also the most accessible, namely the retina. The retina lines the posterior hemisphere of the eye. It consists of two major topographical regions: the macula (the central 18°-wide region specialized for fine spatial resolution) and the peripheral retina. The macula is cone rich whereas the peripheral retina is dominated by rods. Cones are specialized for color vision and fine spatial resolution whereas rods are specialized for low-light levels. The photoreceptors (approximately 120 million rods and 5–8 million cones) are embedded in the retinal pigment epithelium (RPE). The RPE sits on the basement membrane of the retina (Bruch's membrane) and serves as a metabolic "conduit" between the photoreceptor outer segments and the choriocapillary layer on the other side of Bruch's membrane (and the eye–blood barrier). Nerve impulses generated by the rods and cones cascade through a network of bipolar, horizontal, and amicrine cells in the neural layer of the retina and ultimately converge upon the retinal ganglion cells whose axons project directly to the lateral geniculate nucleus (LGN) of the thalmus. From the LGN, visual information ascends to the primary visual cortex located in the occipital lobe of the brain (Bonnel, Mohand-Said, & Sahel, 2003).

1. Retinal Photoreceptors

There is converging evidence that adult aging is accompanied by a dramatic loss in the number of rods (Curcio et al., 1990; Gao & Hollyfield, 1992; Panda-Jonas, Jonas, & Jacobczyk-Zmija, 1995). Curcio and colleagues (1993) reported that rod density in the central retina (3–10°) declined by 30% between 34 and 90 years of age. Despite previous reports that aging was associated with a reduction in cone density as well (Gartner & Henkind, 1981), Curcio et al. (1993) found that cone density remained relatively stable across the same age range. One of the reasons for this inconsistency may be

due to the fact that there are wide individual differences in cone numbers. Given large individual differences in cone count, small but systematic declines with age would be difficult to find given the small number of observations typical of *in vitro* studies of this kind. However, other evidence indirectly supports concomitant age-related losses in cones. For example, foveal cone pigment density appears to decline with age (Kilbride et al., 1986; Eisner et al., 1988). However, electrophysiological evidence has failed to provide consistent evidence regarding macular cone function (Jackson et al., 2002; Seiple et al., 2003). Given that the cones appear to depend on a "survival factor" produced by surrounding rods (Fintz et al., 2003), it would be surprising if the age-related loss of rods did not portend subsequent cone loss at some to-be-determined time lag (see Curcio, Owsley, & Jackson, 2000).

2. Retinal Ganglion Cells

The activity of the photoreceptors is preprocessed in the neural network of retina consisting of interconnected bipolar, amacrine, and horizontal cells. Ultimately, this information converges upon retinal ganglions cells whose axons converge to form the optic nerve and ascend to the brain. Several studies have reported significant age-related reductions in the number of retinal ganglion cells subserving the macular region of the retina (Gao & Hollyfield, 1992; Curcio & Drucker, 1993). Consistent with these findings are reports of age-related losses in the number of axons in the optic nerve (e.g., Repka & Quigley, 1989) and age-related thinning of the neural layer of the retina (Lovasik et al., 2003).

3. Retinal Support Layers

Lipofuscin accumulates in cells of the retinal pigment epithelium (RPE) with advancing age. Lipofuscin is a well-known biomarker of aging and reacts with light to form reactive oxygen species (free radicals) that can damage cell membranes (Bonnel et al., 2003). Abnormal deposits of insoluble material called drusen accumulate between the RPE and Bruch's membrane as people grow older. These drusen may induce local inflammation of retinal tissue and ultimately trigger an autoimmune response and subsequent retinal disease (Anderson et al., 2002). Bruch's membrane also accumulates significant deposits of cholesterol with advancing age, perhaps diminishing the efficient exchange of nutrients and metabolic byproducts between the RPE and the choriocapillary layer (Curcio et al., 2001).

4. Primary Visual Cortex

Initial studies of the human visual cortex reported significant cell loss with advancing age. For example, Devaney and Johnson (1980) reported that the number of cells in the primary visual (striate) cortex declined by 25% as early as age 60. However, subsequent investigations have failed to observe systematic declines of neuron density in the visual cortex with aging (e.g., Haug et al., 1984; Leuba & Garey, 1987). In a comprehensive review of the literature, Spear (1993) concluded there was no consistent histological evidence in the primate to support the hypothesis of senescent cell loss in the ascending visual pathways between the retina and the visual cortex. Rather than general cell loss per se, Kim and co-workers (1997) suggested that age-related neural changes impacting visual function are more likely to involve extrastriate corical areas or "reside on a different level of anatomical analysis, such as the level of synapses or receptors" (p. 126). Indeed, electron microscopy studies have revealed evidence of degenerative changes in dendritic processes and

decreased synaptic density for neurons in the primary visual cortex of "older" rhesus monkeys (Peters, Moss, & Sethares, 2001). Along a similar vein, Leventhal and colleagues (2003) reported age-related degradation of intracortical inhibitory processes related to GABA-receptor insufficiency in the visual cortex of nonhuman primates. Also consistent with the road map of Kim et al. (1997), Park and colleagues (2004) reported that despite histological evidence that neural density in the ventral (i.e., extrastriate) visual cortex is spared with aging, human functional magnetic resonance imaging studies reveal reduced functional efficiency in this region.

III. Visual Impairment and Age-related Pathology

Although the emphasis of this volume focuses on normative changes accompanying adult aging, visual pathology is so common and so potentially debilitating in terms of everyday behavioral function that a brief review of the major age-related visual disorders appears both appropriate and necessary. The Eye Diseases Prevalence Research Group (EDPRG) has estimated that as of the year 2000 approximately 937,000 Americans older than 40 years of age were legally blind (corrected acuity 20/200 or worse in the better eye). Another 2.4 million American adults had low vision (corrected acuity worse than 20/40 but better than 20/200). This means that 1 of 28 adults living in the United States could be described as visually impaired (EDPRG, 2004a). A very large proportion of this age-related increase in the prevalence of visual impairment can be accounted for by three classes of ocular pathology: cataract, age-related maculopathy (ARM), and glaucoma (see Table 7.1). Cataract involves an excessive opacification of the lens and is, by far,

Table 7.1
Prevalence (per 100) of Visual Pathology as
a Function of Age (Years)[a]

Age	Cataract	ARM-Dry	ARM-Wet	Glaucoma
50–54	5.1	0.34	0.23	0.91
60–64	15.5	0.56	0.38	1.57
70–74	36.9	1.66	1.15	2.79
80+	68.3	11.77	8.18	7.74

[a]Data from Eye Diseases Prevalence Research Group (2004 b,c,d).

the leading cause of age-related visual impairment. Fortunately, the deleterious effects of cataract are almost always reversible via outpatient surgical procedures (EDPRG, 2004b). The next most prevalent source of visual impairment among older persons is ARM, which involves a progressive and, as yet, incurable degeneration of central retinal structures. The risk of glaucoma also increases with age and involves the gradual and progressive destruction of the head of the optic nerve due to excessive pressure within the eye. Glaucoma responds reasonable well to drug therapy and much loss of function can be prevented if the disorder is detected early enough.

IV. Age-related Changes in Visual Function

A. Smooth Pursuit and Saccadic Eye Movements

The ability of the visual system to resolve color and fine spatial texture is mediated by the fovea. However, the centrally located fovea represents a very small region of visual space (approximately 2°). Optimal performance on many tasks depends on the ability of the oculomotor system to acquire, track, and maintain stimulus images on the foveal region of the retina. This acquisition and maintenance of the visual stimulus are mediated by two separate but complementary perceptual-motor systems: the *smooth pursuit* and *saccadic* eye movement systems. The smooth pursuit system regulates large-amplitude, continuous motion processes that serve to track moving targets accurately and thus enhance visual performance by extending the functional range of foveal vision across a broader region of visual space. The saccadic eye movement system generates brief, high-velocity, ballistic excursions of the eye, which serve structured visual search (e.g., reading).

Smooth pursuit performance is typically quantified in terms of *pursuit gain* (the ratio of eye velocity divided by target velocity). Ideal smooth pursuit eye tracking performance is signified by unity gain. At increasing target velocities, eye tracking performance begins to lag behind target position/speed and pursuit gain declines proportionately. Previous studies have reported little or no age-related reduction in pursuit gain for target velocities below 5–10°/s but greater rates of decline in pursuit gain as target velocities increased beyond this level (e.g., Sharpe & Sylvester, 1978; Spooner, Sakala, & Baloh, 1980; Kanayama et al., 1994). Of special interest, Kaufman and Abel (1986) demonstrated that age-related declines in smooth pursuit eye movement performance were exacerbated in the presence of competing or distracting objects in the stimulus background. More recently, Moschner and Baloh (1994) measured pursuit gain in a large sample of healthy young ($n = 23$, mean age $= 25$) and older ($n = 57$, mean age $= 79$) adults. The pursuit target oscillated sinusoidally along a $\pm18°$ horizontal meridian at velocities ranging from 11 to $45°/s$ while eye tracking performance was monitored using standard electrooculographic techniques. Age-related declines in smooth pursuit performance were observed at all three target velocities, and the magnitude of this deficit increased significantly with target velocity. Pursuit gain fell to 0.50 in older observers at the highest target velocity, whereas the performance of the young observers at this speed (gain $= 0.87$) was better than that achieved by their older counterparts at the slowest target velocity.

Saccadic eye movements show much less dramatic change with advancing age. Small but significant age-related increases in the latency of saccade onsets have been reported by numerous investigators (e.g., Abel, Troost, & Dell'Osso, 1983; Warabi, Kase, & Kato, 1984; Huaman & Sharpe, 1993; Moschner & Baloh, 1994; Abrams, Pratt, & Chasteen, 1998). The magnitude of this age-related increase in the latency of saccadic eye movements varies from approximately 20 ms (Moschner & Baloh, 1994; Abrams et al., 1998) to 100 ms (Abel et al., 1983), depending on task and stimulus conditions. The peak velocities of saccadic eye movements (which are very fast) have also been shown to slow with age. For example, Pitt and Rawles (1988) reported that saccade velocity decreased by approximately 0.25 % per year from 20 to 68 years of age. Similar findings have been reported by Spooner, Sakala, and Baloh (1980). Despite reports of slowing, there is reasonable agreement that the spatial accuracy of saccadic target acquisition is well maintained into very old age (Warabi et al., 1984; Hotson & Steinke, 1988; Rosenhall et al., 1987; Moschner & Baloh, 1994), but see Sharpe and

Zackon (1987). Related studies have also found that stable fixation accuracy can be maintained by older subjects for task durations of at least 10 s (Kosnik et al., 1987).

Another characteristic of oculomotor function that appears to be affected by aging is the range or extent of upward gaze (i.e., the maximum vertical extent of visual fixation that can be achieved without the benefit of head movement). Chamberlain (1971) reported that the maximum extent of upward gaze declines from $40°$ at 5–14 years of age down to approximately $15°$ by 84 years of age. More recently, Huaman and Sharpe (1993) used a high-resolution magnetic search coil to reassess the maximum extent of upward and downward gaze in young (mean $= 28.3$ years), middle-aged (mean $= 49.8$), and older (mean $= 71.9$) adults. The limits of upward gaze reported were 43.1, 42.0, and $32.9°$ for the young, middle-aged, and older age groups, respectively. Similar findings were reported for downward gaze. An explanation of the differences across studies remains unclear. It should be noted, however, that a more recent study by Clark and Isenberg (2001) yielded results consistent with data of Huaman and Sharpe (1993).

B. Light Sensitivity

The human retina consists of two complementary subsystems that enable it to efficiently process light signals over a remarkable range of stimulus intensities. The *scotopic* system receives input from the rods and performs best under low light levels (10^{-6} to 10^1 cd/m^2). The *photopic* system receives input from cones. Unlike the scotopic system, the photopc system is characterized by keen spatial resolving power and fine color discrimination. However, these enhanced capabilities come at a cost. The photopic system requires much more light (10^0 to

10^7 cd/m^2) in order to respond effectively (Geldard, 1972). When the eye is fully adapted to low light levels (e.g., a darkened hallway or a rural roadway at night), our ability to detect and recognize gross features in the visual environment is ultimately determined by the overall efficiency of the scotopic system. The ability to discriminate fine detail and/or color is dependent on the operating efficiency of the photopic system.

Older adults consistently report problems performing important visual tasks under dim lighting conditions and at night (Kline et al., 1992; Mangione et al., 1998; Owsley et al., 1999). Low illumination levels are related to age-related vehicular crashes and injuries related to falls (Massie, Campbell, & Williams, 1990; McMurdo & Gaskell, 1991). Much of this problem may be attributable to age-related declines in the sensitivity of the scotopic system, as well as the rate at which scotopic sensitivity dynamically adjusts to decreases in background illumination (i.e., dark adaptation). Studies in this area have improved our understanding of the special needs of older observers under low-light levels. Perhaps as important, these studies have enabled investigators to make headway in deciphering the relative roles of optical versus neural factors in mediating age-related declines of visual function.

1. Scotopic Sensitivity

In order to demonstrate the smallest amount of light that can be reliably detected by the human visual system, one must establish special conditions that manifest the ultimate sensitivity of the scotopic system: (1) allow the visual system to adapt to complete darkness for 30–40 min to allow for the full regeneration of rod photopigments necessary for the transduction of light and (2) present the target approximately 10° from central

fixation in order to stimulate the retina in the region of maximum rod density. Classical studies meeting these criteria have revealed age-related reductions in scotopic sensitivity ranging from 0.3 to 2.0 log units in magnitude (e.g., McFarland et al., 1960; Gunkel & Gouras, 1963). However, until very recently, investigators were unable to determine whether these changes were attributable only to age-related optical factors or whether neurophysiological mechanisms might also be involved.

Jackson and colleagues (1997) measured scotopic sensitivity in young (mean = 27 years) and old (mean = 70 years) adults while carefully controlling for optical factors that might contribute to age-related reductions in performance. For example, all participants were carefully screened for manifest ocular disease. Pupils were dilated to a minimum of 6 mm to eliminate the effects of pupillary miosis. Individual differences in lenticular density were measured and used to statistically adjust stimulus dosage at the level of the retina. Finally, all participants were refracted to the test distance to control for refractive error. Even after applying these unprecedented levels of controls to eliminate systematic effects due to optical factors, these investigators still observed a 0.5 log unit loss in scotopic sensitivity in their older group. Similar findings were reported in another carefully controlled study by Sturr and co-workers (1997). In a follow-up study, Jackson and Owsley (2000) replicated and extended these findings in an examination of scotopic and photopic sensitivity in a sample of 94 observers ranging in age from their twenties through eighties (photopic sensitivity data are discussed later). After controlling for all known optical sources of variation in data, they found that scotopic sensitivity declined at a rate of 0.08 log units per decade between 20 and 90 years of age — replicating the same 0.5 log unit (threefold)

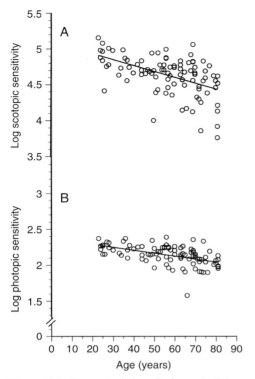

Figure 7.2 Scotopic (A) and photopic (B) sensitivity as a function of age. Source: Jackson and Owsley (2000).

reduction across the observed life span (see Figure 7.2). The authors interpreted these results as strong evidence for the involvement of neural mechanisms in the mediation of age-related losses in visual sensitivity under low luminance conditions. Although they could not rule out involvement of postreceptoral processes involving retinal ganglion cells, optic nerve, or cortical dysfunction given previously noted age-related changes at these levels, these investigators make a strong case for their "retinoid deficiency hypothesis" (see Jackson, Owsley, & Curcio, 2002). This hypothesis suggests that rods are more likely to suffer from the deleterious effects of age-related changes in retinal support structures responsible for satisfying the high metabolic demands of photoreceptor transduction.

2. Photopic Sensitivity

The limits of photopic light sensitivity are typically measured using stimuli delivered to the fovea — the rod-free central region of the retina that sets the limits on form and color vision. Jackson et al. (1997), as described earlier, conducted a carefully controlled assessment of age differences in photopic sensitivity by determining the minimum amount of retinal stimulation needed to detect a brief $1.7°$ light flash presented against a uniform $10 \ cd/m^2$ background. Their results are depicted in Figure 7.2B. Photopic sensitivity declined with age at a rate of 0.04 log units per decade. Thus, age-related declines in photopic sensitivity progress at half the rate observed for scotopic sensitivity. Even greater reductions in the rate of age-related losses of photopic sensitivity have been reported by Coile and Baker (1992). These finding are consistent with the hypothesis put forward by Jackson et al., (2002) that senescent processes differentially affect rod relative to cone function.

C. Spatial Resolution
1. Visual Acuity

Perhaps the best-known index of general visual function, visual acuity is a measure of one's ability to resolve fine spatial detail. Visual acuity is traditionally expressed in terms of the *minimum angle of resolution* (MAR) in minutes of arc. Normal visual acuity for the general population is 1 minarc, namely the smallest spatial contour that can be resolved subtends 1 min of arc (so-called 20/20 vision). It should be noted that many persons demonstrate spatial resolutions better than 1 minarc. In order to achieve optimal reliability, state-of-the-art visual acuity assessment instruments use charts with the same number of

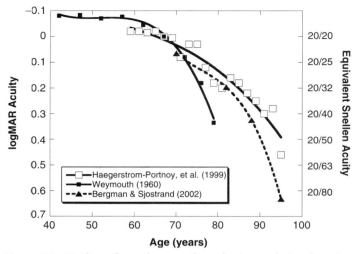

Figure 7.3 Findings from three studies of aging and visual acuity.

letters per line and with letter size and spacing decreasing in 0.1 log unit steps (see Rosser, Laidlaw, & Murdoch, 2001.

Pitts (1982) provided a comprehensive review of the classical literature on age-related changes in visual acuity. Findings across studies revealed a consistent pattern: Corrected visual acuity remained excellent (i.e., 1 minarc) into the sixth decade of life. Beginning in the sixth decade, corrected visual acuity began to decline at an accelerated pace. At this point, however, the consensus among the studies began to break down as the rate of senescent decline varied widely across investigations. Figure 7.3 compares the classical findings of Weymouth (1960) to recent results reported from Europe and North America. The two contemporary studies appear to be consistent and depict an aging visual system that is somewhat more robust than the classical findings (also see Elliott, Yang, & Whitaker, 1995). Both of the contemporary studies used large, representative community-resident samples and modern letter-by-letter scoring criteria. Classical studies, like Weymouth's, typically employed data collected in a clinical setting and used less precise line-by-line scoring

systems — factors that may have contributed to an overly pessimistic estimate of acuity declines expected with advancing adult age. Averaged across studies, the Haegerstrom-Portnoy et al. (1999) and Bergman and Sjostrand (2002) data indicate that representative corrected visual acuity declines from 1.2 minarc (20/24) at age 70 to 3.5 minarc (20/71) at 95 years of age (see Table 7.2).

The estimates presented in Table 7.2 reveal that relatively unimpaired levels of visual acuity can be maintained "for most persons" through the use of eyeglasses and/or contact lenses until 88 years of age. However, "average" values provide little information by which to assess the range of functional impact resulting from age-related declines in visual acuity. Fortunately, Bergman and Sjostrand (2002) provided a detailed breakdown of the distribution of acuity across the range of ages sampled in their study. A summary of their findings is presented in Figure 7.4, where the relative proportion of persons falling into three functional categories of vision are reported across age groups. The three categories of visual acuity, namely 20/25 or better, 20/26-20/66 and 20/66, or worse,

Table 7.2
Representative Corrected Acuity as a Function of Age from Two
Contemporary Studies

Age	Hagerstrom-Portnoy et al. (1999)		Bergman & Sjostrand (2002)		Pooled estimate	
	MAR[a]	Snellen	MAR[a]	Snellen	MAR[a]	Snellen
70	1.2	20/24	1.16	20/23	1.18	20/24
82	1.5	20/30	1.57	20/31	1.54	20/31
88	1.7	20/35	2.08	20/42	1.91	20/38
95	2.9	20/58	4.26	20/85	3.57	20/71

[a]Minimum angle of resolution (minute of arc).

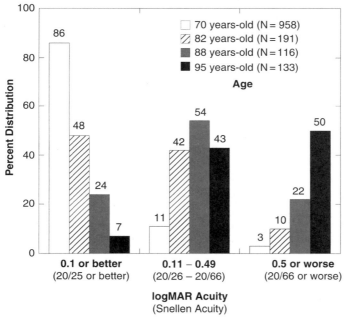

Figure 7.4 Functional levels of visual acuity distributed by age. Data from Bergman and Sjöstrand (2002).

represent levels of general visual function that can be described as "good," "marginal," and "impaired," respectively. Those falling into the "marginal" group would encounter problems reading small text or road signs from a great distance. Many with "marginal" acuity would be challenged when applying for or renewing their driver's license, as the minimum "uncorrected" visual acuity criterion for most state departments of transportation is 20/40 (2 minarc). However, this criterion has gradually been relaxed over the past decade and few drivers with acuities worse than 20/66 will ultimately be denied a driver's

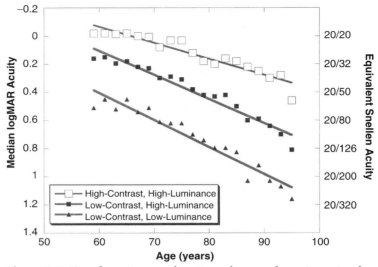

Figure 7.5 Visual acuity as a function of age and varying stimulus contrast and luminance. Source: Haegerstrom-Portnoy, Schneck, and Brabyn (1999).

license (Rosenbloom, 2004). Persons with visual acuities in the "impaired" region would likely have difficulty obtaining a driver's license and could also be expected to be challenged with many activities of daily living.

Several studies have reported that age differences in visual acuity are exacerbated under challenging viewing conditions such as low stimulus contrast and/or low luminance (e.g., Richards, 1977; Sturr, Kline, & Taub, 1990). Haegerstrom-Portnoy, Schneck, and Brabyn (1999) collected acuity data from a large ($N = 900$) sample of healthy older adults while varying background luminance (150 versus 15 cd/m^2) and/or letter contrast (90% versus 16% nominal contrast). Results of this study are summarized in Figure 7.5. Upon inspection of Figure 7.5, it is obvious that acuity declines at low target contrast and falls even farther when luminance is reduced as well. However, what is less apparent is that the slopes of these three

acuity-by-age functions significantly differ from one another. Acuity is lost at a rate of 5.5 letters (0.11 logMAR) per decade for the traditional high-contrast, high-luminance stimulus condition. However, this rate of loss increases to 8 letters (0.16 logMAR) per decade in the low-contrast, high-luminance condition. An even greater rate of loss (9 letters or 0.18 logMAR per decade) is observed when both contrast and luminance are reduced.

In discussing their findings, the authors pointed out an inconsistency in the research literature. Previous studies indicating that age differences in acuity were exacerbated under low-contrast conditions used *binocular* viewing conditions (i.e., Richards, 1977; Taub & Sturr, 1991; Haegerstrom-Portnoy et al., 1999). However, studies using *monocular* viewing conditions failed to observe accelerated age-related loss upon switching from high- to low-contrast stimuli (i.e., Brown & Lovie-Kitchin, 1989; Owsley et al., 1990). Haegerstrom-Portnoy et al. (1999)

concluded that this pattern of results is strongly consistent with the hypothesis that the efficiency of the binocular summation process is compromised with advancing age. This conclusion is also supported by studies of age differences in contrast sensitivity reported previously by Owsley and Sloane (1990) and Pardhan (1996) (see later). Regardless of the theoretical significance, the data presented in Figure 7.5 teach a practical lesson: standard tests of visual acuity under ideal conditions may not be the best indicators of functional status under the more challenging conditions typically encountered in real world settings (Schieber, 1988).

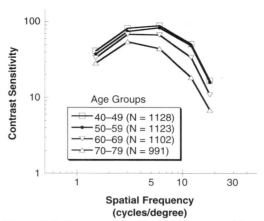

Figure 7.6 Contrast sensitivity functions of four age groups. Source: Nomura et al. (2003).

2. Contrast sensitivity

The ability to detect and recognize objects in the visual environment varies considerably as a function of target size, contrast, and spatial orientation (see Olzak & Thomas, 1985). As a consequence, knowledge about one's visual acuity (the ability to resolve small, high-contrast targets) is not always predictive of real world visual performance involving objects of various size and low-to-moderate contrast (e.g., Ginsburg et al., 1982; Watson, Barlow, & Robson, 1983). The *contrast sensitivity function* (CSF) complements and extends the information provided by simple measures of acuity by assessing an individual's visual efficiency for the detection of targets over an extended range of size and/or orientation. The CSF is determined by measuring the minimum contrast needed to detect idealized spatial targets (sine wave gratings) that vary in their spatial periodicity [cycles per degree of visual angle or (c/deg)]. Contrast thresholds are typically collected using sine wave grating stimuli that vary in spatial frequency from 0.5 c/deg (very wide) to 16–32 c/deg (very narrow). Because high levels of visual sensitivity

are associated with low-contrast thresholds, a reciprocal contrast sensitivity score (1/threshold contrast) is computed and plotted as a function of target spatial frequency, yielding the now familiar inverted U-shaped CSF (e.g., see Figure 7.6).

Numerous studies reveal a consistent pattern of age-related change in the CSF collected under photopic conditions (foveal presentation at moderate to high luminance levels). Contrast sensitivity declines by approximately 0.3 log units across the later half of the adult life span. Large magnitude losses such as these are typically reported for targets of intermediate and high spatial frequency (4–18 c/deg) (Owsley, Sekuler, & Siemsen, 1983; Elliott, 1987; Schieber et al., 1992; Elliott & Whitaker, 1992). However, several studies also report smaller age-related losses at low (less than 2 c/deg) spatial frequencies (Nameda, Kawara, & Ohzu, 1989; Ross, Clarke, & Bron, 1985; Sloane, Owsley, & Alvarez, 1988). Results from a large-scale study of contrast sensitivity reflect this consensus view. Nomura and co-workers (2003) used a clinical contrast sensitivity assessment chart (Vistech VCTS 6500) to assess normative differences in the CSF in a sample of 4344 adults ranging in age from 40 to 79 years of age. Referring to Figure 7.6, observers in their sixties demonstrated a 0.1 log unit loss in contrast sensitivity at intermediate and high spatial frequencies (6, 12, and 18 c/deg). Those in their seventies, the oldest group sampled, demonstrated an even greater loss (0.3 log unit) across the same range of spatial frequency. [Note: The apparent age-related loss in contrast sensitivity at the lowest spatial frequency probably resulted from the small number of stimulus cycles used in the 1.5-c/deg targets on the Vistech chart; see Savoy and McCann, (1975)].

Data of Nomura et al. (2003) also serve to demonstrate the relatively weak correlation between visual acuity and contrast sensitivity that is often observed, especially among older adults. Figure 7.7 shows the distribution of contrast sensitivities required to detect an 18-c/deg target among persons with "good" (20/20 or better) visual acuity. Even among groups of adults screened to preclude problems with visual acuity, large variations in contrast sensitivity performance

remain. It is noteworthy, for example, that 21% of those in their seventies failed to detect the 18-c/deg target at the highest contrast available (i.e., 33%), despite having acuities of 20/20 or better. This pattern of results is consistent with numerous studies that have shown that contrast sensitivity is a good predictor of age differences in visual performance even when subjects are equated for high-contrast visual acuity. For example, Owsley and Sloane (1987) reported that age-related problems in the detection and recognition of human faces could be accounted for by contrast sensitivity losses at intermediate spatial frequencies in observers with good visual acuity. Similar findings have been reported for performance with other domains of real world visual stimuli (e.g., Evans & Ginsburg, 1985; Kline et al., 1990).

Clear evidence shows that much, if not most, of the age-related loss of photopic contrast sensitivity can be explained by changes in the optical properties of the senescent eye. Numerous studies have demonstrated that systematic age differences in the quality of the retinal image due to pupillary miosis, lens opacification, and increased intraocular scatter contribute significantly to age-related reductions in contrast sensitivity (e.g., Owsley et al., 1983; Hemenger, 1984; Guirao et al., 1999). However, much debate remains regarding the relative contribution of neural factors (e.g., changes in the retina, optic nerve, and/or visual cortex) to age differences in contrast sensitivity. Numerous studies that have attempted to isolate the neural contributions to contrast sensitivity change by controlling for senescent changes in preretinal optics (e.g., Elliott, Whitaker & MacVeigh, 1990; Sloane, Owsley & Alvarez, 1988) or through bypassing the optics of the eye altogether by stimulating the retina via laser interferometry (Dressler & Rassow, 1981; Kayazawa, Yamamoto, & Itoi, 1981;

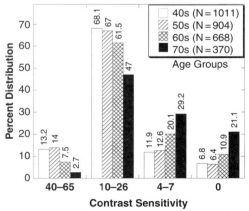

Figure 7.7 Distribution of contrast sensitivity by age for an 18 c/deg target from observers with visual acuity of 20/20 or better. Source: Nomura et al. (2003).

Morrison & McGrath, 1985; Burton, Owsley, & Sloane, 1993) have reported highly inconsistent conclusions. Estimates of the relative contribution of neural mechanisms toward explaining age-related losses in contrast sensitivity range from "zero" (Hemenger, 1984) to "substantial" (Morrison, & McGrath, 1985).

One conclusion that is certain is that the optics versus neural mechanisms debate will continue. It is hoped that, investigators will begin to use more diverse and powerful tools in their attempts to resolve these long-standing questions. In fact, several studies have demonstrated that such developments are already underway. Studies have used structural equation modeling in an attempt to disentangle the relative contributions of optical versus neural mediators of age differences in contrast sensitivity (e.g., Scialfa, Kline, & Wood, 2002). Other investigators have begun using "ideal observer models" of spatial vision together with noise-masking paradigms in an attempt to separate variations due to *internal noise* (which includes senescent optics effects) versus *computational efficiency* (nonoptical factors) (e.g., Pardhan et al., 1996; Bennett, Sekuler, & Ozin, 1999). These approaches hold great potential but will require long-term, programmatic efforts of research to rigorously evaluate the numerous (and yet to be tested) assumptions upon which they are based.

3. Vernier Hyperacuity

Vernier hyperacuity applies to a family of tasks in which the observer is required to detect deviations from perfect linear alignment among two or more suprathreshold visual objects (see Figure 7.8 for sample stimulus configurations). Normal observers are capable of detecting when one of the stimuli deviates from true linear alignment by as little as 5 to

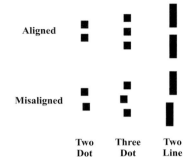

Figure 7.8 Schematic drawing depicting sample vernier acuity alignment stimuli. Stimulus elements are suprathreshold (typical stroke width of 3–5 minarc) separated vertically by a small gap (e.g., 4 minarc). The horizontal alignment of one of the elements is varied. The misalignment is exaggerated for illustration purposes.

10 s of arc. This is a tiny fraction of the smallest spatial gap that can be resolved by a person with 20/20 visual acuity (i.e., 60 s of arc). Hence, this exquisite sensitivity for relative spatial position has been referred to as "hyperacuity" (Westheimer, 1975). Performance on these types of tasks is quantified using two complementary measures: vernier acuity and vernier bias. As classically measured using the method of adjustment, the *vernier acuity* value is an index of the precision of a group of alignment judgments (i.e., the standard deviation). *Vernier bias*, however, refers to the average absolute deviation from true alignment (i.e., a measure of accuracy rather than precision).

Vernier hyperacuity has developed a bit of a mystique among vision researchers interested in aging. It has been claimed that vernier acuity has somehow escaped the deleterious effects of aging, unlike virtually every other measure of spatial vision, and has remained "forever young" (see Enoch et al., 1999). This interpretation is not surprising given the remarkable consensus in the research literature during the 1990s. Numerous studies have consistently reported that vernier acuity remained unchanged throughout the adult life span (e.g., Whitaker, Elliott, & MacVeigh, 1992; Lakshminarayanan, Aziz, & Enoch, 1992; Lakshminarayanan & Enoch, 1995; Vilar et al., 1995; Kline et al., 2001). All of these studies, with the exception of Odom and colleagues (1989), reported that vernier bias also remained stable with advancing adult age. The remarkable stability of vernier hyperacuity across the life span has often been attributed, in part, to its demonstrated insensitivity to optical degradations that might blur or reduce the intensity and/or contrast of the retinal image (Williams, Enoch, & Essock, 1984; Enoch et al., 1999). However, two studies appear to challenge the conclusion that vernier hyperacuity is resistant to aging.

Li, Edwards, and Brown (2000) hypothesized that one possible reason that previous investigations of vernier hyperacuity had failed to observe an age-related decline was because they failed to vary stimulus offset (or misalignment) in fine enough steps to reveal the true sensitivity of their youngest observers. In effect, they suggested that previous studies had systematically underestimated the sensitivity of young observers, thereby masking any true age difference. Indeed, a comparison of the minimum offset increments used in many of these studies reveals that stimuli were manipulated in a relatively crude manner (see Garcia-Suarez et al., 2004). Li et al. (2000) proceeded to measure vernier hyperacuity in a sample of 60 observers equally spaced across the life span between 21 and 75 years of age. Hyperacuity was assessed using a three-line vertical stimulus array in which the alignment of the central stimulus segment was offset between 0 and 18 s of arc (in increments of 6 arc s). The method of constant stimuli was employed using a two-alternative forced-choice procedure in which the observer's task was to report whether the middle line in the vernier stimulus array was displaced to the left or the right. Probit

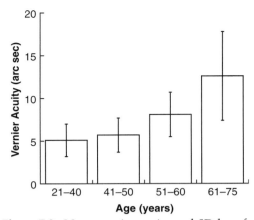

Figure 7.9 Mean vernier acuity and SD bars for four age groups. Source: Li, Edwards, and Brown (2000).

analysis was used to fit a "percent right" psychophysical function to the data. Vernier acuity was defined as half the distance between the 25 and 75% points on this psychophysical function. The "point of subjective equality" (i.e., the 50% point on the psychophysical function) was used as the index of vernier bias. Contrary to many previous studies, the precision of vernier localization was reduced significantly in older observers (see Figure 7.9). Vernier acuity levels remained unchanged between the ages of 21 and 50 but increased significantly between 51 and 75 years of age. A control experiment in which 8 young observers viewed stimuli through a 3-mm artificial pupil and a neutral density filter that reduced light transmission by approximately 60% indicated that expected age-related reductions in retinal illumination could not account for the observed age differences in performance. Finally, mean absolute misalignment error (vernier bias) did not vary as a function of age. Li et al. (2000) concluded that when one uses carefully designed psychophysical procedures and sufficiently small increments of misalignment in the vernier stimulus configuration that age-related declines in vernier acuity will be observed. A more recent study by Garcia-Suarez, Barrett and Pacey (2004) appears to confirm this conclusion. Using a three-point vernier alignment stimulus, the method of constant stimuli, and a very small misalignment increment step size (4.6 s of arc), they assessed vernier acuity in 18 young (mean age = 26.3) and 18 old (mean age = 72.0) highly practiced observers. Like the Li et al. (2000) study, they reported a 0.22 log unit age-related elevation in vernier hyperacuity threshold (7.22 and 11.98 arc s for young and old, respectively). Together, these two studies appear to have dramatically altered the landscape regarding the nature of age-related differences in vernier hyperacuity. Both groups of investigators have attributed these newly discovered age-related declines in spatial hyperacuity to senescent reductions in the efficiency of neural mechanisms. In a follow-up study, Li, Edwards, and Brown (2001) reported electrophysiological evidence consistent with this interpretation.

D. Color Vision

The human visual system is capable of remarkably precise discrimination on the basis of color. Observers with normal vision can distinguish among more than 100,000 hues generated from various combinations of three primary color light sources (Geldard, 1972). Most large-scale investigations of age differences in color discrimination have been based on the *Farnsworth-Munsell 100 Hues Test* (FM-100). The FM-100 is one of a family of color confusion tests in which small (1.4°) color-coated stimuli are arranged by the observer to form a linear sequence in which the most similar stimuli are placed side by side to form a predetermined color gradient. All test colors are of intermediate lightness and color saturation (Munsell value = 5, chroma = 5). The test is scored by counting the number of sequential arrangement errors, as well as noting their placement within each of four regions of color space. A total error score of 100 or more is indicative of anomalous performance (Farnsworth, 1943). Cody, Hurd, and Bootman (1990) demonstrated that older adults with poor FM-100 test scores were more likely to make errors discriminating between medicine capsules with similar color coding especially under relatively low illumination levels. Large-scale studies reported similar patterns of age-related loss in color discrimination performance (Verriest, van Laetham, & Uvijls, 1982; Roy et al., 1991). There is a linear increase in the number of color discrimination errors between 30 and 80 years of age. Much of this age-related change appears to be due to weakness in blue–yellow color mechanisms. That is, the color weakness that emerges with advancing adult age appears to mimic *tritanopia* — a relatively rare form of color anomaly resulting from a weakness in short wavelength (blue) cones. Thus, the typical older observer will tend to have difficulties discriminating between colored surfaces that differ by trace amounts of blue or yellow pigmentation. Representative results from a study of age differences in color discrimination using the FM-100 instrument by Kinnear and Schraie (2002) are presented in Figure 7.10. Note how the proportion of errors due to confusions along the blue–yellow axis of color space increases with age at a faster rate than errors along the red–green axis.

Much of the loss in the capacity for fine color discrimination appears to be related to senescent increases in the density of the ocular media, especially the yellowing and darkening of the crystalline lens. For example, Verriest (1963) reported that the performance of young persons on the FM-100 test became similar to that typically observed in the aged when those younger participants viewed test stimuli through a filter that selectively absorbed short wavelength light. Knoblauch et al. (1987) demonstrated that the tritan-like

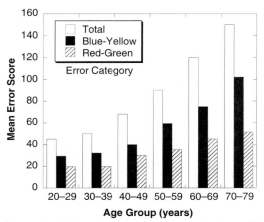

Figure 7.10 Error scores on Farnsworth–Munsell 100 hues test of color discrimination as a function of age. Source: Kinnear and Sahraie (2002).

color discrimination errors of older observers were mimicked in young and middle-aged adults when the FM-100 test was administered under conditions of reduced illumination (i.e., 5.7 lux instead of the traditional test illumination of 200 lux). This suggests that gain in the blue–yellow system may change more rapidly with reductions in the light adaptation level of the retina than gain in the red–green opponent color channel. A large-scale study of age differences in FM-100 color discrimination (Mäntyjärvi, 2001) used an illumination of 1000 lux instead of the conventional 200 lux standard illuminant. Compared to previous large-scale studies, the size of the aging effect appeared to be reduced.

Nonetheless, evidence shows that some of this loss in color discrimination performance may result from senescent changes in cones or postreceptoral processes. Numerous studies have reported age-related declines in the efficiency of the short wavelength (blue) cone system (Eisner et al., 1987; Haegerstrom-Portnoy, Hewlett, & Barr, 1989; Johnson et al., 1988). Other studies report similar rates of age-related loss in sensitivity for middle wavelength (green) and

long wavelength (red) cone systems as well. Werner and Steele (1988) examined age differences (10 to 84 years of age) in the sensitivity of short, medium and long wavelength cones using a chromatic adaptation isolation technique. Increment thresholds for monochromatic light stimuli selected to stimulate one class of cones were collected using a bright chromatic background adaptation field selected to reduce the sensitivity of the remaining two cone types. For example, use of a bright yellow background field suppresses the sensitivity of medium and long wavelength cones, thus allowing the short wavelength cones to set the limits on sensitivity for stimuli with wavelengths under 510 nm (Werner, Peterzell, & Scheetz, 1990). Increment thresholds collected in this fashion revealed similar patterns of age-related loss in sensitivity for all three cone types. More specifically, sensitivity losses of 0.12, 0.14, and 0.14 log units per decade were observed for short, medium, and long wavelength cones, respectively. Most of this loss in cone sensitivity observed across the life span could not be attributed to age-related changes in ocular media density.

Some of the most interesting research conducted recently on the topic of aging and vision has been concerned with the psychophysical scaling of suprathreshold color appearance. For example, Schefrin and Werner (1993) used a psychophysical scaling procedure to examine potential age differences in the appearance of real world broadband stimuli ("color chips") sampled from various regions across color space. Young (mean age = 21.3) and older (mean age = 71.9) participants screened for normal color vision and good ocular health rated the hue and colorfulness (i.e., color saturation) of five representative hues presented at three levels of lightness (i.e., apparent brightness of a reflective surface). Hue scaling was accomplished by rating each sample based on four color components: %-redness, %-green-ness, %-yellowness and %-blueness (the basic dimensions of opponent-color theory, described later). Participants were encouraged to use only two of these components when possible with the constraint that the sum of their hue component ratings for each stimulus must equal 100%. Given some practice, this scaling procedure has been demonstrated to yield reliable results (Gordon & Abramov, 1988). No age differences in hue scaling were observed, indicating that basic color naming performance was maintained through 70+ years of age. However, a different pattern of results was observed for judgments of perceived colorfulness or saturation. In a separate set of trials that followed the hue scaling procedure, these same observers rated each sample on a two component color saturation scale: %-chromatic versus %-achromatic appearance. Again, the sum of these components was constrained to 100%. The older observers consistently reported significant reductions in the strength of the chromatic component of their perceptual experience, especially at the lower lightness levels. In a follow-up study, Kraft and Werner (1999) found that this age-related reduction in the apparent colorfulness of chromatic stimuli was observed only in older adults with remarkable reductions in lens transmittance [i.e., less than 4% transmittance for short (420 nm) wavelength light].

The opponent-process theory, the most broadly supported theory of color vision, holds that output from long wavelength (L) and middle wavelength (M) cones are combined into a single push–pull, or opponent, "red–green" channel. Similarly, a second "blue–yellow" opponent channel is organized by contrasting input from short wavelength ("blue") cones with the summed inputs of L and M cones (to form the "yellow" side of the opponent channel). A simplified

prediction from this opponent-process theory of color vision holds that when activity within the red–green and blue–yellow channels is in equilibrium then no color contrast information is available. Such a condition leads to the perception of an achromatic stimulus. This is the so-called "white point" or "achromatic locus." Because the achromatic locus depends on the relative sensitivity of all three types of cones, as well as the dynamic response of both opponent-color processes, any systematic change in its color space coordinates with age would be indicative of compromised integrity of color perception. Indeed, well-known changes in the senescent lens, such as the differential absorption of short wavelength light, predict specific shifts in the coordinates of the achromatic locus with increasing adult age. That is, the combination of red, green, and blue color primaries needed to yield an achromatic experience would require a greater proportion of blue light to compensate for lens absorption (see Enoch et al., 1999). Yet, remarkably, Werner and Schefrin (1993) have demonstrated that the achromatic locus remains unchanged with advancing adult age. They assessed the position of the "white point" in CIE color space at three levels of retinal illuminance (10, 100, and 1000 Trolands) in 50 observers ranging from 11 to 78 years of age. All observers were determined to be in good ocular health. No reliable age differences in the position of the achromatic locus were observed. The average CIE 1931 coordinates of the achromatic locus was $x = 0.31$, $y = 0.31$ at all three levels of illuminance. Similar results consistent with the interpretation that the overall integrity of color vision is well maintained during senescence had been reported previously by Schefrin and Werner (1990) using a related paradigm to explore the sensitivity of the blue–yellow color contrast coding mechanism.

As noted by Enoch et al. (1999), the stability of the achromatic locus initially suggests that adult aging is not associated with alterations in the basic mechanisms mediating the appearance of colored stimuli. However, upon more careful consideration it becomes obvious that one or more mechanisms must be operating to compensate for lenticular changes in short wavelength opacity. Indeed, it appears that the same mechanisms of local retinal adaptation responsible for the phenomenon of *color constancy* (the invariance of color perception across relatively wide changes in the spectral composition of naturally occurring illumination) may also serve to compensate for systematic age-related changes in the spectral transmission properties of the ocular media. Indeed, Werner and Schefrin (1993) have presented quantitative evidence that modulation of the relative sensitivities of the three cone types could compensate for changes in the spectral content of the retinal image caused by age-related changes in the lens. Enoch et al. (1999) suggested that the mechanisms responsible for everyday color constancy may compensate for a broad range of senescent changes in the visual system in the service of maintaining robust color perception. A recent study by Delahunt et al., (2004) provides additional support for the working hypothesis that color constancy mechanisms contribute to the maintenance of robust color perception in old age. Cataracts tend to differentially absorb short wavelength light but to a much greater extent than normal aging of the lens. Immediately following cataract surgery, patients often report large shifts in color appearance. Predictably, blues and blue–greens are particularly affected. Delahunt et al. (2004) quantified these shifts in color appearance by assessing the achromatic locus (described earlier) before and after cataract surgery in four patients (ranging from 63 to 84 years of age). Prior to surgery, participants reported near-normal achromatic loci in color space, indicating good compensation for short wavelength absorption by their cataracts. However, immediately following surgery the achromatic locus shifted toward the yellow region of color space. Such a shift was consistent with the hypothesized compensation in the blue–yellow mechanisms in response to the alterations in retinal illuminance resulting from cataracts. This postoperative shift in the achromatic locus gradually subsided over the course of the 12-month follow-up assessment. Of particular interest was the fact that the achromatic locus measured in the companion eye of each participant failed to demonstrate any of the postoperative shift or recovery for the achromatic locus. Consistent with the conclusions of Werner and Schefrin (1993), lack of an interocular transfer for the postoperative shift in color appearance suggests that the compensatory processes responsible for maintaining robust senescent color perception occur at the level of the retina rather than in the visual cortex. Also of note, the time course of these adaptation processes occurs on a scale many orders of magnitude longer than that typically associated with classical mechanisms of color constancy such as von Kries adaptation.

E. Temporal Resolution

One of the most fundamental changes in vision that accompanies normal adult aging is the systematic loss of the ability to detect and efficiently process rapid temporal changes in the environment. Temporally contiguous visual events that would be seen as separate and distinct by young observers often appear "fused" or indistinguishable by older individuals (Kline & Schieber, 1982). This loss of temporal resolving power in the visual system manifests itself in the form of apparent age-related slowing in higher order visual processes such as the sequential integration of form (see Kline & Orme-Rogers, 1978; Kline & Schieber, 1980) and backward masking (Kline & Birren, 1975; Walsh, 1976), but is also readily observed in the form of age-related deficits that emerge in rudimentary visual functions such as flicker sensitivity, dynamic visual acuity, speed, and motion perception. Theoretical speculations regarding the mechanism (or mechanisms) mediating this age-related loss in visual temporal resolution are numerous. Some investigators have explained such age differences within the context of general slowing due to random brain cell loss (Cerella, 1990); increased stimulus persistence (Botwinck, 1973); selective loss of transient/magnocellular channel sensitivity (Kline & Schieber, 1981); and, more recently, diminished temporal contrast sensitivity (Shinomori & Werner, 2002).

1. Flicker Sensitivity

The classical method for assessing the temporal resolution of low-level visual processes is the *critical flicker frequency* (CFF) threshold. The CFF represents the minimum frequency of a pulsating (high contrast) light source at which the light appears to be perceptually "fused" into a continuous, rather than flickering, stimulus. Because the stimulus at the CFF threshold is still physically oscillating between "on" and "off" states, it is thought to represent the temporal periodicity at which the visual system can no longer reliably detect rapid changes in scene luminance. There is a well-documented decline in the CFF threshold with advancing age (Brozek & Keys, 1945; McFarland, Warren, & Karis, 1958; Huntington & Simonson, 1965). For example, Wolf and Shaffra (1964) collected CFF thresholds from a sample of 302 observers ranging from 6 to 95

years of age. Flicker sensitivity (and CFF thresholds) decreased gradually between childhood and 60 years of age and declined rapidly thereafter. Experimental manipulations have clearly revealed that much of the age-related decline in the CFF threshold can be attributed to reduced levels of retinal illumination accompanying normal changes in the ocular media and pupillary miosis. However, studies by Weekers and Roussel (1945) and McFarland et al. (1958) support the notion that a significant proportion of the age differences in the CFF may be attributable to senescent changes in the visual nervous system (see Kline & Schieber, 1985).

More contemporary studies of aging and flicker sensitivity have abandoned the CFF threshold paradigm in favor of measuring the *temporal contrast sensitivity function* (tCSF)—a more comprehensive assessment of visual system response in the temporal domain (Wright & Drasdo, 1985; Mayer et al., 1988; Tyler, 1989). When assessing the tCSF, the brightness of a small (2–5°) self-luminous circular target is sinusoidally modulated at a given temporal frequency around a baseline luminance value. Next, the minimum luminance contrast modulation required to detect the presence of flicker is determined for a range of temporal frequencies, which typically extends from 1 to 50 cycles per second (Hz). Wright and Drasdo (1985) collected tCSFs from 70 observers sampled equally across the life span between 10 and 79 years of age. They reported an age-related decrease in temporal contrast sensitivity that grew in magnitude as temporal frequency was increased from 3.3 to 30 Hz. Tyler (1989) measured tCSFs in a large sample of observers ranging from 5 to 75 years of age. He reported a "leftward shift" in the shape of the tCSF among older observers, i.e., a migration of peak temporal contrast sensitivity from higher to lower temporal frequencies. Tyler

(1989) interpreted this age-related leftward shift in the shape of the tCSF as evidence for a generalized slowing in visual information processing and estimated the magnitude of this slowing to approach 20% by 75 years of age. However, Mayer and colleagues (1988) provided evidence that the qualitative difference in the shape of the tCSF for older observers that emerged in these studies could be accounted for primarily on the basis of age-related reductions in retinal illumination.

In a follow-up study, Kim and Meyer (1994) collected tCSF data from 89 observers ranging from 18 to 77 years of age. They used a bright (120 cd/m^2), long wavelength (660 nm) stimulus and statistically controlled for individual differences in pupil size to minimize the influence of any age-related variations in retinal illumination. Upon carefully controlling for differences in retinal illumination, they found a small but statistically significant age-related reduction in temporal contrast sensitivity across the range of temporal frequencies observed. The magnitude of this generalized loss of temporal contrast sensitivity was approximately 0.08 log units per decade beyond 44 years of age. Unlike Tyler's (1989) study, they failed to observe a leftward shift in the overall shape of the tCSF in their older observers and concluded that aging was characterized by a reduction in sensitivity of temporally tuned visual mechanisms rather than a generalized "slowing" in the rate of visual processing. Additional data analyses conducted by Kim and Mayer (1994) provided support for this interpretation of their data. According to linear systems theory, the *impulse response function* (IRF) quantitatively describes the response of the visual system to temporally modulated stimulus input. The classic IRF is biphasic, consisting of an initial excitatory response followed shortly by an inhibitory rebound (see

Figure 7.11B for some examples of an impulse response function). Within constraints, the IRF can be derived via Fourier transformation of the tCSF curve. Upon deriving IRFs in this way for each age group, a clear pattern emerged. Both the peak amplitude and the area of the first (excitatory) lobe of the IRFs for older observers were significantly diminished in magnitude. However, neither the latency of the peak response nor the zero crossing (point of transition between excitatory and inhibitory lobes) slowed with advancing adult age.

Shinomori and Werner (2003) noted that there are some mathematical and conceptual problems associated with the derivation of the temporal impulse response (tIRF) from the temporal contrast sensitivity function (tCSF) using Fourier transformation. tIRFs derived in this manner appear to preserve response amplitude but may not adequately preserve phase (i.e., temporal) information. They proposed that an alternative psychophysical method and modeling approach (see Burr & Morrone, 1993) could be used to assess potential age differences more accurately in the tIRF of the visual system. This approach is based on the *two-pulse contrast detection function* (2PCDF). The 2PCDF is generated by measuring the minimum contrast needed to detect the occurrence of a pair of rapidly presented light pulses as a function of the variable interstimulus interval separating these pulses. The shape of the tIRF can be derived more accurately from 2PCDF data because the autocorrelation function is preserved (for technical details, see Shinomori & Werner, 2003). Two-pulse contrast detection functions were collected from 70 observers between 16 and 86 years of age. Pulses with a duration of 1.2 ms and interstimulus intervals ranging from 6.7 to 180 ms were employed. Representative 2PCDFs and derived tIRFs for a young and an older observer, respectively, are

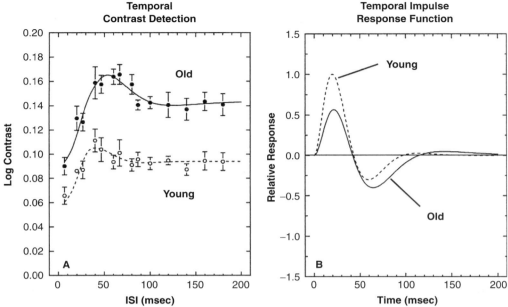

Figure 7.11 Two-pulse contrast detection functions (A) and derived temporal impulse response functions (B) for a representative young and older observer. Source: Shinomori and Werner (2003).

depicted in Figure 7.11. The investigators reported that two-pulse contrast detection thresholds were uniformly elevated with advancing adult age. More interesting, given the current context, was the finding that tIRFs of older observers consistently demonstrated reduced amplitude for the initial excitatory phase with no systematic age differences in the latency of the peak response (or zero crossing between response phases). Hence, Shinomori and Werner (2003) were able to independently confirm the previous conclusion of Kim and Mayer (1994) using an entirely different approach. It would appear, therefore, that age-related changes in flicker sensitivity are indicative of reduced contrast sensitivity within temporally tuned visual mechanisms instead of a more generalized slowing in visual processing. It should be noted, however, that this does not preclude visual slowing as a mediator in other areas of visual perception. Finally, Shinomori and Werner (2003) also noted that the second, or inhibitory, lobe of the tIRF was attenuated greatly or entirely missing in many of their oldest participants. A visual system characterized by such a loss in late, inhibitory processes appears to be consistent with the classical notion of increased "stimulus persistence" in senescent visual information processing (see Kline & Schieber, 1982).

2. Motion Sensitivity

Numerous studies have reported age-related declines in motion detection and discrimination thresholds. One of the most basic approaches to measuring motion sensitivity involves the assessment of the *oscillatory motion displacement threshold* (OMDT). In this paradigm, the spatial position of a stimulus is displaced rhythmically along the horizontal or vertical meridian in a sinusoidal fashion. The minimum amplitude of displacement required to reliably discriminate moving from stationary stimuli is then determined as a function of the temporal frequency of spatial oscillation. Buckingham, Whitaker, and Banford (1987) collected OMDTs from a sample of young (mean age: 20.7), middle-aged (mean age: 48.0), and older (mean age: 69.7) observers using a low spatial-frequency sine wave grating target that oscillated at frequencies ranging from 1 to 20 Hz. Marked and consistent age-related declines in motion sensitivity were observed across the full range of temporal frequencies. For example, at 8 Hz mean OMDTs of 39, 52, and 97 s of arc were observed for the young, middle-aged, and older observers, respectively. Similar findings have been reported by other investigators who have used careful experimental controls indicating that such sizable age differences in OMDT measures of motion sensitivity are independent of age-related changes in retinal illumination and/or refractive error (e.g., Elliott, Whitaker, & Thompson, 1989; Schieber et al., 1990; Kline et al., 1994). As such, OMDT appears to represent a class of hyperacuity phenomena that may provide a uniquely powerful approach to separating the effects of neural versus optical aging in the visual system.

Several groups of investigators have used random dot motion paradigms to study age differences in the sensitivity of *global motion* detection mechanisms. Observers are presented with a large number of small, randomly positioned dots on a computer display. Using basic animation techniques, these dots then take "random walks" across the display during brief stimulus exposures. Under the conditions just described, the observer can not perceive a principal direction of motion in the flow of dots (because there is none). More and more "correlated motion" is gradually added to the stimulus display (by having more and more dots move in a given direction across subsequent frames) until the observer can reliably detect a directional trend in the overall pattern of motion. The amount of correlated motion required to correctly discriminate the direction of flow is the *global motion threshold*. Motion in this case is said to be global, as it represents a statistical trend in the entire population of dot stimuli rather than within any given dot *per se*. Dots contributing to the correlated direction of flow are assigned randomly from one frame of the animation sequence to the next. Trick and Silverman (1991) used this technique to assess age differences in global motion sensitivity. They found that motion sensitivity declined by 50% between 25 and 80 years of age. Gilmore and colleagues (1992) also found sizable age-related declines in global motion sensitivity using a random dot motion paradigm. However, such reductions in global motion sensitivity were limited to the female members of their sample of older observers. Unfortunately, the earlier study by Trick and Silverman (1991) did not report any analyses of their data based on gender. However, two studies using the random dot paradigm that did conduct such analyses have also reported the same interaction, namely global motion sensitivity was reduced in older females but not in older males. Experimental controls in both of these studies indicated that these gender-specific losses were independent of ocular factors, such as differences in retinal illuminance or refractive error (Schieber et al., 1990; Atchley & Anderson, 1998). In the Schieber et al., (1990) study of global motion sensitivity, oscillatory motion detection thresholds (OMDTs) for single dot stimuli were also measured. A strong age-related increase in OMDTs of equal magnitude was observed among both older males and females. This pattern of results suggests that the global motion deficit observed in older females is probably mediated by a reduced efficiency of "spatial pooling" or integration of the motion signal over large regions of space at a location in the nervous system beyond the primary visual cortex. Previous studies using the random dot paradigm indicate that a likely site for this visual processing deficit in older females is the medial temporal (MT) area (see Newsome & Pare, 1988; Zeki et al., 1991).

3. Speed Perception

Clear and compelling evidence shows age-related declines in motion sensitivity under ideal laboratory conditions. What is less clear, however, is how this motion sensitivity deficit scales to real world judgments of absolute and relative speed such as those necessary for safe and efficient operation of a motor vehicle. Scialfa and co-workers (1991) examined age differences in the magnitude estimations of vehicle velocity for actual automobiles traveling around a test track at speeds varying from 15 to 50 mph (24–80 kph). Young (mean age: 22.2) observers tended to underestimate the speed of slowly moving vehicles (15 mph) and overestimate the speed of the most rapidly moving vehicle (50 mph). Older (mean age: 65.3) observers demonstrated a similar, but less severe, slow underestimation/fast overestimation bias. The resulting psychophysical functions relating perceived speed to actual speed suggested that older observers were less sensitive to relative changes in velocity, but, at the same time, demonstrated more accurate absolute judgments of speed at the two ends of the velocity range examined. Staplin, Lococo, and Sim (1993) conducted a series of complementary simulation and field studies that strongly suggested that the perceptual basis of "time-to-collision" and "traffic gap acceptance judgments" changes significantly with advancing adult age.

Relative to younger drivers, older observers seated in a stationary vehicle tended to underestimate the time required for an approaching vehicle to reach their current position. Although less accurate, these judgments erred on the conservative side (i.e., persons making such errors would be less rather than more likely to become engaged in a traffic conflict). Andersen and co-workers (2000) reported similar findings in a part-task visual simulation of vehicular deceleration while approaching a stop sign at an intersection. These authors speculate that such losses in the accuracy of effortless visual perceptual guidance may require compensatory cognitive effort while negotiating intersections. The full costs of such perceptual to cognitive trade-offs remain to be determined.

4. Form from Motion

Spatial vision is principally concerned with the processing and recognition of forms defined by variations in luminance and/or wavelength across space (i.e., luminance and/or color contrast). However, form perception can also be quite robust for motion gradients across space. For example, observers typically have no difficulty perceiving the border between two adjacent regions in a field of random dots moving at sufficiently different angular velocities (Regan & Hong, 1990). Several studies suggest that the ability to perceive motion-defined contours declines dramatically with advancing adult age. For example, Wist, Schrauf, and Ehrenstein (2000) assessed the ability of observers to discriminate between simple geometric forms defined by briefly presented (240 ms) motion gradients (stationary versus moving) in a high-density random dot field. The amount of motion contrast required to discriminate such motion-defined stimuli increased dramatically between 20 and 70 years of age. In fact, half of the observers over the age of 70 were completely unable to discriminate motion-defined form when 100% of the dots in the foreground region moved at a robust level of 1.3°/s. In a related study, Andersen and Atchley (1995) reported that older observers had difficulty perceiving motion-defined, three-dimensional-corrugated surfaces. Similarly, Norman and colleagues (2004) reported that older observers demonstrated difficulty recognizing short animated sequences (6 frames across 240 ms) depicting "biological motion." However, much of this age-related deficit disappeared for longer animated sequences (i.e., 10 frames across 400 ms). The variety of age-related problems observed with the perception of *form-from-motion* stimuli suggests that additional investigations into these phenomena hold great promise for helping to better understand the neurophysiological mechanisms mediating visual aging.

References

Abel, A. L., Troost, B. T., & Dell'Osso, L. F. (1983). The effect of age on normal saccadic characteristics and their variability. *Vision Research, 23,* 33–37.

Abrams, R. A., Pratt, J., & Chasteen, A. L. (1998). Aging and movement: Variability of force pulses for saccadic eye movements. *Psychology and Aging, 13,* 387–395.

Andersen, G. J., & Atchley, P. (1995). Age-related differences in the detection of three-dimensional surfaces from optic flow. *Psychology and Aging, 10,* 650–658.

Andersen, G. J., Cisneros, J., Saidpour, A. & Atchley, P. (2000). Age-related differences in collision detection during deceleration. *Psychology and Aging, 15,* 241–252.

Anderson, D. H., Mullins, R. F., Hageman, G. S., & Johnson, L.V. (2002). A role for local inflammation in the formation of drusen in the aging eye. *American Journal of Ophthalmology, 134,* 411–431.

Artal, P., Berrio, E., Guirao, A., & Piers, P. (2002). Contribution of the cornea and internal surfaces to the change of ocular aberrations with age. *Journal of the Optical Society of America A, 19,* 137–143.

Artal, P., Guirao, A., Berrio, E., Piers, P., & Norrby, S. (2003). Optical aberrations and the aging eye. *International Ophthalmology Clinics, 43,* 63–77.

Atchison, D.A. (1995). Accommodation and presbyopia. *Ophthalmic and Physiological Optics, 15,* 255–272.

Atchley, P., & Andersen, G. J. (1998). The effect of age, retinal eccentricity, and speed on the detection of optic flow components. *Psychology and Aging, 13,* 297–308.

Baldwin, W., & Mills, D. (1981). A longitudinal study of corneal astigmatism and total astigmatism. *American Journal of Optometry and Physiological Optics, 58,* 206–211.

Bennett, P. J., Sekuler, A. B., & Ozin, L. (1999). Effects of aging on calculation efficiency and equivalent noise. *Journal of the Optical Society of America. A., 16,* 654–668.

Bergman, B., & Sjöstrand, J. (2002). A longitudinal study of visual acuity and visual rehabilitation needs in an urban Swedish population followed from the ages of 70 to 97 years of age. *Acta Ophthalmologica Scandanavica, 80,* 598–607.

Bonnel, S., Mohand-Said, S., & Sahel, J. (2003). The aging of the retina. *Experimental Gerontology, 38,* 825–831.

Botwinick, J. (1973). *Aging and behavior.* New York: Springer.

Brown, B., & Lovie-Kitchin, J. E. (1989). High and low contrast acuity and clinical contrast sensitivity tested in a normal population. *Optometry and Vision Science, 66,* 467–473.

Brozek, J., & Keys, A. (1945). Changes in flicker-fusion frequency with age. *Journal of Consulting Psychology, 9,* 87–90.

Buckingham, T., Whitaker, D., & Banford, D. (1987). Movement in decline? Oscillatory movement displacement thresholds increase with age. *Ophthalmic and Physiologic Optics, 7,* 411–413.

Burr, D. C., & Morrone, M. C. (1993). Impulse-response functions for chromatic and achromatic stimuli. *Journal of the Optical Society of America A, 10,* 1706–1713.

Burton, K. B., Owsley, C., & Sloane, M. E. (1993). Aging and neural spatial contrast sensitivity: Photopic vision. *Vision Research*, 33, 939–946.

Chamberlain, W. (1971). Restriction of upward gaze with advancing age. American *Journal of Ophthalmology*, 71, 341–346.

Clark, R. A., & Isenberg, S.J. (2001). The range of ocular movement decreases with aging. *Journal of the American Association of Pediatric Ophthalmology and Strabismus*, 5, 26–30.

Cerella, J. (1990). Aging and information processing rate. In J.E. Birren & K.W. Schaie (Eds.), *Handbook of the psychology of aging* (3rd edition, pp. 201–221). San Diego: Academic Press.

Cody, P. S., Hurd, P. D., & Bootman, J. L. (1990). The effects of aging and diabetes on the perception of medication color. *Journal of Geriatric Drug Therapy*, 4, 113–121.

Coile, D. C., & Baker, H. D. (1992). Foveal dark adaptation, photopigment regeneration and aging. *Visual Neuroscience*, 8, 27–39.

Coren, S., & Girgus, J. S. (1972). Density of human lens pigmentation: In vivo measures over an extended age range. *Vision Research*, 12, 343–346.

Corso, J. F. (1981). *Aging sensory systems and perception*. New York: Praeger.

Curcio, C. A., & Drucker, D. N. (1993). Retinal ganglion cells in Alzheimer's disease and aging. *Annals of Neurology*, 33, 248–257.

Cucio, C. A., Millican, C. L., Allen, K. A. & Kalina, R.E. (1993). Aging and the human photoreceptor mosaic: Evidence for selective vulnerability of rods in central retina. *Investigative Ophthalmology and Visual Science*, 34, 3278–3296.

Curcio, C. A., Millican, C. L., Bailey, T., & Kruth, H.S. (2001). Accumulation of cholesterol with age in human Bruch's membrane. *Investigative Ophthalmology and Visual Science*, 42, 265–274.

Curcio, C. A., Owsley, C., & Jackson, G. R. (2000). Spare the rods, save the cones in aging and age-related maculopathy. *Investigative Ophthalmology and Visual Science*, 41, 2105–2018.

Curcio, C. A., Sloan, K. R., Kalina, R. E., & Hendrickson, A.E. (1990). Human photoreceptor topography. *Journal of Comparative Neurology*, 292, 497–523.

Delahunt, P. B., Webster, M. A., Ma, L., & Werner, J.S. (2004). Long-term

normalization of chromatic mechanisms following cataract surgery. *Visual Neuroscience*, 21, 301–307.

Devaney, K., & Johnson, H. A. (1980). Neuron loss in the aging visual cortex of man. *Journal of Gerontology*, 35, 836–841.

Donders, F.C (1864). *On the anomalies and accommodation and refraction of the eye*. London: The Sydenham Society.

Dressler, M., & Rassow, B. (1981). Neural contrast sensitivity measurement with a laser interference system for clinical screening and application. *Investigative Ophthalmology and Visual Science*, 21, 737–744.

Eisner, A. E., Berk, L., Burns, S. A., & Rosenberg, P. R. (1988). Aging and human cone photopigments. *Journal of the Optical Society of America A*, 5, 2106–2112.

Eisner, A., Fleming, S. A., Klein, M. L., & Mauldin, W. M. (1987). Sensitivities in healthy older eyes with good acuity: Cross-sectional norms. *Investigative Ophthalmology and Visual Science*, 28, 1824–1831.

Elliott, D. B. (1987). Contrast sensitivity decline with aging: A neural or optical phenomenon? *Ophthalmic and Physiological Optics*, 7, 415–419.

Elliott, D. B., & Whitaker, D. (1992). Clinical contrast sensitivity chart evaluation. *Ophthalmic and Physiological Optics*, 12, 275–280.

Elliott, D. B., Whitaker, D., & MacVeigh, D. (1990). Neural contribution to spatiotemporal contrast sensitivity decline in healthy ageing eyes. *Vision Research*, 30, 541–547.

Elliott, D. B., Whitaker, D., & Thompson, P. (1989). Use of displacement threshold hyperacuity to isolate the neural component of senile vision loss. *Applied Optics*, 28, 1914–1918.

Elliott, D. B., Yang, K. C., & Whitaker, D. (1995). Visual acuity changes throughout adulthood in normal, healthy eyes: seeing beyond 6/6. *Optometry and Vision Science*, 72, 186–191.

Enoch, J. M., Werner, J. S., Haegerstrom-Portnoy, G., Lakshminarayanan, V., & Rynders, M. (1999). Forever young: Visual functions not affected or minimally affected by aging: A review. *Journal of Gerontology: Biological Sciences*, 54A, B336–B351.

Evans, D. W., & Ginsburg, A. P. (1985). Contrast sensitivity predicts age differences in highway sign discriminability. *Human Factors, 23,* 59–64.

Eye Diseases Prevalence Research Group (2004a). Causes and prevalence of visual impairment among adults in the United States. *Archives of Ophthalmology, 122,* 477–485.

Eye Diseases Prevalence Research Group (2004b). Prevalence of cataract and pseudo-aphakia/aphakia among adults in the United States. *Archives of Ophthalmology, 122,* 487–494.

Eye Diseases Prevalence Research Group (2004c). Prevalence of open-angle glaucoma among adults in the United States. *Archives of Ophthalmology, 122,* 532–538.

Eye Diseases Prevalence Research Group (2004d). Prevalence of age-related macular degeneration among adults in the United States. *Archives of Ophthalmology, 122,* 564–572.

Farnsworth, D. (1943). The Farnsworth-Munsell 100-Hue and dichotomous tests for color vision. *Journal of the Optical Society of America, 33,* 568–578.

Fintz, A. C., Audo, I., Hicks, D., Mohand-Said, S., Leveillard, T., & Sahel, J. (2003). Partial characterization of retina-derived cone neuroprotection in two culture models of photoreceptor degeneration. *Investigative Ophthalmology and Visual Science, 44,* 818–825.

Fledelius, H. (1988). Refraction and eye size in the elderly. *Archives of Ophthalmology, 66,* 241–248.

Fozard, J. L., & Gordon-Salant, S. (2001). Changes in vision and hearing with age. In J. E. Birren & K. W. Schaie (Eds.), *Handbook of the psychology of aging* (5th edition, pp. 241–266). San Diego: Academic Press.

Gao, H., & Hollyfield, J. G. (1992). Aging of the retina-differential loss of neurons and retinal pigment epithelial cells. *Investigative Ophthalmology and Visual Science, 33,* 1–17.

Garcia-Saurez, L., Barrett, B. T., & Pacey, I. (2004). A comparison of the effects of ageing upon vernier and bisection acuity. *Vision Research, 44,* 1039–1045.

Gartner, S., & Henkind, P. (1981). Aging and degeneration of the human macula. 1. Outer nuclear layer and photoreceptors.

British Journal of Ophthalmology, 65, 23–28.

Geldard, F. A. (1972). *The human senses.* New York: Wiley.

Gilmore, G. C., Wenk, H. E., Naylor, L. A., & Stuve, T. A. (1992). Motion perception and aging. *Psychology and Aging, 7,* 654–660.

Ginsburg, A. P., Evans, D., Sekuler, R., & Harp, S. (1982). Contrast sensitivity predicts pilots' performance in aircraft simulators. *American Journal of Optometry and Physiological Optics, 59,* 105–109.

Gordon, J., & Abramov, I. (1988). Scaling procedures of specifying color appearance. *Color Research and Application, 13,* 146–152.

Guirao, A., Gonzalez, C., Redondo, M., Geraghty, E., Norrby, S., & Artal, P. (1999). Average optical performance of the human eye as a function of age in a normal population. *Investigative Ophthalmology and Visual Science, 40,* 203–213.

Guirao, A., Redondo, M., & Artal, P. (2000). Optical aberrations of the human cornea as a function of age. *Journal of the Optical Society of America A, 17,* 1697–1702.

Gunkel, R.D., & Gouras, P. (1963). Changes in scotopic visibility thresholds with age. *Archives of Ophthalmology, 69,* 38–43.

Haegerstrom-Portnoy, G., Hewlett, S. E., & Barr, S. A. N. (1989). S-cone loss with aging. In B. Drum, & G. Verriest, (Eds.), *Color vision deficiencies IX* (pp. 345–352) Dordrecht: Kluwer.

Haegerstrom-Portnoy, G., Schneck, M. E., & Brabyn, J. A. (1999). Seeing into old age: Vision function beyond acuity. *Optometry and Vision Science, 76,* 141–158.

Haug, H., Kuhl, S., Mecke, E., Sass, N. L., & Wassner, K. (1984). The significance of morphometric procedures in the investigation of age changes in the cytoarchetronic structures of the human brain. *Journal für Hirnforschung, 25,* 353–374.

Hemenger, R.P. (1984). Intraocular light scatter in normal vision loss with age. *Applied Optics, 23,* 1972–1974.

Hofstetter, H. W. (1965). A longitudinal study of amplitude changes in presbyopia. *American Journal of Optometry, 42,* 3–8.

Hotson, J. R., & Steinke, G. W. (1988). Vertical and horizontal saccades in aging and dementia. *Neuroophthalmology*, *4*, 267–273.

Huaman, A. G., & Sharpe, J. A. (1993). Vertical saccades in senescence. *Investigative Ophthalmology and Visual Science*, *34*, 2588–2595.

Huntington, J. M., & Simonson, E. (1965). Critical flicker fusion frequency as a function of exposure time in two different age groups. *Journal of Gerontology*, *20*, 527–529.

Jackson, G. R., Ortega, J., Girkin, C., Rosenstiel, C. E., & Owsley, C. (2002). Age-related changes in the multifocal electroretinogram. *Journal of the Optical Society of America A*, *19*, 185–189.

Jackson, G. R., & Owsley, C. (2000). Scotopic sensitivity during adulthood. *Vision Research*, *40*, 2467–2473.

Jackson, G. R., Owsley, C., Cordle, E. P., & Finley, C. D. (1997). Aging and scotopic sensitivity. *Vision Research*, *38*, 3655–3662.

Jackson, G. R., Owsley, C., & Curcio, C. A. (2002). Photoreceptor degeneration and dysfunction in aging and age-related maculopathy. *Ageing Research Reviews*, *1*, 381–396.

Johnson, C. A., Adams, A. J., Twelker, J. D., & Quigg, J. M. (1988). Age-related changes in the central visual field for short-wavelength sensitive pathways. *Journal of the Optical Society of America A*, *5*, 2131–2139.

Kanayama, R., Nakamura, T., Sana, R., Ohki, M., Okuyama, T., Kimura, Y., & Koike, Y. (1994). Effect of aging on smooth pursuit eye movement. *Acta Octolarygologica*, *(Supplement 511)*, 131–134.

Kaufman, S. R., & Abel, L. A. (1986). The effect of distraction on smooth pursuit in normal subjects. *Acta Otolaryngoloca*, *102*, 57–64.

Kayazawa, G., Yamamoto, T., & Itoi, M. (1981). Clinical measurement of contrast sensitivity function using laser generated sinusoidal grating. *Japanese Journal of Ophthalmology*, *25*, 229–236.

Kilbride, P. E., Hutman, L. P., Fishman, M., & Read, J. S. (1986). Foveal cone pigment density differences in the aging human eye. *Vision Research*, *26*, 312–315.

Kim, C. B. Y., & Mayer, M. J. (1994). Flicker sensitivity in healthy aging eyes. II. Cross sectional aging trends from 18 through 77 years of age. *Journal of the Optical Society of America A*, *11*, 1958–1969.

Kim, C. B. Y., Pier, L. P., & Spear, P. D. (1997). Effects of aging and numbers and sizes of neurons in histochemically defined subregions of monkey striate cortex. *The Anatomical Record*, *247*, 119–128.

Kinnear, P. R., & Sahraie, A. (2002). New Farnsworth-Munsell 100 hue test norms of normal observers for each year of age 5–22 and for age decades 30–70. *British Journal of Ophthalmology*, *86*, 1408–1411.

Kline, D. W., & Birren, J. E. (1975). Age differences in backward dichoptic masking. *Experimental Aging Research*, *1*, 17–25

Kline, D. W., Culham, J. C., Bartel, P., & Lynk, L. (2001). Aging effects on vernier hyperacuity: A function of oscillation rate but not target contrast. *Optometry and Vision Science*, *78*, 676–682.

Kline, D. W., Kline, T. J. B., Fozard, J. L., Kosnik, W., Schieber, F., & Sekuler, R. (1992). Vision, aging and driving: The problems of older drivers. *Journal of Gerontology*: Psychological Sciences, *47*, P27–P34.

Kline, D. W., & Orme-Rogers, C. (1978). Examination of stimulus persistence as the basis for superior visual identification performance among older adults. *Journal of Gerontology*, *33*, 76–81.

Kline, D. W., & Schieber, F. (1980). What are the age differences in visual sensory memory? *Journal of Gerontology*, *36*, 86–89.

Kline, D.W., & Schieber, F. (1981). Visual aging: A transient-sustained shift? *Perception and Psychophysics*, *29*, 181–182.

Kline, D.W., & Schieber, F. (1982). Visual persistence and temporal resolution. In R. Sekuler, D. Kline, & K. Dismukes (Eds.), *Aging and human visual function* (pp. 231–244). New York: Liss.

Kline, D. W., & Schieber, F. (1985). Vision and aging. In J. E. Birren & K. W. Schaie (Eds.) *Handbook of the psychology of aging* (pp. 296–331). New York: Van Nostrand Reinhold.

Kline, D. W., & Scialfa, C. T. (1997). Sensory and perceptual functioning: Basic research and human factors implications. In A. D. Fisk, & W. A. Rogers, (Eds.), *Handbook of human factors and the older adult* (pp. 27–54). San Diego: Academic Press.

Kline, T. J., Ghali, L. A., Kline, D. W., & Brown, S. (1990). Visibility distance of highway signs among young, middle-aged and older observers: Icons are better than text. *Human Factors, 32,* 609–619.

Knoblauch, K., Saunders, F., Kusuda, M., Hynes, R., Podgor, M., Higgins, K. E., & de Monasterio, F. M. (1987). Age and illuminance effects in Farnsworth-Munsell 100-Hue Test. *Applied Optics, 26,* 1441–1448.

Kosnik, W., Kline, D. W., Fikre, J., & Sekuler, R. (1987). Ocular fixation control as a function of age and exposure duration. *Psychology and Aging, 2,* 302–305.

Kraft, J. M., & Werner, J. S. (1999). Aging and the saturation of colors. 2. Scaling of color appearance. *Journal of the Optical Society of America A, 16,* 231–235.

Lakshminarayanan, V., & Enoch, J. M. (1995). Vernier acuity and aging. *International Ophthalmology, 19,* 109–115.

Lakshminarayanan, V., Aziz, S., & Enoch, J. M. (1992). Variation of the hyperacuity function with age. *Optometry and Vision Science, 69,* 423–426.

Leuba, G., & Garey, L. J. (1987). Evolution of neuronal numerical density in the developing and aging human cortex. *Human Neurobiology, 6,* 11–18.

Leventhal, A. G., Wang, Y., Pu, M., Zhou, Y., & Ma, Y. (2003). GABA and its agonists improve visual cortical function in senescent monkeys. *Science, 300,* 721–722.

Li, R. W., Edwards, M. H., & Brown, B. (2000). Variation in vernier acuity with age. *Vision Research, 40,* 3775–3781.

Li, R. W., Edwards, M. H., & Brown, B. (2001). Variation in vernier evoked cortical potential with age. *Investigative Ophthalmology and Visual Science, 42,* 1119–1123.

Loewenfeld, I. E. (1979). Pupillary changes related to age. In. H. S. Thompson & D. R. Frisen (Eds.), *Topics in neuro-ophthalmology.* (pp. 124–150) Baltimore: Williams and Wilkins.

Lovasik, J. V., Kergoat, M. J., Justino, L., & Kergoat, H. (2003). Neuroretinal basis of visual impairment in the very elderly. *Graefe's Archive for Clinical and Experimental Ophthalmology, 241,* 48–55.

Mangione, C. M., Berry, S., Spritzer, K., Janz, N. K., Klein, R., Owsley, C., & Lee, P. P. (1998). Identifying the content area for the 51-item National Eye Institute visual function questionnaire: Results from focus groups with visually impaired persons. *Archives of Ophthalmology, 116,* 227–233.

Mäntyjärvi, M. (2001). Normal test scores on the Farnsworth-Munsell 100 hue test. *Documenta Ophthalmologica, 102,* 73-80.

Massie, D.L., Campbell, K. L., & Williams, A. F. (1990). Traffic accident involvement rates by driver age and gender. *Accident Analysis and Prevention, 27,* 73–87.

Mayer, M. J., Kim, C. B. Y., Svingos, A., & Glucs, A. (1988). Foveal flicker sensitivity in healthy aging eyes. I. Compensating for pupil variation. *Journal of the Optical Society of America A, 5,* 2201–2209.

McFarland, R. A., Domey, R. G., Warren, B. A., & Ward, D.C. (1960). Dark adaptation as a function of age. I. A statistical analysis. *Journal of Gerontology, 15,* 149–154.

McFarland, R. A., Warren, B., & Karis, C. (1958). Alterations in critical flicker frequency as a function of age and light:dark ratio. *Journal of Experimental Psychology, 56,* 529–538.

McMurdo, M., & Gaskell, A. (1991). Dark adaptation and falls in the elderly. *Gerontology, 37,* 221–224.

Mellerio, J. (1971). Light absorption and scatter in the human lens. *Vision Research, 11,* 129–141.

Morgan, M. W. (1993). Normal age related vision changes. In A. A. Rosenbloom, Jr. & M. W. Morgan (Eds.), *Vision and aging (2nd edition.* pp. 178–199). Boston: Butterworth-Heinemann.

Morrison, J. D., & McGrath, C. (1985). Assessment of optical contributions to the age-related deterioration of vision. *Quarterly Journal of Experimental Psychology, 70,* 249–269.

Moschner, C., & Baloh, R. W. (1994). Age-related changes in visual tracking. *Journal of Gerontology: Medical Sciences, 49,* M235–M238.

Nameda, N., Kawara, T., & Ohzu, H. (1989). Human visual spatio-temporal frequency performance as a function of age. *Optometry and Vision Science, 66,* 760–765.

Newsome, W. T., & Pare, E. B. (1988). A selective impairment of motion perception following lesions in the middle temporal visual area. *Journal of Neuroscience, 8,* 2201–2211.

Nomura, H., Ando, F., Niino, N., Shimokata, H., & Miyake, Y. (2003). Age-related change in contrast sensitivity among Japanese adults. *Japanese Journal of Ophthalmology, 47,* 299–303.

Norman, J. F., Payton, S. M., Long, J. R., & Hawkes, L.M. (2004). Aging the perception of biological motion. *Psychology and Aging, 19,* 219–225.

Odom, J. V., Vasquez, R. J., Schwartz, T. L. & Linberg, J. V. (1989). Adult vernier thresholds do not increase with age: Vernier bias does. *Investigative Ophthalmology and Visual Science, 30,* 1004–1008.

Olzak, L. A., & Thomas, J. P. (1985). Seeing spatial patterns. In K. R. Boff, L. Kaufman, & J. P. Thomas (Eds.), *Handbook of perception and human performance* (Chapter 7, pp. 1–56). New York: Wiley.

Owsley, C., Sekuler, R., & Siemsen, D. (1983). Contrast sensitivity throughout adulthood. *Vision Research, 23,* 689–699.

Owsley, C. & Sloane, M. E. (1987). Contrast sensitivity, acuity and the perception of real-world targets. *British Journal of Ophthalmology, 71,* 791–796.

Owsley, C., & Sloane, M. E. (1990). Vision and aging. In R. D. Nebes and S. Corkin (Eds.), *Handbook of neuropsychology, Vol. 4.* New York: Elsevier. (pp. 229–249)

Owsley, C., Sloane, M. E., Skalka, H. W., & Jackson, C. A. (1990). A comparison of the Regan low-contrast letter charts and contrast sensitivity testing in older patients. *Clinical Vision Science, 5,* 325–334.

Owsley, C., Stalvey, B., Wells, J., & Sloane, M.E. (1999). Older drivers and cataract: Driving habits and crash risk. *Journal of Gerontology: Medical Sciences, 54A,* M203–M211.

Panda-Jonas, S., Jonas, J. B., & Jacobczyk-Zmija, M. (1995). Retinal photoreceptor density decreases with age. *Ophthalmology, 102,* 1853–1859.

Pardhan, S. (1996). A comparison of binocular summation in young and older patients. *Current Eye Research, 15,* 315–319.

Pardhan, S., Gilchrist, J., Elliott, D. B., & Beh, G. K. (1996). A comparison of sampling efficiency and internal noise level in young and old subjects. *Vision Research, 36,* 1641–1648.

Park, D. C., Polk, T. A., Park, R., Minear, M., Savage, A., & Smith, M. R. (2004). Aging reduces neural specialization in ventral visual cortex. *Proceedings of the National Academy of Sciences, 101,* 13091–13095.

Peters, A., Moss, M. B., & Sethares, C. (2001). The effects of aging on layer 1 of primary visual cortex in the rhesus monkey. *Cerebral Cortex, 11,* 93–103.

Pitt, M. C., & Rawles, J. M. (1988). The effect of age on saccade latency and velocity. *Neuroophthalmology, 8,* 123–129.

Pitts, D. G. (1982). The effects of aging upon selected visual functions: Dark adaptation, visual acuity, stereopsis, and brightness contrast. In R. Sekuler, D. Kline, & K. Dismukes (Eds.), *Aging and human visual function.* (pp. 131–160). New York: Liss.

Regan, D., & Hong, X. H. (1990). Visual acuity for optotypes made visible by relative motion. *Optometry and Visual Science, 67,* 49–55.

Repka, M. X., & Quigley, H. A. (1989). The effect of age on normal human optic nerve fiber number and diameter. *Ophthalmology, 96,* 26–32.

Richards, O. W. (1977). Effects of luminance and contrast on visual acuity, ages 16 to 90 years. *American Journal of Optometry and Physiological Optics, 54,* 178–184.

Rosenbloom, S. (2004). Mobility of the elderly: Good news and bad news. In Transportation Research Board's *Transportation in an aging society: A decade of experience.* Conference Proceedings 27. (pp. 3–21).

Rosenhall, U., Björkman, G., Pedersen, K., & Hanner, P. (1987). Oculomotor tests in different age groups. In M. D. Graham & J. K. Kemink (Eds.), *The vestibular system: neurophysiologic and clinical research.* (pp. 401–410). New York: Raven.

Ross, J. E., Clarke, D. D., & Bron, A. J. (1985). Effect of age on the contrast sensitivity function: Uniocular and binocular findings. *British Journal of Ophthalmology, 69,* 51–56.

Rosser, D. A., Laidlaw, D. A. & Murdoch, I. E. (2001). The development of a "reduced logMAR" visual acuity chart for use in routine clinical practice. *British Journal of Ophthalmology, 85,* 432–436.

Roy, M. S., Podgar, M. J., Collier, B., & Gunkel, R. D. (1991). Color vision and age in a North American population. *Graefes Archive for Clinical and Experimental Ophthalmology*, 229, 139–144.

Said, F., & Weale, R. A. (1959). Variations with age of the spectral transmissivity of the living human crystalline lens. *Gerontologica*, 3, 1213–1231.

Satchi, K. (1973). Fluorescence in human lenses. *Experimental Eye Research*, 16, 167–172.

Savoy, R. L., & McCann, J. J. (1975). Visibility of low spatial frequency sine wave targets: Dependence on number of cycles. *Journal of the Optical Society of America*, 65, 343–350.

Schefrin, B. E., & Werner, J. S. (1990). Loci of spectral unique hues throughout the life span. *Journal of the Optical Society of America A*, 7, 305–311.

Schefrin, B. E., & Werner, J. S. (1993). Age-related changes in the color appearance of broadband surfaces. *Color Research and Application*, 18, 380–389.

Schieber, F. (1988). Vision assessment technology and the screening of older drivers: Past practices and emerging techniques. National Research Council, *Transportation in an aging society: Improving mobility and safety of older persons. (Special Report 218, Volume 2)*. Washington, DC: Transportation Research Board. (pp. 325–378).

Schieber, F. (2003). Human factors and aging: Identifying and compensating for age-related deficits in sensory and cognitive function. In N. Charness & K.W. Schaie (Eds.), *Impact of technology on successful aging* (pp. 42–84). New York: Springer.

Schieber, F., Hiris, E., White, J., Williams, M., & Brannan, J. (1990). Assessing age differences in motion perception using simple oscillatory displacement versus random dot cinematography. *Investigative Ophthalmology and Visual Science (Supplement)*, 31, 355.

Schieber, F., Kline, D. W., Kline, T. J., & Fozard, J.L. (1992). *Contrast sensitivity and the visual problems of older drivers (SAE Technical Paper No. 920613)*. Warrendale, PA: Society of Automotive Engineers.

Scialfa, C. T., Guzy, L. T., Leibowitz, H. W., Garvey, P. M., & Tyrrell, R. A. (1991). Age differences in estimating vehicle velocity. *Psychology and Aging*, 6, 60–66.

Scialfa, C. T., Kline, D. W., & Wood, P. K. (2002). Structural modeling of contrast sensitivity in adulthood. *Journal of the Optical Society of America A*, 19, 158–165.

Seiple, W., Vajaranant, T. S., Szlyk, J. P., Clemens, C., Holopigian, K., Paliga, J., Badawi, D., & Carr, R. E. (2003). Multifocal electroretinography as a function of age: The importance of normative values for older adults. *Investigative Ophthalmology and Visual Science*, 44, 1783–1792.

Sharpe, J. A., & Sylvester, T. O. (1978). Effect of aging on horizontal smooth pursuit. *Investigative Ophthalmology and Visual Science*, 17, 465–467.

Sharpe, J. A., & Zackon, D. H. (1987). Senescent saccades: Effects of aging on their accuracy, latency and velocity. *Acta Otolarygolica*, 104, 422–428.

Shinomori, K., & Werner, J. S. (2003). Senescence of the temporal impulse response to a luminous pulse. *Vision Research*, 43, 617–627.

Sloane, M. E., Owsley, C., & Alvarez, S. L. (1988). Aging, senile miosis and spatial contrast sensitivity at low luminances. *Vision Research*, 28, 1235–1246.

Spear, P. D. (1993). Neural bases of visual deficits during aging. *Vision Research*, 33, 2589–2609.

Spooner, J. W., Sakala, S. M., & Baloh, R. W. (1980). Effect of aging on eye tracking. *Archives of Neurology*, 37, 575–576.

Staplin, L., Lococo, K., & Sim, J. (1993). *Traffic maneuver problems of older drivers*. Report No. FHWA-RD-92-092. McLean, VA: Federal Highway Administration.

Sturr, J. F., Kline, G. E., & Taub, H. A. (1990). Performance of young and older drivers on a static acuity test under photopic and mesopic luminance conditions. *Human Factors*, 32, 1–8.

Sturr, J.F., Zhang, L., Taub, H.A., Hannon, D.J., & Jackowski,, M. M. (1997). Psychophysical evidence for losses in rod sensitivity in the aging visual system. *Vision Research*, 37, 475–481.

Taub, H. A., & Sturr, J. F. (1991). The effects of age and ocular health on letter contrast sensitivity as a function of luminance. *Clinical Vision Science*, 6, 181–189.

Theodore, F. H. (1975). External eye problems in the elderly. *Geriatrics, 30,* 69–80.

Trick, G. E., & Silverman, S. E. (1991). Visual sensitivity to motion: Age-related changes and deficits in senile dementia of the Alzheimer's type. *Neurology, 41,* 1437–1440.

Tyler, C. W. (1989). Two processes control variations in flicker sensitivity over the lifespan. *Journal of the Optical Society of America A, 6,* 481–490.

van den Berg, T. J. T. P. (1995). Analysis of intraocular stray light, especially in relation to age. *Optometry and Vision Science, 72,* 52–59.

Verriest, G. (1963). Further studies on acquired deficiency of color discrimination. *Journal of the Optical Society of America, 53,* 185–195.

Verriest, G., van Laethem, J., & Uvijls, A. (1982). A new assessment of the normal ranges of the 100 hue total scores. *American Journal of Ophthalmology, 93,* 635–642.

Vilar, E.Y.P., Giraldez-Fernandez, M. J., Enoch, J. M., Lakshminarayana, V., Knowles, R., & Srinivasan, R. (1995). Performance on three-point vernier acuity targets as a function of age. *Journal of the Optical Society of America A, 12,* 2293–2305.

Walsh, D. A. (1976). Age differences in central perceptual processing: A dichoptic backward masking investigation. *Journal of Gerontology, 31,* 178–185.

Warabi, T., Kase, M., & Kato, T. (1984). Effect of aging on the accuracy of visually guided saccadic eye movements. *Annals of Neurology, 16,* 449–454.

Watson, A. B., Barlow, H. B., & Robson, J. G. (1983). What does the eye see best? *Nature, 302,* 419–422.

Weale, R. A. (1963). *The aging eye.* London: Lewis.

Weekers, R., & Roussel, F. (1945). Introduction à l'étude de la fréquence de fusion en clinique. *Ophthalmologica, 112,* 305–319.

Werner, J.S., Peterzell, D.H., & Scheetz, A.J. (1990). Light, vision and aging. *Optometry and Vision Science, 67,* 214–229.

Werner, J. S., & Schefrin, B. E. (1993). Loci of achromatic points throughout the life span. *Journal of the Optical Society of America A, 10,* 1509–1515.

Werner, J. S., & Steele, V. G. (1988). Sensitivity of human foveal cone mechanisms throughout the life span. *Journal of the Optical Society of America A, 5,* 2122–2130.

Westheimer, G. (1975). Visual acuity and hyperacuity. *Investigative Ophthalmology, 14,* 570–572.

Weymouth, F. W. (1960). Effect of age on visual acuity. In M. J. Hirsch & R. E. Wick (Eds.), *Vision of the aging patient: An optometric symposium.* (pp. 37–62). Philadelphia: Chilton.

Whitaker, D., Elliott, D. B., & MacVeigh, D. (1992). Variations in hyperacuity performance with age. *Ophthalmic and Physiological Optics, 12,* 29–32.

Whitaker, D., Steen, R., & Elliott, D. B. (1993). Light scatter in the normal young, elderly and cataractous eye demonstrates little wavelength dependency. *Optometry and Vision Science, 70,* 963–968.

Williams, R. A., Enoch, J. M., & Essock, E. A. (1984). The resistence of selected hyperacuity configurations to retinal image degradation. *Investigative Ophthalmology and Visual Science, 25,* 389–399.

Winn, B., Whitaker, D., Elliott, D. B., & Phillips, N.J. (1994). Factors affecting light-adapted pupil size in normal human subjects. *Investigative Ophthalmology and Visual Science, 35,* 1132–1137.

Wist, E. R., Schruaf, M., & Ehrenstein, W. H. (2000). Dynamic vision based on motion-contrast: Changes with age in adults. *Experimental Brain Research, 134,* 295–300.

Wolf, E., & Shaffra, A. M. (1964). Relationship between critical flicker frequency and age in flicker perimetry. *Archives of Ophthalmology, 72,* 832–843.

Wright, C. E., & Drasdo, N. (1985). The influence of age on the spatial and temporal contrast sensitivity function. *Documenta Ophthamologica, 59,* 385–395.

Zeki, S., Watson, J. D. G., Lueck, C. J., Friston, K. L., Kennard, C., & Frackowiak, R. S. J. (1991). A direct demonstration of the functional specialization in the human visual cortex. *Journal of Neuroscience, 11,* 641–649.

Eight

Aging, Complexity, and Motor Performance

Karl M. Newell, David E. Vaillancourt, and Jacob J. Sosnoff

I. Introduction

The capacity of the human system for physical work and skilled motor performance tend to decline over the aging years of adulthood. Research emphasis of the extant sensory-motor literature on motor control and aging has been captured in three relatively distinct areas of study: (1) physical fitness aspects such as strength, flexibility, and endurance (Shepard, 1998); (2) the information processing activities that relate variables such as reaction time and movement time (Cerella, 1990) as factors that mediate the reduced motor performance with aging (Rogers, Fisk, & Walker, 1996); and (3) the neurophysiological control of posture, locomotion, and the fine motor control of finger force production (Enoka et al., 2003). These three areas have not been integrated to any significant degree (although see Spirduso, 1995), but growing evidence shows that enhanced physical capacity facilitates sensory-motor functioning and the performance of posture, locomotion, and manipulation in the context of daily living (Colcombe et al., 2004).

Since the early 1990s, there has been a concerted effort to introduce a new view to understanding the problems of aging that is formulated around the general construct of self-organization (Glass & Mackey, 1988; Yates, 1987, 1988) and the related and emergent construct of complexity (Lipsitz & Goldberger, 1992; Lipsitz, 2002; Vaillancourt & Newell, 2002). The construct of self-organization in behavior is intimately tied to the emergent dynamics and their change over the life span and the contribution of different time scales to this process (Newell, Liu, & Mayer-Kress, 2001). This chapter considers the influence and progress of this complexity orientation to the theory and practice of aging within the behavioral context of physical activity and skilled motor performance.

II. Aging and Movement Complexity

A central and traditional hypothesis from theorizing on complexity and aging holds that aging necessarily involves a loss of complexity in physiology and behavior (Lipsitz, 2002; Lipsitz & Goldberger, 1992). That is, as individuals age, they are less capable of producing behavior that can be viewed as complex and that this loss of complexity is an index of morbidity and mortality. The loss of complexity hypothesis is, in many respects, a subset of the more encompassing view of dynamical disease (Glass & Mackey, 1988) in which behavioral and physiological systems change as a consequence of aberrations in the temporal organization of the evolving dynamics. Complexity theory, methods, and analysis techniques have been applied distinctly to healthy aging and disease states with the anticipation that there is a unique dynamical signature related to specific population groups and disease states.

The general concept of complexity has long been a backdrop to theories of aging (cf. Arking, 1991), but introduction of the concept of self-organization (Yates, 1987), together with the methods, tools, and principles of nonlinear dynamics, provides direct approaches to examining the concept of complexity in aging (Goldberger & West, 1987). For example, there have now been a number of studies on heart rate variability and other microbiological processes in aging that show that the organization of the respective system output is structured with lower complexity (Goldberger & West, 1987; Lipsitz & Goldberger, 1992) and, as a consequence, lacks the natural adaptive variability of younger individuals. The loss of complexity with aging has also been shown at the behavioral level of the motor output in a variety of tasks (e. g., Newell, 1998; Vaillancourt & Newell, 2002).

Complexity has proved to be a slippery concept in all domains of inquiry but here we take a straightforward view of it and consider as a signature feature the number of dimensions (dynamical degrees of freedom) of behavior that can be regulated independently (Newell & Vaillancourt, 2001; Vaillancourt & Newell, 2002). The loss of complexity of a physiological or behavioral control system is hypothesized to result from either a reduction in the number of individual structural components of the system or a restriction in the couplings between those components (Lipsitz & Goldberger, 1992; Vaillancourt & Newell, 2002). The age-related changes in the complexity of behavior can be approached by considering the multiple timescales in the organization of movement output.

In human motor behavior the complexity of measured output arises from the interaction of the individual with the environment in the pursuit of a task goal (Newell, 1986). In this view, the complexity should not be interpreted merely as something that is within or arises from within the body, but rather a property of the behavior that is emergent from a number of sources of constraint in action. The significance of recognizing this confluence of constraints to action is that it is difficult to tease out the independent roles of the organism or environment in the measures of behavior. Furthermore, we show that the goals and intentions of behavior play an important role in mediating the degree and direction of change in the complexity of behavior as a function of aging.

Understanding the complexity of movement in action requires an unraveling of the structure of movement and postural variability. Traditionally, the distribution of outcomes that came from the within-subject repetition of movement in discrete, serial, and continuous tasks was assumed implicitly and, on occasions explicitly, to reflect white Gaussian noise. This position was a particular assumption of information processing accounts of human performance (Broadbent, 1958) following the foundational information theory of Shannon and Weaver (1949), but the white noise interpretation of variability was rarely examined directly by experimental work. For example, Welford (1981) hypothesized that aging-related differences in the speed and variability of performance were mediated by enhanced neural noise in the aging system, but there were no attempts to provide direct tests of the age-related structure of variability. Indeed, most studies of variability in human movement and performance have focused on the *amount* of variability using the standard deviation as an index, without measures of the *structure* of the variability, including those that reflect the change in behavior over time.

Introduction of the principles and techniques of nonlinear dynamics and chaos theory has opened the door to the search for dynamic patterns of complexity in the variance of movement output (Newell & Sliflkin, 1998; Riley & Turvey, 2002; Slifkin & Newell, 1999). A growing collection of recent studies on aging has shown that there is substantial and systematic structure in the variability of movement that is very sensitive to system and output changes as a function of healthy aging and disease states (Lipsitz, 2002; Vaillancourt & Newell, 2002). This emphasis on the structure of within-subject variability in movement control is timely because, in general, intraindividual variability has been a neglected theme in research on the psychology of aging that is only now beginning to be addressed (Hultsch & MacDonald, 2004; Martin & Hofer, 2004; Nesselroade & Salthouse, 2004).

Finally, it should be recognized that the complexity approach to the study of behavior tends to use very different measures than are usual in experimental psychology or the psychology of aging (mean and standard deviation). This reflects the importance in this new approach to considering the time-dependent properties of behavior and psychological processes. Time series analysis is not new to psychology (e.g., Gottman, 1981), but it has not gained prominence in the theoretical work of most subfields of study, including the

psychology of aging. Introductions to the dynamical principles and many of the dependent variables used in the studies reported here may be found in recent books on nonlinear dynamics, cognition, and psychology (Heath, 2000; Ward, 2002).

III. Complexity in Posture, Locomotion, and Manipulation

This section presents selected studies that have investigated the relationships among aging, the complexity of the motor output, and the level of performance outcome. We will review this work by considering experimental data within the action categories of posture, locomotion, and manipulation. To anticipate the findings, there is growing evidence in the aging adult that there is a strong relationship between the complexity of movement output and the skill level of performance as a function of task. Much of this work shows a positive correlation between complexity and performance level, and a negative relation between both of these variables and aging, all features that are consistent with the loss of complexity with aging hypothesis (Lipsitz & Goldberger, 1992). However, not all movement studies are consistent with the loss of complexity hypothesis and it appears that the task goal plays a large role in driving the organization of the motor output and the nature of the differences in complexity that arise with aging (Vaillancourt & Newell, 2002, 2003).

A. Posture

Postures require the maintenance of a position of a body segment or segments either with respect to the environment (as in standing) or with respect to other body segments (as in running). There are many acts of posture in their own right, such as standing, sitting, and holding ones arm and/or hand in a particular orientation, but postures of one kind or another are typically embedded in the other action categories of communication, locomotion, and manipulation. Thus, posture is fundamental to human action and is the product of an interplay between central and peripheral systems (including sensory systems, e.g., vision, proprioception, cutaneous, vestibular) over multiple timescales of control.

It has long been established that there is a decrement in postural control with advanced age, as indexed by an increase in the area, length, or velocity of the center of pressure profile (Hasselkus & Shambes, 1975; Sheldon, 1963). This decline in postural control has been reported to begin as early as the third decade and to progress slowly but systematically over the remainder of the life span (Du Pasquier et al., 2003; Rogind et al., 2003). There is also typically an even greater postural sway in a number of disease states of the aging adult, including Parkinson's disease (Adkin, Frank, & Jog, 2003) and Alzheimer's disease (Elble & Leffler, 2000). In general, the amplitude of sway and its standard deviation tend to increase as a function of aging, although enhanced fitness and physical capacity can mediate the degree and rate of this decrement in postural control (Rosano et al., 2004; Woollacott, 2000). In the complex systems viewpoint it would be hypothesized that a healthy life style reduces the rate of the decrement of the functioning degrees of freedom, either by preserving the integrity of individual components or their couplings with other components, and, at a larger scale, the complexity of the dynamics of subsystem interactions.

There is a boundary to the stability of upright standing posture that, if the center of mass of the body traverses, will require the individual to take a step to maintain stability or, in the more

severe case, it will lead to a fall (King, Judge, & Wolfson, 1994). The stability boundary can be estimated through the center of pressure by having the individual move the torso to the extremes of stable posture in all directions without changing the postural mode or taking a step. The stability of postural control in aging has been investigated with reference to this stability boundary.

Slobounov and colleagues (1998) examined the virtual time to contact to the stability boundary in quiet upright standing as a function of aging. The virtual time-to-contact variable is calculated at every point in the center of pressure time series and is the time it would take the center of pressure to reach the boundary of stability if it were to continue on its pathway with the *same* dynamic properties. This variable was called virtual because contact with this boundary is not what the individual wants, as it would indicate a loss of stability, thus requiring the subject to take a step or maybe even fall.

The experiment showed that in older adults (60–80 years olds) the potential area within the stability boundary for upright standing was reduced and also that the time to contact of the center of pressure with this stability boundary was reduced with age (see Figure 8.1). This reduced time to contact with the stability boundary as a function of aging points to the tighter constraints on the stability of posture with advancing age and suggests some temporal limits on the perceptual control of posture. Van Wegen and colleagues (2002) have shown similar findings with slightly different measures of time to contact as a function of healthy aging.

The increase in the amplitude of postural sway is related to the reduced frequency of the sway, as would be predicted by a pendulum-like model of posture (Mergner, Maurer, & Peterka, 2003). Spectral analysis, a technique that

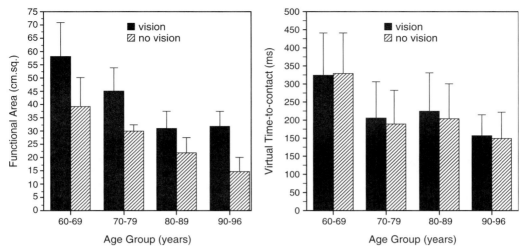

Figure 8.1 (Left) Area (cm^2) of the functional stability region (with between subject standard deviations) as a function of age group and vision condition. (Right) Mean VTC (ms) calculated against the functional stability region as a function of age group and vision condition. Adapted from Slobounov et al., (1998), with permission.

decomposes a signal into its relative contribution of different frequencies (Gottman, 1981), has shown that there is a modal frequency of ~0.6 Hz in the standing posture of humans (Bensel & Dzendolet, 1968), but until more recently, other dynamic properties of the dynamics of the center of pressure profile had not been investigated. Several age-related dynamic properties of the center of pressure have been revealed that, when viewed collectively, can be interpreted as supporting the hypothesis that the stability of the posture of the older adult continues to decline. Furthermore, as reviewed in a subsequent section, this reduced stability is realized through a reduction in the complexity of the postural system that leads to greater postural sway and, it is hypothesized, an increase in the probability of falling.

Newell (1998) contrasted the complexity of postural sway in children aged 3 and 5 years, young adults aged 20–29 years, and older adults aged 65–75 years. The complexity of the sway output was indexed by nonlinear dynamic measures

of the correlation dimension and approximate entropy (a measure of irregularity) of the center of pressure time series. Results of this study clearly showed that the increase in sway of the older subjects was matched by a simultaneous decrease in the complexity or irregularity of the signal. In other words, the amount of sway of older adults was increased but at the same time it became more regular or rhythmic. The inverse relationship between amount of sway and complexity is consistent with the hypothesis that there is a loss of complexity or dynamical degrees of freedom in the regulation of posture with aging (Newell, 1998) and supports the general idea that aging is associated with a loss of complexity (Lipsitz & Goldberger, 1992).

Another approach to the examination of the time-dependent properties of the center of pressure as a function of aging was initiated by Collins and De Luca (1993, 1995). They modeled the center of pressure as a two-process random walk using the square of the displacement increment as a function of increasing time intervals between the center of pressure data points. Collins and De Luca found that the initial open-loop diffusion process for older adults (71–80 years old) was a more positively correlated random walk than that of the normal healthy young control group (age 19–30 years old), whereas the closed-loop component was a more negatively correlated random walk than that of the young adults. Thus, the aging group had a greater tendency to drift away initially from the equilibrium point but in the closed-loop phase had a greater tendency to provide corrective adjustments back toward the equilibrium point. This greater emphasis of the older adults on open loop control is consistent with findings of a lower dimension to the attractor dynamic and more generally a loss of complexity of the postural dynamics due to reduced involvement of more rapid feedback loops. Thus, the loss of faster time scales of control in aging reduces the adaptive capacity of the postural system to minimize the motion in posture.

The idea that the level of complexity of the motor output mediates postural control has been tested by inducing noise in balance control to enhance the detection and transmission of weak signals in aging adults. Here noise is seen as a mechanism that enhances the signal amplitude so that the complexity of system interactions of postural control can be preserved. It has been shown that the postural sway of young and elderly adults during quiet standing can be reduced by applying subsensory mechanical noise to the feet (Priplata et al., 2003) and to the knee (Gravelle et al., 2002). Indeed, the postural sway of the aging group was reduced to the levels of young adults with this intervention. These tests, based on the ideas of stochastic resonance (Wiesenfeld & Moss, 1995) where noise can enhance the detection of weak signals, may lead to the development of therapeutic devices that will help the elderly

overcome the functional difficulties in action due to age-related sensory loss.

Postural stability has also been investigated in limb postures such as the clinical protocol of finger, hand, or arm postural tremor. In postural finger tremor, for example, the individual supports the arm on a table and forms a fist with the hand to hold the index finger still and parallel to the ground. In postural arm tremor the protocol is that of holding the arms out straight, parallel and still to the ground while standing. Postural tremor is one of the most studied clinical actions and has been shown to be influenced by aging and disease states (Elble & Koller, 1990; Findley & Capildeo, 1984). Clearly, however, losing stability of an index finger posture has a different clinical and personal consequence for the individual than losing stability of standing posture, but there are common theoretical perspectives to the performance and complexity changes across these actions with aging.

There are a number of central and peripheral processes that contribute to the change in tremor dynamics across the life span, including healthy aging and disease states (Marsden, 1984). It has traditionally been thought that there is an increase in the amplitude of postural tremor with aging that is associated with a small but systematic slowing of the modal frequency of finger tremor (Marshall & Walsh, 1956). However, studies with more careful subject exclusion criteria and sensitive modern technology for measurement show that the effect of healthy aging on the modal frequency of physiological tremor is negligible to nonexistent (Elble, 2003; Raethjen et al., 2000), but there still remain measurable changes in the complexity of tremor in the aging adult (Sturman et al., 2005). The modal frequency is even lower in Parkinson's disease where tremor is one of the primary markers of the disease state (Beuter et al., 2003; Elble &

Koller, 1990). Chronic stimulation of the thalamus for patients with essential tremor (Vaillancourt et al., 2003) and subthalamus nucleus for patients with Parkinson's disease (Sturman et al., 2004) increases the modal frequency, reduces tremor amplitude, and increases tremor complexity "close" to healthy physiological levels.

In summary, studies on the complexity of postural control in aging adults have shown that the dimension of control tends to be reduced systematically with advancing age and that this reduction in dimension is related to a decrement in motor performance as measured in properties of the outcome of the action. Thus, behavioral postural studies provide strong support for the central tenet of the loss of complexity with aging hypothesis (Lipsitz & Goldberger, 1992). Reduction in the dimension of posture with aging is linked to a reduction in the contribution of shorter (faster) timescale feedback processes to postural control (Newell et al., 1997; Collins & De Luca, 1995). This finding complements the traditional notion that information processing is slowed with advancing age (Welford, 1988; Salthouse, 1985), but places the slowness and aging relation in a different theoretical orientation to that of information theory.

B. Locomotion

Locomotion is that class of physical activities that transport the body from one spatial location to another, including walking, running, hopping, swimming, and climbing stairs. It is well established that a variety of factors lead to declines in the efficiency and effectiveness of gait patterns in aging (Masdeu, Sudarsky, & Woldson, 1997). Human walking is the most studied locomotory action, and recent experiments have examined the structure of the variability of the gait cycle as a function of aging.

Walking is, in effect, made up of a sequential series of steps that move the individual through the dynamics of the stability, instability, and stability spiral but within a single action. There have been very few studies of a single step, but Johnston, Mahalko, and Newell (2003) examined the time it took young (20–29 years) and older adults (60–89 years) to regain postural stability after taking just a single step forward that varied as a percentage of the preferred step length. They measured the time from contacting the force platform on taking a step to the regaining of stability as measured by the velocity of the center of pressure being below the criterion of 4 cm/s.

Figure 8.2 shows that there is a systematic increase in the time it takes to regain stability as a function of increasing age. Thus, older adults need more time to reacquire stability following the self-induced perturbation of taking even just a single step. This increasing difficulty of reacquiring stability having lost stability on taking a step may be a factor in the prevalence of falls in aging. Many falls in aging take place around the house where the transition between posture and locomotion is taking place continually, as opposed to the relatively steady-state dynamics that occur in standing or even walking from one location to another (Blake et al., 1988).

The walking patterns in healthy old people show systematic differences when contrasted with those of young adults. Modal features of the aging gait cycle are the slowing of the preferred walking speed, a reduction in stride length, and a broadening of the footfall pattern (Murray, Kory, & Clarkson, 1969; Winter et al., 1990). Importantly for the context of this chapter is also the case that although the amount of variability of stride frequency and length seems to be uninfluenced by age (Gabel & Nayak, 1984), the variability of the step width span increases with age in older adults (Grabiner, Biswas, &

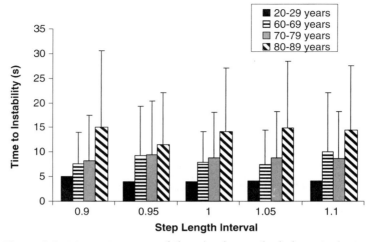

Figure 8.2 Mean time to stability (with standard deviation) as a function of age group and step length (expressed as a ratio of preferred step length). Adapted from Johnson, Mihalko, and Newell, (2003), with permission.

Grabiner, 2001; Owings & Grabiner, 2004). Thus, the increments in variability of step properties with increasing age of older adults exist both in the isolated case of a single step and the more cyclical activity of walking from one location to another.

The structure of the increased variability of the walking pattern in aging adults has been studied by Hausdorff and colleagues (e.g., 1997). They have used spectral analysis and detrended fluctuation analysis to reveal structure in the gait cycle as a function of age and disease state. Their general finding was that temporal fluctuations in the variability of the gait cycle are self-similar. That is, fluctuations of the gait cycle exhibit long-range correlations such that the stride properties of any given cycle are dependent on a cycle that occurred previously at rather remote times, perhaps hundreds of cycles earlier in the locomotion sequence. Their analyses show that the dependence of the stride interval decays as a function of a power law, suggesting a fractal pattern to the structure of the variability of the gait cycle over time. In other words,

the variability of the gait cycle is not that of a signal plus white noise process, as has been viewed traditionally in studies of gait variability.

Of particular relevance here is that the long-range correlations of walking have been shown to break down as a function of aging and disease (Hausdorff et al., 1997). The sequential dependence as revealed through the long-range correlations was lower in elderly as opposed to young adult subjects. Furthermore, it was shown that this long-range dependency was even lower in older subjects with Huntington's disease. Similar findings have been shown in a comparison of normal and diabetic neuropathic walking patterns (Dingwell & Cusumano, 2000). Thus, the structure of gait variability is influenced by aging and disease states, a finding that is consistent with earlier studies reporting on the nonlinear dynamics of postural variability. Again, it is instructive to note that these age-related findings from the nonlinear analysis of gait were not apparent with the traditional techniques to examine the amount of variability in the step cycle.

The structure of gait variability has also been investigated by the application of nonlinear analysis to selected kinematic properties of the lower leg in walking (Buzzi et al., 2003; Dingwell & Cusumano, 2000). The local stability of the gait cycle was assessed through the nonlinear measure of the largest Lyapunov exponent (a measure of dynamical stability) with surrogate data techniques. Results showed that fluctuations in the gait cycle may reflect deterministic processes. Moreover, Buzzi et al. (2003) revealed that the elderly (71–79 years) had larger Lyapunov exponents and correlation dimension, indicating lower local stability in walking as a function of aging.

In closing this section on aging and gait variability, it should be noted that the *direction* of change in the structure of variability as a function of aging is *opposite* in the actions of posture and locomotion. Postural studies showed a loss of complexity with aging, whereas walking studies showed an increase in the dynamical degrees of freedom, as indexed by the reduction in the long range correlations. Hausdorff and colleagues (1997) did not discuss the theoretical significance of this difference in the directional change in the degrees of freedom as a function of the action, but this contrast provides an indication that loss of complexity is not such a universal phenomenon in aging as implied by Lipsitz and Goldberger (1992). Vaillancourt and Newell (2002) have used these contrasting findings, together with others, to propose that the general behavioral feature of aging in human action is loss of adaptation rather than loss of complexity. That is, the reduced ability to change the dynamical degrees of freedom is what is reduced (or lost) with aging whether the task-dependent change requires an increase or decrease in the dynamical degrees of freedom to realize the task goal. This contrasting theoretical position to the loss of complexity hypothesis is developed more fully in the closing section of this chapter.

C. Manipulation

The complexity of behavior in aging has also been studied in manipulation tasks that typically involve the arms, hand, and fingers in task-oriented actions. These kinds of tasks have also been called fine motor tasks in the behavioral literature because they emphasize the role of the smaller muscle groups in more precision oriented actions, including the speed and accuracy of the motor output. There is a systematic relationship between performance level and complexity of the motor output as a function of aging in a range of manipulation tasks.

Vaillancourt, Slifkin, and Newell (2002) examined fluctuations in the control of grip force to determine if force variability increased or decreased in relation to the degree of interdigit individuation. Interdigit individuation reflects the degree of independent force output of the digits in control of the grasping action. The degree of interdigit individuation was viewed as an index of the complexity of the system on the grounds that greater interdigit variation is a reflection of a higher dimension to behavioral output. This relation was examined in young (21–29 years) and elderly (68–80 years) participants and in participants diagnosed with Parkinson's disease (68–80 years). Force was produced under different force levels (5, 25, 50% MVC) with and without visual feedback. Force variability was assessed using the standard deviation and root mean square error, and interdigit individuation was examined using cross-approximate entropy.

Force variability increased with the force level, the removal of visual feedback, and also in patients with Parkinson's disease compared to the young and elderly matched control participants. There was a reduction in the degree of interdigit individuation, with increases in force level, the removal of visual feedback, and in Parkinson's disease participants compared to the matched controls. Overall, there was a negative correlation between the degree of interdigit individuation and the amount of force variability. The force fluctuations in precision grip, shown in

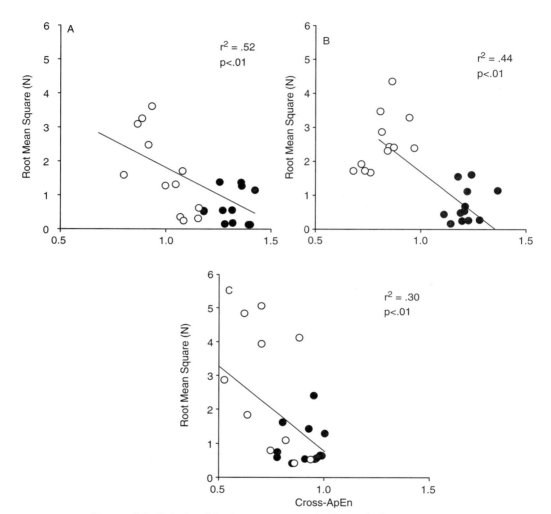

Figure 8.3 Relationship between cross-ApEn and the root mean square (RMS) of total force for young (**A**), elderly (**B**), and Parkinson's disease (**C**) participants. Cross-ApEn and the RMS index the relationships between the degree of interdigit individuation and force variability. Each data point represents the participant average at each specific force and visual feedback condition in the experiment. The r^2 and the fit from the linear regression analysis are shown for each group. ○, no-visual feedback condition; and •, visual feedback condition. In all three groups, there was a significant negative relationship between the degree of interdigit individuation and force variability. Adapted from Vaillancourt, Slifkin, and Newell, (2002), with permission.

Figure 8.3, revealed a continuum for the degree of interdigit individuation in which task constraints, aging, and Parkinson's disease alter the coupling between the digits in controlling grip force. Thus, there was an inverse relationship between the amount of force variability and the complexity of the structure of the force signal that was magnified with the aging process and the presence of Parkinson's disease.

The linear fit drawn through the complexity and performance data of the population groups of Figure 8.3 is probably missing the interesting interaction that is present through the manipulation of vision. Indeed, more recent work from our group shows that the age complexity interaction is only present when the quality of visual information is manipulated. The age by complexity by performance interaction is not present under no vision conditions in this kind of tracking task. A closer inspection of data in Figure 8.3 shows that this trend is also evident in that a best-fitting linear fit through vision data alone for each group will probably yield a horizontal line and hence no relation. This outcome highlights the important role of information in driving the age by complexity by performance interaction in force control tasks.

The influence of aging on the inverse performance and complexity relationship in force variability has also been studied with intramuscular electromyography (EMG) to examine a physiological correlate of the greater force variability with aging (Vaillancourt, Larsson, & Newell, 2003). Young (mean 22 ± 1 years), old (mean 67 ± 2 years), and older-old (mean 82 ± 5 years) adult humans produced isometric, index finger abduction force in both constant and sinewave tasks at 5, 10, 20, and 40% of their maximal voluntary contraction. Force and fine-wire intramuscular EMG were recorded from the first dorsal interosseous muscle.

Analyses of the amount and time-dependent structure of the discharge rate of single motor units and Fourier analysis of the rectified intramuscular EMG were performed.

As anticipated, the amount of force output variability increased across the young, old, and older-old groups. The amount and time-dependent structure of the discharge rate variability of single motor units did not differ between the young and the older groups. However, there was a progressive decrease in the relative power of ~40-Hz EMG activity from the young > old > older-old subjects across the 5, 10, 20, and 40% MVC force levels. There was also a progressive increase in the relative power of the ~10-Hz EMG activity from young < old < older-old subjects at each target force level. Findings showed that a shift in the relative contribution of ~40- to ~10-Hz neural activity was related to the reduced capacity of older adults to maintain optimal force control and the appropriate task-dependent complexity.

A subsequent study examined the influence of aging on the oscillatory activity of a population of motor units during rhythmical force production (Sosnoff, Vaillancourt, & Newell, 2004). It was hypothesized that more rapid force contractions would reverse the established finding of reduced high- and greater low-frequency EMG activity to greater high- and reduced low-frequency EMG activity in older adults. Intramuscular EMG activity and effector force were recorded while 45 human subjects (20–31 years and 60-88 years of age) rhythmically produced force at four distinct frequencies (1, 2, 3, and 4 Hz) and two force levels (5 and 25% MVC). Spectral and coherence analyses were performed on the force output and EMG activity. In young adults, the dominant peak of EMG activity shifted to lower frequencies at faster contractions. In the 2- to 4-Hz targets the older adults had greater 35- to 50-Hz and reduced 0- to 5-Hz EMG activity compared to the young adults. There was greater EMG-force coherence in the 0–5 Hz bandwidth for the young subjects. Thus, higher frequency force contractions reversed the previously established aging diffe-rences in the relative contribution of low- and high-frequency EMG activity. Collectively, these findings show that aging humans lose the adaptive capability to modulate and balance the excitatory and inhibitory activity of multiple neural oscillators required to meet task demands.

Additional research examining the effect of aging on force control has shown that older adults have a stronger correlation between concurrently active motor units, which was referred to as a greater common drive with aging (Erim et al., 1999). Other literature that exam-ined the correlated discharge of action potentials from pairs of motor units in the time domain did not find an age-related increase in motor unit synchroni-zation (Kamen & Roy, 2000; Semmler et al., 2000). In contrast, a separate study by Semmler and colleagues (2003) using the same sample of individuals and motor units where no differences in motor unit synchronization were found did find a difference in the correlated discharge of action potentials from pairs of motor units between young and elderly adults in the frequency domain using motor unit–motor unit coherence. These find-ings from Erim et al (1999) and Semmler et al. (2003) were in the context of a constant force level task, and thus the increased common drive and motor unit–motor unit coherence in older adults may not be found when sinusoidal force production is considered.

In summary, findings from these studies on the complexity–performance relationship in manipulation tasks are consistent with those shown in the earlier sections on posture and locomotion.

There is a reduced capacity for adaptive change in the motor output in the aging adult that is reflected in the output of a single effector, the coordination dynamics between effectors, and in the relationships of the output of different levels of the system (e.g., EMG—move-ment dynamics). We have characterized the adaptive control in aging and its change under task constraints by consid-ering the dynamical degrees of freedom that are regulated as an index of complex-ity in control of the motor output. Over-all, studies show a strong relationship between complexity of the motor output and the performance level achieved for the motor task.

IV. Aging and Loss of Adaptation in Motor Performance

In the general motor control literature, a central issue is the question of how the many active degrees of freedom of the system at all levels of analysis are harnessed (coordinated) to produce the structure and form of movement output to realize the task goals of everyday actions. This has become known as the degrees of freedom problem (Bernstein, 1967; Turvey, 1990). In this literature there is considerable support for the idea that as an individual becomes more skilled, he or she learns to regulate independently a larger number of degrees of freedom, thus, in essence, enhancing the complexity of the motor output. In short, improvement in realizing a task goal or learning is accompanied by an increment in the dynamical degrees of freedom regulated. This central finding and its associated theoretical proposi-tions are consistent with the aging and loss of complexity literature cited earlier in that if one becomes more skilled by increasing dynamical degrees of freedom, it might naturally follow then that the performance decrement of aging is associated with a loss of dynamical degrees of freedom or reduction in complexity (Newell & Vaillancourt, 2001).

Experiments conducted in our laboratory have examined the universality of the notion of the increase in active degrees of freedom with motor learning (Newell et al., 2003). The view that we are pursuing builds on the proposition that performance outcome is the product of a concurrence of constraints to action that fall under the three major categories of organism, environment, and task (Newell, 1986). In this view, the outcome of action is an emergent property of the constraints that are channeling the dynamics of performance at that moment in time (Kugler & Turvey, 1987). One significant element of this formulation is that it brings directly into center place the importance of task constraints in driving motor output.

Our current view is that while an *increment* to the dynamical degrees of freedom is common in motor learning, it does not follow that the *increment* in complexity is a universal principle of learning (Newell & Vaillancourt, 2001). Learning is associated with an increment in degrees of freedom, enhancement of complexity if you will, because that is the way in which the task constraints are often driving adaptation of the natural motor output (intrinsic dynamic) to the system. However, we postulate that a more general hypothesis is that task constraints can also drive a reduction in the degrees of freedom regulated and demonstrate an adaptive loss of complexity in learning of the given motor task. In other words, the general problem of learning is one of *changing* the degrees of freedom from the natural dynamic that people can produce (the intrinsic dynamic where there are minimal task constraints) because whether they have to increase or decrease the degrees of freedom regulated from the current state of system output is task specific.

The significance of a demonstration of this increase and decrease view of active degrees of freedom from the learning literature to the aging problem of complexity is that it suggests that the loss of complexity data cited earlier for posture and aging is not reflective of a universal aging principle regarding complexity of behavior and aging. The problem is that demonstration of a loss of complexity in aging is likely to be task specific. It should be emphasized that we are not arguing that there are not examples of a loss of complexity in behavior with aging, but rather we are proposing that in tasks where a reduction of dynamical degrees of freedom is required that aging individuals will be less adaptive in realizing these same task demands by showing higher complexity than is adaptive for the task goal. This then leads to the general theoretical proposition that the problem of complexity in aging is not one simply of the loss of complexity as proposed originally by Lipsitz and Goldberger (1992), but rather the loss of the ability to *adapt* the degrees of freedom regulated from the current state of the system (Vaillancourt & Newell, 2002). On this view then, aging would be reflected by a reduced ability to *change* the degrees of freedom either in an increment or a decrement according to task demands.

Vaillancourt and Newell (2003) conducted a direct test of the task-dependent nature of the direction of change in the dynamical degrees of freedom as a function of aging. Healthy young (20–24 years), old (60–69 years), and older-old (75–90 years) humans produced isometric force contractions in separate conditions to constant and sine wave force targets that also varied in level of force output. As would be predicted from previous work, the force variability on each force task increased with advancing age. Furthermore, both time and frequency analyses showed that the structure of the force output in the old and older-old adults was less complex in the constant force level task and more complex in the sine wave force task. Figure 8.4 shows that this trend was evident for analyses of ApEn, detrended fluctuation analysis (DFA), and spectral degrees of freedom. These alterations in force output with aging were due primarily to the activity in the low-frequency bands below 4 Hz. Overall, then, these results support the postulation that the observed increase or decrease in physiological complexity with aging is influenced by the relatively fast timescale of

external task demands (Vaillancourt & Newell, 2002). This finding was confirmed with several measures of complexity and was not an artifact of the limits of a single dynamical measure (Vaillancourt, Sosnoff, & Newell, 2004).

The demonstration that older adults can have reduced or enhanced complexity of motor output compared to younger adults is counter to the notion that loss of complexity is the universal direction of change in the dynamics of aging (Newell & Vaillancourt, 2001; Vaillancourt & Newell, 2002). This potential for a bidirectional difference in

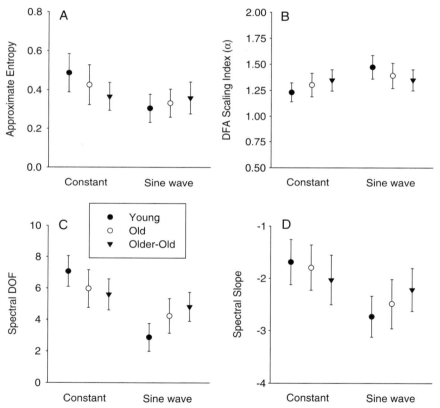

Figure 8.4 Structure of force output variability. Time and frequency analysis using ApEn (A), detrended fluctuation analysis (B), spectral degrees of freedom (C), and spectral slope analysis (D), •, young; ○, old; and ▼, older-old group. Each symbol represents the average of all 10 subjects collapsed across all four force levels, and error bars represent the standard deviation. Adapted from Vaillancourt and Newell (2003), with permission.

the number of dynamical degrees of freedom regulated as a function of aging invites the hypothesis that it is the loss of adaptation of the intrinsic dynamics that is the key feature of change as a function of age. It appears that the amount and rate of change of the dynamical degrees of freedom are reduced in aging no matter the direction, increase, or decrease that is required (implicitly usually) by the task demand.

As a generalization, postures require an increase in degrees of freedom regulated to minimize the amount of motion, even though in task space the dimension by definition is zero (Newell et al., 2003). In these tasks the aging adult, due to adaptation losses, cannot increase sufficiently the degrees of freedom regulated, revealing by comparison to younger adults a reduction or loss of the complexity. The loss of adaptation is in the regulation of the faster timescale components, which leads to less compensation in the frequencies of force output and a stronger modal frequency and higher amplitude of sway motion. In contrast in the highly rhythmical but low dimensional oscillatory tasks the aging adult cannot reduce the complexity of the output sufficiently and, therefore, displays in contrast to the younger adults, an enhanced complexity that is not adaptive to the task demands. Thus, although behavior is a product of the confluence of environmental, organismic, and task constraints, it is the case that the independent manipulation of task demands can produce both qualitative and quantitative differences in the motor output and the direction of change in the complexity of behavior in aging that arises in the control of the dynamical degrees of freedom.

Finally, it is interesting to note that the time-dependent measure of irregularity (ApEn–Pincus, 1991) has also been shown to be more sensitive to detecting the onset of Parkinson's disease than the traditional modal frequency and amplitude measures (Vaillancourt & Newell, 2000). That is, a reduction in complexity in the finger tremor time series was observed while there were no differences in the modal frequency and mean amplitude of tremor in a group of aging adults diagnosed with mild stage 1 Parkinson's disease. The potential of complexity measures in behavioral assessment as a prospective screening or diagnostic tool is an area of research that deserves more emphasis. This finding and approach are consistent with the idea of dynamical disease (Glass & Mackey, 1988) and aberrations in the time-dependent properties of the evolving dynamics.

V. Concluding Comments

This chapter has shown that there is a substantial body of experimental work in motor control that has tested aspects of the aging and complexity relationship. Across a range of posture, locomotion, and manipulation tasks it has been shown that there is a strong link between the complexity of the motor output and the level of task performance. In many tasks, particularly postural tasks, the enhanced sway or loss of performance is related to a significant loss of complexity in the output over the aging years. The complexity–performance relationship is not limited to postural tasks, as many movement tasks have a relatively high-dimension movement solution and it is hypothesized that they would be influenced similarly by the processes of aging.

Our work suggests, however, that there is not a unidirectional relationship between complexity and performance, and hence the necessity or universality of a loss of complexity in behavioral outcome with aging (Newell et al., 2003; Vaillancourt & Newell, 2003). The nature of the change in complexity with aging is task dependent and reflects the role of intentions and goals in organizing the dynamics of the output. It is, however, likely that a loss of complexity with aging will be most prevalent in behavioral output because many tasks require an increase in the dimension from the intrinsic dynamics of the system if the task goal is to be realized. Thus, the age-related change in behavior often may be reflected in a loss of complexity but it does not have to be; the direction and degree of difference in organization of the dynamical degrees of freedom between young and older adults are task dependent. This perspective leads to the more general hypothesis that aging mediates the adaptive change in the dimension of the movement dynamics to realize tasks goals (Vaillancourt & Newell, 2002).

There are many timescales of influence to the complexity of posture, locomotion, and manipulation and the changes that occur in these actions through the aging process. The examination here of the complexity of within-subject variability has emphasized the relatively shorter timescales of motor control, ones that are strongly influenced by information and feedback control. Clearly, there is a need for a fuller and broader examination of the role of timescales in the complexity of the invariance of movement variance. Such an approach would need to embrace elements of longitudinal designs to investigate the contribution of a broader range of timescales to aging, complexity, and motor performance.

There needs to be more experimental work that pursues the rate of change of posture and movement complexity in aging and its relation to the rate of change in the performance outcome. The experiments reported here show that such a relationship exists, but the formal nature of it has yet to be elucidated. It is well known that the functions and exponents of change in aging are different for different systems (Arking,

1991; Austad, 2001), and we might anticipate that the same will be the case for the change in complexity.

Acknowledgments

The preparation of this chapter was supported in part by Grants RO1 HD046918, RO3 AG023259, and RO1 NS052310. The authors thank John Challis and Scott Hofer for helpful comments on an earlier version of the chapter.

References

Adkin, A. L., Frank, J. S., & Jog, M. S. (2003). Fear of falling and postural control in Parkinson's disease. *Movement Disorders, 18*, 496–502.

Arking, R. (1991). *Biology of aging: Observations and principles*. Englewood Cliffs, N.J.: Prentice Hall.

Austad, S. N. (2001). Concepts and theories of aging. In E. J. Masoro & S. N. Austad (Eds.), *Handbook of the biology of aging (5th Edition* pp.3–22). New York: Academic Press.

Bensel, C. K., & Dzendolet, E. (1968). Power spectral density analysis of the standing sway of males. *Perception and Psychophysics, 4*, 285–288.

Bernstein, N. A. (1967). *The co-ordination and regulation of movements*. New York: Pergamon Press.

Beuter, A., Edwards, R., & Titcombe, M. S. (2003). Data analysis and mathematical modeling of human tremor. In A. Beuter, L. Glass, M. C. Mackey, & M. S. Titcombe (Eds.), *Nonlinear dynamics in physiology and medicine (pp. 303–355)*. New York: Springer.

Blake, A. J., Morgan, K., Bendall, M. J., Dallosso, H., Ebrhaim, S. B., Arie, T. H., Fentem, P. H., & Bassey, E. J. (1988). Falls by elderly at home: Prevalence and associated factors. *Age and Ageing, 17*, 365–372.

Broadbent, D. E. (1958). *Perception and communication*. London: Pergamon Press.

Buzzi, U. H., Stergiou, N., Kurz, M. J., Hageman, P. A., & Heidel, J. (2003). Nonlinear dynamics indicates aging affects variability during gait. *Clinical Biomechanics, 18*, 435–443.

Cerella, J. (1990). Aging and information processing rate. In J. Birren & K. W. Schaie (Eds.), *Handbook of psychology and aging (pp. 201–221)*. New York: Academic Press.

Colcombe, S. J., Kramer, A. F., Erickson, K. I., et al. (2004). Cardiovascular fitness, cortical plasticity, and aging. *Proceedings of the National Academy of Science USA, 101*, 3316–3321.

Collins, J. J., & De Luca, C. J. (1993). Open-loop and closed-loop control of posture: A random-walk analysis of center-of-pressure trajectories. *Experimental Brain Research, 95*, 308–318.

Collins, J. J., & De Luca, C. J. (1995). Upright, correlated random walks: A statistical-biomechanics approach to the human postural control system. *Chaos, 5*, 57–63.

Dingwell, J. B., & Cusumano, J. P. (2000). Non-linear time series of normal and pathological human walking. *Chaos, 10*, 848–963.

Du Pasquier, R. A., Blanc, Y., Sinnreich, M., Landis, T., Burkhard, P., & Vingerhoets, F. J. (2003). The effect of aging on postural stability: A cross sectional and longitudinal study. *Clinical Neurophysiology, 33*, 213–218.

Elble, R. J. (2000). Essential tremor frequency decreases with time. *Neurology, 55*, 1547–1551.

Elble, R. J. (2003). Characteristics of physiologic tremor in young and elderly adults. *Clinical Neurophysiology, 114*, 624–635.

Elble, R. J., & Koller, W. C. (1990). *Tremor.* Baltimore: Johns Hopkins University Press.

Elble, R. J., & Leffler, K. (2000). Pushing and pulling with the upper extremities while standing: the effects of mild Alzheimer dementia and Parkinson's disease. *Movement Disorders, 15*, 255–168.

Enoka, R. M., Christou, E. A., Hunter, S. K., Kornatz, K. W., Semmler, J. G., Taylor, A. M., & Tracy, B. L. (2003). Mechanisms that contribute to differences in motor performance between young and old adults. *Journal of Electromyography and Kinesiology, 13*, 1–12.

Erim, Z., Beg, M. F., Burke, D. T., & DeLuca, C. J. (1999). Effects of aging on motor-unit control properties. *Journal of Neurophysiology, 82*, 2081–2091.

Findley, L. J., Gresty, M. A., & Halmagyi, G. M. (1981). Tremor, the cogwheel phenomenon and clonus in Parkinson's disease. *Journal of Neurology, Neurosurgery and Psychiatry, 44*, 534–546.

Findley, L. J., & Capildeo, R. (Eds.). (1984). *Movement disorders: Tremor.* New York: Oxford University Press.

Gabell, A., & Nayak, U. S. (1984). The effect of age on variability in gait. *Journal of Gerontology, 39*, 662–666.

Glass, L., & Mackey, M. C. (1988). *From clocks to chaos.* New Jersey: Princeton University Press.

Goldberger, A. L., & West, B. J. (1987). Fractals in physiology and medicine. *Yale Journal of Biological Medicine, 60*, 421–435.

Gottman, J. M. (1981). *Time-series analysis: A comprehensive introduction for social scientists.* New York: Cambridge University Press.

Grabiner, P. C., Biswas, S. T., & Grabiner, M. D. (2001). Age-related changes in spatial and temporal gait variables. *Archives of Physical Medicine and Rehabilitation, 82*, 31–35.

Gravelle, D. C., Laughton, C. A., Dhruv, N. T., Katdare, K. D., Niemi, J. B., Lipsitz, L.A., & Collins, J. J. (2002). Noise-enhanced balance control in older adults. *Neuroreport, 13*, 1853–1856.

Hasselkus, B. R., & Shambes, G. M. (1975). Aging and postural and sway in women. *Journal of Gerontology, 30*, 661–667.

Hausdorff, J. M., Mitchell, S. L., Firtion, R., Peng, C. K., Cudkowicz, M. E., Wei, J. Y., & Goldberger, A. L. (1997). Altered fractal dynamics of gait: Reduced stride interval correlations with aging and Huntington's disease. *Journal of Applied Physiology, 82*, 262–269.

Heath, R. A. (2000). *Nonlinear dynamics: Techniques and applications to psychology.* Mahwah, N.J.: Lawrence Erlbaum Associates.

Hultsch, D. F., & MacDonald, S. W. S. (2004). Intraindividual variability in performance as a theoretical window onto cognitive aging. In R. A. Dixon, L. Backman, & L-G. Nilsson (Eds.), *New frontiers in cognitive aging (pp. 63–88)*. Oxford: Oxford University Press.

Johnston, C. B., Mihalko, S. L., & Newell, K. M. (2003). Aging and the time needed to reacquire postural stability. *Journal of Aging and Physical Activity, 11*, 419–429.

Kamen, G., & Roy, A. (2000). Motor unit synchronization in young and elderly adults. *European Journal of Applied Physiology, 81*, 403–410.

King, M. B., Judge, J. O., & Wolfson, L. (1994). Functional base of support decreases with age. *Journal of Gerontology: Medical Sciences, 49*, M258–M263.

Kugler, P. N., & Turvey, M. T. (1987). *Information, natural law, and the self-assembly of rhythmic movement.* Hillsdale, NJ: L. Erlbaum Associates.

Liebovitch, L. S. (1998). *Fractals and chaos simplified for the life sciences.* New York: Oxford University Press.

Lipsitz, L. A. (2002). Dynamics of stability: the physiologic basis of functional health and frailty. *Journal of Gerontology A: Biological Science and Medical Science, 57*, B115–25.

Lipsitz, L. A., & Goldberger, A. L. (1992). Loss of "complexity" and aging: Potential applications of fractals and chaos theory to senescence. *Journal of the American Medical Association, 267*, 1806–1809.

Marsden, C. (1984). Origins of normal and pathological tremor. *In* L. Findley, & R. Capildeo (Eds.), *Movement Disorders: Tremor.* (pp. 37–84). London: Butterworth.

Marshall, J., & Walsh, G. (1956). Physiological tremor. *Journal of Neurology, Neurosurgery, and Psychiatry, 19*, 260–267.

Martin, M., & Hofer, S. M. (2004). Intraindividual variability, change, and aging: conceptual and analytical issues. *Gerontology, 50*, 7–11.

Masdeu, J. C., Sudarsky, L., & Wolfson, L. (Eds.) (1997). *Gait disorders of aging: Falls and therapeutic strategies.* Philadelphia: Lippincott-Raven

Mergner, T., Maurer, C., & Peterka, R. J. (2003). A multisensory posture control model of human upright stance. *Progress in Brain Research, 142*, 189–201.

Murray, M., Kory, P., & Clarkson, B. H. (1969). Walking patterns in healthy old men. *Journal of Gerontology, 24*, 169–178.

Nesselroade, J. R., & Salthouse T. A. (2004). Methodological and theoretical implications of intraindividual variability in perceptual-motor performance. *Journal of Gerontology B: Psychological Science and Social Science, 59*, P49–P55.

Newell, K. M. (1986). Constraints on the development of coordination. In M. G. Wade & H. T. A. Whiting (Eds.), *Motor skill acquisition in children: Aspects of coordination and control.* Amsterdam: Martinies NIJHOS.

Newell, K. M. (1998). Degrees of freedom and the development of postural center of pressure profiles. In K. M. Newell & P .C. M. Molenaar (Eds), *Applications of nonlinear dynamics to developmental process modeling (pp. 63–84).* New Jersey: Lawrence Erlbaum Associates.

Newell, K. M., Broderick, M. P., Deutsch, K. M., & Slifkin, A. B. (2003). Task goals and change in dynamical degrees of freedom with motor learning. *Journal of Experimental Psychology: Human Perception and Performance, 29*, 379–387.

Newell, K. M., Liu, Y. T., & Mayer-Kress, G. (2001). Time scales in motor learning and development. *Psychological Review, 108*, 57–82.

Newell, K. M., & Slifkin, A. B. (1998). The nature of movement variability. In J. Piek (Ed.). *Motor Control and human skill: A multidisciplinary perspective.* Champaign, IL: Human Kinetics.

Newell, K. M., Slobounov, S. M., Slobounova, E. S., & Molenaar, P. C. (1997). Stochastic processes in postural center-of-pressure profiles. *Experimental Brain Research, 113*, 158–164.

Newell, K. M., & Vaillancourt, D. E. (2001). Dimensional change in motor learning. *Human Movement Science, 20*, 695–715.

Owings, T. M., & Grabiner, M, D. (2004). Variability of step kinematics in young and older adults. *Gait & Posture, 20*, 26–29.

Priplata, A. A., Niemi, J. B., Harry, J. D., Lipsitz, L. A., & Collins, J. J. (2003). Vibrating insoles and balance control in elderly people. *Lancet, 362*, 1123–1124.

Pincus, S. M. (1991). Approximate entropy as a measure of system complexity. *Proceedings of the National Academy of Science, USA, 88*, 2297–2301.

Raethjen, J., Pawlas, F., Lindemann, M., Wenzelburger, R., & Deuschl, G. (2000).

Determinants of physiologic tremor in a large normal population. *Clinical Neurophysiology, 111*, 1825–1837.

Riley M. A., & Turvey, M. T. (2002). Variability of determinism in motor behavior. *Journal of Motor Behavior, 34*, 99–125.

Rogers, W. A., Fisk, A. D., & Walker, N. (1996). *Aging and skilled performance: Advances in theory and application.* Mahwah, NJ: Erlbaum.

Rogind, H., Lykkegaard, J. J., Bliddal, H., & Danneskiold-Samsoe, B. (2003). Postural sway in normal subjects aged 20–70 years. *Clinical Physiology and Functional Imaging, 23*, 171–176.

Rosano, C., Simonsick, E. M., Harris, T. B., Kritchevsky, S. B., Brach, J., Visser, M., Yaffe, K., & Newman, A. B. (2004). Association between physical and cognitive function in healthy elderly: The health, aging and body composition study. *Neuroepidemiology, 24*, 8–14.

Salthouse, T. A. (1985). Speed of behavior and its implications for cognition. In J. E. Birren & K. W. Schaie (Eds.), *Handbook of the psychology and aging (pp. 400–426).* New York: Van Nostrand Reinhold.

Semmler, J. G., Steege, J. W., Kornatz, K. W., & Enoka, R. M. (2000). Motor-unit synchronization is not responsible for larger motor-unit forces in old adults. *Journal of Neurophysiology, 84*, 358–366.

Semmler, J. G., Kornatz, K. W., & Enoka, R. M. (2003). Motor-unit coherence during isometric contractions is greater in a hand muscle of older adults. *Journal of Neurophysiology, 90*, 1346–1349.

Shannon, C. E., & Weaver, W. (1949). *The mathematical theory of communication.* Urbana-Champaign: University of Illinois Press.

Sheldon, J. H. (1963). The effect of age on the control of sway. *Gerontology Clinics, 5*, 129–138.

Shephard, R.J. (1998). Aging and exercise. In T.D.Fahey (Ed.) *Encyclopedia of sports medicine and science*, Internet Society for Sport Science: http://sportsci.org. 7 March 1998.

Slifkin, A. B., & Newell, K. M. (1999). Is variability in human performance a reflection of system noise? *Current Directions in Psychological Science, 7*, 170–176.

Slobounov, S. M., Moss, S. A., Slobounova, E. S., & Newell, K. M. (1998). Aging and time to instability in posture. *Journal of Gerontology A: Biological Science and Medical Science, 53*, B71–B78.

Sosnoff, J. J., Vaillancourt, D. E., & Newell, K. M. (2004). Aging and force output performance: Loss of adaptive control of multiple neural oscillators. *Journal of Neurophysiology, 91*, 172–181.

Spirduso, W. W. (1995). *Physical dimensions of aging.* Champaign, IL: Human Kinetics.

Sturman, M.M., Vaillancourt, D.E., & Corcos, D.M. (2005). Effects of aging on the regularity of physiological tremor. *Journal of Neurophysiology, 93*, 3064–3074.

Sturman, M. M., Vaillancourt, D. E., Metman, L. V., Bakay, R. A., & Corcos, D. M. (2004). Effects of subthalamic nucleus stimulation and medication on resting and postural tremor in Parkinson's disease. *Brain, 127*, 2131–2143.

Turvey, M.T. (1990). Coordination. *American Psychologist, 45*, 938–953.

Vaillancourt, D. E., Larsson, L., & Newell, K. M. (2003). Effects of aging on force variability, motor unit discharge patterns, and the structure of 10, 20 and 40 Hz EMG activity. *Neurobiology of Aging: Experimental and Clinical Research, 24*, 25–35.

Vaillancourt, D. E., & Newell, K. M. (2000). The dynamics of resting and postural tremor in Parkinson's disease. *Clinical Neurophysiology, 111*, 2042–2052.

Vaillancourt, D. E., & Newell, K.M. (2002). Changing complexity in human behavior and physiology through aging and disease. *Neurobiology of Aging, 23*, 1–11.

Vaillancourt, D. E., & Newell, K. M. (2003). Aging and the time and frequency structure of force output variability. *Journal of Applied Physiology, 94*, 903–912.

Vaillancourt, D. E., Slifkin, A. B., & Newell, K. M. (2002). Inter-digit individuation and force variability in precision grip. *Motor Control, 6*, 113–128.

Vaillancourt, D. E., Sosnoff, J. J., & Newell, K. M. (2004). Age-related changes in complexity depend on task dynamics. *Journal of Applied Physiology, 97*, 454–455.

Vaillancourt, D. E., Sturman, M. M., Metman, L. V., Bakay, R. A., & Corcos, D. M. (2003). Deep brain stimulation of the VIM thalamic nucleus modifies several features of essential tremor. *Neurology, 61,* 919–925.

Van Wegen, E. E. H., Van Emmerik, R. E. A., & Riccio, G. E. (2002). Postural orientation: Age-related changes in variability and time-to-boundary. *Human Movement Science, 21,* 61–84.

Ward, L. M. (2002). *Dynamical cognitive science.* Cambridge, MA: MIT Press.

Welford, A. T. (1981). Signal, noise, performance, and age. *Human Factors, 23,* 97–109.

Welford, A. T. (1988). Reaction time, speed of performance, and age. *Annals of the New York Academy of Science, 515,* 1–17.

Wiesenfeld, K., & Moss, F. (1995). Stochastic resonance and the benefits of noise; from

ices ages to crayfish and SQUIDS. *Nature, 373,* 33–36.

Winter, D. A., Patla, A. E., Frank, J. S., & Walt, S. E. (1990). Biomechanical walking pattern changes in the fit and healthy elderly. *Physical Therapy, 70,* 340–347.

Woollacott, M. H. (2000). Systems contributing to balance disorders in older adults. *Journals of Gerontology: A Biological Sciences and Medical Sciences, 55,* M424–M428.

Yates, F. E. (1987). *Self-organizing systems: The emergence of order.* New York: Plenum Press.

Yates, F. E. (1988). The dynamics of aging and time: How physical action implies social action. In J. E. Birren & V. L. Bengtson (Eds), *Emergent theories of aging.* New York: Springer.

Nine

Changing Role of the Speed of Processing Construct in the Cognitive Psychology of Human Aging

Alan Hartley

Arguably, the concept of speed of processing with its related measures and constructs has had more influence on research into the cognitive psychology of aging than any other over the nearly 30 years from the first edition of the *Handbook of the Psychology of Aging* (Birren & Schaie, 1977) to the current edition. The ranges of discourse have been the same throughout that period, although the emphasis has changed along with a paradigm shift in the research. One range of discourse has been the increased slowness of behavioral and cognitive processes with advancing adult age as a phenomenon to be explained. The second range of discourse has been the reduced speed of processing as a construct to explain age differences in various areas of cognitive functioning. A persistent side issue has been the use of response latency or reaction time as a dependent measure. As we shall see, speed of processing evolved from a term that conveniently summarized a ubiquitous finding into a construct that was a leading candidate for the principal cause of age-related difference and

change. The construct moved out of the foreground as slowing came to be seen as one of many indicators of some single, unidentified common factor underlying most age-related change. The most recent evidence points to the existence of at least several and possibly many underlying factors, leaving the future of the speed of processing construct open to debate.

I. Earlier Reviews

In the earlier editions of the *handbook* and in reviews that preceded those, efforts were primarily to explain the origins of the phenomenon and to describe the accumulated results with precision and parsimony. More recently the emphasis has been on whether slowing can account for age-related differences in cognitive functions, either as a direct cause or as a marker for the general intactness of the central nervous system. One underlying question is how speed of response should be measured, and the answers to that question have depended on the theoretical questions being asked.

A. The First Edition of the Handbook

The outlines of the empirical phenomenon have long been clear both to observant laypersons who noted the longer time needed for older adults to complete almost any task and to scientists who noted the increase in the measured time to respond to almost any stimulus — the reaction time (RT). Reflecting on earlier summaries, Birren and Renner (1977) said, "one of the most clearly established phenomena of aging is the tendency toward slowness of perceptual, motor, and cognitive processes" (p. 28). In 1985, Salthouse collected 15 different superlative adjective phrases used by 20 different groups of authors to convey that reduction of speed with age is an unquestioned laboratory result. Because slowing is so pervasive, it is attractive both as a target and as a tool for theory. It is an attractive target because it is plausible that it might be the result of relatively few underlying changes, allowing for a parsimonious account of a large body of findings. It is an attractive tool because it is plausible that age-related differences in many different complex behaviors might be described parsimoniously as resulting from changes in basic speed and timing of cognitive operations.

If slowing is a central feature of age-related differences, what causes the slowing? The answers have important consequences for both theory and practice. If, on the one hand, the slowing is due to changes in the structure and functioning of the central or peripheral nervous systems, then speed of response could serve as a valid, reliable, and inexpensive marker for *primary aging* (Birren & Schroots, 1996). Primary aging refers to irreversible changes that are intrinsic to the aging process, changes that can be thought of as *normal* or *usual*.

Interventions would tend to be medical and pharmaceutical. If, on the other hand, the slowing is due to differences in arousal, engagement, practice, or strategy that simply accompany differences in age or cohort — whether reversible or not — then speed of response would not be a marker for primary aging and interventions would tend to be environmental or psychosocial.

In the earliest summaries of research on behavioral slowing with age, Birren proposed that it was the result of fundamental changes in the central nervous system (Birren, 1974; Birren & Renner, 1977). He considered but rejected the hypothesis that slowing of the frequency of electrical activity in the brain, demonstrated, for example, by slowing of the alpha rhythm in the EEG, was responsible for behavioral slowing. Birren and Renner (1977) suggested that the slowing might be the result of degenerative change in one neuroanatomical system, the basal ganglia. The basal ganglia are richly connected in feedback–feedforward circuits with large parts of the cortex (Graybiel, 2000), as are the thalami (LaBerge, 1995). These circuits serve to select some stimuli for processing while suppressing others and to select some lines of action to be carried out and others inhibited. Damage to or dysfunction of these circuits could affect most, if not all, cortical processing.

In a review of motor performance that also appeared in the first *Handbook*, Welford (1977) pointed out that a reaction time, Y, could be thought of as resulting from three parameters: $Y = a + bx$, where x reflected the inherent difficulty or complexity of the task. He argued that age-related slowing in Y could be attributed to changes in a, b, or both. These changes could be the result of fundamental changes in the central nervous system. However, Welford argued that changes in a could also result from changes in signal strength (i.e., impaired transduction of signals from the physical world into neural events) but they could also result from changes in general level of arousal, in strategies adopted, or in criteria set for judgment. Similarly, changes in b could result from increased caution or an increased likelihood of monitoring and rechecking results of mental operations.

B. The Second Edition of the Handbook

In the second *handbook*, Salthouse (1985) reasserted the strength and pervasiveness of the basic phenomenon, reporting that the correlation between chronological age and RT averaged 0.45 (with a range from 0.15 to 0.64) over 50 correlations from 39 separate studies with substantial age ranges, implying that 20% of the variance among individuals in RT is accounted for by their age. Because some of the variance in RT must be noise, he argued that the proportion of reliable variance accounted for by age is likely greater than 0.20. Salthouse extended Welford's (1977) analysis of possible explanations for age-related slowing, using the information processing metaphor of the time. Salthouse suggested that slowing could be due to (a) a slowed rate of input and output in older adults; (b) strategic differences, including poorer preparation or inefficient use of stimulus information by older adults or positioning themselves at a different point in the trade-off of accuracy for speed; (c) less well-integrated or compiled or automated control processes; (d) a smaller capacity of working memory; (e) greater concurrent processing demands (perhaps due to under- or overarousal); or (f) hardware differences such as greater neural noise, slowing of fundamental neural events, or a slowed cycle time. Salthouse also cautioned that at least some of the age differences in speed of response could be

due to artifacts in the measurement of RT. Older adults might be less practiced at tasks similar to those used to measure RT. Variability in RT tends to increase with the mean RT, and variability is greater in older adults, making reliable measurement of RT less likely in older adults. Studies using RT as a measure typically have high levels of accuracy. Models of the speed–accuracy trade-off indicate that there will be large costs in RT for small gains in accuracy at high levels of performance. Thus, relatively small differences between younger and older adults in their response criteria could produce substantial differences in RT. Tasks that produce relatively long response latencies allow the possibility that different age groups may use different sequences of operations to carry out the task or that individuals may use different sequences on different trials. As a result, age differences in overall RT will be less informative than they appear. Finally, transformations may be applied to RTs to correct for violations of normality, particularly positive skew, in the process losing the original real-time metric. Salthouse concluded that it was difficult to find many published studies that avoided all of these possible pitfalls and argued that, as a result, there was little reliable evidence for deciding among the possible theoretical mechanisms for age-related slowing that he elaborated. His pessimistic conclusion was that "temporal variables may not be as well suited for developmental investigations of cognitive processes as for those involving more homogeneous populations" (p. 421). Nevertheless, he also proposed, looking forward, that "it is reasonable to expect that other cognitive processes will share some of the causes, and perhaps be influenced by the consequences of, age-related slowing" (p. 421). That is to say, age-related slowing could serve as a construct to explain age-related differences in behaviors presumed to reflect other and various cognitive processes.

C. The Third Edition of the Handbook

Given Salthouse's (1985) pessimistic warning about methodological and interpretive problems, it is reasonable to ask why research on age-related slowing continued at all, much less why its value as an explanatory construct was explored. The answers to those questions are instructive and lead to the developments summarized in the chapters on speed of processing in the third edition (Cerella, 1990) and the fifth edition (Madden, 2001) of the *handbook*. [There was no chapter devoted specifically to age-related differences in speed of processing in the fourth edition of the *handbook*, although Birren and Schroots (1996) mentioned continuing developments later elaborated and summarized by Madden (2001).]

What is not in doubt is that longer latencies and slower speeds of responses have been reported routinely in all manner of tasks. The age-related differences can be lower in aerobically conditioned older adults and in those who are elite athletes (e.g., Clarkson-Smith & Hartley, 1989, 1990), can be reduced but not eliminated by practice (e.g., Salthouse & Somberg, 1982), and are lower when responses are vocal rather than manual (e.g., Nebes, 1978). Nevertheless, these are relatively minor qualifications of the general result. What is also not in doubt is that response latency is theoretically overdetermined — many different constructs can be plausibly seen as influencing RT, including sensory limitations (Li & Lindenberger, 2002), increased cautiousness or other strategy differences (Salthouse & Hedden, 2002), focal changes in the nervous system (Rubin, 1999), or diffuse changes in the nervous system (Birren, 1974). As a result, the interpretation of age-related slowing is in doubt.

The most parsimonious interpretation is that there are one or a few differences or changes that have widespread effects on virtually all behaviors. Call this the *few causes hypothesis*. The least parsimonious interpretation is that there are a large number of differences or changes that have significant effects on speed of responses, that those effects may be different in different individuals or that those effects may be different even within the same individuals at different times. Call this the *many causes hypothesis*. Between these two extremes lie a large number of families of possible interpretations, each with an impossibly large number of specific instantiations.

Arguing from plausibility or from logical necessity, we can rule out some of the possible changes as few causes. A simple diminution of sensory input would slow older adults relative to younger adults and the slowing would be evident in most tasks, but the effect would not be exaggerated as the complexity of the task is increased (in Welford's formulation, sensory impairment would affect the intercept, a, but not the slope, b, in the formula for RT: $Y = a + bx$). An increase in RT with increasing complexity is observed routinely. It is implausible that age differences in RT due to differences in arousal, outlook, or specific strategy would be relatively unaffected by changes in task or task demands, in instruction, in incentive, or in motivation if there were few causes. Nevertheless, manipulations of these variables have little effect and may affect younger adults as much or more than older adults (for a summary, see Salthouse, 1985). Only changes in the nervous system — either focal changes in systems that broadly affect nervous system functioning or diffuse but reasonably uniform changes — seem attractive as candidates for the few causes hypothesis.

If instead the many causes hypothesis is correct, age differences may be seen in most tasks but there should be no systematicity to the differences that are seen. This appears to provide an empirical and descriptive way around the theoretical conundrum. If there is only one cause, then the same systematic relation between response times for younger adults and response times for older adults should be observed across all tasks and individuals. The specific task should not matter. If there are a few principal causes, then there would be systematic relations within families of tasks (requiring similar processes) or within similar individuals (utilizing similar processes). If there are many causes and particularly if there are different causes affecting different situations and individuals differently, there should be no systematic relation between the RTs of younger and older adults. Is there, in fact, a systematic relationship? This question was addressed by a number of researchers and Cerella (1990) summarized the relevant findings in the third *handbook*.

Cerella (1990) concluded that there were indeed highly systematic, even lawful, relationships between the RTs of younger adults and those of older adults across a wide range of tasks. Data summarized in his review were the mean latencies for younger adults and for older adults in each of a large number of cognitive tasks. These pairs of mean RTs are often presented graphically in what has come to be called a Brinley plot (after Brinley, 1965). The question he asked was this: "Do these pairs of points show a systematic relationship across tasks and, if so, what is the nature of the relationship?" This renders moot the methodological concerns about RT raised by Salthouse (1985). If RTs are inherently unreliable or if they have routinely been collected in ways that render them unreliable, systematic relationships will not be found. If they are

not found, then the question will rearise whether the lack of systematicity is due to the measurement of RT or to the presence of multiple causes of age differences in RT.

Cerella (1990) considered a variety of functions for their fit to existing data. The simplest described the latency for older adults (L_{OLD}) as a multiple of the latency on the same task for younger adults (L_{YOUNG}):

$$L_{OLD} = mL_{YOUNG} \qquad (1)$$

Cerella described this as the *classical model*, which provided a good fit to data in earlier summaries (Cerella, Poon, & Williams, 1980; Salthouse, 1985). The striking implication of this model is that the only relevant aspect of a task is the relative time required for completion; the nature of the task is otherwise irrelevant. As tasks take longer, differences in latency between younger and older adults will be multiplied. Such a generalized slowing would result if there were diffuse changes in a network structure such as the nervous system. A typical value of the multiplier, m, might be about 1.50. This would result if each synaptic transmission in an older adult required 50% longer than the same transmission in a younger adult. Alternatively, the same outcome would result if only 1/1.50 or 67% of the neural connections remained intact.

Cerella also considered a variant of the multiplicative model (Cerella, 1985), prompted by a reanalysis of data summarized in Cerella et al. (1980). This model proposed two processing stages: one fixed across tasks of a particular type (of duration S_1) and one varying with the complexity of the specific task of that type (of duration S_2). Cerella suggested that the fixed stage, S_1, might include perceptual-motor operations necessary to register and, later, give an effector response to the stimulus, whereas the variable-duration stage, S_2, would include central computational operations. Because the total latency for young adults would be $L_{YOUNG} = S_1 + S_2$, latencies for older adults would then be given by

$$L_{OLD} = m_{S_1}S_1 + m_{S_2}(L_{YOUNG} - S_1) \quad (2)$$

In such a multilayer model, operations in the fixed stage would have a constant penalty for older adults, whereas operations in the variable stage would show an overhead cost for each operation (precisely, each unit of time) that would increase as the number of operations increased. The result is a nonlinear function with two parts, each itself linear.

Cerella (1990) described a model proposed by Hale and Myerson (Hale, Myerson, & Wagstaff, 1987; Meyerson et al., 1990) that also resulted in a nonlinear function. This model supposed that there is information loss with each operation, e.g., each synaptic transmission, such that a proportion, p, of the information is transmitted. The model supposed further that the proportions could be different for older adults (p_{OLD}) and younger adults (p_{YOUNG}). Response latency for older adults would then be given as

$$L_{OLD} = cL_{YOUNG}^{P_{OLD}/P_{YOUNG}} \quad (3)$$

where c is a constant dependent only on p_{OLD}/p_{YOUNG}.

Cerella (1990) concluded that all of the models described aggregate data well and did not settle on any one as definitive. All of the models he explored could be considered as following from a neural network metaphor, and he considered their good fit to data to be an indication that a small number of assumptions about degeneration in the central nervous system could economically replace a large number of task-specific explanations of age-related differences in RT. He considered alternative explanations for age-related slowing including increased cautiousness or a shift in the speed–accuracy trade-off, lack of practice, and adoption of different task strategies by younger and older adults. He rejected these as both not consistent with available data and not parsimonious theories.

Cerella's conclusions must be taken with caution. Clear evidence shows that the slope of the L_{OLD}/L_{YOUNG} functions—captured by the multiplier, m, or information loss parameter, p—differs for different types of tasks (e.g, Hale, Lima, & Myerson, 1991; Lima, Hale, & Myerson, 1991) or even for different measures of response latency in the same task (Bashore, Osman, & Heffley, 1989). This means that the changes underlying the slowing are not uniform and diffuse but rather must be different for different operations or combinations of operations, consistent with the few causes hypothesis. Fisher and Glaser (1996) showed formally that there is a relatively high likelihood of accepting the hypothesis of common, generalized slowing when in fact there is different slowing in different processes. In addition, the fact that data are well fit by models derived from simple neural network assumptions does not mean that other, very different models deriving from other metaphors would not also provide good fits. That is, it is possible and plausible that age-related slowing is due to fundamental and pervasive changes in central nervous system structure or function, but it is not necessary. Finally, Ratcliff, Spieler, and McKoon (2000, 2004) have questioned whether the slope of the L_{OLD}/L_{YOUNG} functions might be a statistical artifact rather than a reflection of underlying differences in structure or function. They noted that these functions are very similar to quantile–quantile functions, in which the plotted points are the data value at a particular quantile of one distribution paired with the data value for a second distribution at the same quantile. The slope of a quantile–quantile function is determined by the ratio of the variability in the first distribution to that in the second. If it is stipulated that the mean performance for older adults across a set of tasks is more variable than that of younger adults, the slope will differ from one and no assumption about relative speed of processing is necessary. Although L_{OLD}/L_{YOUNG} functions may not always meet the strict definition of a quantile–quantile function (Myerson et al., 2003), they are sufficiently similar that this conclusion also holds for functions relating younger and older adult RTs (Ratcliff et al., 2004). Only if a model assumes sequential, serial processing will the slope reflect differences in processing speed. All of the models entertained by Cerella (1990) made this assumption.

D. The Fifth Edition of the Handbook

In the fifth edition of the *handbook*, Madden (2001) recapitulated the attempts to fit L_{OLD}/L_{YOUNG} functions, an approach he termed the *method of systematic relations*. He identified a newly emerging research approach, *mediational models*, that grew out of Salthouse's (1985) call to explore the possibility that changes in speed of response might account for changes in complex cognitive tasks. The questions are to what extent the age-related variance in cognitive tasks is shared across tasks and to what extent that shared variance can be explained by individual differences in speed of processing (Salthouse 1992a, 1996a,b). In addition to these *macroapproaches*, Madden (2001) also reviewed *microapproaches* including quasi-experimental studies in the areas of memory, attention, and mental arithmetic, some of whose findings appear inconsistent with models that predict general slowing with age. He also described various approaches taken to adjust the results of these studies to compensate for general age-related slowing of speed of processing. Madden's distinction between microapproaches and macroapproaches remains a very useful way to parse the field. We will return to the issues he raised and resummarize some of the research he reviewed as we examine current work concerned with age-related slowing.

II. Current Research

With mediational approaches, the emphasis shifted from explaining age-related differences in speed of processing to using those differences as an explanation for other phenomena. The mediational approach itself has evolved, and with that evolution the role of speed of processing in explaining age-related differences in cognitive performance has shifted.

A mediational approach does not require that one take a position on whether differences in speed of processing are causal or are simply correlates of changes in task performance. It is possible that slowing plays a causal role either because more basic processes are lengthened, taking necessary time away from higher level processes, or because slowing of some operations means that their output will not be available to later operations at a critical point (Salthouse, 1996b). However, it is also possible that slowing is simply a correlate of or marker for other changes (Rabbitt et al., 2004a). For example, because responses in most speeded tasks require a large number of component operations performed under time pressure, RT may reflect the general intactness of the nervous system, tapping the aggregate effect of many small and disparate age-related changes.

A. Mediation Models

The simplest mediation models hold that age differences in performance on

a. Independence Model

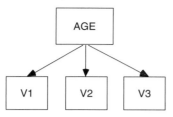

b. Mediation Model (Version 1)

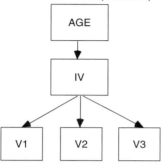

c. Mediation Model (Version 2)

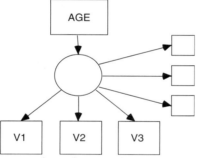

Figure 9.1 Independence and mediation models of the influence of chronological age on measured cognitive performance. After Salthouse (2001b) with the permission of the author and Elsevier.

initially presumed to be speed of response. This could be a single measured variable as in Figure 9.1b or it could be a latent variable inferred from several observed measures as in Figure 9.1c. The methods used to test mediation models have evolved from partial correlations — in which variance in the cognitive variables is adjusted for speed before exploring correlations of age and cognitive performance — to hierarchical linear regression — in which the effects of age are compared when stepped in as the first predictor and when stepped in after speed — to structural equation models in which all relevant variables and their causal or correlational connections are dealt with simultaneously.

In one example of research using a mediational approach, Salthouse and Fristoe (1995; also see Salthouse et al., 2000) analyzed performance on both the standard version of the Trailmaking Test and a computerized version. In the simpler version of the task, Trails A, the participant must link numbered nodes on a sheet in numeric order; in the more complex version of the task, trails B, the participant must maintain two lists — numeric and alphabetic — shifting between sequences with each successive connection: A to 1 to B to 2, and so on. A large portion of the variance in trails B performance was accounted for by measures of speed, either speed as measured by the time to complete the simpler trails A or as measured by a composite variable from two computerized reaction time tasks based on the WAIS-R digit symbol substitution subtest. Using trails A to predict trails B is the model shown in Figure 9.1b, whereas using the composite is the model shown in Figure 9.1c. Salthouse (2001b) explored whether constructs at the same level of analysis as speed of processing, such as working memory, inhibitory functioning, or attentional capacity, mediated age differences in performance. Salthouse's

cognitive tasks can be explained by age differences in speed of processing (e.g., Salthouse, 1993, 1994, 2001b). Versions of the mediation model are shown in Figure 9.1b and 9.1c, distinguished from the independence model shown in Figure 9.1a, which allows for independent effects of age on each of the cognitive variables (V). The intervening variable mediating the effect of age (IV) was conclusion was that these constructs could account for significant portions of the variance in cognitive performance, but that measures of speed typically accounted not only for more of the variance in cognitive performance, but also for much of the variance in the other construct.

Other investigators explored whether observed or latent variables from other levels of analysis could be mediating age differences in performance. From results of the Berlin Aging Study (BASE), Lindenberger and Baltes (1994) and Baltes and Lindenberger (1997) found that measures of visual and auditory acuity predicted significant portions of the variance in a battery of cognitive tests designed to assess intelligence. Controlling for individual differences in sensory acuity was about as effective in reducing age-related variance in cognitive measures as was controlling for speed. Lindenberger, Scherer, and Baltes (2003) later showed that the impairment of sensory input alone was not responsible for poorer performance, as degrading input for younger adults did not reproduce the poorer performance of the older adults. Anstey, Luszcz, and Sanchez (2001) obtained results similar to those of Lindenberger and Baltes (1994) in a large-scale study in the Australian Longitudinal Study of Aging (ALSA), finding that a larger portion of the age-related variance in cognitive performance was shared with sensory function than was shared with speed.

Other noncognitive mediators have also been explored, including balance, grip strength, respiratory function (forced expiratory lung volume, FEV), and blood pressure (e.g., Anstey et al., 2004; Christenson et al., 2001; Hofer, Berg, & Era, 2003). Other putative mediators have been even more basic physiological measures, including cortical area, global brain volume, cerebral blood flow, cerebral white matter volume, and presence of apolipoprotein E (APOE) alleles (e.g., Anstey & Christensen, 2000; Christensen et al., 2001; Deary et al., 2003; Madden et al., 2004; Rabbitt et al., 2005; Rabbitt et al., 2004a; Rodrigue & Raz, 2004). Because many of these measures account for a significant portion of the variance in cognitive variables, one interpretation is that the underlying cause for age-related differences is a general reduction in the functional intactness of the central nervous system (e.g., Salthouse & Caja, 2000).

B. Common Cause Models

A very different conceptualization of the finding that both cognitive and noncognitive variables share substantial variance is that age can be modeled as affecting whatever is common to many different types of variables (Salthouse & Ferrer-Caja, 2003). Models of this type are called common cause or shared influence models, the simplest form of which is shown in Figure 9.2. Note that Figure 9.2 closely resembles Figure 9.1c, in which the effects of age were mediated by an intervening construct. In shared

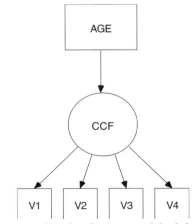

Figure 9.2 Shared influence model of the influence of chronological age on measured cognitive performance. After Salthouse (2001b) with the permission of the author and Elsevier.

influence models, there is no assumption that any particular construct serves as the principal mediator. The association between speed or sensory acuity and cognitive variables might simply be an artifact of the relationship each of these variables has with age (Christensen et al., 2001; Salthouse, 1998, 2001b). In shared influence models the construct that intervenes between age and specific measures of behavior is simply capturing the variance that is shared by all of the measured variables. Christensen et al. (2001) call this a *common cause factor* (CCF) to emphasize the fact that it is an empirically determined latent variable. They reserve the term *common cause* to refer to the underlying processes that are postulated to be responsible for the decline with age in a large number of observed variables. Age is modeled as affecting the common cause. Measures of speed are no longer privileged as causally prior to other variables or constructs; they are simply variables that share age-related variance with other variables. In a structural modeling approach, the question whether it is necessary to add a specific connection from age to performance on a particular task beyond the indirect connection via the CCF can be answered empirically by testing whether the fit of the model with only a single, common latent variable can be improved by adding specific paths. Relationships among the variables that do not involve age can also be accommodated in hierarchical models such as those proposed by Salthouse and Ferrer-Caja (2003), two of which are shown in Figure 9.3. In Figure 9.3a, the effects of age are mediated through the component cognitive factors, whereas in Figure 9.3b, the effects of age, through the common factor, on the measured variables are independent of the structural composition of the measures.

One example of an investigation exploring common cause models was carried out

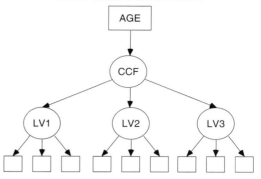

a. CCF affects first-order factors

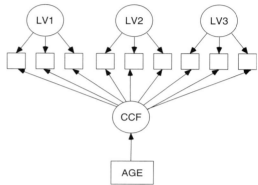

b. CCF affects measured variables

Figure 9.3 Shared influence models allowing first-order factor structure among the measures of cognitive performance. After Salthouse and Ferrer-Caja (2003) with the permission of the authors.

by Christensen et al. (2001) on 374 Australian participants, in four age cohorts with average ages ranging from 80 to 94 years (see also Anstey, Luszcz, & Sanchez, 2001). The measures included blood pressure, grip strength, visual acuity, FEV, simple and choice RT, crystallized intelligence measures (vocabulary and similarities from the WAIS-R, the National Adult Reading Test, Nelson, 1982), and memory measures of recognition and recall. Speed was measured by a variant of the digit symbol substitution test in which the participant translated symbols into letters using a key. A multiple indicator, multiple cause (MIMIC) model as shown in Figure 9.4 was fit to the data. In addition to age, the MIMIC

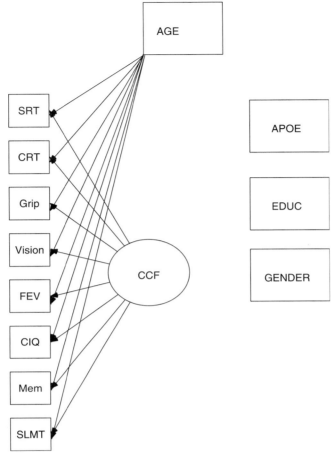

Figure 9.4 Multiple indicator, multiple cause model with effects of covariates both through the common cause factor and through individual influences on measures of performance. Links are shown only for the age covariate, but were explored for presence of the APOE allele, years of education, and gender as well. SRT, simple reaction time; CRT, choice reaction time; Grip, grip strength; Vision, visual acuity; FEV, forced expiratory lung volume; CIQ, crystallized intelligence score; Mem, memory score; SLMT, symbol letter modalities test (similar to the digit symbol substitution test from the WAIS-R). After Christensen et al. (2001) with the permission of the authors.

model included demographic and genetic predictors such as gender, education, and APOE genotype. The existence of connections from every predictor to every variable was assessed, although Figure 9.4 shows the connections only for age. The final model, which provided a good fit to data, included significant loadings on the CCF for every measured variable except blood pressure. The estimated value of the CCF declined as age increased. In addition, there were direct effects of age on grip strength and visual acuity beyond those mediated by the CCF. For the other predictors, CCF was significantly lower for women than men but it was not affected significantly by education or presence of the APOE genotype. As with age, gender showed significant direct effects on measured variables. Grip strength and FEV were lower in women than in men and crystallized intelligence, memory, and speed were higher when CCF was held constant. Consistent with an earlier hypothesis by Salthouse (1998), Christensen et al. (2001) speculated that the common factor might represent the individual's conscious understanding of her or his situation, as blood pressure was unrelated to the CCF and it was the only measure that did not require the participant to follow instructions for the measure to be obtained. Simultaneous modeling of covariates other than age allowed some conclusions about the underlying common cause. The common cause is probably not a form of general intelligence, as education does not significantly affect the CCF. Similarly, brain disorders associated with the APOE ε4 allele are not the common cause, although this does not rule out the possibility that other indicators of central nervous system intactness such as white matter lesions or cortical atrophy might affect the CCF.

Another example of an investigation guided by the common cause conception illustrates other extensions to the approach (Salthouse & Ferrer-Caja, 2003). Multiple measures of spatial ability, reasoning, memory, and speed were obtained from 204 individuals, aged 20 to 91 years. In addition to models of the CCF such as those described earlier, Salthouse and Ferrer-Caja (2003) also explored models that allowed for the existence of interrelations among the measured variables other than those due to the common cause. One such model shown in Figure 9.3a (model C in Salthouse & Ferrer-Caja) allows a hierarchical structure of cognitive abilities in which the CCF is a second-order factor hypothesized to exist at a level above first-order factors on which the measured variables load. Additional layers could also intervene between the lowest level factors and the highest level CCF. With this model it was also possible to explore whether there were significant paths from age to either the first-order factors or the measured variables beyond the effects mediated by the CCF. The best-fitting model is shown in Figure 9.5. Estimated values of the CCF declined with age. Beyond the effects mediated by the CCF, factor scores for speed and memory also declined

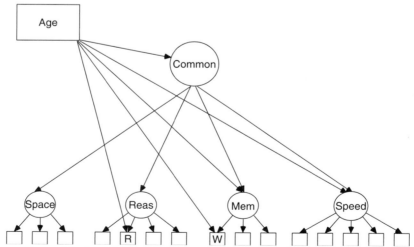

Figure 9.5 Best-fitting model from Salthouse and Ferrer-Caja (2003). Reas, reasoning; R, Raven progressive matrices; Mem, memory; W, Wechsler logical memory scale.

significantly with increasing age. In addition for individual measured variables, there was a significant negative connection of age with reasoning performance on Raven's progressive matrices and a positive connection of age with memory performance on the Wechsler memory scale logical memory subscale. Further analyses showed the best-fitting model to be highly robust. The same model fit well when fit simultaneously to data of participants over and under 50 years of age; it also fit well to the relationships among the measured variables with variance due to age partialled out. The model also fit well when fit simultaneously to three data sets: data that were collected and two previously collected data sets.

An investigation by Salthouse, Atkinson, and Berish (2003) highlighted the relationship between earlier mediational models in which some ability or aspect of processing was given causal primacy in explaining cognitive performance and common cause models in which the CCF captures variance common to many measures, without giving causal primacy to any. In recent years there has been considerable interest in the possibility that many observed age differences are mediated by age-related decrements in executive functioning, those control processes responsible for planning, coordinating, and monitoring other cognitive processes (Salthouse, 2001b; Salthouse et al., 2003). Further, many variables measuring executive functioning had been grouped together because they were sensitive to damage to the frontal lobes of the cortex, particularly prefrontal regions. Two constructs often presumed to require executive contributions are switching between tasks (task switching) and carrying out two tasks simultaneously (time sharing). In earlier investigations, Salthouse and Miles (2002) and Salthouse and colleagues (1998) had found that latent variables measuring task switching and time sharing could be distinguished from

other constructs, although the relationships between these constructs, age, and other constructs were largely shared. Following a research strategy described by Salthouse (2001a), Salthouse et al. (2003) tested whether age-related variance in various measures was mediated through a second-order construct of executive function, which in turn comprised distinct constructs of updating (similar to switching), time sharing, and inhibition of distracting information. In addition, Salthouse et al. (2003) also included a number of neuropsychological instruments used commonly to assess executive function, presumably reflecting frontal lobe functioning. The model of executive function is shown in Figure 9.6. The model in which executive function mediates the effects of age is shown in Figure 9.7. Tasks were constructed to yield 11 measures of executive function, augmented by five common neuropsychological measures. Fifteen other tasks assessed other cognitive constructs: crystallized and fluid intelligence as well as episodic memory and perceptual speed. The tasks were administered to 261 individuals, aged 18 to 84 years. The executive function factor did mediate significant variance in the cognitive variables. However, there was little evidence that updating, time sharing, and inhibitory function were distinguishable aspects of executive function or that the executive function construct could be distinguished from fluid intelligence. Salthouse et al. (2003) concluded that executive function did not have sufficient discriminant validity to warrant exploration as a cause of age-related differences.

C. Alternatives to Cross-Sectional Designs

Juxtaposing these examples of investigations taking a common cause approach raises a number of issues. One, however,

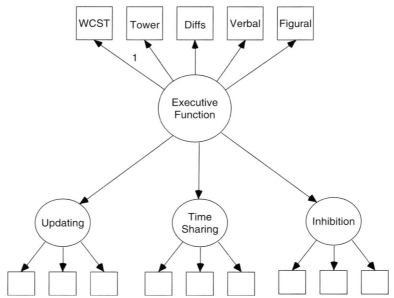

Figure 9.6 Model of executive functioning with neuropsychological measures (top) and experimental measures (bottom). WCST, Wisconsin card sorting test; Tower, Tower of Hanoi; Diffs, connections test (a variant of the trail making test); Verbal, verbal fluency; Figural, figural fluency. After Salthouse et al. (2003) with the permission of the authors.

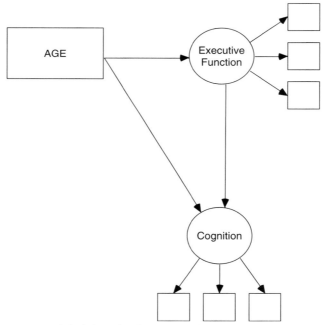

Figure 9.7 Model of the role of executive functioning in mediating the effects of chronological age on cognitive performance. After Salthouse et al. (2003) with the permission of the authors.

is central. All of these investigations have used cross-sectional designs over a range of ages. Hofer (Hofer & Sliwinski, 2001; Hofer, Sliwinski, & Flaherty, 2002) demonstrated that mean differences between age groups can result in nonzero covariance between variables even when the underlying association between the variables is zero. This is a specific instance of a previously known general problem that combining distinct groups in which differences in the two variables to be associated are both correlated with group membership can result in a spurious correlation. Put simply, this means that the presence of the CCF may be a statistical artifact.

Hofer, Berg, and Era (2003) proposed one solution to this problem: *narrow age cohort designs*, in which all the participants fall in a very narrow age range. In their case, the 1,041 participants from the Nordic Research on Aging Study (Schroll e al., 1993; Heikkenen et al., 1997) were all 75 years of age. The assumption is that there have been age-related changes both within and between individuals and so the covariation of individual differences across measured variables will, to a large degree, reflect covariation in rates of aging. They assessed performance on cognitive measures, proximal age-related variables (visual and auditory acuity), and distal age-related variables (balance; hand, arm, and leg strength; FEV; and number of teeth). The term distal reflects that supposition that the variable bears no apparent direct relation to cognitive function. Results showed moderate-to-strong associations across variables within each of the domains, but weak and inconsistent associations across domains. They concluded that a common factor model would have provided a poor fit. The fact that variables distal to cognition, especially number of teeth, correlated as well with cognitive performance, as did measures of sensory function, suggested that the covariation

may be due more to the effects of changes due to health and socioeconomic status than to a common cause such as aging of the central nervous system.

Longitudinal designs provide even stronger tests of the common cause hypothesis, and results from such studies have begun to become available (Anstey, Hofer, & Luszcz, 2003a,b; Christensen et al., 2001, 2004; Sliwinski & Buschke, 1999; Sliwinski, Hofer, & Hall, 2003; Sliwinski et al., 2003; Zimprich & Martin, 2002). If individual differences in the rate of change are governed by a common factor, then changes over time in the levels of latent variables reflecting cognitive and sensory function should be strongly correlated. For example, Anstey et al. (2003a) modeled data collected from 1823 individuals from the Australian Longitudinal Study of Aging who had participated in at least one of three waves of measurement over an 8-year period. Measures of cognitive performance included verbal ability, memory, and processing speed. Visual and auditory acuity were also assessed. In addition to chronological age, measurements were obtained for gender, education, depression, medical conditions, and self-reported health. Preliminary analysis showed that the factor structure for the cognitive and sensory latent variables was stable over time. With this established, latent growth curves for the latent variables could then be examined. A latent growth curve specifies both the level of the latent variable at the outset of measurement (the latent mean) and the rate of change, or slope, in the variable over the longitudinal period. Consistent with the earlier, cross-sectional evidence for a common cause factor, the initial levels of the latent variables — verbal, memory, speed, vision, and hearing — were strongly correlated. In the analysis of rates of change, slopes for the two cognitive variables — memory and speed — were strongly correlated ($r = 0.62$); those for cognitive and sensory variables were moderately correlated $(0.15 \leq r \leq 0.54)$; those for the two sensory variables — vision and hearing — were only weakly correlated $(r=0.16)$. (The estimated slopes for verbal ability did not have sufficient variance to permit analysis.) Adjusting for age and other covariates reduced the correlations substantially, leaving only significant correlations of speed with memory $(r=0.52)$, vision with memory $(r=0.22)$, and vision with hearing $(r=0.16)$. Adjusting for age removes that portion of the observed association among variables that is due to a shared statistical association with age. At the same time, it would also remove the effects of unmeasured common causes. Nevertheless, longitudinal analyses of the rates of change in the values of the latent constructs were not consistent with a single, monolithic, common process underlying age-related changes in sensation and cognition. Rather, there appear to be independent processes that affect some abilities but not others.

Sliwinski et al. (2003a) analyzed data from 488 participants in the Bronx Aging Study who were tested up to 12 times during a 16-year period. The average age at the first assessment was 80 years; at the last assessment, 85 years. They measured free recall memory, category fluency, and speed. As did Anstey et al. (2003a), Sliwinski et al. (2003a) found moderately strong correlations both among the initial levels of the latent variables $(0.47 \leq r \leq 0.62)$ and among the slopes giving the rates of change $(0.56 \leq r \leq 0.61)$. These correlations are interindividual or between persons. Sliwinski et al. (2003a) also computed intraindividual or within-person correlations across occasions. Intraindividual correlations between the latent variables were only about half the magnitude of the interindividual correlations. A unique feature of the study by Sliwinski et al.

(2003a) was that every participant was followed until an outcome was obtained: (a) a clinical diagnosis of dementia, (b) a dropout from participation in the study, or (c) death. When results for those who never developed dementing disease were compared to those for the full sample, the rates of decline were lower and the intercorrelations of both the initial levels and slopes were attenuated. The group that later developed dementia is particularly important. Although dementing disorders have differential effects on different parts of the brain at different stages of the disease, it should be approximately correct to think of the underlying disease as a common cause. If this is so, then change is modeled more appropriately with respect to disease progression than with respect to chronological age. This was done by indexing measures not by the chronological age at which they were collected, but rather by the number of years before a diagnosis of dementia was made. When this was done, no reliable variance remained in the individual rates of change over the 5 years prior to the diagnosis of dementia; the interindividual correlations were not significantly larger than zero. The intraindividual correlations were robust $(0.45 \leq r \leq 0.51)$. Sliwinski et al. (2003a) offered the counterintuitive conclusion that the lack of interindividual correlations among abilities is not evidence against a single common cause, rather it is evidence that the loss of cognitive abilities due to a common cause will be essentially uniform across individuals when change is specified correctly relative to the time course of the common cause. Operation of a common cause does not necessitate high between-persons correlations among rates of change in cognitive variables. Sliwinski et al. (2003a) demonstrated, both empirically and analytically, that spurious correlations of rates of change can be generated by mixing of subgroups with different average rates of change (such as dementing and nondementing individuals).

D. Evaluating Common Cause Approaches

Where does the common cause hypothesis stand? Let us review our steps. Evidence from cross-sectional studies generally supported the existence of a common cause factor through which age affected most cognitive and noncognitive constructs. There was some evidence for direct connections from age to constructs and even to specific measures. Nevertheless, most of the age-related variance was shared, consistent with the operation of a common cause. The high proportion of shared variance was used as an argument against considering certain constructs, particularly executive function, as separable constructs when attempting to explain age-related differences. There are practical concerns. The standardized coefficient for the regression of the CCF onto age was higher when all of the variables measured cognitive performance, using primarily psychometrically devised measures [e.g., in Salthouse & Ferrer-Caja, (2003) $\beta = -.51$] than when there was a mix of cognitive and noncognitive variables [e.g., in Anstey et al., (2003), $\beta = -.28$]. The proportion of shared variance may be inflated when the measures used are relatively homogeneous. There are also methodological limitations. Correlational methods are relatively weak approaches for testing causality, and variance that is apparently associated with age may be the artifactual result of intercorrelations of other factors (Lindenberger & Pötter, 1998). Moreover, the methods are relatively weak at finding associations beyond those due to a CCF even when data sets are constructed with such associations present (Allen et al., 2001).

Critical evidence against the common cause hypothesis, however, comes from the results of longitudinal studies. Anstey et al. (2003a) and Sliwinski et al. (2003a) found that rates of change were correlated only moderately among cognitive variables such as speed, memory, and fluid intelligence. Sliwinski et al. (2003a) demonstrated that correlations were attenuated when individuals who were later diagnosed with dementia were removed. Because the natural history of the dementia is tied only loosely to chronological age, mixing dementing and nondementing individuals together would inflate the apparent correlations in rates of change. It is still possible that there is a common cause operating in individuals without dementia (noncases), that the cause is tied only loosely to chronological age as is diagnosis of dementia, and that the smearing that results when change is indexed by age produces nonzero correlations. Presumably, if it were possible to find a good marker for the progression of the common cause and it were possible to index change to that marker, interindividual correlations might be close to zero. However, if there is a common cause, then intraindividual correlations should be high and should be elevated by selecting an appropriate marker. Sliwinski et al. (2003a) found this for individuals later diagnosed as demented. For the noncases, however, the magnitude of intraindividual correlations was about half that of interindividual correlations.

Longitudinal studies are not without methodological limitations, such as participant selection at the outset and selective attrition over the course of the study (Christensen et al., 2004) as well as test–retest effects (Ferrer et al., 2004). Salthouse (2005) suggested that longitudinal studies must span decades to capture change adequately, so the low correlations among rates of change in constructs that have been observed may be the result of time spans that are too short. Nevertheless, there are two plausible interpretations of the low correlations.

One, multiple, independent causes may be operating to produce age-related change (Anstey et al., 2003a,b; Anstey, Luszcz, & Sanchez, 2001; Christensen et al., 2004; Sliwinski et al., 2003a,b; Zimprich & Martin, 2002). Two, there may be only one or a few causes, but those causes are related only very weakly to chronological age. If there is no common cause, this implies that an age-related change in speed of processing cannot be the principal cause of age-related change in cognitive function. If there is a common cause, linked weakly to age, speed of processing might be an indicator for its effects.

III. Summary

The earliest invocation of the speed of processing construct was as a parsimonious way to summarize a large body of findings that older adults were slower to execute tasks than younger adults over a wide range of tasks. The relationship was lawful, although there was debate about the nature of the most appropriate law. Hope was expressed that the lawful relationship would point the way to the identification of a single underlying cause for age-related slowing. It did not. A fact that was sometimes noted but usually accorded little attention was that the precise nature of the lawful relationship, the specific parameter value fit to a group of studies, was different within different domains of speeded cognitive tasks. The asserted homogeneity of the findings was greater than the actual homogeneity, probably because of a strong desire to find a parsimonious explanation for age-related differences. The evidence was consistent with, at least, the few causes hypothesis and, possibly, the many causes hypothesis.

Even without knowing the underlying cause of slowing, it was still possible to speculate that a wide variety of other changes in cognitive function with age might be either correlated with or sequelae of changes in speed of processing. Speed of processing, whether as a measured variable or an inferred latent variable, accounted for a large portion of the age-related variance in a wide range of cognitive tasks. A fact that was sometimes noted but usually accorded little attention was that the measures of speed of processing that were most effective in accounting for variance in cognitive tasks were not relatively pure measures such as simple reaction time but, rather, were complex psychometric measures that tapped a variety of functions, including not just speed but also attention, working memory, and executive function. Not only is the WAIS digit-symbol substitution subscale widely used to measure speed, but Salthouse (1985) even argued at one point that it would be a good candidate for a universal measure to allow comparisons of groups. However, variation in paper-and-pencil digit symbol performance reflects not only differences in the speed of determining the appropriate symbol digit link, but also in the organization and monitoring of the process of working across and down the page, the extent to which the pairings are kept available in working memory, the efficiency of the scan through the key if they are not, the extent to which the motor movements of responding require higher level monitoring, and other factors beyond pure speed of processing. Simple reaction time, which ought to be a very pure marker for speed, is not as effective at accounting for variance in cognitive performance. Once again, the asserted homogeneity of the findings was greater than the actual homogeneity, probably because of a strong desire to find a parsimonious explanation for age-related differences.

Speed of processing lost primacy of place as a cause of age-related decline when it became clear that other, noncognitive variables, such as sensory acuity, could also account for a large portion of the age-related variance in cognitive performance. Whereas speed of processing had been treated as a primitive cognitive process in explaining more complex processes, it was now treated either as one of several possible markers for the physiological intactness of the organism or, more frequently and simply, as one of many cognitive processes. Instead of looking for a single, underlying cause that mediated change in cognitive performance, researchers proposed that there was some deeper underlying change that in turn explained strongly associated changes across a variety of tasks, including tasks that measured speed of processing. The common cause models that resulted largely provided very good fits to data collected on cognitive performance across a wide cross-sectional range of adult ages. Speed of processing was no longer the leading candidate for a common cause. The common cause hypothesis foundered on longitudinal data that showed weak intraindividual correlations between measured or latent variables over time. What remains is a presumption that age-related change is driven at least by a few and possibly by many causes. Further, we must entertain the possibility that a single cause could appear to be a few causes or that a few causes could appear to be many causes if cognitive changes are linked tightly to underlying processes that are themselves only moderately linked to age. The clear example of this was the finding by Sliwinski et al. (2003a) that cognitive change was linked tightly to the progress of dementia, whereas the occurrence and progression of dementia are related only moderately to chronological age.

A. Searching for Causes

What might those causes be and how might we identify them? Concerning what the causes might be, Salthouse (2004; Salthouse, Atkinson, & Berish, 2003; Salthouse & Czaja, 2000; Salthouse & Ferrer-Caja, 2003) suggested insightfully that possible causes can be sought at many different levels of analysis. Even if we can no longer hope for a single cause, both the ubiquity of age-related differences and parsimony suggest it is worthwhile to look for a few causes that could have broad affects on many aspects of functioning. At the level of cognitive constructs, possible causes might be changes in various executive functions such as maintaining goals, switching between tasks, or preserving internal representations despite distraction. Alternatively, they might be differential loss in different working memory systems. At the level of neuroanatomy, the causes might be changes in specific brain regions, such as the prefrontal cortex, medial temporal cortex, or caudate nucleus, or they might be changes in the brain white matter that subserves communication between brain regions. At the level of neurochemistry, they might be changes in neurotransmitter systems such as dopaminergic systems. Although it is tempting to assume that reductionist approaches will bring us closer to the level of the ultimate causes (Salthouse, 2005), there is no way to know in advance which will be the most productive avenues to follow. The success of a construct depends on how close it comes to capturing the underlying cause or causes, to what extent emergent properties may make one or another level of analysis more productive, and how comfortably it fits with currently popular constructs.

The other important questions concern methodology, how the causes can be identified. As Lindenberger and Pötter (1998) have noted, experiments provide the best evidence for causality, although designs involving age are, of course, only quasi-experimental. A salient difficulty is that most experiments are done in isolation. It is difficult to aggregate results and conclusions across experiments, which works against identifying a relatively few common causes. In contrast, correlational designs are inherently weaker, but they can provide information about strength and interrelationships or contexts of effects. As we have seen, they may convey the impression of causality when there is none. It is probably a historical accident that correlational methods have tended to use instruments that tap a number of basic abilities, in contrast to experimentally driven manipulations that target certain hypothetical constructs quite specifically. A combination of techniques used in the past may provide a promising line of attack. When results of similar reaction time experiments were aggregated in L_{OLD}/L_{YOUNG} functions, the functions were well fit by simple functions. The parameters of the functions differed for different experimental domains (e.g., Hale et al., 1991; Lima et al., 1991). Attempts to derive a taxonomy of domains might prove profitable (cf. Hartley, 1992). What is likely to be more productive, however, is to look for covariates that account for large portions of the age-related variance in tasks that share parameter values for the L_{OLD}/L_{YOUNG} function. However, these functions need not be limited to reaction time. Accuracy, activation levels from neuroimaging, peak locations from EEG, or other measures might be used profitably. Moreover, the theoretical issue raised by Ratcliff et al. (2000, 2004) is largely moot. It is not necessary to assume that the slopes of the L_{OLD}/L_{YOUNG} functions reflect differences in the underlying speed of processing or even to limit the functions to reaction time. Even if the driving factor is the relative variability of performance across conditions between age groups, it is likely that the clustering of experimental procedures that have

similar slopes could provide useful direction to tasks that reflect operation of a similar ensemble of causes. Particularly promising results occur when a single covariate accounts for much of the variation in disparate tasks. For example, Bäckman et al. (2000) found that dopamine receptor (D_2) binding in the caudate, putamen, and cerebellum as measured by positron emission tomography not only accounted for age-related variance in measures of speed measures and accuracy measures of episodic memory, but also accounted for substantial variance beyond that accounted for by age. In the search for causes, parsimony can be a helpful heuristic, but it should not be used to justify putting aside evidence that the number of causes is more than we had hoped.

B. Implications for Reaction Time as a Dependent Variable

In the third Edition of the *handbook*, Salthouse (1985) offered the opinion that measures of speed or reaction time might not be well suited to the investigation of age-related differences. They continue to be used actively and it is likely that use will continue. Should we abandon such measures as dependent variables? No. RT is highly sensitive, is measured easily and inexpensively, and provides at least the basis for a common metric aggregating across studies. Should we be sure that participants of all ages are at comparable levels of practice and motivation? Yes. Should we worry that younger and older adults are choosing different speed–accuracy trade-offs. No. First, it is unlikely that different groups across many experimental procedures would choose the same, although different, trade-off points. More important, Salthouse (1998) demonstrated empirically that all portions of the reaction time distribution contain qualitatively similar individual difference information. Thus modest differences in speed–accuracy trade-offs are unlikely to introduce substantial artifacts and distort conclusions. Although it is possible that variability in performance might be a useful predictor, Salthouse and Berish (2005) showed that mean reaction times are more powerful predictors of cognitive performance than either between-person or within-person variability.

For a number of years it has been judged essential to adjust reaction time results to compensate for effects of general age-related slowing. Madden (2001) reviewed both rudimentary methods and sophisticated methods for accomplishing this compensation. Should we routinely compensate for slowing? When we do this we are asking the extent to which results are not explained by the common cause of age-related change, slowed speed of processing. If slowing is not the common cause, or even a principal cause, of age-related differences, then we should not adjust for it. If we do so, we may be removing variance that could guide us to the possibly multiple causes of age-related differences.

Compensating for general slowing is in fact a simple example of attempting to fit a formal model to data that we gather. Other, more complex and elaborate models have been proposed, some which have the attractive feature of simultaneously modeling both speed and accuracy. One example is the *diffusion model* proposed by Ratcliff (1978). The diffusion model holds that evidence gradually collects favoring one of two possible responses. Parameters include both the rate of evidence collection, which may be lower in older adults, and the criteria for a decision, which may be more stringent in older adults. Such models have been fit successfully to age-related differences in sensation, perception, and cognition (e.g., Ratcliff, Thapar, & McKoon, 2004). Another example is the *executive process*

interactive control (EPIC) architecture developed by Meyer and Kieras (1997a,b), which holds that the individual can flexibly set controls on the processing of information to optimize task and environmental demands. Glass et al. (2000) successfully accounted for age-related differences in managing overlapping tasks with EPIC-based models with age differences in parameters for accumulating perceptual evidence and for unlocking the second task once the first task was underway or completed. Because these efforts proceed from strong theoretical bases, they offer interesting possibilities. It is important to remember, however, that interpretations of elements in a formal theory are psychological constructs assigned to them by the theorist. Their true meaning is more abstract and underdetermined; it is simply their role in the formalism.

References

Allen, P. A., Hall, R. J., Druley, J. A., Smith, A. F., Sanders, R. E., & Murphy, M. D. (2001). How shared are age-related influences on cognitive and noncognitive variables? *Psychology and Aging, 16*, 532–549.

Anstey, K., & Christensen, H. (2000). Education, activity, health, blood pressure and apolipoprotein E as predictors of cognitive change in old age: A review. *Gerontology, 46*, 163–177.

Anstey, K. J., Hofer, S. M., & Luszcz, M. A. (2003a). A latent growth curve analysis of late-life sensory and cognitive function over 8 years: Evidence for specific and common factors underlying change. *Psychology and Aging, 18*, 714–726.

Anstey, K. J., Hofer, S. M., & Luszcz, M. A. (2003b). Cross-sectional and longitudinal patterns of dedifferentiation in late-life cognitive and sensory function: The effects of age, ability, attrition, and occasion of measurement. *Journal of Experimental Psychology: General, 132*, 470–487.

Anstey, K. J., Luszcz, M. A., & Sanchez, L. (2001). A reevaluation of the common factor theory of shared variance among age, sensory function, and cognitive function in older adults. *Journals of Gerontology: Series B: Psychological Sciences & Social Sciences, 56B*, P3-P11.

Anstey, K. J., Windsor, T. D., Jorm, A. F., Christensen, H., & Rodgers, B. (2004). Association of pulmonary function with cognitive performance in early, middle and late adulthood. *Gerontology, 50*, 230–234.

Bäckman, L., Ginovart, N., Dixon, R. A., Wahlin, T-B. R., Wahlin, Å, Halldin, C., & Farde, L. (2000). Age-related cognitive deficits mediated by changes in the striatal dopamine system. *American Journal of Psychiatry, 157*, 635–637.

Baltes, P. B, & Lindenberger, U. (1997). Emergence of a powerful connection between sensory and cognitive functions across the adult life span: A new window to the study of cognitive aging? *Psychology and Aging, 12*, 12–21.

Bashore, T. R., Osman, A., & Heffley, E. F., III (1989). Mental slowing in elderly persons: A cognitive psychophysiological analysis. *Psychology and Aging, 4*, 235–244.

Birren, J. E. (1974). Translations in gerontology: From lab to life: Psychophysiology and speed of response. *American Psychologist, 29*, 808–815.

Birren, J. E., & Renner, V. J. (1977). Research on the psychology of aging: Principles and experimentation. In J. E. Birren & K. W. Schaie (Eds), *Handbook of the psychology of aging* (pp. 3–38). New York: Van Nostrand Reinhold.

Birren, J. E., & Schaie, K. W. (1977). *Handbook of the psychology of aging*. New York: Van Nostrand Reinhold.

Birren, J. E, & Schroots, J. J. F. (1996). History, concepts, and theory in the psychology of aging. In J. E. Birren & K. W. Schaie (Eds), *Handbook of the psychology of aging* (4th edition, pp. 3–23). San Diego: Academic Press.

Brinley, J. F. (1965). Cognitive sets, speed, and accuracy of performance in the elderly. In A. T. Welford & J. E. Birren (Eds.), *Behavior, aging, and the nervous system* (pp. 114–149). Springfield, IL: Charles C. Thomas.

Cerella, J. (1985). Information processing rates in the elderly. *Psychological Bulletin, 98*, 67–83.

Cerella, J. (1990). Aging and information-processing rate. In J. E. Birren & K. W. Schaie (Eds), *Handbook of the psychology of aging* (3rd edition, pp. 201–221). San Diego: Academic Press.

Cerella, J., Poon, L. W., & Williams, D. M. (1980). Age and the complexity hypothesis. In L. W. Poon (Ed.), *Aging in the 1980s: Psychological issues* (pp. 332–340). Washington, DC: American Psychological Association.

Christensen, H., Hofer, S. M., Mackinnon, A. J., Korten, A. E., Jorm, A. F., & Henderson, A. S. (2001). Age is no kinder to the better educated: Absence of an association investigated using latent growth techniques in a community sample. *Psychological Medicine, 31*, 15–28.

Christensen, H., Mackinnon, A., Jorm, A. F., Korten, A., Jacomb, P., Hofer, S. M., & Henderson, S. (2004). The Canberra longitudinal study: Design, aims, methodology, outcomes and recent empirical investigations. *Aging, Neuropsychology, & Cognition, 11*, 169–195.

Christensen, H., Mackinnon, A. J., Korten, A., & Jorm, A. F. (2001). The "common cause hypothesis" of cognitive aging: Evidence for not only a common factor but also specific associations of age with vision and grip strength in a cross-sectional analysis. *Psychology and Aging, 16*, 588–599.

Clarkson-Smith, L., & Hartley, A. A. (1989). Relationships between physical exercise and cognitive abilities in older adults. *Psychology and Aging, 4*, 183–189.

Clarkson-Smith, L., & Hartley, A. A. (1990). Structural equation models of relationships between exercise and cognitive abilities. *Psychology and Aging, 5*, 437–446.

Deary, I. J., Leaper, S. A., Murray, A. D., Staff, R. T., & Whalley, L. J. (2003). Cerebral white matter abnormalities and lifetime cognitive change: A 67-year follow up of the Scottish mental survey of 1932. *Psychology and Aging, 18*, 140–148.

Ferrer, E., Salthouse, T. A, Stewart, W. F, & Schwartz, B. S. (2004). Modeling age and retest processes in longitudinal studies of cognitive abilities. *Psychology and Aging, 19*, 243–259.

Fisher, D. L., & Glaser, R. A. (1996). Molar and latent models of cognitive slowing: Implications for aging, dementia, depression, development, and intelligence. *Psychonomic Bulletin & Review, 3,* 458–480.

Glass, J. M., Schumacher, E. H., Lauber, E. J., Zurbriggen, E. L., Gmeindl, L., Kieras, D. E., & Meyer, D. E.(2000). Aging and the psychological refractory period: Task-coordination strategies in young and old adults. *Psychology & Aging, 15,* 571–595.

Graybiel, A. M. (2000). The basal ganglia. *Current Biology, 10,* R509–R511.

Greenwood, P. M. (2000). The frontal aging hypothesis evaluated. *Journal of the International Neuropsychological Society, 6,* 705–726.

Hale, S., Lima, S. D., & Myerson, J. (1991). General cognitive slowing in the nonlexical domain: An experimental validation. *Psychology and Aging, 6,* 512–521.

Hale, S., Myerson, J., & Wagstaff, D. (1987). General slowing of nonverbal information processing: Evidence for a power law. *Journal of Gerontology, 42,* 131–136.

Hartley, A. A. (1992). In search of a theory of the aging of intelligence. *Contemporary Psychology, 37,* 1009–1010.

Heikkenen, E., Berg, S., Schroll, M., Steen, B., & Viidik, A. (Eds.) (1997). Functional status, health, and aging: The NORA study. *Facts, research, and intervention in geriatrics.* Paris: Serdi.

Hofer, S. M., Berg, S., & Era, P. (2003). Evaluating the interdependence of aging-related changes in visual and auditory acuity, balance, and cognitive functioning. *Psychology and Aging, 18,* 285–305

Hofer, S. M., Christensen, H., Mackinnon, A. J., Korten, A. E., Jorm, A. F., Henderson, A. S., & Easteal, S. (2002). Change in cognitive functioning associated with ApoE genotype in a community sample of older adults. *Psychology & Aging, 17,* 194–208.

Hofer, S. M., & Sliwinski, M. S. (2001). Understanding ageing. *Gerontology, 47,* 341–352.

Hofer, S. M., Sliwinski, M. J., & Flaherty, B. P. (2002b). Understanding ageing: Further commentary on the limitations of cross-sectional designs for ageing research. *Gerontology, 48,* 22–29.

LaBerge, D. (1995). *Attentional processing.* Cambridge, MA: Harvard University Press.

Li, K. Z. H. & Lindenberger, U. (2002). Relations between aging sensory/sensorimotor and cognitive functions. *Neuroscience & Biobehavioral Reviews, 26,* 777–783.

Li, S.-C. (2002). Connecting the many levels and facets of cognitive aging. *Current Directions in Psychological Science, 11,* 38–43.

Lima, S. D., Hale, S., & Myerson, J. (1991). How general is general slowing? Evidence from the lexical domain. *Psychology and Aging, 6,* 416–425.

Lindenberger, U., & Baltes, P. B. (1994). Sensory functioning and intelligence in old age: A strong connection. *Psychology and Aging, 9,* 339–355.

Lindenberger, U., & Pötter, U. (1998). The complex nature of unique and shared effects in hierarchical linear regression: Implications for developmental psychology. *Psychological Methods, 3,* 218–230.

Lindenberger, U., Scherer, H., & Baltes, P. B. (2003). The strong connection between sensory and cognitive performance in old age: Not due to sensory acuity reductions operating during cognitive assessment. *Psychology & Aging, 16,* 196–205.

Madden, D. J. (1990). Adult age differences in the time course of visual attention. *Journals of Gerontology: Psychological Sciences, 45,* P9–P16.

Madden, D. J. (2001). Speed and timing of behavioral processes. In J. E. Birren & K. W. Schaie (Eds.), *Handbook of the psychology of aging* (5th edition, pp. 288–312). San Diego: Academic Press.

Madden, D. J., Whiting, W. L., Huettel, S. A., White, L. E., MacFall, J. R., & Provenzale, J. M. (2004). Diffusion tensor imaging of adult age differences in cerebral white matter: Relation to response time. *Neuroimage, 21,* 1174–1181.

Meyer, D. E., & Kieras, D. E. (1997a). A computational theory of executive cognitive processes and multiple-task performance. Basic mechanisms. *Psychological Review, 104,* 3–65.

Meyer, D. E., & Kieras, D. E. (1997b). A computational theory of executive cognitive processes and multiple-task performance. Accounts of psychological refractory-period phenomena. *Psychological Review, 104,* 749–791.

Myerson, J., Adams, D. R., Hale, S., & Jenkins, L. (2003). Analysis of group differences in processing speed: Brinley plots, Q-Q plots, and other conspiracies. *Psychonomic Bulletin & Review, 10,* 224–237.

Myerson, J., Hale, S., Wagstaff, D., Poon, L. W., et al. (1990). The information-loss model: A mathematical theory of age-related cognitive slowing. *Psychological Review, 97,* 475–487.

Nebes, R. D. (1978). Vocal versus manual response as a determinant of age differences in simple reaction time. *Journal of Gerontology, 33,* 884–889.

Nelson, H. E. (1982). *National adult reading test (NART).* Berkshire, UK: NFER.

Rabbitt, P. M., Lowe, C., Scott, M., Thacker, N., Horan, M., Pendleton, N., et al. (2004a). Balance as a marker for global brain atrophy, blood flow, and cognitive changes in old age. Unpublished manuscript.

Rabbitt, P. M., Lowe, C., Thacker, N., Scott, M., Jackson, A., Horan, M., et al., (2004b). Age-related losses in gross brain volume and cerebral blood flow and in cognition. Unpublished manuscript.

Ratcliff, R. (1978). A theory of memory retrieval. *Psychological Review, 85,* 59–108.

Ratcliff, R., Spieler, D., & McKoon, G. (2000). Explicitly modeling the effects of aging on response time. *Psychonomic Bulletin & Review, 7,* 1–25.

Ratcliff, R., Spieler, D., & McKoon, G. (2004). Analysis of group differences in processing speed: Where are the models of processing? *Psychonomic Bulletin & Review, 11(4),* 755–769.

Ratcliff, R., Thapar, A., & McKoon, G. (2004). A diffusion model analysis of the effects of aging on recognition memory. *Journal of Memory & Language, 50,* 408–424.

Rodrigue, K. M., & Raz, N. (2004). Shrinkage of the entorhinal cortex over five years predicts memory performance in healthy adults. *Journal of Neuroscience, 24,* 956–963.

Rubin, D. C. (1999). Frontal-striatal circuits in cognitive aging: Evidence for caudate involvement. *Aging, Neuropsychology, and Cognition, 6,* 241–259.

Salthouse, T. A. (1985). Speed of behavior and its implications for cognition. In J. E. Birren & K. W. Schaie (Eds.), *Handbook of the psychology of aging* (2nd edition, pp. 400–426). New York: Van Nostrand Reinhold.

Salthouse, T. A. (1992a). *Mechanisms of age-cognition relations in adulthood.* Hillsdale, NJ: Lawrence Erlbaum.

Salthouse, T. A. (1992b). Shifting levels of analysis in the investigation of cognitive aging: Reply. *Human Development, 35,* 355–360.

Salthouse, T. A. (1993). Speed mediation of adult age differences in cognition. *Developmental Psychology, 29,* 722–738.

Salthouse, T. A. (1994). The nature of the influence of speed on adult age differences in cognition. *Developmental Psychology, 30,* 240–259.

Salthouse, T. A. (1996a). The processing-speed theory of adult age differences in cognition. *Psychological Review, 103,* 403–428.

Salthouse, T. A. (1996b). Where in an ordered sequence of variables do independent age-related effects occur? *Journals of Gerontology: Series B: Psychological Sciences & Social Sciences, 51,* P166–P178.

Salthouse, T. A. (1998). Relation of successive percentiles of reaction time distributions to cognitive variables and adult age. *Intelligence, 26,* 153–166.

Salthouse, Timothy A. (2000). Aging and measures of processing speed. *Biological Psychology, 54,* 35–54.

Salthouse, T. A. (2001a). A research strategy for investigating group differences in a cognitive construct: Application to ageing and executive processes. *European Journal of Cognitive Psychology, 13,* 29–46.

Salthouse, T. A. (2001b). Structural models of the relations between age and measures of cognitive functioning. *Intelligence, 29,* 93–115.

Salthouse, T. A. (2004). Localizing age-related individual differences in a hierarchical structure. *Intelligence, 32,* 541–561.

Salthouse, T. A. (2005). From description to explanation in cognitive aging. In R. J. Sternberg & J. E. Pretz (Eds.), *Cognition and intelligence: Identifying the mechanisms of mind* (pp. 288–305). Cambridge, UK: Cambridge University Press.

Salthouse, T. A., Atkinson, T. M., & Berish, D. E. (2003). Executive functioning as a potential mediator of age-related cognitive decline in normal adults. *Journal of Experimental Psychology: General, 132,* 566–594.

Salthouse, T. A., & Berish, D. E. (2005). Correlates of within-person (across-occasion) variability in reaction time. *Neuropsychology, 19,* 77–87.

Salthouse, T. A, & Caja, S. J. (2000). Structural constraints on process explanations in cognitive aging. *Psychology & Aging, 15,* 44–55.

Salthouse, T. A, & Ferrer-Caja, E. (2003). What needs to be explained to account for age-related effects on multiple cognitive variables? *Psychology & Aging, 18,* 91–110.

Salthouse, T. A, & Fristoe, N. M. (1995). Process analysis of adult age effects on a computer-administered trail making test. *Neuropsychology, 9,* 518–528.

Salthouse, T. A, Fristoe, N., McGuthry, K. E., & Hambrick, D. Z. (1998). Relation of task switching to speed, age, and fluid intelligence. *Psychology & Aging, 13,* 445–461.

Salthouse, T. A., Hambrick, D. Z., & McGuthry, K. E. (1998). Shared age-related influences on cognitive and noncognitive variables. *Psychology and Aging, 13,* 486–500.

Salthouse, T. A, & Hedden, T. (2002). Interpreting reaction time measures in between-group comparisons. *Journal of Clinical & Experimental Neuropsychology, 24,* 858–872.

Salthouse, T. A, & Miles, J. D. (2002). Aging and time-sharing aspects of executive control. *Memory & Cognition, 30,* 572–582.

Salthouse, T. A., & Somberg, B. L. (1982). Time-accuracy relationships in young and old adults. *Journal of Gerontology, 37,* 349–353.

Salthouse, T. A, Toth, J., Daniels, K., Parks, C., Pak, R., Wolbrette, M., & Hocking, K. J. (2000). Effects of aging on efficiency of task switching in a variant of the trail making test. *Neuropsychology, 14,* 102–111.

Schroll, M., Steen, B., Berg, S., Heikkenen, E., & Viidik, A. (1993). NORA—Nordic Research on Aging: Functional capacity of 75-year-old men and women in three Nordic localities. *Danish Medical Bulletin, 40,* 618–624.

Sliwinski, M., & Buschke, H. (1999). Cross-sectional and longitudinal relationships among age, cognition, and processing speed. *Psychology and Aging, 14,* 18–33.

Sliwinski, M. J., Hofer, S. M., Hall, C. (2003a). Correlated and coupled cognitive change in older adults with and without preclinical dementia. *Psychology and Aging, 18,* 672–683.

Sliwinski, M. J., Hofer, S. M., Hall, C., Buschke, H., & Lipton, R. B. (2003b). Modeling memory decline in older adults: The importance of preclinical dementia, attrition, and chronological age. *Psychology and Aging, 18,* 658–671.

Verhaeghen, P., & Salthouse, T. A. (1997). Meta-analyses of age-cognition relations in adulthood: Estimates of linear and nonlinear age effects and structural models. *Psychological Bulletin, 122,* 231–249.

Welford, A. T. (1977). Motor performance. In J. E. Birren & K. W. Schaie (Eds). *Handbook of the psychology of aging* (pp. 450–496). New York: Van Nostrand Reinhold.

Zimprich, D., & Martin, M. (2002). Can longitudinal changes in processing speed explain longitudinal age changes in fluid intelligence? *Psychology and Aging, 17,* 690–695.

Ten

Memory Aging

William J. Hoyer and Paul Verhaeghen

I. Introduction

The term memory is used broadly to refer to the various operations of mind that involve the encoding, retention, and retrieval of information and experiences. Behavioral and biological events and processes that occur during the passage of time determine memory aging. The objective of this chapter is to provide an overview and review of the current status of research and theory on this topic. We review age-performance relations for several forms of memory, including recollection, episodic memory, prospective memory, and working memory, for which there are age-related deficits, and we consider the recent theoretical and empirical advances that bear on the explanation of age-related effects on memory. We give special consideration to age effects that seem to involve the extent to which there is individual control over basic processes of memory.

The coverage is necessarily selective. We say too little about current work on aging and priming, perceptual learning, autobiographical memory, everyday memory, and meta-memory. Also, we say too little about some of the antecedents known to affect memory aging, especially genetic factors, dementia and disease influences, sensory and perceptual influences, social and contextual influences, emotional influences, and circadian influences (for reviews or key findings on these topics, see Charles, Mather, & Carstensen, 2003; Deary et al., 2004; Hertzog & Hultsch, 2000; Hess, 2005; Isaacowitz, Charles, & Carstensen, 2000; Madden, Whiting, & Huettel, 2005; Mather, 2004; Reynolds et al., 2005; Rogers & Fisk, 2001; Small et al., 2004; Winocur & Hasher, 2002).

This chapter is intended to serve as an update to the chapters on aging and memory found in previous editions of this *Handbook* (Bäckman, Small, & Wahlin, 2001; Craik, 1977; Hultsch & Dixon, 1990; Poon, 1985; Smith, 1996). Our coverage builds on some of the material found in those chapters and in recently published reviews and overviews (e.g., Craik & Jennings, 1992; Light et al., 2000; Parkin & Java, 2000; Raz, 2005; Zacks, Hasher, & Li, 2000). We begin by summarizing patterns in data that indicate the principal differences in the effects of aging on measures of memory. Then we discuss macro-level and micro-level explanations of memory aging.

Finally, we consider the effects of memory interventions.

II. Varieties of Memory Aging

It is generally accepted that there are different forms of memory and multiple systems of memory. As discussed by Roediger, Marsh, and Lee (2002), forms of memory can be distinguished on the basis of temporal characteristics (e.g., sensory memory, short-term memory, long-term memory, remote memory), processing requirements at encoding and retrieval (e.g., recollection, familiarity), and stimulus domain (e.g., visual–spatial, verbal). Most early reviews of the memory aging literature emphasized data showing differences in short-term and long-term tasks and processes, data bearing on the relative inefficiencies in encoding, storage, and retrieval, and the differential aging of visual–spatial processing relative to verbal processing. More recent work has been strongly guided by models of multiple memory systems and the distinction between the processes of recollection and familiarity, on the one hand (cf. microlevel research); and multivariate models and mediator and shared variance models applied to large cross-sectional and longitudinal data sets, on the other hand (cf. macro-level research).

At the micro level, different memory systems can be distinguished on the basis of neuroanatomical as well as behavioral evidence from patients and healthy adults. One taxonomy for which a considerable amount of evidence has accumulated is shown in Figure 10.1, taken from Squire (2004). This framework serves as a useful scheme for guiding research as well as for organizing data bearing on the aging of different memory systems. The well-known findings of age-related deficits in declarative episodic memory (memory for events) in contrast to much smaller or negligible age effects in nondeclarative forms of memory (e.g., repetition priming) are consistent with the relations between distinct memory functions and their neural substrates indicated in this scheme. Impaired recall and other forms of declarative memory are associated with age-related changes in the brain that affect the medial temporal area, encompassing the hippocampus and surrounding cortical regions (perirhinal, entorhinal, and parahippocampal cortices). Note that medial temporal lobe is implicated in declarative memory for both events and facts, yet age deficits are

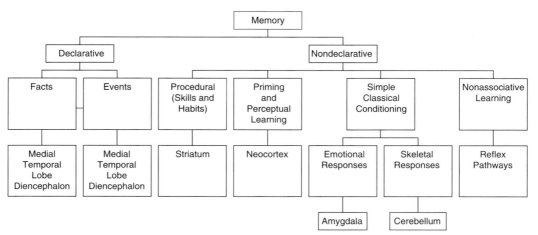

Figure 10.1 A composite taxonomy of memory systems (based on Squire, 2004).

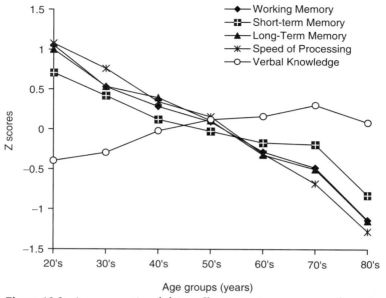

Figure 10.2 A cross-sectional data collection using measures of speed of processing, short-term memory, working memory, and long-term memory. Adapted from Park et al. (2002), with permission.

known to be much greater for declarative retrieval of *particular* events and facts than for declarative retrieval of *general* events and facts. The extent to which the hippocampus supports the formation, organization, and retrieval of richly detailed memories and their distinctive contexts probably diminishes with aging (e.g., Prull, Gabrieli, & Bunge, 2000; Raz, 2000, 2005).

As a first introduction to the varieties of memory aging, Figure 10.2 shows data from a comprehensive cross-sectional study by Park and colleagues (2002) that included composite measures of many aspects of memory: episodic long-term memory (free recall, cued recall, Rey auditory verbal learning test, and the Benton test), short-term memory (forward corsi blocks, backward corsi blocks, forward digit span, and backward digit span), working memory (line span, letter rotation, reading span, and computation span), processing speed (pattern comparisons, letter comparisons, and digit symbol substitution), and semantic

memory (three vocabulary tests). It can be seen that episodic memory, speed of processing, short-term memory, and working memory all decline (and to about the same amount) over the course of the adult life span. In contrast to these negative age trends, the measures of verbal knowledge show a flat profile (see also Allen et al., 2002; Rönnlund et al., 2005; Verhaeghen & Salthouse, 1997). Other aspects of memory that evidence little or no age-related decline include (1) measures influenced by the process of familiarity as opposed to recollection and (2) measures of implicit memory and priming as opposed to explicit memory, as discussed below.

A. Recollection and Familiarity

A substantial amount of recent evidence supports the view that many varieties of memory are subserved by two distinct processes, recollection and familiarity (see Yonelinas, 2002). Recollection involves the retrieval of contextual information about a past event (e.g., time and place), and familiarity involves a feeling of recognition or "oldness" about the event in the absence of retrieval of contextual information. Increasing evidence suggests that recollection and familiarity map to different neural substrates. Yonelinas and colleagues (2005), in a fMRI study, showed that the neural signature of recollection was distinct from variations in familiarity across four brain regions. First, in the hippocampus, recollection was directly related to hippocampal activation, whereas familiarity was inversely related to hippocampal activity. Second, in the prefrontal cortex, recollection was related to an anterior medial region, and familiarity was related to lateral regions, including the anterior and dorsolateral prefrontal cortex. Third, along the lateral parietal cortex, recollection was related to the temporal region, and familiarity was related to a more superior region. Fourth, in the medial parietal region, recollection was related to the posterior cingulate, and familiarity was related to the precuneus. In another study bearing on the neural sustrates of recollection and familiarity, Kensinger, Clarke, and Corkin (2003) reported fMRI data suggesting that detailed (recollective) information and less-detailed (familiarity-based) information are lateralized. The left prefrontal cortex is specialized for recollective memories, and the right prefrontal cortex is specialized for familiarity-based traces. Behaviorally, there is strong support for a dissociation between recollection and familiarity. Support comes from a large variety of studies examining the effects of selected task conditions on memory performance. Task factors such as test-phase divided attention and response deadlines affect recollection performance but not familiarity, and task factors such as perceptual fluency of test stimuli and changes in the appearance of stimuli from study to test

affect familiarity but not recollection (see Yonelinas, 2002).

At least three different methods have been used to estimate the contributions of recollection and familiarity processes to memory performance in younger and older adults. Across methods, young–old comparisons generally reveal that recollection is substantially impaired with normal aging but the status of familiarity appears to be method sensitive (for a meta-analysis, see Prull et al., 2003). One method for distinguishing the contributions of recollection and familiarity is Jacoby's (1991) process dissociation procedure (PDP). In this procedure, subjects typically study two lists (A and B) and are then given two types of instructions for a recognition or recall test. Under the inclusion instruction, the subject selects or recalls words from either list; under the exclusion instruction, the subject selects or recalls only words from list A (or B), not B (or A). In the inclusion condition, memory performance is based on both recollection and familiarity; in the exclusion condition, only recollection will lead to correct exclusions. Prull et al. (2003) found nine experiments that used the PDP procedure with younger and older adults, and this set of studies contained 13 young–old comparisons. Estimates of recollection were lower for older adults than for younger adults in 12 of the 13 comparisons. Estimates of familiarity were lower for older adults in 7 comparisons and higher for older adults in 5 comparisons. Overall, for young and old, respectively, the average recollection estimates were .49 and .29, and the average familiarity estimates were .41 and .48 for young and old.

Another procedure for distinguishing the processes of recollection and familiarity is the remember–know paradigm. For each item that is recognized, the participant is asked whether she remembers contextual information about the original study situation or whether she just has a sense of familiarity for the item absent of contextual information. Prull et al. (2003) located 19 studies that used the remember–know procedure with younger and older adults, and 24 young–old comparisons could be made. Of these, 19 estimates of recollection were lower in older adults than in younger adults. For the estimates of familiarity, 18 of the 24 comparisons were lower for older adults. Overall, for studies using the remember–know procedure, that average recollection estimates were .52 and .37, and the average familiarity estimates were .49 and .37 for young and old, respectively.

A third approach to the study of recollection and familiarity is to fit estimates of these processes in receiver operating characteristic (ROC) space (e.g., Yonelinas, 1997). This procedure yields a highly constrained picture because recollection and familiarity are estimated across an entire range of confidence levels. To gather data needed for fitting ROC curves, items are first presented in a study phase and then study participants give confidence ratings in a test phase both for items that were presented in the study phase and for nonpresented probes. The quality of recognition memory is a joint function of hit rates (the probability of correctly endorsing previously presented items as "old") and false alarm rates (probability of incorrectly endorsing not-presented probes as "old"). Recollection and familiarity can accrue differently, and different combinations of the estimates for recollection and familiarity derive asymmetric ROC plots. Light and co-workers (2000) estimated functions for recollection and familiarity using data from a study by Harkins, Chapman, and Eisdorfer (1979) that reported a full range of recognition ROCs for 8 young adults and 16 older adults and found that both recollection and familiarity were lower for older adults than for younger adults.

Results from several new studies using ROCs also reveal large age-related deficits in recollection (e.g., Healy, Light, & Chung, 2005; Howard et al., 2006).

B. Declarative and Nondeclarative Forms of Memory

In reference to Figure 10.1, operations of the declarative memory system involve conscious access to (1) episodic information about events and experiences and/or (2) accumulated knowledge about the general characteristics of things or places or people in the world. Operations of the nondeclarative memory system are revealed in the performance of various tasks such as repetition priming, procedural learning, simple classical conditioning, and habituation — tasks that do not involve conscious access to item information. For example, perceptual and motor learning benefits accrue primarily through repetitions of instances and/or repeated movements or responses, such as learning to row a boat or play a musical instrument skillfully or speak a language.

Perhaps the most robust age–memory relationship is the well-known decline in declarative memory for episodic information over the course of the adult life span. Representative data showing age-related declines on standardized measures of immediate and delayed memory for information in stories, for lists of unrelated words, for paired associates (using unrelated words as stimuli), and for faces are depicted in Figure 10.3. These data, expressed as z scores across age groups, are taken from the normative sample for the Wechsler memory scale III (Wechsler, 1997; as summarized by Salthouse, 2003). Numerous studies in the 1990s and earlier using laboratory measures (for meta-analyses, see La Voie & Light, 1994; Verhaeghen, Marcoen, & Goossens, 1993; Verhaeghen & Salthouse, 1997), as

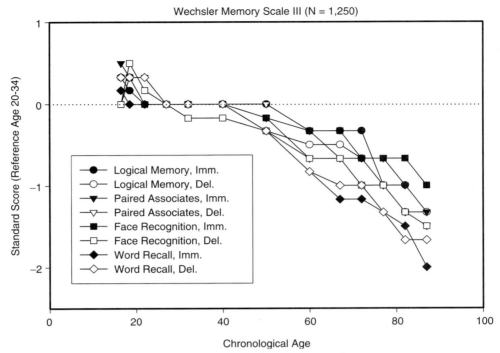

Figure 10.3 Standard scores for eight measures of memory: Cross-sectional data from the standardization groups for the Wechsler Memory Scale III [Wechsler, (1997); adapted from Salthouse, (2003), with permission].

well as standardized memory scales (e.g., Hulicka, 1966; Margolis & Scialfa, 1984; Wechsler, 1997), reported just these trends. In contrast, studies of age–performance relations using nondeclarative measures of memory reveal only mild negative effects of age (Fleischman et al., 2004; Rodrigue, Kennedy, & Raz, 2005; Rybash, 1996; for a meta-analysis on repetition priming, see La Voie & Light, 1994).

C. Episodic Memory and Semantic Memory

Older adults have much more trouble than younger adults in tasks that involve conscious or declarative retrieval of specific events located in time and place and/or retrieval of the context of experienced events. This form of memory is referred to as episodic memory, and its

status depends largely but not entirely on the process of recollection (Li, Morcom, & Rugg, 2004; Mark & Rugg, 1998). Performance in tasks that tap the conscious recollection of prior episodes declines substantially with advancing age (e.g., for excellent reviews, see Bäckman et al., 2001; Light et al., 2000; Zacks et al., 2000). Meta-analysis indicates that the size of the age-related effect in cross-sectional studies of episodic memory (using measures of list recall, paired-associate recall, recall for narrative text) is about −1.0 SD (Verhaeghen, Marcoen, & Goossens, 1993). Longitudinal data from the Betula study, however, give a much more positive description of the age trends for episodic memory (Rönnlund et al., 2005). As shown in Figure 10.4, practice-adjusted (top) and education-adjusted (bottom) estimates of change scores indi-

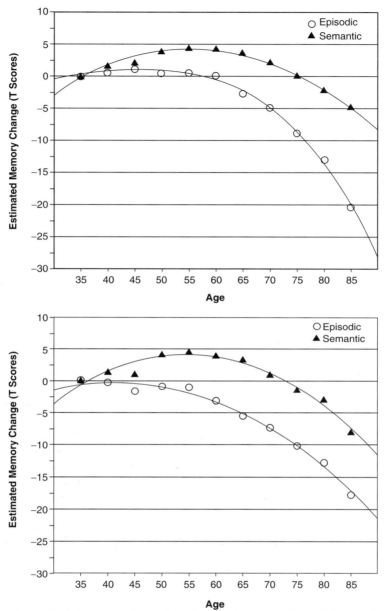

Figure 10.4 Practice-adjusted (top) and education-adjusted (bottom) estimates of longitudinal change in semantic memory and episodic memory. From Rönnlund et al. (2005), with permission.

cate that measures of episodic memory are largely unaffected by aging until after age 60.

Age-related deficits in episodic memory are known to reflect weakly formed associations at encoding, conceptualized as age-related associative deficits or binding deficits (e.g., Li, Naveh-Benjamin, & Lindenberger, 2005; Naveh-Benjamin, 2000), or the age-sensitive consequences of attentional demands at either encoding or retrieval (Castel & Craik, 2003;

Naveh-Benjamin, 2001; Naveh-Benjamin et al., 2005).

In contrast to memory for particular events that are precisely tied to their context and source, semantic memory refers to the retrieval or use of accumulated knowledge about people, places, and things without an explicit appraisal of when or where the information was experienced. In other words, measures of semantic memory tap the contents of an individual's cumulative knowledge without reference to the source, temporal context, or the experience that produced that knowledge. Although the formation and organization of both semantic and episodic information is subserved by the hippocampus and the parahippocampal regions of the medial temporal lobe (Figure 10.1), retrieval of general information from memory is likely to be widely distributed over the cortical areas (e.g., Eichenbaum, 2003). Particular kinds of semantic information such as color may engage different cortical regions (e.g., Martin et al., 1995). Thus, generally, tests of retrieval of general knowledge depend on the intactness of distributed representations, whereas assessments of memories for particular episodes depend much more heavily on the status of newly built associations and the integrity of hippocampal functions (e.g., Eichenbaum, 2003; Howard et al., 2006).

One way to assess semantic memory is through tests for vocabulary. Older adults do not show a deficit on these tasks, but rather an advantage of about 0.80 SD (Verhaeghen, 2003, see also the data from Park et al., 2002). Part of the advantage is due to differences in the educational characteristics of the samples typical used in young–old comparative research. The age advantage is larger for verification or recognition measures than for production measures of vocabulary, probably because retrieval requires more resources in production tasks. However, vocabulary measures probably

underestimate the breadth and depth of knowledge the development of word meanings and language accumulated through years of experience and use. Longitudinal research confirms this picture of an increase or stability in word knowledge (e.g., Schaie, 1996), with a possible decline after age 90 (Singer et al., 2003). In the Betula study (Rönnlund et al., 2005), measures of semantic memory showed gains up to about age 60. The negative age trends for semantic memory after age 60 paralleled those for episodic memory, with similar slopes (see also Dixon et al., 2004; Lövdén et al., 2004).

D. Source Memory and Item-Context Associations

Older adults show deficits in remembering source information (for a meta-analysis, see Spencer & Raz, 1995), and these deficits are larger than those for content information. Age-related deficits on measures of episodic memory and source memory probably involve failures to adequately associate target items with other items or target items with their contexts (Chalfonte & Johnson, 1996; Naveh-Benjamin, 2000; Naveh-Benjamin et al., 2003, 2004). Several fMRI and structural MRI studies and PET studies have affirmed the role of the left prefrontal cortex and the hippocampus in age-related associative deficits or feature-binding deficits in memory for source (e.g., Mitchell et al., 2000a,b).

Research on age-related differences in susceptibility to false memories and misinformation effects gives some leverage to the task of understanding the processes that contribute to age-deficits in episodic memory and source memory (e.g., Balota et al., 1999; Karpel, Hoyer, & Toglia, 2000; Kensinger & Schacter, 1999; McCabe & Smith, 2002; Watson, McDermott, & Balota, 2004). Jacoby and colleagues (2005) reported that older adults are substantially more vulnerable to interference effects produced by a misleading prime. In one of the experiments conducted by Jacoby et al. (2005), older adults were 10 times more likely to falsely remember misleading information than younger adults, even when original learning was equated. A plausible interpretation for these findings and other results from Jacoby's laboratory (e.g., Jacoby, 1999) is that an impoverished memory for the details of actual episodes renders older adults more vulnerable than younger adults to falsely accepting misinformation, such as in scams.

A number of studies have pointed to the importance of giving more attention to details at encoding as a way to minimize false memory in older adults (Koutstaal et al., 1998, 1999, 2003). For example, postevent review has beneficial effects for both younger adults and older adults in terms of accessibility to the details of complex everyday events (Koutstaal et al., 1998). Watson et al. (2004) examined whether older adults would benefit from a warning to reduce false memories in the Deese–Roediger–McDermott paradigm and found that warnings served to eliminate false memories for younger adults but not for older adults. Older adults did show some effect of warnings on trial 1 and were more likely to reduce false memories at a slower presentation rate. Watson et al. (2004) attributed these findings to an age-related breakdown in spontaneous, self-initiated source monitoring, but age-related differences in working memory capacity could also account for these effects (i.e., see Watson et al., 2005).

E. Working Memory

Working memory is involved in tasks that require the individual to simultaneously store and actively transform information (e.g., Baddeley, 1986; Reuter-Lorenz & Sylvester, 2005; Wager & Smith, 2003).

Relatively small age differences are already found in the performance of short-duration memory tasks that do not require much concurrent or controlled processing, such as digit span tasks. Comparatively, age-related deficits in working memory, as measured by tasks such as reading span, listening span, or operation span, are demonstrably larger (Bopp & Verhaeghen, 2005; Verhaeghen & Salthouse, 1997). Laboratory measures of working memory likewise reveal reliable and large age-related deficits (Byrne, 1998; Oberauer & Kliegl, 2001; Oberauer, Wendland, & Kliegl, 2003; Reuter-Lorenz & Sylvester, 2005; Zelinski & Burnight, 1997).

The nature of age-related deficits in working memory has received much research attention, perhaps because working memory captures cognitive operations that are fundamentally involved in a wide variety of complex cognitive tasks. Significant relationships have been demonstrated between fluid intelligence and short-term memory capacity, between fluid intelligence and working memory capacity, and between spatial and language abilities and working memory (e.g., Conway et al., 2002; Engle, Kane, & Tuholski, 1999; Kemper, Herman, & Lian, 2003; Kyllonen, 1996).

F. Prospective Memory

Prospective memory refers to a person's intentions for actions to be carried out in the future. In the laboratory, prospective memory has been found to be reliably less age sensitive than episodic memory (Henry et al., 2004). The size of the age effect is about −0.75 SD, regardless of whether the task is time based (i.e., remembering to do something at a particular time) or event based (i.e., remembering to do something when a particular event occurs). Age differences in event-based tasks are larger when the demands on prospective memory are higher (e.g., when cues are not particularly salient, when the association between cue and action is weak, or when the embedded task is highly engaging). Interestingly, older adults dramatically outperform younger adults in naturalistic prospective studies, where they are, for instance, asked to mail back postcards at regular intervals or telephone the experimenter at specified times. The effect size is about 0.70 SD for event-based studies and 1.20 SD for time-based studies. This old–age advantage is probably due to optimized strategy use, such as the use of effective external devices, possibly driven by long years of experience with a declining episodic memory. Carrying the higher-risk genotype for Alzheimer's disease, apolipoprotein E, seems to be associated with greater difficulties in prospective memory tasks (Driscoll, McDaniel, & Guynn, 2005).

III. Explanations of the Aging of Memory

A comprehensive treatment of age-related differences in memory involves the description and explanation of (1) age–performance relations that cut across various forms of memory and (2) the effects of aging on selected memory systems or forms of memory aging that are of theoretical or practical import. As noted elsewhere (Madden, 2001; Salthouse, 2000; Zacks, Hasher, & Li, 2000), advances in the understanding of memory aging depend on analysis of age–memory relationships at both micro and macro levels. This section, reviews two types of explanations. First, at the macro level, we review the role of across-the-board factors, including the insidious effects of slowing of the speed of processing and the consequences of age-related changes in perceptual and sensory factors on memory performance (e.g., Lindenberger & Baltes, 1994; Cerella,

1990; Fisher, Duffy, & Katsikopoulos, 2000; Madden, 2001; Salthouse, 1996; Madden, Whiting, & Huettel, 2005). Second, we review explanations that emphasize the consequences for memory performance of age deficiencies in executive control processes in working memory processes (e.g., Braver & Barch, 2002; Verhaeghen & Cerella, 2002). Additionally, at a more micro level, researchers have emphasized more specific processes, such as age-related deficits in binding or associative processes in selected forms of memory (e.g., Chalfonte & Johnson, 1996; Mitchell et al., 2000; Naveh-Benjamin, 2000; Naveh-Benjamin et al., 2004). These explanations and approaches to explanation are not mutually exclusive. Rather, memory aging has multiple antecedents, with some being task general and some being process specific (e.g., Perfect & Maylor, 2000).

A. Task-General Influences on Memory Performance

A large amount of research on memory aging addresses the extent to which age-related declines can be accounted for by task-general cognitive aging mechanisms. One approach for exploring the role of task-general factors in age–performance relationships across measures of memory involves using the tools of multivariate statistics (e.g., Anstey, Hofer, & Luszcz, 2003; Hofer, Sliwinski, & Flaherty, 2002; Lemke & Zimprich, 2005; Salthouse, 2004; Schmiedek & Li, 2004). Two such mechanisms have been proposed: a neointegration between sensory and cognitive functions and an age-related decline in processing speed.

Although findings from many early studies indicated a strong relationship between performance on various tests of cognition and the status of visual and auditory information processing systems (e.g., Chown & Heron, 1965; Welford, 1965), work by Lindenberger and Baltes (1994) is notable for advancing the notion of a "common cause" to account for age-related deficits across a wide range of basic and higher order information processing and cognitive functions. Lindenberger and Baltes (1994) examined relationships among visual and auditory acuity and 14 tests of five cognitive factors (speed, reasoning, memory, knowledge, and fluency) in an age-stratified sample of 156 old and very old individuals. The status of visual and auditory acuity accounted for 93% of the age-related reliable variance in the cognitive factors, suggesting that sensory functioning is a strong late-life predictor of individual differences in cognitive function. Results from cross-sectional studies have provided solid support for the hypothesis that age-related sensory and cognitive declines are attributable to a common cause — a general or distributed decline in the functional integrity of the brain (e.g., Anstey, Hofer, & Luszcz, 2003; Christensen et al., 2001; Lövdén & Wahlin, 2005; Salthouse et al., 1996). Between 50 and 100% of all the age-related variance in general cognitive functioning can be explained by tests of vision and hearing. Similarly, results from two large longitudinal studies, the Australian Longitudinal Study of Ageing and the Maastricht Longitudinal Ageing Study, have provided support for a common factor or common cause, reflected in a moderately strong relation between age declines in visual acuity and age declines in memory (Anstey et al., 2003; Valentijn et al., 2005). One difficulty in interpreting associations between sensory and cognitive measures is that sensory and cognitive measures are by themselves both highly associated with age. Also, estimates of shared age-related variance are computed differently in cross-sectional and longitudinal data. Shared age-related variance in cross-sectional analyses represents only the reliable variance that is shared, whereas estimates of shared variance in the relationship between two change scores in longitudinal analyses are proportions of the total variance that include error variance. Further, because the age range is usually much larger in cross-sectional comparisons than in longitudinal comparisons, narrow age-cohort data collection strategies are useful for minimizing the potential problem of shared age effects in the associations between sensory and cognitive variables (Hofer, Sliwinski, & Flaherty, 2002).

Birren (1965) was one of the first researchers to point to the importance of speed of processing as a general factor in cognitive aging. Salthouse (e.g., 1991, 1996) proposed the theory that slowing of basic information processing might have insidious consequences for higher order cognition. In studies of the relationships between age and measures of associative learning and associative memory (Dunlosky & Salthouse, 1996; Salthouse, 1994), between 44 and 80% age variance is associated with processing speed. In a large meta-analysis, Verhaeghen and Salthouse (1997) found that processing speed explained 93% of the age-related variance in short-term memory and working memory measures and 71% of the age-related variance in episodic memory measures. Longitudinal estimates of shared variance between speed and memory declines are much more modest, ranging between 8% and 46% (Hultsch et al., 1998; Lempke & Zimprich, 2005; Sliwinski & Buschke, 1999). The underlying source of age-related slowing in speed of processing is still unclear. Brain mechanisms that have been advanced to account for slowing include increased neural noise (e.g., Li, 2005), depletion of dopamine receptors (e.g., Bäckman, & Farde, 2005), frontal lobe dysfunction (West, 1996), and white matter abnormalities (e.g., Deary et al., 2003; Gunning-Dixon & Raz, 2000).

B. Cognitive Control and Executive Control Functions

A second category of explanations aims for more resolution than task-general accounts. Theories in this category postulate age-related deficits that are specific to particular basic control processes in working memory, over and beyond the effects of sensory impairments or general age-related slowing. These deficits would have a direct impact on working memory and an indirect impact on episodic memory and source memory and on the process of recollection.

Three types of control processes have been researched extensively in the field of cognitive aging (for a classification of control processes, see Miyake et al., 2000). First, *resistance to interference*, also known as inhibitory control, has been a central explanatory construct in aging theories throughout the 1990s (e.g., Hasher et al., 2001; Hasher & Zacks, 1988; Hasher, Zacks, & May, 1999; Lövdén, 2003; for a computational approach, see Braver & Barch, 2002). Inhibition theory casts resistance to interference as a true cognitive primitive and posits an age-related breakdown in this resistance. A breakdown with aging would lead to mental clutter in older adult's working memory, thereby limiting its functional capacity, and perhaps also its speed of operation. Second, age-related deficits have been posited in the ability to *coordinate* distinct tasks or distinct processing streams. Some of the attendant literature pertains to dual-task and task-switching performance (Kramer, Hahn, & Gopher, 1999; Verhaeghen et al., 2003), but the concept has also received some attention in the working memory literature (e.g., Braver, Gray, & Burgess, 2005; Fisk & Sharp, 2004; Verhaeghen & Basak, 2005; Verhaeghen & Hoyer, 2005;

Verhaeghen, Kliegl, & Mayr, 1997). This theory typically sees age differences in coordination as independent of age differences in speed. That is, coordination is considered a mechanism that operates over and above the effects of mere slowing and is presumably necessary to explain age-related differences in more complex tasks. Third, the late 1990s and early 2000s have seen a surge in the number of publications devoted to aging and *task switching* (e.g., Mayr, Spieler, & Kliegl, 2001). Much like the coordination theory, this work considers age differences in task switching as additional to other age-related deficits that might exist in the cognitive system. A fourth factor, working memory *updating*, has been investigated relatively rarely in an aging context (e.g., Fisk & Sharp, 2004; Van der Linden, Brédart, & Beerten, 1994). Some of the studies in this area of research emphasize the neuropsychological bases of cognitive and executive control and call attention to associations between selected memory deficits and the consequences of brain aging on specific functions associated with the prefrontal and midfrontal regions of the human cortex (e.g., Moscovitch & Winocur, 1995; West, 1996). Alternatively, some researchers take a more integrated view of brain aging effects that includes the integration of multiple brain regions and distributed brain functions (e.g., Adcock et al. 2000; Braver et al. 2001; Rosen et al., 2003; Small et al., 2002).

Verhaeghen and Cerella (2002) pooled the available aging literature on resistance to interference (namely, the Stroop effect and negative priming), dual-task performance and task switching, using different techniques to control for the effects of general slowing. They found that age effects were absent in tasks measuring resistance to interference and in local task-switching costs (i.e., the comparison, within a block of task-switching trials, between trials in which task switching is actually required with trials in which the task did not switch). In contrast, age effects were seen in dual-task performance and global task switching (i.e., the comparison between reaction times in blocks with only single tasks with reaction times in blocks when the participant has to switch between tasks). One possible interpretation is that age differences only emerge in tasks that involve the maintenance of two distinct mental task sets and not in tasks that involve active selection of relevant information. In other words, the perceived executive control deficits might not be related to control after all, but may be due to a smaller capacity of the mental workspace for information processing.

Other researchers have pointed to the effects of cognitive control at a more global level. Early studies on the role of contextual support (or the lack of it) were among the first to implicate subject-controlled factors in age-related deficits in memory. Craik and Jennings (1992) suggested that the magnitude of age-related deficits in memory is inversely related to the amount of contextual support provided by task factors. Studies showing that age differences are larger in tasks that require recall of unprimed stimuli than in tasks that support retrieval by priming (e.g., Fleischman et al., 2004; La Voie & Light, 1994; Prull, 2004) are consistent with this view (as well as with the distinction between declarative and nondeclarative memory systems). Item retrieval in tasks lacking support depends mostly on the individual's initiation or use of optimal processing strategies, and age-related reductions in processing resources constrain the use of processing strategies that require more initiative. Older adults are then at a disadvantage in generating or producing strategies, and thereby must deploy extra resources or more effort for their performance to match the performance of younger adults in tasks that provide less

contextual support. Findings that point to strategy production deficiencies as a source of memory deficits are also consistent with this view (e.g., Dunlosky, Kubat-Silman, & Hertzog, 2003; Onyper, Hoyer, & Cerella, 2006; Rogers, Hertzog, & Fisk, 2000; Touron & Hertzog, 2004; Verhaeghen & Marcoen, 1994). Verhaeghen and Marcoen (1994), for example, showed a connection between age-related limitations in the availability of general processing resources and efficient strategy use.

Meta-analytic summaries of memory aging data support the contention that effect sizes for age-related deficits in memory performance correspond to the cognitive control demands associated with effective task performance. La Voie and Light (1994) reported mean weighted effect sizes of 0.97 for free recall and 0.50 for recognition memory, and Verhaeghen, Marcoen, and Goosens (1993) reported mean weighted effect sizes of 0.99 for list recall and 0.67 for prose recall.

IV. Memory Interventions

Memory functioning throughout the adult life span is affected by health status and health-related behavior and by a variety of social or environmental factors (e.g., Birnbaum et al. 2004; Cotman, 2000; Raz, Rodrigue, & Acker, 2003; Reynolds et al., 2005; Sliwinski et al., 2003). This section considers cardiovascular fitness, memory training, and cognitive enrichment as illustrations of interventions that seem to have positive effects on the memory performance of older adults.

A. Cognitive Plasticity and Cardiovascular Fitness

A meta-analysis of 18 intervention studies examining the relationship between cognitive vitality and physical fitness training showed a robust effect of fitness training on measures of executive function, cognitive control, visual–spatial information processing, and speed of processing (Colcombe & Kramer, 2003). Such benefits must be mediated by changes in neural activation, and a study by Colcombe, et al. (2004) showed what seems to be a general relationship between cardiovascular fitness and cortical plasticity. Colcombe et al. (2004) conducted a cross-sectional assessment of fitness effects on brain activation and behavioral measures of attentional control and conflict monitoring and a randomized clinical trial assessing the prepost benefits of aerobic exercise on the same brain and behavioral measures; their findings suggest that cardiovascular fitness has general benefits on cognitive plasticity. Increased aerobic fitness was associated with reduced age-related differences in regions of the brain known for their vulnerability to aging. These investigators suggested that the relationship between cardiovascular fitness and cortical plasticity could be attributed to increased blood flow to the brain or to increased synaptic interconnectivity in the frontal lobes as a result of cardiovascular fitness.

B. Memory Training and Plasticity

Because the strategies that people use to remember and retrieve information contribute to the effectiveness of memory functioning, it is important to understand the extent to which the memory performance of older adults can be improved through training and instruction. Programs designed to improve the memory of older adults produce some benefits (Willis, 2000). For example, in a recent large-scale clinical trial examining the effects of a 10-session group training intervention for verbal episodic memory, 26% of the 711 older adults

given memory training demonstrated reliable memory improvements compared with baseline (Ball et al., 2002). The participants in this study were taught strategies for remembering lists of words and items, text material, and themes and details in stories and were then given exercises and performance feedback in both laboratory-like and everyday-like memory tasks. The improvements were observed immediately after the intervention and were found to be durable for 2 years.

In a meta-analysis of 33 studies, based on data from 1539 persons, Verhaeghen, Marcoen, and Goossens (1992) reported that mnemonic training benefited the memory performance of older adults. Memory performance was boosted by about 0.75 SD, compared to a 0.40 SD boost from mere retesting. Meta-analysis has also demonstrated that intervention programs aimed at alleviating memory complaints indeed enhance the subjective memory functioning of older adults (Floyd & Scogin, 1997).

Although these results show that there is a clear potential for behavioral plasticity in the later years (Nyberg, 2005) the evidence is unequivocal that plasticity of cognitive functions declines with advancing age (e.g., Singer, Lindenberger, & Baltes, 2003; Verhaeghen & Marcoen, 1996) and that observed benefits of training or interventions of any sort depend on the mental status and health status of the trainees (Colcombe et al. 2004; Nyberg, 2005). Generally, compared with younger adults, older adults are less able to benefit from training designed to optimize performance on memory tasks and other types of cognition.

C. Enrichment Effects on Memory

Related to the understanding of age-related differences in behavioral plasticity and intervention effects on memory is the general question of whether an individual's memory function benefits from lifelong participation in relatively more cognitively complex and challenging environments. The effects of cognitive stimulation in everyday life and performance on markers of cognitive function have been examined in a number of studies (e.g., Salthouse, Berish, & Miles, 2002; Schooler & Mulatu, 2001; Wilson et al., 2002). Salthouse et al. (2002) investigated the role of cognitive stimulation as a potential moderator of cognitive performance by asking adults ranging in age from 20 to 91 to complete an activity inventory and a variety of cognitive tests, including measures of episodic memory and associative learning; they found no relationship between self-reported cognitive stimulation and the measures of cognition. However, Hultsch and coworkers (1999) found a positive and possibly reciprocal relationship between level of cognitive activity and cognitive measures. In regard to reciprocity, high levels of cognitive activity may afford the opportunity to participate in and benefit from enriching experiences, enriching activities may serve to buffer cognitive decline, or both. Wilson et al. (2002) showed that frequent participation in cognitively stimulating activities is associated with a lower risk of developing Alzheimer's disease. Wilson et al. (2002) reported that even a small increase in cognitive activity scores was predictive of a 33% reduction in the risk of developing Alzheimer's. It is also the case that educational attainment is associated with a lower risk of developing Alzheimer's disease and with less age-related decline in memory and related cognitive functions (Springer et al., 2005).

V. Summary and Conclusions

The aim of this chapter was to provide an overview and review of the current status of description and explanation of age trends for various forms of memory. Strong evidence suggests age-related dissociations in memory functions, and findings are consistent with the recollection–familiarity distinction and with multiple systems models of memory. In just the past decade, results from literally hundreds of studies demonstrated age-related deficits in tasks that involve recollection, declarative memory, episodic memory, and working memory in contrast to much more mild age-related deficits or declines in tasks measuring familiarity, use of semantic knowledge, and nondeclarative systems of memory. This general pattern implicates the importance of examining age–memory relationships in terms of the neural substrates most affected by aging, especially regions of the prefrontal cortex and the medial temporal lobe and their mappings to regions engaged by the task domain and response requirements.

The most challenging issue facing researchers working in the area of memory aging is how to explain age-related memory phenomena. Memory aging and various cognitive aging phenomena can be interpreted and explained at relatively micro- or macro-levels. At the macro-level, a large portion of the age variance observed in memory performance is attributable to task-general effects of slowing that add overhead to any speeded measures of responding. Further, age-related sensory and perceptual changes that impair processing of stimulus information add task-general overhead. Because the consequences of slowing effects and of stimulus processing impairments are a direct function of task complexity, variance associated with task-general aging effects should be taken into account as a baseline before resorting to process-specific explanations. At a more micro-level, questions arise regarding the aging of specific cognitive processes and specific neurocognitive mechanisms that reliably account for behavioral data on memory aging. Many studies have aimed to identify memory "primitives" or the key variables that influence the cognitive function without themselves being attributable to other constructs. In regard to control processes in memory, good evidence suggests that executive demands related to multiple-task contexts (global task switching and dual task performance) may be important for the understanding of a wide range of memory aging phenomena that involve loading and maintaining multiple task sets. New research calls for a shift away from static descriptions of memory systems at different ages and toward models that give emphasis to cognitive control and attention in memory aging and to the understanding of the interventions that affect change.

Acknowledgment

Preparation of this chapter was supported by research grants AG11451 and AG16201.

References

Adcock, R. A., Constable, R. T., Gore, J. C., & Goldman-Rakic, P. S. (2000). Functional neuroanatomy of executive processes involved in dual-task performance. *Proceedings of the National Academy of Sciences, 97,* 3567–3572.

Allen, P. A., Sliwinski, M., Bowie, T., & Madden, D. J. (2002). Differential age effects in semantic and episodic memory. *Journal of Gerontology: Psychological Sciences, 57B,* P173-P186.

Anstey, K. J., Hofer, S. M., & Luszcz, M. A. (2003). Cross-sectional and longitudinal patterns of dedifferentiation in late-life cognitive and sensory function: The effects of age, ability, attrition, and occasion of measurement. *Journal of Experimental Psychology: General, 132,* 470–487.

Bäckman, L., & Farde, L. (2005). The role of dopamine systems in cognitive aging.

In R. Cabeza, L. Nyberg, & D. Park (Eds.), *Cognitive neuroscience of aging* (pp. 58–84). New York: Oxford University Press.

Bäckman, L., Small, B. J., & Wahlin, Å. (2001). Aging and memory: Cognitive and biological perspectives. In J. E. Birren & K. W. Schaie (Eds.), *Handbook of the psychology of aging* (pp. 349–377). San Diego: Academic Press.

Baddeley, A. D. (1986). *Working memory.* New York: Oxford University Press.

Ball, K., Berch, D. B., Helmers, K. F., Jobe, J. B., Leveck, M. D., Marsiske, M., Morris, J. N., Rebok, G. W., Smith, D. M., Tennstedt, S. L., Unverzagt, F. W., & Willis, S. W. (2002). Effects of cognitive training interventions with older adults. *Journal of the American Medical Association, 288,* 2271–2281.

Balota, D. A., Cortese, M. J., Duchek, J. M., Adams, D., Roediger, H. L., III, McDermott, K. B., & Yerys, B. E. (1999). Veridical and false memories in healthy older adults and in dementia of the Alzheimer's type. *Cognitive Neuropsychology, 16,* 361–384.

Bastin, C., & Van der Linden, M. (2003). The contribution of recollection and familiarity to recognition memory: A study of the effects of test format and aging. *Neuropsychology, 17,* 14–24.

Birnbaum, S. G., Yuan, P. X., Wang, M., Vijayraghavan, S., Bloom, A. K., Davis, D. J., Gobeske, K. T., Sweatt, J. D., Manji, H, K., & Arnsten, F. T. (2004). Protein kinase C overactivity impairs prefrontal cortical regulation of working memory. *Science, 306,* 882–884.

Birren, J. E. (1965). Age changes in speed of behavior: Its central nature and physiological correlates. In A. T. Welford & J. E. Birren (Eds.), *Behavior, aging, and the nervous system* (pp. 191–216). Springfield, IL: Charles C. Thomas.

Bopp, K. L., & Verhaeghen, P. (2005). Aging and verbal memory span: A meta-analysis. *Journal of Gerontology: Psychological Sciences, 60B,* P223–P233.

Braver, T. S., Gray, J. R., & Burgess, G. C. (2005). Explaining the many varieties of working memory variation: Dual mechanisms of cognitive control. In A. R. A. Conway, C. Jarrold, M. Kane, A. Miyake, & J. Towse (Eds.), *Variation in working memory.* New York: Oxford University Press.

Braver, T. S., & Barch, D. M. (2002). A theory of cognitive control, aging cognition and neuromodulation. *Neuroscience and Biobehavioral Reviews, 26,* 809–817.

Braver, T. S., Barch, D. M., Keys, B., et al. (2001). Context processing in older adults: Evidence for a theory relating cognitive control to neurobiology in healthy aging. *Journal of Experimental Psychology: General, 130,* 746–763.

Buckner, R. L. (2005). Three principles for cognitive aging research: Multiple causes and sequelae, variance in expression and response, and the need for integrative theory. In R. Cabeza, L. Nyberg, & D. Park (Eds.), *Cognitive neuroscience of aging* (pp. 267–285). New York: Oxford University Press.

Byrne, M. D. (1998). Taking a computational approach to aging: The SPAN theory of working memory. *Psychology and Aging, 13,* 309–322.

Castel, A. D., & Craik, F. I. M. (2003). The effects of aging and divided attention on memory for item and associative information. *Psychology and Aging, 18,* 873–885.

Cerella, J. (1990). Aging and information processing rate. In J. E. Birren & K. W. Schaie (Eds.), *Handbook of the psychology of aging* (3rd edition, pp. 201–221). San Diego: Academic Press.

Chalfonte, B. L., & Johnson, M. K. (1996). Feature memory and binding in young and older adults. *Memory & Cognition, 24,* 403–416.

Charles, S. T., Mather, M., & Carstensen, L. L. (2003). Aging and emotional memory: The forgettable nature of negative images for older adults. *Journal of Experimental Psychology: General, 132,* 310–324.

Chown, S. M., & Heron, A. (1965). Psychological aspects of aging in man. *Annual Review of Psychology, 16,* 417–450.

Christensen, H., Mackinnon, A. J., Korten, A., & Jorm, A. F. (2001). The "common cause hypothesis" of cognitive aging: Evidence for not only a common factor but also specific associations of age with vision and grip strength in a cross-sectional analysis. *Psychology and Aging, 16,* 588–599.

Colcombe, S. J., & Kramer, A. F. (2003). Fitness effects on the cognitive function of older adults. *Psychological Science, 14,* 125–130.

Colcombe, S. J., Kramer, A. F., Erickson, K. I., Scalf, P., McAuley, E., Cohen, N. J., Webb, A., Jerome, G. J., Marquez, D. X., and Elavsky, S. (2004), Cardiovascular fitness, cortical plasticity, and aging. *Proceedings of the National Academy of Sciences, 101,* 3316–3321.

Conway, A. R. A., Cowan, N., Bunting, M. F., Therriault, D. J., & Minkoff, S. R. B. (2002). A latent variable analysis of working memory capacity, short-term memory capacity, processing speed, and general fluid intelligence. *Intelligence, 30,* 163–183.

Cotman, C. W. (2000). Homeostatic processes in brain aging: The role of apoptosis, inflammation, and oxidative stress in regulating healthy neural circuitry in the aging brain. In P. C. Stern & L. L. Carstensen (Eds.), *The aging mind* (pp. 114–143). Washington, DC: National Academy of Sciences.

Craik, F. I. M. (1977). Age differences in human memory. In J. E. Birren & K. W. Schaie (Eds.), *Handbook of the psychology of aging* (pp. 384–420). New York: Van Nostrand Reinhold.

Craik, F. I. M., Govoni, R., Naveh-Benjamin, M., & Anderson, N. D. (1996). The effects of divided attention on encoding and retrieval processes in human memory. *Journal of Experimental Psychology: General, 125,* 159–180.

Craik, F. I. M., & Jennings, J. (1992), Human memory. In F. I. M. Craik & T. A. Salthouse (Eds.), *Handbook of aging and cognition* (pp. 51–110). Hillsdale, NJ: Erlbaum.

Deary, I. J., Leaper, S. A., Murray, A. D., Staff, R. T., & Whalley, L. J. (2003). Cerebral white matter abnormalities and life-time cognitive change: A 67 year follow-up of the Scottish Mental Survey 1932. *Psychology and Aging, 18,* 140–148

Deary, I. J., Wright, A. F., Harris, S. E., Wally, L. J., & Starr, J. M. (2004). Searching for genetic influences on normal cognitive aging. *Trends in Cognitive Sciences, 8,* 178–184.

D'Esposito, M., Detre, J. A., Alsop, D. C., Shin, R. K., Atlas, S., & Grossman, M. (1995). The neural basis of the central executive of working memory. *Nature, 378,* 279–281.

Dixon, R. A., Wahlin, Å., Maitland, S. B., Hultsch, D. F., Hertzog, C., & Bäckman, L. (2004). Episodic memory change in late adulthood: Generalizability across samples and performance indices. *Memory & Cognition, 32,* 768–778.

Driscoll, I., McDaniel, M. A., & Guynn, M. J. (2005). Apolipoprotein E and prospective memory in normally aging adults. *Neuropsychology, 19,* 28–34.

Dunlosky, J. Kubat-Silman, A., & Hertzog, C. (2003). Training monitoring skills improves older adults' self-paced associative learning. *Psychology and Aging, 18,* 340–345.

Dunlosky, J., & Salthouse, T. A. (1996). A decomposition of age-related differences in multitrial free recall. *Aging, Neuropsychology, and Cognition, 3,* 2–14.

Eichenbaum, H. (2003). How does the hippocampus contribute to memory? *Trends in Cognitive Science, 7,* 427–429.

Engle, R. W., Kane, M. J., & Tuholski, S. W. (1999). Individual differences in working memory capacity and what they tell us about controlled attention, general fluid intelligence, and functions of the prefrontal cortex. In A. Miyake & P. Shah (Eds.), *Models of working memory: Mechanisms of active maintenance and executive control* (pp. 102–134). New York: Cambridge University Press.

Fisher, D. L., Duffy, S. A., & Katsikopoulos, K. V. (2000). Cognitive slowing among older adults: What kind and how much? In T. J. Perfect & E. A. Maylor (Eds.), *Models of cognitive aging* (pp. 87–124). Oxford, England: Oxford University Press.

Fisk, J. E., & Sharp, C. A. (2004). Age-related impairment in executive functioning: Updating, inhibition, shifting, and access. *Journal of Clinical and Experimental Neuropsychology, 26,* 874–890.

Fleischman, D. A., Wilson, R. S., Gabrieli, J. D. E., Bienias, J. L., & Bennett, D. A. (2004). A longitudinal study of implicit and explicit memory in old persons. *Psychology and Aging, 19,* 617–625.

Floyd, M., & Scogin, F. (1997). Effects of memory training on the subjective memory functioning and mental health of older adults: A meta-analysis. *Psychology and Aging, 12,* 150–161.

Gunning-Dixon, & Raz, N. (2000). The cognitive correlates of white matter abnormalities in normal aging: A quantitative review. *Neuropsychology, 14,* 224–232.

Harkins, S. W., Chapman, C. R., & Eisdorfer, C. (1979). Memory loss and response bias in senescence. *Journal of Gerontology, 34,* 66–72.

Hasher, L., Tonev, S. T., Lustig, C., & Zacks, R. T. (2001). Inhibitory control, environmental support, and self-initiated processing in aging. In M. Naveh-Benjamin, M. Moscovitch, & R. L. Roediger, III (Eds.), *Perspectives on human memory and cognitive aging: essays in honour of Fergus Craik* (pp. 286–297). East Sussex, UK: Psychology Press.

Hasher, L., & Zacks, R. T. (1988). Working memory, comprehension, and aging: A review and a new view. In G. H. Bower (Ed.), *The psychology of learning and motivation* (Vol. 22, pp. 193–225). San Diego: Academic Press.

Hasher, L., Zacks, R. T., & May, C. P. (1999). Inhibitory control, circadian arousal, and age. In D. Gopher & A. Koriat (Eds.), *Attention and performance, XVII, Cognitive regulation of performance: Interaction of theory and application* (pp. 653–675). Cambridge, MA: MIT Press.

Healy, M. R., Light, L. L., & Chung, C. (2005). Dual–process models of associative recognition in young and older adults: Evidence from receiver operating characteristics. *Journal of Experimental Psychology: Learning, Memory, and Cognition, 31,* 768–787.

Henry, J. D., MacLeod, M. S., Phillips, L. H., & Crawford, J. R. (2004). A meta-analytic review of prospective memory and aging. *Psychology and Aging, 19,* 27–39.

Hertzog, C., & Hultsch, D. F. (2000). Metacognition in adulthood and old age. In F. I. M. Craik & T. A. Salthouse (Eds.), *Handbook of aging and cognition* (2nd edition, pp. 417–466). Mahwah, NJ: Erlbaum.

Hess, T. (2005). Memory and aging in context. *Psychological Bulletin, 131,* 383–406.

Hofer, S. M., Sliwinski, M. J., & Flaherty, B. P. (2002). Understanding ageing: Futher commentary on the limitations of cross-sectional designs for ageing research. *Gerontology, 48,* 22–29.

Howard, M. W., Bessette-Symons, B., Zhang, Y., & Hoyer, W. J. (2006). Aging selectively impairs recollection in recognition memory for pictures: Evidence from modeling ROC curves. *Psychology and Aging*.

Hulicka, I. M. (1966). Age differences in Wechsler Memory Scale scores. *Journal of Genetic Psychology, 109*, 134–145.

Hultsch, D. F., & Dixon, R. A. (1990). Learning and memory in aging. In J. E. Birren & K. W. Schaie (Eds.), *Handbook of the psychology of aging* (3rd edition, pp. 258–274). San Diego: Academic Press.

Hultsch, D. F., Hertzog, C., Dixon, R. A., & Small, B. J. (1998). *Memory change in the aged*. New York: Cambridge University Press.

Hultsch, D. F., Hertzog, C., Small, B., & Dixon, R. A. (1999). Use it or lose it: Engaged lifestyle as a buffer of cognitive decline in aging? *Psychology and Aging, 14*, 245–263.

Isaacowitz, D. M., Charles, S. T., & Carstensen, L. L. (2000). Emotion and cognition. In F. I. M. Craik & T. A. Salthouse (Eds.), *Handbook of aging and cognition* (2nd edition, pp. 593–632). Mahwah, NJ: Erlbaum.

Jacoby, L. L. (1991). A process dissociation framework: Separating automatic from intentional uses of memory. *Journal of Memory and Language, 30*, 513–541.

Jacoby, L. L. (1999). Ironic effect of repetition: Measuring age-related differences in memory. *Journal of Experimental Psychology: Learning, Memory, and Cognition, 25*, 3–22.

Jacoby, L. L., Bishara, A. J., Hessels, S., & Toth, J. P. (2005). Aging, subjective experience, and cognitive control: Dramatic false remembering by older adults. *Journal of Experimental Psychology: General, 134*, 131–148.

Kahn, I., Davachi, L., & Wagner, A. D. (2004). Functional neuroanatomic correlates of recollection: Implications for models of recognition memory. *The Journal of Neuroscience, 24*, 4172–4180.

Kemper, S., Herman, R. E., & Lian, C. H. T. (2003). The costs of doing two things at once for young and older adults: Talking while walking, finger tapping, and ignoring speech noise. *Psychology and Aging, 18*, 181–192.

Karpel, M. E., Hoyer, W. J., & Toglia, M. P. (2001). Accuracy and qualities of real and suggested memories: Non-specific age differences. *Journal of Gerontology: Psychological Sciences, 56B*, 103–110.

Kensinger, E. A., Clarke, R. J., Corkin, S. (2003). What neural correlates underlie successful encoding and retrieval? A functional magnetic resonance imaging study using a divided attention paradigm. *The Journal of Neuroscience, 23*, 2407–2415.

Kensinger, E. A., & Schacter, D. L. (1999). When true memories suppress false memories: Effects of aging. *Cognitive Neuropsychology, 16*, 399–415.

Koutstaal, W., Reddy, C., Jackson, E. M., Prince, S., Cenden, D. L., & Schacter, D. L. (2003). False recognition of abstract versus common objects in older adults and younger adults: Testing the semantic categorization account. *Journal of Experimental Psychology: Learning, Memory, & Cognition, 29*, 499–510.

Koutstaal, W., Schacter, D. L., Galluccio, L., & Stofer, K. A. (1999). Reducing gist-based false recognition in older adults: Encoding and retrieval manipulations. *Psychology and Aging, 14*, 220–237.

Koutstaal, W., Schacter, D. L., Johnson, M. K., Angell, K. E., & Gross, M. S. (1998). Post-event review in older and younger adults: Improving memory accessibility of complex everyday events. *Psychology and Aging, 13*, 277–296.

Kramer, A. F., Hahn, S., & Gopher, D. (1999). Task coordination and aging: Explorations of executive control processes in the task switching paradigm. *Acta Psychologica, 101*, 339–378.

Kyllonen, P. C. (1996). Is working memory capacity Spearman's g? In I. Dennis & P. Tapsfield (Eds.), *Human abilities: Their nature and measurement* (pp. 49–75). Mahwah, NJ: Erlbaum.

La Voie, D. J., & Light, L. L. (1994). Adult age differences in repetition priming: A meta-analysis. *Psychology and Aging, 9*, 539–553.

Lempke, U., & Zimprich, D. (2005). Longitudinal changes in memory performance and processing speed in old age. *Aging, Neuropsychology, and Cognition, 12*, 57–77.

Li, J., Morcom, A. M., & Rugg, M. D. (2004). The effects of age on the neural correlates of successful episodic retrieval: An ERP study.

Cognitive, Affective, and Behavioral Neuroscience, 4, 279–293.

Li, S.-C. (2005). Neurocomputational perspectives linking neuromodulation, processing noise, representational distinctiveness, and cognitive aging. In R. Cabeza, L. Nyberg, & D. Park (Eds.), *Cognitive neuroscience of aging* (pp. 354–379). New York: Oxford University Press.

Li, S.-C., Naveh-Benjamin, M., & Lindenberger, U. (2005). Aging neuromodulation impairs associative binding: A neurocomputational account. *Psychological Science, 16,* 445–450.

Light, L. L., Prull, M. W., La Voie, D. J., & Healy, M. R. (2000). Dual-process theories of memory in old age. In T. J. Perfect & E. A. Maylor (Eds.), *Models of cognitive aging* (pp. 238–300). Oxford, England: Oxford University Press.

Lindenberger, U., & Baltes, P. B. (1994). Sensory functioning and intelligence in old age: A strong connection. *Psychology and Aging, 9,* 339–355.

Lövdén, M. (2003). The episodic memory and inhibition accounts of age-related increases in false memories: A consistency check. *Journal of Memory and Language, 49,* 268–283.

Lövdén, M. Rönnlund, M., Wahlin, Å., Bäckman, L. Nyberg, L., & Nilsson, L.-G. (2004). The extent of stability and changes in episodic and semantic memory in old age: Demographic predictors of level and change. *Journal of Gerontology: Psychological Sciences, 59B,* P130–P134.

Lövdén, M., & Wahlin, Å. (2005). The sensory-cognition association in adulthood: Different magnitudes for processing speed, inhibition, episodic memory, and false memory? *Scandinavian Journal of Psychology, 46,* 253–262.

Madden, D. J. (2001). Speed and timing of behavioral processes. In J. E. Birren & K. W. Schaie (Eds.), *Handbook of the psychology of aging* (5th edition, pp.288–312). San Diego: Academic Press.

Madden, D. J., Whiting, W. L., & Huettel, S. A. (2005). Age-related changes in neural activity during visual perception and attention. In R. Cabeza, L. Nyberg, & D. Park (Eds.), *Cognitive neuroscience of aging*

(pp. 157–185). New York: Oxford University Press.

Margolis, R. B., & Scialfa, C. T. (1984). Age differences in Wechsler Memory Scale performance. *Journal of Clinical Psychology, 40,* 1442–1449.

Mark, R. E., & Rugg, M. D. (1998). Age effects on brain activity associated with episodic memory retrieval: An electrophysiological study. *Brain, 121,* 861–873.

Martin, A., Haxby, J. V., Lalonde, F. M., Wiggs, C. L., & Ungerleider, L. G. (1995). Discrete cortical regions associated with knowledge of color and knowledge of action. *Science, 270,* 102–105.

Mather, M. (2004). Aging and emotional memory. In D. Reisberg & P. Hertel, (Eds.) *Memory and emotion* (pp. 272–307). New York: Oxford University Press.

Mayr, U., Spieler, D. H., & Kliegl, R. (2001). *Aging and executive control.* New York: Routledge.

McCabe, D. P., & Smith, A. D. (2002). The effect of warnings on false memories in young and older adults. *Memory & Cognition, 30,* 1065–1077.

Mitchell, K. J., Johnson, M. K., Raye, C. L., & D'Esposito, M. D. (2000a). fMRI evidence of age-related hippocampal dysfunction in feature binding in working memory. *Cognitive Brain Research, 10,* 197–206.

Mitchell, K. J., Johnson, M. K., Raye, C. L., Mather, M., & D'Esposito, M. (2000b). Aging and reflective processes of working memory: Binding and test load deficits. *Psychology and Aging, 15,* 527–541.

Miyake, A., Friedman, N. P., Emerson, M. J., Witzki, A. H., Howerter, A., & Wager, T. D. (2000). The unity and diversity of executive functions and their contributions to 'frontal lobe' tasks: A latent variable analysis. *Cognitive Psychology, 41,* 49–100.

Moscovitch, M., & Winocur, G. (1995). Frontal lobes, memory, and aging. In J. Grafman, K. J. Holyoak, & F. Boller (Eds.), *Structure and functions of the human prefrontal cortex* (pp. 119–150). New York: New York Academy of Sciences.

Naveh-Benjamin, M. (2000). Adult-age differences in memory performance: Tests of an associative deficit hypothesis. *Journal of*

Experimental Psychology: Learning, Memory and Cognition, 26, 1170–1187.

Naveh-Benjamin, M. (2001). The effects of divided attention on encoding processes: Underlying mechanisms. In M. Naveh-Benjamin, M. Moscovitch, & H. L. Roediger, III (Eds.), *Perspectives on human memory and cognitive aging: Essays in honour of Fergus Craik* (pp. 193–207). Philadelphia, PA: Psychology Press.

Naveh-Benjamin, M., Craik, F. I. M., Guez, J., & Kreuger, S. (2005). Divided attention in younger and older adults: Effects of strategy and relatedness on memory performance and secondary task costs. *Journal of Experimental Psychology: Learning, Memory, and Cognition, 31,* 520–537.

Naveh-Benjamin, N., Guez, J., Bilb, A., & Reedy, S. (2004). The associative memory deficit in older adults: Further support using face-name associations. *Psychology and Aging, 19,* 541–546.

Naveh-Benjamin, M., Hussain, Z., Guez, J., & Bar-On, M. (2003). Adult age differences in episodic memory: Further support for an associative-deficit hypothesis. *Journal of Experimental Psychology: Learning, Memory and Cognition, 29,* 826–837.

Nilsson, L.-G., Adolfsson, R., Bäckman, L., Cruts, M., Edvardsson, H., Nyberg, L., & Van Broeckhoven, C. (2002). Memory development in adulthood and old age: The Betula prospective-cohort study. In P. Graf & N. Ohta (Eds.), *Lifespan development of human memory* (pp. 185–204). Cambridge, MA: MIT Press.

Nilsson, L.-G., Bäckman, L., Erngrund, K., Nyberg, L., Adolfsson, R., Bucht, G., Karlsson, S., Widing, G., & Wilblad, B. (1997). The Betula prospective cohort study: Memory, health, and aging. *Aging, Neuropsychology, and Cognition, 4,* 1–32.

Nyberg, L. (2005). Cognitive training in healthy aging: A cognitive neuroscience perspective. In R. Cabeza, L. Nyberg, & D. Park (Eds.), *Cognitive neuroscience of aging: Linking cognitive and cerebral aging* (pp. 309–321). New York: Oxford University Press.

Nyberg, L., Maitland, S. B., Rönnlund, M., Bäckman, L., Dixon, R. A., Wahlin, Ä., et al. (2003). Selective adult age differences in an age-invariant multifactor model of declarative memory. *Psychology and Aging, 18,* 149–160.

Oberauer, K., & Kliegl, R. (2001). Beyond resources: Formal models of complexity effects and age differences in working memory. *European Journal of Cognitive Psychology, 13,* 187–215.

Oberauer, K., Wendland, M., & Kliegl, R. (2003). Age differences in working memory: The roles of storage and selective access. *Memory & Cognition, 31,* 563–569.

Onyper, S. V., Hoyer, W. J., & Cerella, J. (2006). Determinants of retrieval solutions during cognitive skill training: Source confusions. *Memory & Cognition.*

Park, D. C., Lautenschlager, G., Hedden, T., Davidson, N. S., Smith, A. D., & Smith, P. K. (2002). Models of visuospatial and verbal memory across the adult life span. *Psychology and Aging, 17,* 299–320.

Parkin, A. J., & Java, R. I. (2000). Determinants of age-related memory loss. In T. J. Perfect & E. A. Maylor (Eds.), *Models of cognitive aging* (pp. 188–203). Oxford, UK: Oxford University Press.

Parkin, A. J., & Walter, B. M. (1992). Recollective experience, normal aging, and frontal dysfunction. *Psychology and Aging, 7,* 290–298.

Perfect, T. J., & Maylor, E. A. (2000). Rejecting the dull hypothesis: The relation between method and theory in cognitive aging research. In T. J. Perfect & E. A. Maylor (Eds.), *Models of cognitive aging* (pp. 1–18). Oxford, UK: Oxford University Press.

Poon, L. W. (1985). Differences in human memory with aging. In J. E. Birren & K. W. Schaie (Eds.), *Handbook of the psychology of aging* (2nd edition, pp. 427–462). New York: Van Nostrand Reinhold.

Prull, M. W. (2004). Exploring the identification-production hypothesis of repetition priming in young and older adults. *Psychology and Aging, 19,* 108–124.

Prull, M. W., Crandell, L. L., Martin, A. M., III, Backus, H. F., & Light, L. L. (2003). *Adult age differences in familiarity depend on which process estimation method is used.* Poster presented at the meetings of the Psychonomic Society, Vancouver.

Prull, M. W., Gabrieli, J. D. E., & Bunge, S. A. (2000). Age-related changes in memory: A cognitive neuroscience perspective. In F. I. M. Craik & T. A. Salthouse (Eds.), *Handbook of aging and cognition* (2nd edition, pp. 91–153). Mahwah, NJ: Erlbaum.

Raz, N. (2000). Aging of the brain and its impact on cognitive performance: Integration of structural and functional findings. In F. I. M. Craik & T. A. Salthouse (Eds.), *Handbook of aging and cognition* (2nd edition, pp. 1–90). Mahwah, NJ: Erlbaum.

Raz, N. (2005). The aging brain observed in vivo: Differential changes and their modifiers. In R. Cabeza, L. Nyberg, & D. Park (Eds.), *Cognitive neuroscience of aging* (pp. 19–57). New York: Oxford University Press.

Raz, N., Rodrigue, K., & Acker, J. (2003). Hypertension and the brain: Vulnerability of the prefrontal regions and executive functions. *Behavioral Neuroscience, 17,* 1169–1180.

Reuter-Lorenz, P. A., & Sylvester, C-Y. C. (2005). The cognitive neuroscience of working memory and aging. In R. Cabeza, L. Nyberg, & D. Park (Eds.), *Cognitive neuroscience of aging* (pp. 186–218). New York: Oxford University Press.

Reynolds, C. A., Finkel, D., McArdle, J. J., Gatz, M., Berg, S., & Pedersen, N. L. (2005). Quantitative genetic analysis of latent growth curve models of cognitive abilities in adulthood. *Developmental Psychology, 41,* 3–16.

Rodrigue, K. M., Kennedy, K. M., & Raz, N. (2005). Aging and longitudinal change in perceptual-motor skill acquisition in healthy adults. *Journal of Gerontology: Psychological Sciences, 60B,* P174–P181.

Roediger, H. L., III, Marsh, E. J., & Lee, S. C. (2002). Kinds of memory. In Stevens' handbook of experimental psychology. (3rd edition, vol. 2, pp. 1–41). New York: Wiley.

Rogers, W. A., & Fisk, A. D. (2001). Understanding the role of attention in cognitive aging research. In J. E. Birren & K. W. Schaie (Eds.), *Handbook of the psychology of aging* (Fifth edition, pp. 267–287). San Diego: Academic Press.

Rogers, W. A., Hertzog, C., & Fisk, A. D. (2000). An individual differences analysis of ability and strategy influences: Age-related differences in associative learning. *Journal of Experimental Psychology: Learning, Memory, and Cognition, 26,* 359–394.

Rönnlund, M., Nyberg, L., Bäckman, L., & Nillson, L-G. (2005). Stability, growth, and decline in adult life span development of declarative memory: Cross-sectional and longitudinal data from a population-based study. *Psychology and Aging, 20,* 3–18.

Rosen, A. Prull, M. W., Gabrieli, J. D. E., Stoub, T., O'Hara, R., Friedman, L., Yesavage, J. A., & deToledo-Morrell, L. (2003). Differential associations between entorhinal and hippocampal volumes and memory performance in older adults. *Behavioral Neuroscience, 117,* 1150–1160.

Rybash, J. M. (1996). Implicit memory and aging: A cognitive neuropsychological perspective. *Developmental Neuropsychology, 12,* 127–179.

Salthouse, T. A. (1991). *Theoretical perspectives on cognitive aging.* Hillsdale, NJ: Erlbaum.

Salthouse, T. A. (1992). Shifting levels of analysis in the investigation of cognitive aging. *Human Development, 35,* 321–342.

Salthouse, T. A. (1994). Aging associations: Influence of speed on adult age differences in associative learning. *Journal of Experimental Psychology: Learning, Memory, and Cognition, 20,* 1486–1503.

Salthouse, T. A. (1996). The processing speed theory of adult age differences in cognition. *Psychological Review, 103,* 403–428.

Salthouse, T. A. (2000). Steps toward the explanation of adult age differences in cognition. In T. J. Perfect & E. A. Maylor (Eds.), *Models of cognitive aging* (pp. 19–49). New York: Oxford University Press.

Salthouse, T. A. (2003). Memory aging from 18 to 80. *Alzheimer's Disease and Associated Disorders, 17,* 162–167.

Salthouse, T. A. (2004). From description to explanation in cognitive aging. In R. Sternberg, J. Davidson, & J. Pretz (Eds.), *Cognition and intelligence* (pp. 288–305). New York: Oxford University Press.

Salthouse, T. A., Berish, D. E., & Miles, J. D. (2002). The role of cognitive stimulation on the relations between age and cognitive functioning. *Psychology and Aging, 17,* 548–557.

Salthouse, T. A., Hancock, H. E., Meinz, E. J., & Hambrick, D. Z. (1996). Interrelations of age, visual acuity, and cognitive functioning. *Journal of Gerontology: Series B: Psychological Sciences and Social Sciences, 51B*, P317-P330.

Schaie, K. W. (1996). *Intellectual development in adulthood: The Seattle longitudinal study.* New York: Cambridge University Press.

Schmiedek, F., & Li, S.-C. (2004). Toward an alternative representation for disentangling age-associated differences in general and specific cognitive abilities. *Psychology and Aging, 19*, 40–5.

Schooler, C., & Mulatu, M. S. (2001). The reciprocal effects of leisure time activities and intellectual functioning in older people: A longitudinal analysis. *Psychology and Aging, 16*, 466–482.

Singer, T., Lindenberger, U., & Baltes, P. B. (2003). Plasticity of memory for new learning in very old age: A story of major loss? *Psychology and Aging, 18*, 306–317.

Singer, T., Verhaeghen, P., Ghisletta, P., Lindenberger, U., & Baltes, P. B. (2003). The fate of cognition in very old age: Six-year longitudinal findings in the Berlin Aging Study (BASE). *Psychology and Aging, 18*, 318–331.

Sliwinski, M., & Buschke, H. (1999). Cross-sectional and longitudinal relationships among age, cognition, and processing speed. *Psychology and Aging, 14*, 18–33.

Sliwinski, M. J., Hofer, S. M., Hall, C., Buschke, H., & Lipton, R. B. (2003). Modeling memory decline in older adults: The importance of preclinical dementia, attrition, and chronological age. *Psychology and Aging, 18*, 658–671.

Small, B. J., Rosnick, C. B., Fratiglioni, L., & Bäckman, L. (2004). Apolipoprotein E and cognitive performance: A meta-analysis. *Psychology and Aging, 19*, 592–600.

Small, S. A., Tsai, W. Y., deLaPaz, R., Mayeux, R., & Stern, Y. (2002). Imaging hippocampal function across the human life span. Is memory decline normal or not? *Annals of Neurology, 51*, 290–295.

Smith, A. D. (1996). Memory. In J. E. Birren & K. W. Schaie (Eds.), *Handbook of the psychology of aging* (4th edition, pp. 236–250). San Diego: Academic Press.

Spencer, W. D., & Raz, N. (1995). Differential effects of aging on memory for content and context: A meta-analysis. *Psychology and Aging, 10*, 527–539.

Springer, M. V., McIntosh, A. R., Winocur, G., & Grady, C. L. (2005). The relation between brain activity during memory tasks and years of education in young and older adults. *Neuropsychology, 19*, 181–192.

Squire, L. R. (2004). Memory systems of the brain: A brief history and current perspective. *Neurobiology of Learning and Memory, 82*, 171–177.

Touron, D. R., & Hertzog, C. (2004). Distinguishing age differences in knowledge, strategy use, and confidence during strategic skill acquisition. *Psychology and Aging, 19*, 452–466.

Valentijn, S. A., van Boxtel, M. P., van Hooren, S. A., Bosma, H., Beckers, H. J., et al. (2005). Change in sensory functioning predicts change in cognitive functioning: Results from a 6-year follow-up in the Maastricht Aging Study. *Journal of the American Geriatrics Society, 53*, 374–380.

Van der Linden, M., Brédart, S., & Beerten, A. (1994). Age-related differences in updating working memory. *British Journal of Psychology, 85*, 145–152.

Verhaeghen, P. (2003). Aging and vocabulary scores: A meta-analysis. *Psychology and Aging, 18*, 332–339.

Verhaeghen, P., & Basak, C. (2005). Aging and switching of the focus of attention in working memory: Results from a modified N-Back task. *Quarterly Journal of Experimental Psychology, 58A*, 134–154.

Verhaeghen, P., & Cerella, J. (2002). Aging, executive control, and attention: A review of meta-analyses. *Neuroscience and Biobehavioral Reviews, 26*, 849–857.

Verhaeghen, P., & Hoyer, W. J. (2005). Aging, focus switching, and task switching in a continuous calculation task: Further evidence toward a new working memory control process. *Aging, Neuropsychology, and Cognition.*

Verhaeghen, P., Kliegl, R., & Mayr, U. (1997). Sequential and coordinative complexity in time-accuracy function for mental arithmetic. *Psychology and Aging, 12*, 555–564.

Verhaeghen, P., & Marcoen, A. (1993). Memory aging as a general phenomenon: Episodic recall of older adults is a function of episodic recall of the young. *Psychology and Aging, 8,* 380–388.

Verhaeghen, P., & Marcoen, A. (1994). The production deficiency hypothesis revisited: Adult age differences in strategy use as a function of processing resources. *Aging and Cognition, 1,* 323–338.

Verhaeghen, P., & Marcoen, A. (1996). On the mechanisms of plasticity in young and older adults after instruction in the method of loci: Evidence for an amplification model. *Psychology and Aging, 11,* 164–178.

Verhaeghen, P., Marcoen, A., & Goossens, L. (1992). Improving memory performance in the aged through mnemonic training: A meta-analytic study. *Psychology and Aging, 7,* 242–251.

Verhaeghen, P., Marcoen, A., & Goossens, L. (1993). Fact and fiction about memory aging: A quantitative integration of research findings. *Journal of Gerontology: Psychological Sciences, 48,* P157–P171.

Verhaeghen, P., & Salthouse, T. A. (1997). Meta-analyses of age-cognition relations in adulthood: Estimates of linear and non-linear age effects and structural models. *Psychological Bulletin, 122,* 231–249.

Verhaeghen, P., Steitz, D. W., Sliwinski, M. J., & Cerella, J. (2003). Aging and dual-task performance: A meta-analysis. *Psychology and Aging, 18,* 443–460.

Wager, T. D., & Smith, E. E. (2003). Neuroimaging studies of working memory: A meta-analysis. *Cognitive, Affective, & Behavioral Neuroscience, 3,* 255–274.

Watson, J. M., Bunting, M. F., Poole, B. J., & Conway, A. R. A. (2005). Individual differences in susceptibility to false memory in the Deese-Roediger-McDermott paradigm. *Journal of Experimental Psychology: Learning, Memory, and Cognition, 31,* 76–85.

Watson, J. M., McDermott, K. B., & Balota, D. A. (2004). Attempting to avoid false memories in the Deese-Roediger-McDermott paradigm: Assessing the combined influence of practice and warnings in young and older adults. *Memory & Cognition, 32,* 135–141.

Wechsler, D. (1997). *Wechsler Memory Scale (WMS III): Administration and scoring manual.* San Antonio, TX: The Psychological Corporation.

Welford, A. T. (1965). Performance, biological mechanisms, and age: A theoretical sketch. In A. T. Welford & J. E. Birren (Eds.), *Behavior, aging, and the nervous system* (pp. 3–20). Springfield, IL: Thomas.

West, R. L. (1996). An application of prefrontal cortex function theory to cognitive aging. *Psychological Bulletin, 120,* 272–292.

Willis, S. L. (2001). Methodological issues in behavioral intervention research with the elderly. In J. E. Birren & K. W. Schaie (Eds.), *Handbook of the psychology of aging* (Fifth edition, pp. 78–108). San Diego: Academic Press.

Wilson, R. S., et al. (2002). Participation in cognitively stimulating activities and risk of incident Alzheimer's disease. *Journal of the American Medical Association, 287,* 742–748.

Winocur, G., & Hasher, L. (2002). Circadian rhythms and memory in aged humans and animals. In L. R. Squire and D. L. Schacter (Eds.), *Neuropsychology of memory* (3rd edition, pp. 273–285). New York: Guilford.

Yonelinas, A. P. (1997). Recognition memory ROCs for item and associative information: Evidence for a single-process signal-detection model. *Memory & Cognition, 25,* 747–763.

Yonelinas, A. P. (2002). The nature of recollection and familiarity: A review of 30 years of research. *Journal of Memory and Language, 46,* 441–517.

Yonelinas, A. P., Otten, L. J., Shaw, K. N., & Rugg, M. D. (2005). Separating the brain regions involved in recollection and familiarity in recognition memory. *The Journal of Neuroscience, 25,* 3002–3008.

Zacks, R. T., Hasher, L., & Li, K. Z. H. (2000). Human memory. In F. I. M. Craik & T. A. Salthouse (Eds.), *Handbook of aging and cognition* (2nd edition, pp. 293–357). Mahwah, NJ: Erlbaum.

Zelinski, E. M., & Burnight, K. P. (1997). Sixteen year longitudinal and time lag changes in memory and cognition in older adults. *Psychology and Aging, 12,* 503–513.

Eleven

Applied Learning and Aging: A Closer Look at Reading

Bonnie J. F. Meyer and Carlee K. Pollard

I. Introduction

Learning and knowledge acquisition across the life span depend in part on engagement of reading in various domains (e.g., Ackerman & Rolfhus, 1999; Johnson, 2003; Stanovich, West, & Harrison, 1995). New learning for adults often comes from reading prose from newspapers, magazines, technical materials, documents, or books via traditional text or e-learning online. Reading comprehension is an important skill for older adults to employ in maintaining functional independence and quality of life. Understanding and remembering written information are useful in managing health and finances, enjoying leisure and recreational activities, and continued learning in a variety of areas. For many older adults, reading, itself, is a favorite leisure activity (e.g., Meyer, Talbot, Poon, & Johnson, 2001; Smith, 2000). Proficient older readers have years of experience reading large quantities of text, resulting in a store of rich background knowledge, including knowledge

about different types of texts and genres (Meyer & Rice, 1989).

Mixed findings for age effects in discourse comprehension and memory have been reported. Some studies have reported age deficits (e.g., Cohen, 1979; Dixon, Hultsch, Simon, & von Eye, 1984; Hartley, Stojack, Mushaney, Annon, & Lee, 1994; Spilich, 1983; Stine, 1990; Zelinski & Burnight, 1997), whereas others have not (e.g., Mandel & Johnson, 1984; Meyer & Poon, 2001; Meyer & Rice, 1981; Stine-Morrow, Milinder, Pullara, & Herman, 2001; Stine-Morrow, Gagne, Morrow, & DeWall, 2004; Tun, 1989). Some of the disparity in findings is due to the complexity of the interaction among text, task, reader, and strategy variables involved in reading (Meyer & Rice, 1983, 1989). Individual differences in basic cognitive processes as well as more crystallized abilities, such as word knowledge and reading skills, contribute to both between-group and within-group variability in learning from text (e.g., Johnson et al., 1997; Hartley, et al., 1994; Hultsch, Hertzog, & Dixon, 1990; Rice & Meyer, 1986).

II. Summary of Past Reviews of Aging and Learning and Memory from Text

Numerous reviews have attempted to bring order to this growing research domain with divergent findings (e.g., Hartley, 1989; Hultsch & Dixon, 1984; Meyer, 1987; Meyer & Rice, 1983; 1989; Meyer & Talbot, 1998; Verhaeghen, Marcoen, & Goossens, 1993; Wingfield & Stine-Morrow, 2000; Zelinski & Gilewski, 1988). Johnson (2003) produced a capstone, meta-analytic review of 194 studies published from 1941 to mid-1997. He computed 1385 effect sizes from studies comparing healthy young and older adults with varied assessments of learning and memory from text including both verbatim and substantive free recall, cued recall, recognition, and true–false sentence verification and latency. Significant age deficits resulted for all comparisons and subclassifications. The magnitude of age differences was found to vary as a function of the types of learners, kinds of texts, learning instructions, procedures, and type of scoring of text remembered.

Age differences were magnified when young adults were compared to old–old adults (70 and older) rather than young–old adults. Young adults' performance surpassed that of middle-aged adults, who in turn outperformed older adults. When older adults had an advantage in vocabulary or intelligence over younger adults, age differences were smaller. Contrary to past meta-analytic comparisons of young and older adult learners (Zelinski & Gilewski, 1988; Verhaeghen et al., 1993), Johnson (2003) reported the greatest age differences comprehending and remembering newspaper articles followed by narratives with expository text showing the smallest age differences. The magnitude of age differences for descriptive text was similar to narratives,

and age differences for any of these text genres were smaller than age differences in learning and remembering lists of unrelated sentences. In contrast to prior meta-analytic reviews examining length of passage, age effects were minimized with longer text selections versus short ones. Longer texts may call for reading skills used more frequently in the lives of older adults that focus on gist recall and integration of ideas with interpretive contexts based on familiar text schemata and other prior knowledge schemata (Meyer, Young, & Bartlett, 1989; Wingfield & Stine-Morrow, 2000). Johnson also reported that age effects were reduced when participants were told in advance that gist scoring of performance would be used rather than verbatim scoring. Similarly, age deficits were smaller when gist scoring was actually used to score responses rather than verbatim scoring. Age deficits were also reduced when mode of presentation was written or written and aural rather than aural via a taped presentation of a text. Age deficits were reduced under self-paced versus experimenter-paced presentations of text as well as self-paced performance on the criterion task versus experimenter-imposed time limits. Greater age effects were found for tasks requiring manual reaction-time responses versus tasks requiring yes or no judgments or selecting a response, but no differences in the magnitude of age deficits were found for written versus oral response modes. Increasing the number of passages to be learned in a testing session magnified age effects, as did experimenter-imposed strategies. Age deficits were minimized when scoring focused on meaning of idea units or pausal units allowing scoring for equivalent paraphrases of similar meaning rather than more verbatim word recall of single, undivided propositions. In summary, Johnson's (2003) comprehensive meta-analysis of studies conducted through mid-1997 clearly showed age deficits in prose learning and memory, but also showed learner, task, text, and strategy variables that can lessen differences in performance between young and older adults.

A limitation of this important meta-analysis was the focus on cross-sectional studies. Schaie (2004, 2005) demonstrated different trajectories of decline for vocabulary comprehension when studies examined age differences with cross-sectional design versus longitudinal designs. Conclusions drawn from cross-sectional designs would paint a steady, grim decline in word understanding after about 40 years of age, whereas conclusions based on longitudinal data following the same individuals over time would yield a picture of growth until late middle age with only modest declines through the early eighties. Longitudinal studies (MacDonald, Hultsch, & Dixon, 2003) have shown no declines in recall of narratives by younger groups of older adults, but declines for groups of old–old adults. Specifically, in a 6-year longitudinal study, recall of information after reading 300-word stories about lives of older people for a maximum of 4 min. decreased for old–old adults, but not for young–old adults. Longitudinal studies of memory from text over a 3-year delay showed no decline for older adults (Hultsch, Hertzog, Dixon, & Small, 1998; Hultsch, Hertzog, Small, McDonald-Miszczak, & Dixon, 1992; Zelinski, Gilewski, & Schaie, 1993), but Zelinski and Burnight (1997) reported declines in text recall over a 16-year period. Zelinski and Stewart (1998) reported that declines in text recall over the 16-year interval could be best predicted by declines in reasoning ability (28% of the variance) with age adding another 7% of variance explained.

Johnson (2003) reviewed only studies with samples of both young and older adults so data from longitudinal studies composed of only older adults were not included. A limitation of cross-sectional designs is the inability to distinguish between cohort effects and aging effects. However, Johnson's meta-analysis does shed some insight relevant to potential cohort effects. Johnson compared studies published during different time spans. Approximately equivalent numbers of effect sizes were calculated from research published within three time periods of unequal duration: 1941 to 1985 ($n = 242$ from 64 studies), 1986 to 1990 ($n = 209$ from 55 studies), and 1991 to 1997 ($n = 244$ from 65 studies). The time intervals of the spans are disparate, limiting the usefulness of the analysis, but demonstrate the growth of research concerned with aging and learning and remembering text. Overall, Johnson found that the difference between younger and older learners has changed relatively little over the time spans analyzed. On average, an older learner performed at the 22nd percentile of the distribution of performances from the younger group. However, considerable heterogeneity in effect sizes for old compared to young groups was reported in this meta-analysis, as well as an earlier meta-analysis, presented by Verhaeghen et al. (1993).

III. Aging: Cognitive and Motivational Changes and How They May Impact Reading

Age-related changes differ across individuals, and some cognitive functions are primarily spared, whereas others show different trajectories of decline (e.g., Hultsch et al., 1998; Schaie, 1996). Some changes attributed to aging result from disease (e.g., Verhaghan, Borchelt, & Smith, 2003) whereas others reflect cohort differences (Schaie, 1996). For example, contemporary older adults attain more years of formal schooling (Bass, 1995) and score higher on vocabulary tests (Uttl & Van Alstine, 2003) than previous cohorts of older adults. Additionally, today's older adults have less experience with computers than older adults are expected to have in the future (Crow, 2002; Willis, 2004).

A. Sensory Changes

Aging commonly brings losses of peripheral sensory functions critical to reading or listening — vision and hearing (see Fozard & Gordon-Salant, 2001; Stuen & Faye, 2003; Schaie, 2004). For example, the aging cornea decreases in curvature and pupil size gets smaller and the lens becomes thicker, stiffer, more yellow, and more opaque as well as pulled out of shape by the ciliary muscle (Arking, 1998). As a result, older adults need more light to enter the eye, but more light yields greater haze or blurring due to a more opaque lens. The yellowing of the lens leads to more difficulty in blue/violet/green discriminations after age 70. Some studies (Baltes & Lindenberger, 1997; Baltes & Mayer, 1999) indicate that after statistically controlling for sensory differences, aging effects on cognitive performance are decreased dramatically.

Compensation for some of the sensory loss resulting from aging can be provided by technology in such forms as eyeglasses, zoom menus, computerized eyeglasses, laser surgery, hearing aids, books on tape, and text telephones (see Czaja & Moen, 2004). Future adaptations of technology and telecommuting hold challenges and potential solutions for remedying some of the sensory and everyday needs of older adults (Patrickson, 2002; Pew & Van Hemel, 2004; Sharit et al., 2004).

Additionally, older adults show a greater benefit from contextual support than younger adults (see meta-analysis of Laver & Burke, 1993). Speranza, Daneman, and Scheider (2000) had young and older adults read sentences where the last word in the sentence was either very predictable from the context of the sentence or not. They also varied visual noise, making the sentences more difficult to read. Sensory age deficits were noted in that young and older adults could identify the same number of target final words only when visual noise was diminished. The difference in the number of correct identifications between the predictable context and the low-context conditions was higher for older adults than younger ones, suggesting that older learners used context more in an attempt to compensate for their sensory decline.

B. Changes in Processing of Information

With aging, time increases on tasks (e.g., Birren, 1974; Salthouse, 1996) and the number of items immediately accessible in memory (working memory) decreases (e.g., Just & Carpenter, 1992). Due to changes in processing speed, one would expect reading speed to be slower with aging, as was confirmed by Johnson's meta-analysis, but this is not always the case (see Meyer & Talbot, 1998; Hartley et al., 1994) and again appears to be dependent on reader, task, strategy, and text variables. Speed of processing, working memory, attention-switching abilities (McDowd & Shaw, 2000), and other fluid intelligence measures peak in early midlife and begin to decline around 60. In contrast, crystallized intelligence, including verbal abilities closely related to reading, usually peaks in the fifties, starts to decline in the seventies, and often shows only marginal declines in the eighties (Backman et al., 2000; Schaie, 1996). These crystallized abilities focus on skills and knowledge learned in a culture.

Two main components in models of reading are working memory and prior knowledge; the former shows substantial decline with aging and the latter often shows growth across the life span and stability into late life. For prior knowledge to facilitate reading, it needs to be related to the reading material. In addition, the related knowledge must be retrieved and integrated with incoming information. Age deficits have been found in retrieval of information from long-term memory, particularly when cues or environment supports are reduced. The magnitude of age differences has been shown to increase with effortful processing/explicit memory rather than automatic processing/implicit memory (Graf & Masson, 1993). A reader routinely and unconsciously activates background knowledge during the reading process (e.g., Kintsch, 1988). Longer passages may reduce aging effects due to additional elaborations of a text topic that increase the explicit and implicit cueing of relevant prior knowledge. Models of reading comprehension often posit automatic processes for basic decoding skills and activation of background knowledge that is associated with what they read (e.g., McKoon & Ratcliff, 1992) or necessary for understanding (e.g., van den Broek, Rohleder, & Narvaez, 1996).

The primary theories posited to explain the preponderance of extant research showing declines in processing ability over the life span focus on age differences in working memory capacity (e.g., Kwong, Sheree, & Ryan, 1995; Park & Hedden, 2001), inhibition (e.g., Hasher & Zacks, 1988), and speed (e.g., Birren & Fisher, 1995; Salthouse, 1991, 1996). The general slowing hypothesis (Cerella, 1990; MacKay & Burke, 1990; Myerson et al., 1990; Salthouse, 1982) predicts that as the complexity of tasks increases, the decline with aging increases. Evidence involving declines in working memory resources in later life support this prediction (Salthouse, 1982). Age differences are often found with increases with task complexity (e.g., McDowd & Craik, 1988), but some recent investigations using more everyday problem solving or job-related tasks rather than laboratory tasks have failed to find predicted age by task complexity interactions (Finucane, Mertz, Slovic, & Schmidt, 2005; Taylor, O'hara, Mumenthaler, Rosen, & Yesavage, 2005).

Reading is also a complex, everyday activity. The great number of subsystems working together to form a cohesive understanding of extended discourse might be expected to create a substantial decrease in the processing speed and proficiency of older readers. The problem, however, comes when research attempts to isolate the relationship between reading and the declines resulting from aging. One of the reasons is that reading offers so many variables, such as topic interest, text length, text structure, readability, presentation method, and purpose. On top of text and task characteristics there are differences in the reading strategies used by readers that may cause some readers to process different types of information or process information at different rates. In everyday life, adults can use strategies to compensate for processing declines, such as altering their reading speed or rereading (see Harris, Rogers, & Qualls, 1998; Stine-Morrow et al., 2004). Tasks used in the laboratory to study the reading process may alter the manner in which reading occurs. For instance, while in everyday life both young and old adults are able to adjust their reading strategies and rates according to the requirements of the task before them, often in experimental settings participants are asked to read unfamiliar texts in unfamiliar modes and then asked to perform unfamiliar tasks. The question raised by this discrepancy between real life and the laboratory is to what extent are young and old adults able to adjust their reading patterns to fit the requirements of the research tasks? To what extent can those readers who are subject to a decline in processing abilities compensate via slowing or some other strategy? What types of information are then processed and stored in these tasks and to what extent are they available to be integrated into a solution for some decision task? The latter question addresses the issue of proficiency with aging readers. Many studies have shown that there is a discrepancy between the amount of information young and old adults can acquire from text. However, it is the nature of the information remembered that is most important. Often research participants are required to recall all they remember from text they have just read when in everyday reading the most important information is the gist.

C. Improvement Through Instruction

Another aspect of cognitive aging research relevant to reading is that instruction can make a positive difference for older learners (Ball et al., 2002; Schaie & Willis, 1994; Schaie, 1996, 2004; Willis, 1989). Schaie reported that 5 hr. of training in spatial orientation or inductive reasoning resulted in substantial gains in these abilities. Meyer and colleagues (Meyer et al., 1989; Meyer & Poon, 2001) found equivalent gains in recall by young and older adults after 7.5 to 9 hr. of training with a reading comprehension strategy. Rogers (2000) provided a summary of training recommendations for older adults; they include (a) self-paced learning, (b) easy access to assistance, (c) well-organized training materials with emphasis provided for the most important components, (d) practice on components, (e) "hands-on" practice, and (f) settings free from distractions. When experimenters provide reading strategies to participants, care is required to follow such training guidelines to ensure learning, as the outcome is often disappointing (e.g., Johnson, 2003). Because both young and old

improve from instruction, any pretraining age deficits are usually not eliminated through training (e.g., Baltes & Kliegl, 1992).

D. Advantages, Disadvantages, and Adaptations of Older Adults

The older reader can be characterized as having advantages as well as disadvantages in comparison to the younger reader. Often cognitive aging research has focused on the disadvantages of processing declines, but despite these declines, older adults are resilient and able to productively use information gathered from text (Meyer & Talbot, 1998). Sinnott (1989) identified three processing styles related to age. The first was a "youthful" style focusing on learning, intense data gathering, and bottom–up processing. The individual using this style was characterized as possessing few relevant knowledge structures. The second was a "mature" style focusing on data gathering and both bottom–up and top–down processing. This mature solver balanced the use of a rich relevant knowledge structure and more expertise with information seeking. The third was an "old" style involving little attention to data and reliance on top–down processing. Sinnott explained that this style was suited for fast low-energy demand solutions done by an experienced solver with many available structures of knowledge. Talbot (2004) involved men across the adult life span in a hypothetical, Web-based prostate cancer treatment decision that unfolded as they proceeded through various stages of the decision process. He found that younger men and those with greater verbal abilities sought more information on which to base a treatment decision.

Aging people are often successful in using their capacities to make adaptations through selection of areas to let go and other areas to optimize (e.g., Marsiske, Lang, Baltes, & Bates, 1995) as well as environmental supports to buffer effects of declines in processing efficiency. In the area of motivation, aging adults also adapt (Carstensen, 1995). Carstensen described the different trajectories for information seeking and emotional regulation. Information seeking starts at a moderate point in infancy, grows into adolescence, and then levels off and declines into late life, whereas emotional regulation is high in infancy, drops to a low in adolescence, and rises again for older adults. Older adults appear to be saving their emotion for the most important people in their lives (Carstensen, 1995) and their energies for their most valued activities (Lawton et al., 2002). These motivational factors may be related to the types of reading materials selected by older adults and the time they spend reading, as well as the reading goals and standards for understanding they set and follow as participants in research studies. Additionally, these factors may relate to the generally poor performance of older adults reading short texts in the laboratory with little relevance to their interests, particularly when judged by nearly verbatim standards. Meyer and colleagues (1998) reported that older adults displayed greater interest in the topic of trusts (vehicle for wealth distribution) than young adults; 21% of the older adults rated the topic of trusts as of extreme interest, whereas this level of interest was only given by 6% of the young adults. A comparable text in terms of structure, number of words, and difficulty on the topic of schizophrenia was of more interest to younger adults than older adults. Meyer et al. (1998) found a significant interaction between age group and passage topic for the amount of information remembered with older adults remembering significantly and substantially more information from the trust text than young

adults, but young adults tending to remember more information from the schizophrenia text than older adults.

The remainder of this chapter focuses on general models of reading comprehension, their development, and how these cognitive and motivational changes that accompany aging may affect these models. Most of the research studies about aging and reading comprehension discussed in relation to the models focus on studies appearing in the literature after mid-1997, those not included in Johnson's (2003) comprehensive meta-analysis.

IV. Aging and Models of Reading Comprehension

A. Three Strands of Cognitive Research on Reading Comprehension

Historically cognitive research on reading comprehension has seen three major thrusts, but all continue as active areas of research today (see van den Broek et al., 1999). In the 1970s the focus of research was on memory representations and what readers remembered after reading (e.g., Crothers, 1972; Kintsch & van Dijk, 1978; Mandler & Johnson, 1977, Meyer, 1975; Meyer & McConkie, 1973). For example, the logical structure of a text was specified with some ideas high in a hierarchy of importance with many ideas connected to them, whereas other ideas were peripheral and low in the structure with few connections to other ideas (Meyer & McConkie, 1973). Effects of this logical structure were seen in (a) the kinds of ideas that were remembered (more high-level information than low-level information — the levels effect), (b) intraindividual stability in ideas recalled, and (c) clustering of recall, suggesting that the structure was related to constructed cognitive structures (if a particular idea was recalled, the idea above it in logical structure recalled 70% of the time, rather than average 23% recall of all ideas). The logical structure accounted for much of the variance that might ordinarily be attributed to other variables: serial position effects and rated importance. Aging research examined the levels effects in the 1980s (e.g., Meyer & Rice, 1981; Dixon et al., 1984). Overall, young and older adults show similar levels effects remembering more main ideas than details, but reader, text, task, and strategy variables can impact types of information remembered (see Meyer & Rice, 1989).

A new focus in reading comprehension research during the 1980s was on-line processes in reading using gaze durations with eye-tracking techniques, reading times for words and parts of sentences, lexical-decision latencies on tested words, recognition latencies, probing techniques, and so on. Models focused on cognitive processes that take place on-line, such as what ideas are activated, which inferences are made, and how processing relates to limited working memory capacity (e.g., Kintsch, 1988; McKoon & Ratcliff, 1992; Graesser, Singer, & Trabasso, 1994). Because working memory capacity is limited, a reader can only pay attention at one time to a subset of words, concepts, or relationships. This subset is thought to be the text currently being processed, some ideas from the preceding cycle of processing, and possibly reactivation of important ideas from earlier cycles of processing, as well as activated background knowledge. Limitations in older adults working memory capacities impact such processing as shown in the work of Spilich (1983). However, many of these processes are often automatic, such as activation of background knowledge, reducing potential aging difficulties.

The construction portion of Kintsch's (1988, 2004) construction–integration (CI) model is an example of bottom–up processing models used to understand on-line processes in reading. Instead of trying to find only one correct meaning of a sentence, the CI model constructs several possible meanings in parallel and later sorts out the best meaning of the sentence. The sorting is accomplished by an integration process that inhibits constructions that do not fit well with the emerging context of the text and strengthens the constructions that do. Activation is spread around an incoherent propositional network with contradictory assumptions that is then cleaned up by the integration process that results from the stabilizing of spreading activation, eventually settling on those nodes in the structure that hang together. The outliers and isolated nodes become deactivated in this bottom–up integration process. The model was based in part on data from Till, Mross, and Kintsch (1988) using the lexical decision technique. Participants read sentences such as "A beautiful sight in downtown Denver is the mint." Immediately after reading the sentence response times were short for both "money" and "tea," exemplifying the construction portion of the CI model. This is a passive, implicit low priming of long-term memory called resonance by some theorists (e.g., Myers & O'Brien, 1998). Most research indicates that older adults do not have problems with this type of implicit memory (e.g., Graf & Masson, 1993). Delaying the lexical decision task by 350 ms yielded short times for "money," but not "mint;" the differential priming after the delay gives evidence for the integration portion of the model. However, little research has focused on how the more top–down, inference-generation process of integration actually works (Long & Lea, 2005).

Due to aging limitations related to ineffective inhibitory mechanisms in working memory (e.g., Hasher & Zacks, 1988; Hedden & Park, 2001), one would expect reading problems for older adults within the operating system posited by the CI model. Radvansky and co-workers (2001) used computer simulation of the CI model as a possible explanation for age deficits in processing and memory of text-based information, but not higher level, more top–down representations of text meanings.

The most recent focus of cognitive research on reading comprehension is an integration between the former two approaches of memory representation and comprehension processes and how the two relate. An example of this approach is the computational model called the landscape model of reading (e.g., van den Broek et al., 1999; van den Broek, Rapp, & Kendeou, 2005). The model incorporates both bottom–up activation (automatic spread of activation for associated concepts in the reader's long-term knowledge base) and top–down processes aimed at seeking coherence (strategic, goal-directed searches for meaning, e.g., Graesser et al., 1994).

A major source of individual differences in reading comprehension is background or prior knowledge, often an asset of the older reader. In the associative simulation models, such as the landscape model, background knowledge strongly influences activation of the vectors driving the activation model. Background knowledge from a reader with much knowledge that is richly interconnected will be automatically activated during reading through associative processes. A central component of the landscape model is that attending to the referent/concept behind a word read in the text results in a process called cohort activation. When a concept is activated, the concepts related to it in prior knowledge (i.e., the concept's cohorts) are, to some degree, also activated through implicit memory processes, another strength of older adults, so the more interconnected the knowledge of the reader, the more

resulting cohort activation. This in turn affects the activation vectors that affect the final representation in long-term memory. Van den Broek et al. (2005) conducted three simulations of reading expository text to see if both cohort activation and a top–down focus on major causal and referential connections among ideas, called coherence, were required to predict what readers recall. With both the cohort activation and coherence retrieval processes, accumulated node strength in the model correlated strongly with ideas recalled ($r = .70$); when cohort activation was removed, predictive power decreased ($r = .60$), but when coherence-based processes were removed, the simulation's predictions fell further ($r = .50$). This finding indicates the importance of coherence-based processing and also the usefulness of both hypothesized processes in the reading comprehension; that is, both the strategic and goal-direction search for meaning and overall logical structure and the more autonomous and passive processes. Zelinski and Burnight's (1997) findings related to the importance of reasoning ability in predicting reading comprehension for older adults relates to these coherence-based processes.

Readers' standards of coherence (van den Broek et al., 1999) affect processing in the landscape model and are influenced by learner, task, text, and strategy variables. This model is well suited for studying individual differences, such as aging. Although aging research has not worked specifically with this theory, research (e.g., Miller & Stine-Morrow, 1998; Radvansky, Copeland, & Zwaan, 2003; Radvansky et al., 2001; Stine-Morrow, Loveless, & Soederberg, 1996) has examined both bottom–up on-line processing and its relationship to hypothesized mental representations, often called the situational model (Johnson-Laird, 1983; van Dijk & Kintsch, 1983; Radvanky & Zacks, 1991).

B. Establishing Coherence

Most contemporary models of good comprehension posit readers to (a) parse sentences at syntactic boundaries and buffer incoming semantic information, represented as propositions in working memory; (b) develop a network of associated propositions drawn both from explicit text information and from existing prior knowledge network of the reader; and (c) integrate these propositions into a coherent, reasonable meaning structure that fits the context (e.g., Kintsch & van Dijk, 1978; Kintsch, 1988, 1998; VanderVeen, 2004). These processes are driven by a search for making meaning that satisfy a reader's goals, establish coherence, and explain why information, such as actions, events, and states, are relayed by the author in the text (e.g., Bartlett, 1932; Stein & Trabasso, 1985; Graesser et al., 1994; van den Broek et al., 1999).

Reading results in cognitive representations showing connectedness are characterized by coherence (Sanders & Gernsbacher, 2004). Coherence includes the overall logical structure of the text (Meyer, 1975), as well as cohesion, how well the parts between clauses and sentences of the text stick together (e.g., Halliday & Hasan, 1976). Texts that are coherent are characterized by interrelationships among concepts and easily linked recurrent concepts. In order for a reader to build a coherent mental representation, they must be able to follow the explicit and implicit logical structure of the text and to identify recurring concepts. Robertson et al. (2000) studied tracking of recurring concepts by comparing definite articles (the), indicating prior discussion of the concept, versus indefinite articles (a). The former results in more coherent text and also led to differential brain activity as tracked by Functional Magnetic Resonance Imaging (fMRI) technology.

Knowledge about the structure strategy and text structures can help the reader establish both global and local coherence. According to this strategy, authors utilize hierarchical, logical text structures to organize their writing (Meyer, 1982). The reader can then make use of this structure to build a coherent mental representation.

1. Local Text Coherence

Readers' efforts toward establishing local coherence focus on instantiating and organizing referents of adjacent clauses or short sequences of clauses. Words used by text authors trigger in readers' minds the concepts that are these referents requiring organization. If readers have limited vocabularies, they are handicapped by not knowing what concept or idea the author is referring to in the text. Even comprehension of young adults is reduced if writers use different words for the same concept instead of using the same words repeatedly (e.g., Britton & Gulgoz, 1991). Readers without rich vocabularies to identify paraphrased words are even at a greater disadvantage. Thus, a rich vocabulary that has grown over the life span (Schaie, 1996) is a strong resource for competent reading and a way that highly verbal older adults can compensate for slower processing. Older adults with poor verbal skills and processing limitations are doubly disadvantaged in reading (see Meyer & Rice, 1983, 1989).

One example of readers establishing cohesion at this local textbase level is by inferring a common referent between an antecedent noun and a subsequent pronoun (e.g., Gernsbacher, 1989). Also, at the local level of coherence, verb phrases and verb modifiers help readers establish relationships among instantiated referents. Readers infer case structure roles (Fillmore, 1968) to structure semantic referents, including identifying whether a referent serves as an agent, patient, instrument, etc. Readers also organize at this local level by seeing that ideas in one clause are related to another by various text structures, such as cause and effect or comparison.

2. Global Coherence

The structure strategy is particularly helpful in teaching readers how to establish coherence globally. This involves organizing local chunks of texts into large chunks, e.g., seeing that ideas in two adjacent paragraphs are related to each other by comparison or a problem and responding solution, identifying a shift in topic. The essential property of these relationships is that they establish coherence in the cognitive representation readers create while reading. These relationships have been called various names in the literature: rhetorical predicates or relationships (Grimes, 1975; Mann & Thompson, 1986; Meyer, 1975), top-level structures (e.g., Meyer, 1985; Meyer, Brandt, & Bluth, 1980; Meyer & Poon, 2001), and coherence relations (Sanders & Noordman, 2000).

At the global coherence level, readers infer an author's purposes and goals for writing the article and what rhetorical and pragmatic strategies underlie the way the author has put the article together. Prior knowledge can help these processes; e.g., among both younger and older readers, prior knowledge of the heart was shown to facilitate the processing of topic shifts in passages about the structure and functioning of the heart (Miller et al., 2004). Miller and colleagues (2001, 2003, 2004) found that older adults with prior knowledge spent more time integrating and organizing concepts relative to their low-knowledge counterparts. Although these data suggest that older learners must work at making inferences and applying prior knowledge during reading, they also show that this extra time pays off in terms of increased memory performance.

3. Processing for Local and Global Coherence All at Once

Although local and global processing are distinct processes, readers are thought to process texts at multiple levels in parallel. Information from the different levels informs the processing of the other levels. Added to these processes are meta-cognitive processes for management and reasoning. Meta-cognitive processes help readers figure out efficient reading strategies for the task demands and types of texts. Strengths in some areas can offset weaknesses in another. For example, relevant schemata can balance deficits in speed or capacity of working memory. Support for this notion can be found in research examining age differences in the effects of schematic knowledge on reading. Miller and Stine-Morrow (1998) found that older relative to younger readers were particularly facilitated by schematic knowledge during reading as measured by time allocated to conceptual organization and integration. Similarly, Miller, Cohen, and Wingfield (2004) found that schematic knowledge increased reading efficiency (defined as the time spent per unit of recall) among young, middle-aged, and older readers, but that the increase was most pronounced among older readers with reduced working memory spans. Thus, knowledge appears to reduce demands on working memory, which is particularly beneficial for older readers.

Other data suggest that rich word knowledge often associated with increased age can also mitigate age-related declines in capacity. Stine-Morrow et al. (2001) found that older readers demonstrated conceptual integration at sentence boundaries just like young adults, and older adults were even more responsive to task demands than younger adults.

a. Signals Help Search for Coherence Authors often convey important ideas and relationships in text through the use of signals. Signals are stylistic writing devices that highlight aspects of semantic content or structural organization in text without communicating additional semantic content (Lorch & Lorch, 1995; Meyer, 1975, 1985). Such devices may include headings, preview statements, summary statements, pointer words, or words that explicitly state the relational structure among main propositions of the text (Meyer, 1975, 1985). For example, expository texts can be characterized by their top-level structures: description, sequence, cause and effect, problem and solution, comparison, and listing. Each structure has unique signaling words. For example, the cause/effect structure uses "caused, led to, consequence, thus," and signals like these within the text.

Numerous studies (e.g., Lorch & Lorch, 1995; Mandler & Johnson, 1977; Meyer, 1975; Meyer et al., 1980; Meyer & Poon, 2001) have pointed to the importance of looking at the organization in text and clearly signaling this organization to readers from elementary school through retirement. The factors of text organization and signaling of this organization are important when looking at the interaction between the reader and the text in the reading process. Ideally, the text will be well organized with signaling emphasizing this organization, and the readers will possess strategies to find and use this organization to facilitate their understanding and memory. Signals influence the processes of selecting and organizing information in text by readers (Meyer et al., 1980; Lorch & Lorch, 1995; Loman & Mayer, 1983). Britton and colleagues (1982) found that signaling in text

reduced the load on working memory during the processing of text.

In one study (Meyer & Rice, 1989), young and older adults read with signaling or without signaling versions of text and answered questions focused on the major relationships among the main ideas. The participants in each age group were divided in half on the basis of their scores on a vocabulary test. The signaling words helped both younger and older adults with high verbal ability understand the logical relationships among the main ideas in the text. However, older adults with low verbal skills were not able to take advantage of the signaling words to aid in their selection and organizing of ideas in the text. Further investigations showed that they did not know how to use the structure strategy or the purpose of signaling words, but they could be taught these skills with good success in about 8 hr. of training (Meyer et al., 1989). Additionally, Meyer et al. (2001) trained a group of African–American older adults with low vocabulary and reading comprehension test scores. Prior to instruction, education was the only reader variable predicting use of the structure strategy. After training in use of the structure strategy only scores on the MMSE (Folstein, 1983) predicted strategy usage; participants with high scores (30) on the MMSE and low levels of education made large improvements in strategy usage and remembering what they read, whereas those with lower scores (26) tended to make little improvement. Interestingly, global coherence is affected earlier in the progression of dementia than local coherence and cohesion (Dijkstra, Bourgeois, Petrie, Burgio, & Allen-Burge, 2002).

Meyer et al. (1998) found that signaling had its largest effect on older adult readers who had low interest in a topic. When structural relations in text are explicitly signaled for the readers, it is no longer incumbent upon them to actively seek out or infer such relations on their own, thereby making the motivating influence of topic interest less critical. Because older adults will have to read about topics of little interest (i.e., medical forms), it is important that such readers with little interest in critical topics be provided with clearly organized and clearly signaled reading materials.

McNamara and colleagues (1996; Kintsch, 1998) have reported findings that signaling actually hurts the performance of young adult readers with high prior knowledge. They thus have argued for text with reduced signaling and coherence for high knowledge readers to increase their engagement and processing during reading (see Kintsch, 1998). Meyer et al. (1998) data were reexamined to look at signaling and prior knowledge scores. The group of older adults with high prior knowledge who read text with signaling performed significantly higher on main idea questions than the group of older adults with high prior knowledge who read text without signaling. Thus, the findings that McNamara and colleagues reported for young adults do not appear to hold for older adults. With simpler learning materials, Taconnat and Isingrini (2004) found the generation effect (generated words better memorized than read words) less effective for older adults than younger adults when self-initiated processing was required. Because everyday reading often involves multiple tasks, such as reading an article for the purpose of comparing its findings to another article in an effort to make a wise decision, it seems unreasonable to produce text purposely with low coherence and little signaling. The often complex contexts of reading in everyday life make reducing cognitive demands with coherent, clearly signaled text desirable, particularly for older adults. In addition, McNamara (2004) reported that by looking at another reader variable, reading comprehension skills, in addition to prior knowledge, the

picture changes. The presence of signaling did not hinder the reading performance of skilled readers with high knowledge about a topic, but only diminished performance of high knowledge readers who had poor reading comprehension skills. Basically, these findings corroborate those of Meyer and Rice (1989) that signaling devices only help readers who know how to take advantage of them.

Reasoning is needed to make inferences about text and to understand it adequately (Zelinski & Stewart, 1998). For example, if not explicitly signaled, a reader needs to figure out the cause of an event or problem. Meyer and Rice (1989) found that highly verbal older adults were capable of inferring such implicit relationships in complex expository text and could perform as well as highly verbal young adults under certain conditions. When signaling was missing and older readers needed to infer relationships at the global coherence level, they were successful when distracting names and dates were removed and replaced with more general terms (e.g., 1879 replaced with late in the 19th century). When the specific details were present, they picked up the details, but missed the implicit global coherence relationships. However, comparable highly verbal young adults could generate these interrelationships and still pick out the specific details. Meyer and Rice (1989) recommended dropping unimportant details and signaling important interrelationships when writing important information for older adults.

b. Structure Strategy Training Helps Search for Coherence The structure strategy (e.g., Bartlett, 1978; Carrell, 1985; Cook & Mayer, 1988; Englert & Hiebert, 1984; Meyer et al., 1989; Meyer & Poon, 2001) teaches readers to identify the structure of expository text, such as cause and effect or comparison, and to use that structure to find global coherence markers in text and to construct a globally coherent memory representation (e.g., Meyer, 1975). The structure strategy is important in improving reading comprehension skills because it enhances the ability to "[use and analyze] text structure to abstract main ideas" (Pressley & McCormick, 1995, p. 480), a functionally important everyday skill for older adults.

Meyer and Poon (2001) found that a group of young and older adults trained for six 1.5-hr. sessions in the structure strategy outperformed a group trained with a motivational strategy receiving equivalent practice in reading the same texts and a no contact control group. Young adults in this study performed substantially better than older adults on tests of reaction time, working memory, and a timed reading comprehension test; older adults performed similarly on an untimed version of the test, but substantially better on a vocabulary test. Both age groups in their everyday lives read approximately the same number of hours per day, but varied in the types of materials read, with older adults reading more for their own interests and pleasure than younger adults. The structure strategy instruction increased trained participants' total recall, recall of the most important information, correspondence between recall and the text's logical structure, and consistent use of the structure strategy across five articles. Information in the five expository texts came from everyday materials found in magazine articles and informative brochures. For both young and older adults, structure strategy instruction plus signaling had an additive effect on consistently using the strategy for all passages. In contrast to Meyer et al. (1998), who reported an interaction between signaling and age group 6 months after training with the strategy, signaling had equivalent effects on young and older adults immediately after training. Meyer and Poon (2001) found no age differences in reading performances or training gains. Also, Meyer and Poon (2001) found that training in the structure strategy generalized to remembering information from an informational video and multiple sources of medical information in a simulated health decision-making task. With this highly educated sample of older adults, there were no age differences in total recall except on the medical decision-making task. The medical decision-making task involved multiple demands and may have more severely taxed older adults' resources. Alternatively, the older adults may have understood the task demands differently and focused more on the decision and affect surrounding it rather than focusing on recall of information.

In more recent research, older adults, who learned the structure strategy, trained fifth-grade students to use the same strategy via the Internet (Meyer et al., 2002). Both tutors and students showed enhanced performance on recall tasks as well as self-efficacy following the program. For example, one tutor when 66 years old volunteered for instruction with the structure strategy. Through the training she more than doubled her ability to remember information from her reading and after training demonstrated mastery of the strategy. Over 6 subsequent years she helped teach the strategy to other older adults and then children via the Internet. Over this time period she maintained her mastery of the strategy and high level of text recall.

B. Levels of Representation

Currently there is wide agreement that text comprehension leads to multiple levels of representation (Halldorson & Singer, 2002). There is much concordance that there are at least three levels of representation: (a) the actual text—its surface form; (b) the idea network or hierarchy—the "textbase," and (c) the situation to which the text is referring—the situation model. Thus, studies of aging and prose learning have compared old and young on textbase versus situation model processing and performances (e.g., Radvansky et al., 2001).

1. Idea Network/Hierarchy—The Textbase

In Kintsch's work related to establishing the textbase (Kintsch, 1974; Kintsch & van Dijk, 1978), working memory played a central role with information together in a working memory cycle linked in a growing textbase; repetition of ideas in a text was a critical factor for linking ideas in working memory. According to Kintsch and van Dijk's (1978) model, propositions from text are organized by the reader in cycles that move information out of working memory and into long-term memory. Some propositions are chosen to stay in working memory as important aspects to interpret and organize the information to be processed in the next cycle. The exact size and characteristics of individual cycles and the propositions held over or stored vary with the individual reader and the text being read. In determining the probability of certain propositions being recalled, Kintsch and van Dijk (1978) considered the maximum number of idea units that can be stored in the working memory buffer for carryover to the next cycle. By varying this number, most commonly ranging from one to four, the propositions differentially vie for retention. A reader who can hold four propositions is more likely to find the necessary proposition overlap for comprehension than a reader who can only carry over one such proposition. By including more propositions, there is an additional increase in the

likelihood of any one proposition participating in the threshold number of cycles necessary for more permanent storage, and subsequent recall. In testing the relationship between Kintsch's model, working memory size, and aging, Spilich (1983) found that the differences between young and old adults indicate that the young are operating with a larger working memory space in which to hold and manipulate incoming text than older adults.

Additionally, Kintsch and van Dijk, (1978, p. 371) stated that "in effect, lowering the speed of scanning and matching operations would have the same effect as decreasing the capacity of the buffer." Thus, very slow reading rates were thought to lower comprehension through limiting working memory capacity. Similarly, Smith (1994) pointed out that when reading too slowly (below 200 wpm, p. 80), the reader is probably trying to read word by word, therefore seeing isolated words without any context. He explained that this would result in making the text meaningless and consequently put an additional burden on memory, thus impairing comprehension. Because older adults have greater limitations in working memory than younger adults, the devastation of a slow rate of reading as posited by these investigators should be greater for older adults than for younger adults. Some support for this comes from studies by Hartley et al. (1994) and Stine and Hindman (1994) that found gain in recall, resulting from more time available for reading (slower reading times), was less for the older age groups than for the younger groups.

Meyer, Talbot, and Florencio (1999) investigated these questions of rate, comprehension, and working memory with computer presentation of text at 90 and 130 wpm to young and older adults. Older adults showed diminished working memory capacities in comparison to young adults, but even the older adults with less resources functioned better at the slow presentation rate. No evidence was found for the theory that limitations in working memory pose a lower limit to reading rate for effective prose recall. In fact, in a study by Legge, Ross, Maxwell, & Leubker, 1989, young adults were found to show increased comprehension as presentation rates decreased all the way down to 10 wpm. Fortunately, the information bottleneck of working memory does not doom slow readers (e.g., some low-vision readers) or readers with working memory deficits (e.g., some older readers) to poor understanding and memory for what they read.

Meyer and Talbot (1998) reported findings from young and older adults reading texts of varying lengths, in varying presentation units (one sentence at a time, one page at a time, and the whole text), and in various modes (print and computer). Average group reading rates under these various conditions ranged from 76 to 198 wpm. Reading times fluctuated dramatically depending on the text and task factors. There appears to be no simple relationship between comprehension and natural reading speed (also see Carlson, 1949 as cited in Legge et al., 1989; Hartley et al., 1994). There were no significant age differences in self-paced reading times from print, but there were age differences in self-paced reading from computers. Meyer and Poon (1997) reported less familiarity with computers and less efficient reading comprehension when reading from computers than print for older adults than younger adults. In fact, there was a significant interaction between age group and mode of presentation with older adults recalling more information per time spent reading from a printed page than younger adults, and younger adults reading more efficiently from computers than older adults. These findings no doubt reflect cohort effects in familiarity

with computers. Readers appear to engage in an array of reading strategies, such as integration, elaboration, and rereading, to different degrees of efficiency. As a result, reading times will vary greatly according to characteristics of the reader as well as characteristics of the reading material and the reading task.

Due to the contrast between the predictions of the Kintsch and van Dijk (1978) model related to the short-term memory buffer and actual performances of readers, Ericsson and Kintsch (1995) added the theory of long-term working memory (LT-WM). The original model involved resource-consuming reinstatement searches from long-term memory, but the theory of LT-WM does away with this resource drain, as the cost is only 400 ms for a single retrieval from LT-WM that brings up an entire mental structure from long-term memory (Kintsch, 1998). The new model makes efficient and effective reading comprehension by older adults much more plausible than the original model.

It is important to clarify differences between the textbase in Kintsch's model (1998) used for scoring recall in aging studies and the content structure following Meyer's procedures (1975, 1985) used by others. The differences may relate to some of the disparate findings, such as Johnson's (2003) finding for lessened age deficits for expository text, often analyzed with Meyer's system in the aging literature. Although at the propositional level both systems are identical because they are based on case grammar, how the propositions are related together in a coherent structure is very different. Kintsch's textbase is linked by argument repetition. Once a schema (like a restaurant schema) is used to interpret the linked propositions, it becomes a situation model in his approach. Similarly, if a causal link is inferred between two propositions, it is a situation model (Kintsch, 1998, pp. 106).

In contrast, the Meyer approach, based on earlier empirical work (Meyer & McConkie, 1973) and Grimes' (1975) work in linguistics, links propositions by subordination or coordination rules based on the major, logical, or rhetorical relationships explicit or inferred in the text. Thus, the resulting structure contains ideas to score that would have commonalities to Kintsch's textbase, but also his situational model, as causal, time, comparative, and other relationships are specified. Older adults often perform better or as well as young adults on the situation model. Thus, the equivalent recall by highly verbal young and older adults on expository texts reported in the extant literature (Johnson, 2003) may result from use of the different scoring structures as well as gist scoring criteria as pointed out in Johnson's review.

Before leaving the textbase and examining situation models more fully, a recent development related to the textbase needs mentioning. Similar to propositional analyses of text that lay out the concepts related to a particular text, latent semantic analysis (LSA) uses computer technology to provide a fully automatic method to look at semantic coherence (e.g., Foltz, Kintsch, & Landauer, 1998), looking at repetition of words, but also synonyms, antonyms, and other words that tend to be used in similar contexts. LSA is a model of how human knowledge is represented as well as an extremely useful tool that has been applied to produce automated strategy trainers (e.g., iSTART: McNamara, Levinstein, & Boonthum, 2004; ITTS: Wijekumar & Meyer, in press). Such training could be of use in teaching comprehension strategies to older readers. Although LSA provides a good account of associative basis of human verbal knowledge, it does not account for analytic, logical thought, or global aspects of coherence.

2. Situation Model

The situation model is an elaborated representation in which the ideas from a text are elaborated, embellished, and integrated with information from the reader's prior knowledge. Most research dealing with situation models has focused on narrative texts (e.g., Graesser et al., 1994; Zwaan, 1999; Zwaan, Langston, & Graesser, 1995). Organizing referents by case structure (Fillmore, 1968, e.g., who is the agent in an action?) helps readers build a referential situation model. This is a mental representation of people, setting, actions, and events such as a little play set up in each reader's mind and based on explicit text statements or inferences based on world knowledge. The situation model serves as a mental situation of what is going on in the world of the text characters and events. The situation is somewhat different for expository or persuasive text in that often the ideas are more abstract and characters are not moving around in spatial orientation. For expository text (see Stine-Morrow et al., 2004) the situation model has been examined in terms of following the logic of arguments (Britton, 1994; Meyer & Poon, 2001), figuring out important elements from detail (Millis, Simon, & tenBroek, 1998), or developing a working model of how a system works (Bayman & Mayer, 1984).

Knowledge structures applied to produce a situation model include schemata (e.g., Rumelhart & Ortony, 1977), well-learned and established sequences of events of networks of propositions abstracted from familiar experiences. Good readers who frequently read stories have developed story schemata just as frequent readers of journal articles know the top-level structure of a journal article with its problem and related research, research questions or hypotheses, methods, results, and discussion. Older adult readers, who developed good reading skills in their early years and have practiced them reading a variety of genres, have another strong resource by having repertoires of relevant knowledge structures for building good situation models of text. Soederberg and Stine (1995) showed that older adults are qualitatively similar to younger readers in the representation of emotion in text during on-line reading. In addition, older adults reading narrative texts with familiar story structures exhibited no differences in recall from that of young adults in an early study (Mandel & Johnson, 1984) and a more recent study (Stine-Morrow, Miller, & Leno, 2001).

Radvansky and colleagues (2001) reported that younger adults showed superior memory for the surface form and textbase knowledge, whereas older adults showed superior or equivalent for information related to a situation model. However, Stine-Morrow et al. (2001) found no age deficits in textbase performance for highly verbal older adults with short expository texts when reading for recall or comprehension.

Radvansky and colleagues' studies (Radvansky et al. 2001; Radvansky & Copeland, 2003, 2004) are particularly important in that they help explain the paradox between older adults poor performances on laboratory measures of speed and working memory and productive and competent performance in the workplace or other everyday contexts (Czaja, 2001). Radvansky et al. (2001) conducted two studies looking at both reading times (procedures from Zwaan, Magliano, & Graesser, 1995) and recognition performance (procedures from Schmalhofer & Glavanov, 1986). On-line reading times collected focused on traditional readability indices such as word frequency and number of syllables in words, as well as shifts in the text related to situational dimensions, such as time, space, intentionality, entity, and causality. Young and older adults read a clause at a time

from four counterbalanced texts read from a computer screen under self-paced conditions. After reading all the texts, participants read verbatim, paraphrased, correct inference, or incorrect inference statements and clicked "Yes" or "No" about whether they had read the sentences. The Johnson (2003) meta-analysis showed diminished age deficits for such tasks. The texts in the first study were actual historical events and written with dates and time marker, such as "then," typical of expository text following the sequence structure (Meyer, 1985).

To understand this study it is necessary to see an example of the materials. For example, in the text about the Dutch tulip craze in the 17th century, a verbatim sentence from the text was "It is said that a sailor mistook a tulip bulb worth several thousand florins for an onion." (The immediately preceding sentence in the text was "People who had been away from Holland and then returned during the craze sometimes made mistakes.") The paraphrase sentence kept the textbase the same but used paraphrases for most words in the text and some also changed the order of words in the sentence, e.g., "It is said that a sailor accidentally thought that a tulip bulb worth several thousand florins was an onion." The correct inference matching a reasonable situation model for the text and related to this target sentence was "Tulip bulbs often resemble other bulbs, such as onions and garlic," whereas an incorrect inference was "People often stored the bulbs in secure places." A signal detection paradigm was used to obtain a surface form measure (verbatim = hit; paraphrase = false alarm), a textbase measure (paraphrase = hit; inferences = false alarms), and a situation model measure (correct inference = hit; incorrect inference = false alarms).

Findings reported by the authors showed that younger adults performed better at remembering what the text was, both its surface form and textbase, whereas older adults were better at remembering what the text was about, its situation model. Additionally, reading time data showed similar patterns for young and older adults with some indication that younger adults reading times were more affected by the surface level of the text, whereas older adults were more affected by changes related to the situation. An unexpected finding was that older adults' processing indicated greater attention than younger adults' processing to names, dates, and time markers that fit the discourse schema of sequence, the most frequent structure for organizing historical texts; these data are similar to Meyer and Rice's (1989) finding that proficient older readers are more likely to change their processing schema to a sequence structure when a history is related with time-ordered dates and names than younger adults. Another unexpected finding was that self-assessed prior knowledge related to the historical events of the texts facilitated performance on the surface form measure only and not the situation measure as expected.

Radvansky et al. (2001) and Radvansky and Copeland (2003) with narrative texts found similar findings regarding the differential textbase versus situation model processing of young and older adults as Radvansky et al. (2001) with historical expository texts. Findings from all three studies examining on-line reading and recognition memory suggest that older adults devote greater effort in reading comprehension and memory to processing at the situation model level than at the textbase or surface model levels. There were not age deficits at the situation level either at immediate testing or testing a week later; in some cases, older adults scored higher than younger adults at the situation model level. The findings suggest that there is little age-related change in processing at the situation model level in comprehension and memory, although there are declines at the textbase level. Also, some of the findings (older adults greater attention to new entities and dates in histories and functional spatial relations in narratives) are consistent with the view that older adults are better than younger adults at selecting ideas that are more pertinent to understanding a described situation (also see Hess & Auman, 2001).

How can older adults who manifest declines in processing speed, working memory, or inhibition maintain this strength at the situation level? Older adults have been shown to work with more inferences during comprehension than younger adults (Hamm & Hasher, 1992), and older adults' more interesting stories (James et al., 1998) are a likely result. More inferences could be a result of less inhibitory control (Hasher & Zacks, 1988; von Hippel, Silver, & Lynch, 2000). Radvansky and Copeland (2004) demonstrated that measures of working memory related to textbase performance, but not performance at the situation level. Fuzzy-trace theories of memory (Brainerd, Reyna, & Mojardin, 1999) explain that information is stored in at least two levels of representation: an item-specific trace level corresponding to the textbase and a gist-based representation corresponding to the situation model. Older adults' strength is the gist-based representation, but whether this is due to greater expertise in reading, greater functionality and use in everyday life, or deficits in processing at the textbase level is currently unclear. Radvansky et al. (2001) discussed such explanations and explained that they are not mutually exclusive, but may work in concert. Younger adults may work harder to preserve the textbase due to its functionality in formal schooling (i.e., multiple choice testing), but such testing is a rare occurrence in the everyday life of the older adult. Older adults may employ the textbase as scaffolding in the creation of a functional situation model and then let the textbase go. Older adults may have more expertise in reading and are better able to select ideas pertinent to the construction and memory of a situation model. They may have less raw processing resources, but they marshal those they have to focus on the most important information for construction of the situation model as an effective compensatory strategy. Meyer and Rice (1989) saw some evidence for this in that older, high-verbal readers were more sensitive to the emphasis patterns in text for altering their differential selection and memory of ideas than younger, high-verbal readers. Meyer and colleagues (Meyer & Rice, 1989, 1983; Meyer & Talbot, 1998) also pointed to large age deficits in reading comprehension found for older adults with lower verbal skills; adults with little expertise in reading comprehension lack the skills to adequately compensate for reduced processing resources.

Van den Broek et al. (1999) explained that individuals differ in the extent to which they relate their prior knowledge to text while reading. One reader attempted to stay as close to the text as possible, trying to augment their memory representation with little prior knowledge, whereas others attempted to connect every aspect of the text to prior knowledge. They explained that most readers fall between these two extremes in mixing text information with prior knowledge. Clearly aging is an individual difference that places older adults toward the end of the continuum representing a fully expanded situation model. The problem arises in how to adequately evaluate the quality of a situation model, as each person's model varies on the basis of their unique prior knowledge and how much they integrate it with incoming text. Crothers' (1972) early approach to prose analysis focused on an integration of semantic information related to concepts in text, as well those not in the text, and inferred relationships with no regard to the text's organizational structure. Little research used the method, as his structures did not relate to what people remembered after reading. However, his work may have displayed the ideal situation model for a text.

A practical way to assess the quality of a person's situation model resulting from reading a text might be to look at problems solved or decisions made. Thornton and Dumke (2005) examined age differences in the effectiveness of everyday problem solving and decision making. Age differences were found, but were reduced by aspects of rating criteria, interpersonal nature of the content, and with highly educated samples. Meyer, Russo, and Talbot (1995) found that older adults sought less information, recalled less information, and systematically used less information in their decision rationale than younger adults [latter measure used in Thornton and Dumke's (2005) meta-analysis]. However, young and older adults did not differ in the actual choices they made for treatments of breast cancer. The situation models created by the young and older adults were equally as effective for selecting a second lumpectomy versus any of the other viable, five treatment options. Again, older adults showed resilience, capability, and ways to compensate for basic processing declines. Some research questions remain to be answered, but in the meantime, older adults with well-practiced, effective reading comprehension skills will continue to function effectively and those with poorer skills can improve their skills through instruction and practice.

References

Ackerman, P. L., & Rolfhus, E. L. (1999). The locus of adult intelligence: Knowledge, abilities, and nonability traits. *Psychology and Aging, 14*, 314–330.

Arking, R. (1998). *Biology of Aging: Observations and principles*. (2nd edition). Sunderland, MA: Sinauer Associates.

Backman, L., Small, B. J., Wahlin, A., & Larsson, M. (2000). Cognitive functioning in very old age. In T. A. Salthouse & F. I. M. Craik, (Eds.), *The handbook of aging and cognition* (2nd edition, pp. 499–558). Mahwah, NJ: Lawrence Erlbaum Associates.

Ball, K., Berch, D. B., Helmers, K. F., Jobe, J. B., Leveck, M. D., Marsiske, M., Morris, J. N., Rebok, G. W., Smith, D. M., Tennstedt, S. L., Unverzagt, F. W., & Willis, S. L. (2002). Effects of cognitive training intervention with older adults: A randomized controlled trial. *Journal of the American Medical Association, 288*, 2271–2281.

Baltes, P. B., & Kliegl, R. (1992). Further testing of limits of cognitive plasticity: Negative age differences in a mnemonic skill are robust. *Developmental Psychology, 28*, 121–125.

Baltes, P. B., & Lindenberger, U. (1997). Emergence of a powerful connection between sensory and cognitive functions across the adult life span: A new window to the study of cognitive aging? *Psychology and Aging, 12*, 12–21.

Baltes, P. B., & Mayer, K. U. (Eds.) (1999). *The Berlin Aging Study: Aging from 70 to 100*. New York: Cambridge University Press.

Bartlett, F. C. (1932). *Remembering*. Cambridge, UK: Cambridge University Press.

Bartlett, B. J. (1978). *Top-level structure as an organizational strategy for recall of classroom text*. Unpublished doctoral dissertation, Arizona State University.

Bass, S. A. (Ed.) (1995). *Older and active: How Americans over 55 are contributing to society*. New Haven: Yale University Press.

Bayman, P., & Mayer, R. E. (1984). Instructional manipulation of users' mental models for electronic calculators. *International Journal of Man Machine Studies, 20*, 189–199.

Birren, J. E. (1974). Translations in gerontology: From lab to life: Psychophysiology and speed of response. *American Psychologist, 29*, 808–815.

Birren, J. E., & Fisher, L. M. (1995). Aging and speed of behavior: Possible consequences for psychological functioning. *Annual Review of Psychology, 46*, 329–353.

Brainerd, C. J., Reyna, V. F., & Mojardin, A. H. (1999). Conjoint recognition. *Psychological Review, 106*, 160–179.

Britton, B. K. (1994). Understanding expository text: Building mental structures to induce insights. In M. A. Gernsbacher (Ed.), *Handbook of psycholinguistics* (pp. 641–674). San Diego: Academic Press.

Britton, B. K., Glynn, S. M., Meyer, B. J. F., & Penland, M. J. (1982). Effects of text structure on use of cognitive capacity during reading. *Journal of Educational Psychology, 74*, 51–61.

Britton, B. K., & Gulgoz, S. (1991). Using Kintsch's computational model to improve instructional text: Effects of repairing inference calls on recall and cognitive structure. *Journal of Educational Psychology, 83*, 329–345.

Carrell, P. L. (1985). Facilitating ESL reading by teaching text structure. *TESOL Quarterly, 19*, 727–752.

Carstensen, L. L. (1995). Evidence for a life-span theory of socioemotional selectivity. *Current Directions in Psychological Science, 4*, 151–156.

Cerella, J. (1990). Aging and information-processing rate. In K. W. Schaie & J. E. Birren (Eds.), *Handbook of the psychology of aging* (3rd edition, pp. 201–221). San Diego: Academic Press.

Cohen, G. (1979). Language comprehension in old age. *Cognitive Psychology, 11*, 412–429.

Cook, L. K., & Mayer, R. E. (1988). Teaching readers about the structure of scientific text. *Journal of Educational Psychology, 80*, 448–456.

Crothers, E. J. (1972). Memory structure and the recall of discourse. In J. B. Carroll & R. O. Freedle (Eds.), *Language comprehension and the acquisition of knowledge*, (pp. 247–283). Washington, DC: V. H. Winston & Sons, Inc. Publishers.

Crow, A. (2002). Computers and aging: Marking raced, classed and gendered inequalities. *Journal of Technical Writing and Communication, 32*, 23–44.

Czaja, S. J. (2001). Technological change and the older worker. In J. E. Birren (Ed.),

Handbook of the psychology of aging (5th edition, pp. 547–568). San Diego: Academic Press.

Czaja, S. J., & Moen, P. (2004). Technology and employment. In R. Pew & S. Van Hamel (Eds.), *Technology and adaptive aging* (pp. 150–178). Washington, DC: National Research Council.

Dijkstra, K., Bourgeois, M., Pertrie, G., Burgio, L., & Allen-Burge, R. (2002). My recaller is on vacation: Discourse analysis of nursing-home residents with dementia. *Discourse Processes, 33*, 53–76.

Dixon, R. A., Hultsch, D. F., Simon, E. W., & von Eye, A. (1984). Verbal ability and text structure effects on adult age differences in text recall. *Journal of Verbal Learning and Verbal Behavior, 23*, 569–578.

Englert, C. S., & Hiebert, E. H. (1984). Children's developing awareness of text structures in expository materials. *Journal of Educational Psychology, 76*, 65–74.

Ericsson, K. A., & Kintsch, W. (1995). Long-term working memory. *Psychological Review, 102*, 211–245.

Fillmore, C. J. (1968). The case for case. In E. Bach & R. Harms (Eds.), *Universals in linguistic theory* (pp. 1–81). New York: Holt, Rhinehart, and Winston.

Finucane, M. L., Mertz, C. K., Slovic, P., & Schmidt, E. S. (2005). Task complexity and older adults' decision-making competence. *Psychology and Aging, 20*, 71–84.

Folstein, M. (1983). The Mini-Mental State Exam. In T. Crook, S. Farris, & R. Bartus (Eds.), *Assessment in geriatric psychopharmacology* (pp. 47–51), New Canaan, CT: Mark Powley.

Foltz, P. W., Kintsch, W., & Landauer, T. K. (1998). The measurement of textual coherence with latent semantic analysis. *Discourse Processes, 25*, 285–307.

Fozard, J. L., & Gordon, S. S. (2001). Changes in vision and hearing with age. In J. E. Birren (Ed.), *Handbook of the psychology of aging* (5th edition, pp. 241–266). San Diego: Academic Press.

Gernsbacher, M. A. (1989). Mechanisms that improve referential access. *Cognition, 32*, 99–156.

Graesser, A. C., Singer, M., & Trabasso, T. (1994). Constructing inferences during narrative text comprehension. *Psychological Review, 101*, 371–395.

Graf, P., & Masson, M. E. J. (Ed.) (1993). *Implicit memory: New directions in cognition, development, and neuropsychology.* Hillsdale, NJ: Lawrence Erlbaum Associates.

Grimes, J. E. (1975). *The thread of discourse.* The Hague: Mouton.

Halldorson, M., & Singer, M. (2002). Inference processes: Integrating relevant knowledge and text information. *Discourse Processes, 34*, 145–161.

Halliday, M. A. K., & Hasan, R. (1976). *Cohesion in English.* London: Longman.

Hamm, V. P., & Hasher, L. (1992). Age and the availability of inferences. *Psychology and Aging, 7*(1), 56–64.

Harris, J. L., Rogers, W. A., & Qualls, C. D. (1998). Written language comprehension in younger and older adults. *Journal of Speech, Language, and Hearing Research, 41*, 603–617.

Hartley, A. A. (1989). The cognitive ecology of problem solving. In L. W. Poon, D. C. Rubin, & B. A. Wilson (Eds.), *Everyday cognition in adulthood and late life* (pp. 300–329). Cambridge, England: Cambridge University Press.

Hartley, J. T., Stojack, C. C., Mushaney, T. J., Annon, T. A., & Lee, D. W. (1994). Reading speed and prose memory in older and younger adults. *Psychology and Aging, 9*, 216–223.

Hasher, L., & Zacks, R. T. (1988). Working memory, comprehension, and aging: A review and a new view. In G. H. Bower (Ed.), *The psychology of learning and motivation: Advances in research and theory* (Vol. 22, pp. 193–225). San Diego: Academic Press.

Hedden, T., & Park, D. (2001). Aging and interference in verbal working memory. *Psychology and Aging, 16*, 666–681.

Hess, T. M., & Auman, C. (2001). Aging and social expertise: The impact of trait-diagnostic information on impressions of others. *Psychology and Aging, 16*, 497–510.

Hultsch, D. F., & Dixon, R. A. (1984). Memory for text materials in adulthood. In P. B. Baltes & O. G. Brim, Jr. (Eds.), *Life-span development and behavior* (Vol.6, pp. 77–108). New York: Academic Press.

Hultsch, D. F., Hertzog, C., & Dixon, R. A. (1990). Ability correlates of memory performance in adulthood and aging. *Psychology and Aging, 5,* 356–368.

Hultsch, D. F., Hetzog, C., Dixon, R. A., & Small, B. J. (1998). *Memory change in the aged.* New York: Cambridge University Press.

Hultsch, D. F., Hertzog, C., Small, B. J., McDonald-Miszczak, L., & Dixon, R. A. (1992). Short-term longitudinal change in cognitive performance in later life. *Psychology and Aging, 7,* 571–584.

James, L. E., Burke, D. M., Austin, A., & Hulme, E. (1998). Production and perceptions of "verbosity" in younger and older adults. *Psychology and Aging, 13,* 355–367.

Johnson, M. M., Elsner, R. J. F., Poon, L. W., Meyer, B. J. F., Yang, B., Smith, G., Noble, C. A., Talbot, A. P., Hetrick, C. J., Stubblefield, R. A., Puskar, D., Edmondson, J., & Shaffer, S. C. (1997, April). Building a model to test the capacity-speed hypotheses. In C. A. Noble & R. J. F. Elsner (Eds.), *An odyssey in aging* (pp. 123–141). Athens, GA: University of Georgia Gerontology Center.

Johnson, R. E. (2003). Aging and the remembering of text. *Developmental Review, 23,* 261–346.

Johnson-Laird, P. N. (1983). *Mental models: Towards a cognitive science of language, inference, and consciousness.* Cambridge, MA: Harvard University Press.

Just, M. A., & Carpenter, P. A. (1992). A capacity theory of comprehension: Individual differences in working memory. *Psychological Review, 99,* 122–149.

Kintsch, W. (1974). *The representation of meaning in memory.* Oxford, England: Lawrence Erlbaum.

Kintsch, W. (1988). The use of knowledge in discourse processing: A construction-integration model. *Psychological Review, 95,* 165–182.

Kintsch, W. (1998). *Comprehension: A paradigm for cognition.* New York: Cambridge University Press.

Kintsch, W. (2004). The construction-integration model of text comprehension and its implications for instruction. In R. Ruddell & N. Unrau (Eds.) *Theoretical models and processes of reading.* (5th edition). International Reading Association.

Kintsch, W., & van Dijk, T. A. (1978). Toward a model of text comprehension and production. *Psychological Review, 85,* 363–394.

Kwong, S., Sheree, T., & Ryan, E. B. (1995). Cognitive mediation of adult age differences in language performance. *Psychology and Aging, 10,* 458–468.

Laver, G. D., & Burke, D. M. (1993). Why do semantic priming effects increase in old age: A meta-analysis. *Psychology and Aging, 8,* 34–43.

Lawton, M. P., Moss, M. S., Winter, & Hoffman, C. (2002). Motivation in later life: Personal projects and well-being. *Psychology and Aging, 17,* 539–547.

Legge, G. E., Ross, J. A., Maxwell, K. T., & Luebker, A. (1989). Psychophysics of reading. VII. Comprehension in normal and low vision. *Clinical Vision Science, 4,* 51–60.

Loman, N. L., & Mayer, R. F. (1983). Signaling techniques that increase the understandability of expository prose. *Journal of Educational Psychology, 75,* 402–412.

Long, D. L., & Lea, R. B. (2005). Have we been searching for meaning in all the wrong places? Defining the "search after meaning: Principle in comprehension. *Discourse Processes, 39,* 279–298.

Lorch, R. F., Jr., & Lorch, E. P. (1995). Effects of organizational signals on text-processing strategies. *Journal of Educational Psychology, 87,* 537–544.

MacDonald, S. W. S., Hultsch, D. F., & Dixon, R. A. (2003). Performance variability is related to change in cognition: Evidence from the Victoria longitudinal study. *Psychology and Aging, 18,* 510–523.

MacKay, D. G., & Burke, D. M. (1990). Cognition and aging: A theory of new learning and the use of old connections. In T. M. Hess (Ed.), *Aging and cognition: Knowledge organization and utilization* (pp. 213–263). Oxford, England: North-Holland.

Mandel, R. G., & Johnson, N. S. (1984). A developmental analysis of story recall and comprehension in adulthood. *Journal of Verbal Learning and Verbal Behavior, 23,* 643–659.

Mandler, J. M., & Johnson, N. S. (1977). Remembrance of things parsed: Story structure and recall. *Cognitive Psychology, 9,* 111–151.

Mann, W. C., & Thompson, S. A. (1986). *Rhetorical structure theory: Description and construction of text structures.* Marina del Rey, CA: Information Sciences Institute.

Marsiske, M., Lang, F. B., Baltes, P. B., & Baltes, M. M. (1995). Selective optimization with compensation: Life-span perspectives on successful human development. In L. Backman & R. A. Dixon (Eds.), *Compensating for psychological deficits and declines: Managing losses and promoting gains* (pp. 35–79). Hillsdale, NJ: Erlbaum.

McDowd, J. M., & Craik, F. I. (1988). Effects of aging and task difficulty on divided attention performance. *Journal of Experimental Psychology: Human Perception and Performance, 14,* 267–280.

McDowd, J. M., & Shaw, R. J. (2000). Attention and aging: A functional perspective. In T. A. Salthouse & Craik, F. I. M. (Ed.), *The handbook of aging and cognition* (2nd edition, pp. 221–292). Mahwah, NJ: Erlbaum.

McKoon, G., & Ratcliff, R. (1992). Inference during reading. *Psychological Review, 99,* 440–466.

McNamara, D. S. (2004, January*) Coh-Metrix: Automated cohesion and coherences scores to predict test readability and facilitate comprehension.* Paper presented at the Reading Comprehension Principal Investigators Meeting of the Institute of Educational Sciences in Washington, DC.

McNamara, D., Kintsch, E., Songer, N., & Kintsch, W. (1996). Are good texts always better? Interactions of text coherence, background knowledge, and levels of understanding in learning from text. *Cognition and Instruction, 14,* 1–43.

McNamara, D. S., Levinstein, I. B., & Boonthum, C. (2004). iSTART: Interactive strategy trainer for active reading and thinking. *Behavioral Research Methods, Instruments, and Computers, 36,* 222–233.

Meyer, B. J. F. (1975). Identification of the structure of prose and its implications for the study of reading and memory. *Journal of Reading Behavior, 7,* 7–47.

Meyer, B. J. F. (1982). Reading research and the composition teacher: The importance of plans. *College Composition and Communication, 33,* 37–49.

Meyer, B. J. F. (1985). Prose analysis: Purposes, procedures, and problems. In B. K. Britton & J. Black (Eds.), *Analyzing and understanding expository text* (pp. 11–64, 269–304). Hillsdale, NJ: Erlbaum.

Meyer, B. J. F. (1987). Reading comprehension and aging. In K. W. Schaie (Ed.), *Annual review of gerontology and geriatrics* (Vol. 7, pp. 93–115). New York: Springer.

Meyer, B. J. F., Brandt, D. M., & Bluth, G. J. (1980). Use of top-level structure in text: Key for reading comprehension of ninth-grade students. *Reading Research Quarterly, 16,* 72–103.

Meyer, B. J. F., & McConkie, G. W. (1973). What is recalled after hearing a passage? *Journal of Educational Psychology, 65,* 109–117.

Meyer, B. J. F., Middlemiss, W., Theodorou, E., S., Brezinski, K. L., McDougall, J., & Bartlett, B. J. (2002). Older adults tutoring fifth-grade children in the structure strategy via the Internet. *Journal of Educational Psychology, 94,* 486–519.

Meyer, B. J. F., & Poon, L. W. (1997). Age differences in efficiency of reading comprehension from printed versus computer-displayed text. *Educational Gerontology, 23,* 789–807.

Meyer, B. J. F., & Poon, L. W. (2001). Effects of structure strategy training and signaling on recall of text. *Journal of Educational Psychology, 93,* 141–159.

Meyer, B. J. F., & Rice, G. E. (1981). Information recalled from prose by young, middle, and old adults. *Experimental Aging Research, 7,* 253–268.

Meyer, B. J. F. & Rice, G. E. (1983). *Effects of discourse type on recall by young, middle and old adults with high and average vocabulary scores.* Paper presented at the National Reading Conference, Austin, TX.

Meyer, B. J. F., & Rice, G. E. (1989). Prose processing in adulthood: The text, the reader, and the task. In L. W. Poon, D. C. Rubin, & B. A. Wilson (Eds.), *Everyday cognition in adulthood and later life* (pp. 157–194). New York: Cambridge University Press.

Meyer, B. J. F., Russo, C., & Talbot, A. (1995). Discourse comprehension and problem solving: Decisions about the treatment of breast cancer by women across the life span. *Psychology and Aging, 10*(1), 84–103.

Meyer, B. J. F., & Talbot, A. P. (1998). Adult age differences in reading and remembering text and using this information to make decisions in everyday life. In T. Pourchot & M. C. Smith (Eds.), *Adult learning and development: Perspectives from educational psychology* (pp. 179–199). Mahwah, NJ: Erlbaum.

Meyer, B. J. F., Talbot, A. P., & Florencio, D. (1999). Reading rate and prose retrieval. *Scientific Studies of Reading, 3,* 303–329.

Meyer, B. J. F., Talbot, A. P., Poon, L. W., & Johnson, M. M. (2001). Effects of structure strategy instruction on text recall of older African American Adults. In J. L. Harris, A. Kamhi, & K. Pollock (Eds.), *Literacy in African Americans Communities* (pp. 233–263). Mahwah, NJ: Erlbaum.

Meyer, B. J. F., Talbot, A. P., Stubblefield, R. A., & Poon, L. W. (1998). Interest and strategies of young and old readers differentially interact with characteristics of texts. *Educational Gerontology, 24,* 747–771.

Meyer, B. J. F., Young, C. J., & Bartlett, B. J. (1989). *Memory improved: Reading and memory enhancement across the life span through strategic text structures.* Hillsdale, NJ: Lawrence Erlbaum.

Miller, L. M. S. (2001). Effects of real-world knowledge on text processing among older adults. *Aging, Neuropsychology, and Cognition, 8,* 137–148.

Miller, L. M. S. (2003). The effects of age and domain knowledge on text processing. *Journal of Gerontology: Psychological Sciences, 58B,* 217–223.

Miller, L. M. S., Cohen, J. A., & Wingfield, A. (2004). *Knowledge reduces demands on working memory during reading.* Paper presented at the Cognitive Aging Conference, Atlanta.

Miller, L. M. S., & Stine-Morrow, E. A. L. (1998). Aging and the effects of knowledge on on-line reading strategies. *Journal of Gerontology: Psychological Sciences, 53B,* P223–P233.

Miller, L. M., Stine-Morrow, E. A. L., Kirkorian, H. L., & Conroy, M. L. (2004). Adult age differences in knowledge- driven reading. *Journal of Educational Psychology, 96,* 811–821.

Millis, K. K., & Simon, S., & tenBroek, N. S. (1998). Resource allocation during the rereading of scientific texts. *Memory and Cognition, 26,* 232–246.

Myers, J. L., & O'Brien, E. L. (1998). Accessing the discourse representation during reading. *Discourse Processes, 26,* 131–157.

Myerson, J., Hale, S., Wagstaff, D., Poon, L. W., & Smith, G. A. (1990). The information loss model: A mathematical theory of age-related cognitive slowing. *Psychological Review, 97,* 475–487.

Park, D. C. & Hedden, T. (2001). Working memory and aging. In M. Naveh-Benjamin, M. Moscovitch, & R. L. Roediger (Eds.), *Perspective on human memory and cognitive Aging: Essays in honour of Fergus Craik* (pp. 148–161). East Sussex, UK: Psychology Press.

Patrickson, M. (2002). Teleworking: Potential employment opportunities for older workers? *International Journal of Manpower, 23,* 704–715.

Pew, R. W., & Van Hamel, S. B. (Eds.), (2004). *Technology and adaptive aging.* Washington, DC: National Research Council.

Pressley, M., & McCormick, C. B. (1995). *Advanced educational psychology for educators, researchers, and policymakers.* New York: Harper Collins.

Radvansky, G. A. & Copeland, D. E. (2003). Mental models. In J. W. Gutherie (Ed.) *Encyclopedia of education:* (2nd edition, pp. 1600–1602). New York: Macmillian.

Radvansky, G. A., & Copeland, D. E. (2004). Working memory span and situation model processing. *American Journal of Psychology, 117,* 191–213.

Radvansky, G. A., Copeland, D. E., & Zwaan, R. A. (2003). Brief report: Aging and functional spatial relations in comprehension and memory. *Psychology and Aging, 18,* 161–165.

Radvansky, G. A., & Zacks, R. T. (1991). Mental models and the fan effect. *Journal of Experimental Psychology: Learning, Memory, and Cognition, 17,* 940–953.

Radvansky, G. A., Zwaan, R. A., Curiel, J. M., & Copeland, D. E. (2001). Situation models and aging. *Psychology and Aging, 16,* 145–160.

Rice, G. E., & Meyer, B. J. F. (1986). Prose recall: Effects of aging, verbal ability, and reading behavior. *Journal of Gerontology, 41*, 469–480.

Robertson, D. A., Gernsbacher, M. A., Guidotti, S. J., Robertson, R. R. W., Irwin, W., Mock, B. J., & Campana, M. E. (2000). Functional neroanatomy of the cognitive process of mapping during discourse comprehension. *Psychological Science, 11*, 255–260.

Rogers, W. A. (2000). Attention and aging. In D. Park & N. Schwarz (Eds.), *Cognitive aging: A primer.* Philadelphia, PA: Psychology Press.

Rumelhart, D. E., & Ortony, A. (1977). The representation of knowledge in memory. In R. C. Anderson, R. J. Spiro, & W. E. Montague (Eds.), *Schooling and the acquisition of knowledge* (pp. 99–135). Hillsdale, NJ: Erlbaum.

Salthouse, T. A. (1982). Duration estimates of two information processing components. *Acta Psychologica, 52*, 213–226.

Salthouse, T. A. (1991). Mediation of adult age differences in cognition by reductions in working memory and speed of processing. *Psychological Science, 2*, 179–183.

Salthouse, T. A. (1996). The processing-speed theory of adult age differences in cognition. *Psychological Review, 103*, 403–428.

Sanders, T. J. M., & Gernsbacher, M. A. (2004). Accessibility in text and discourse processing. *Discourse Processes, 37*(2), 79–89.

Sanders, T. J. M., & Noordman, L. G. M. (2000). The role of coherent relations and their linguistic markers in text processing. *Discourse Processes, 29*, 37–60.

Schaie, K. W. (1996). *Intellectual development in adulthood: The Seattle longitudinal study.* New York: Cambridge University Press.

Schaie, K. W. (2004). Cognitve Aging. In R. W. Pew & S. B. Van Hemel (Eds.), *Technology for adaptive aging* (pp. 43–63). Washington, DC: The National Academies Press.

Schaie, K. W. (2005). *Developmental influence on adult intelligence: The Seattle longitudinal study.* London: Oxford University Press.

Schaie, K. W., & Willis, S. L. (1994). Assessing the elderly. In C. B. Fisher & R. M. Lerner (Eds.), *Applied developmental psychology* (pp. 339–372). New York: McGraw Hill.

Schmalhofer, F., & Glavanov, D. (1986). Three components of understanding a programmer's manual: Verbatim, propositional, and situational representations. *Journal of Memory and Language, 25*, 279–294.

Sharit, J., Czaja, S. J., Hernandez, M., Yang, Perdomo, D., Lewis, J., Lee, C. C., and Nair, S. S (2004). *An evaluation of performance by older persons on a simulated telecommuting task.* Submitted for publication.

Sinnott, J. D. (1989). A model for solution of ill-structured problems: Implications for everyday and abstract problem solving. In J. D. Sinnott (Ed.), *Everyday problem solving: Theory and applications* (pp. 72–99). New York: Praeger.

Smith, F. (1994). Understanding reading (5th ed.). Hillsdale, NJ: Erlbaum.

Smith, M. C. (2000). The real-world reading practices of adults. *Journal of Literacy Research, 32*, 25–52.

Soederberg, L., & Stine, E. A. L. (1995). Activation of emotion information in text among younger and older adults. *Journal of Adult Development, 2*, 23–36.

Speranza, F., Daneman, M., & Schneider, B. A. (2000). How aging affects the reading of words in noisy backgrounds. *Psychology and Aging, 15*, 253–258.

Spilich, G. J. (1983). Life-span characteristics of text processing: Structural and procedural differences. *Journal of Verbal Learning and Verbal Behavior, 22*, 231–244.

Stanovich, K. E., West, R. L., & Harrison, M. R. (1995). Knowledge growth and maintenance across the life span: The role of print exposure. *Developmental Psychology, 31*, 811–826.

Stein, N. L., & Trabasso, T. (1985). The search after meaning: Comprehension and comprehension monitoring. In F. J. Morrison, C. Lord, & D. Keating (Eds.), *Applied developmental psychology* (Vol. 2, pp. 33–58). San Diego: Academic Press.

Stine, E. L. (1990). On-line processing of written text by younger and older adults. *Psychology and Aging, 5*, 68–78.

Stine-Morrow, E. A. L., Gagne, D. D., Morrow, D. G., & DeWall, B. (2004). Age differences in re-reading. *Memory and Cognition, 32*, 696–710.

Stine, E. A. L., & Hindman, J. (1994). Age differences in reading time allocation for propositionally dense sentences. *Aging, Neuropsychology, and Cognition, 1,* 2–16.

Stine-Morrow, E. A. L., Loveless, M. K., & Soederberg, L. M. (1996). Resource allocation in on-line reading by younger and older adults. *Psychology and Aging, 11,* 475–486.

Stine-Morrow, E. A. L., Milinder, L., Pullara, O., & Herman, B. (2001). Patterns of resource allocations are reliable among younger and older readers. *Psychology and Aging, 16,* 69–84.

Stine-Morrow, E. A. L., Miller, L. M. S., & Leno, R., III (2001). Patterns of on-line resource allocation to narrative text by younger and older readers. *Aging, Neuropsychology and Cognition, 8,* 36–53.

Stuen, C., & Faye, E. E. (2003). Vision loss: Normal and not normal changes among older adults. *Generations, 27,* 8–14.

Taconnat, L., & Isingrini, M. (2004). Cognitive operations in the generation effect on a recall test: Role of aging and divided attention. *Journal of Experimental Psychology: Learning, Memory, and Cognition, 30,* 827–837.

Talbot, A. P. (2004). *How much information do men really want? Information search behavior and decision rationale in a medical decision-making task for men.* Unpublished doctoral dissertation, The Pennsylvania State University.

Taylor, J. L., O'Hara, R., Mumenthaler, M. S., Rosen, A. C., & Yesavage, J. A. (2005). Cognitive ability, expertise, and age differences in following air-traffic control instructions. *Psychology and Aging, 20,* 117–133.

Thornton, W. J. L., & Dumke, H. A. (2005). Age differences in everyday problem-solving and decision-making effectiveness: A meta-analytic review. *Psychology and Aging, 20,* 85–99.

Till, R. E., Mross, E. F., & Kintsch, W. (1988). Time course of priming for associate and inference words in a discourse context. *Memory and Cognition, 16,* 283–298.

Tun, P. A. (1989). Age differences in processing expository and narrative text. *Journals of Gerontology, 44,* P9–P15.

Uttl, B., & Van Alstine, C. L. (2003). Rising verbal intelligence scores: Implications for research and clinical practice. *Psychology and Aging, 18,* 616–621.

van den Broek, Rapp, D. N., & Kendeou, P. (2005). Integrating memory-based and constructionist processes in accounts of reading Comprehension. *Discourse Processes, 39,* 299–316.

van den Broek, P., Rohleder, L., & Narvaez, D. (1996). Causal inferences in the comprehension of literary texts. In M. S. MacNealy & R. J. Kreuz (Eds.), *Empirical approaches to literature and aesthetics* (pp. 179–200). Westport, CT: Ablex Publishing.

van den Broek, P., Young, M., Tzeng, Y., & Linderholm, T. (1999). The landscape model of reading: Inferences and the online construction of memory representations. In S. R. Goldman & H. van Oostendorp (Eds.), *The construction of mental representations during reading* (pp. 71–98). Mahwah, NJ: Lawrence Erlbaum Associates.

VanderVeen, A. A. (2004, April). *Toward a construct of critical reading for the new SAT.* Paper presented at the annual meeting of the National Council on Measurement in Education in San Diego, CA.

Van Dijk, T. A., & Kintsch, W. (1983). *Strategies of discourse comprehension.* New York: Academic Press.

Verhaeghen, P., Borchelt, M., & Smith, J. (2003). Relation between cardiovascular and metabolic disease and cognition in very old age: Cross-sectional and longitudinal findings from the Berlin aging study. *Health Psychology, 22,* 559–569.

Verhaeghen, P., Marcoen, A., & Goossens, L. (1993). Facts and fiction about memory aging: A quantitative integration of research findings. *Journals of Gerontology, 48,* P157–P171.

Von Hippel, W., Silver, L. A., & Lynch, M. E. (2000). Stereotyping against your will: The role of inhibitory ability in stereotyping and prejudice among the elderly. *Personality and Social Psychology Bulletin, 26,* 523–532.

Wijekumar, K., & Meyer, B. J. F. (in press). Design and pilot of a web-based intelligent tutoring system to improve reading comprehension in middle school students. *Journal of Computers in Schools: Special Issue on Intelligent Agents in Education.*

Willis, S. L. (1989). Improvement with cognitive training: Which old dogs learn what trick? In L. W. Poon, D. C. Rubin, & B. A. Wilson (Eds) .*Everyday cognition in adulthood and late life* (pp. 545–569). Cambridge: Cambridge University Press.

Willis, S. L. (2004). Technology and learning in current and future older cohorts. In R. W. Pew & S. B. Van Hemel (Eds.) *Technology for adaptive aging* (pp. 209–229). Washington, DC: The National Academies Press.

Wingfield, A., & Stine-Morrow, E. A. L. (2000). Language and speech. In T. A. Salthouse & Craik, F. I. M. (Eds.), *The handbook of aging and cognition* (2nd edition, pp. 359–416). Mahwah, NJ: Lawrence Erlbaum Associates.

Zelinski, E. M., & Burnight, K. P. (1997). Sixteen-year longitudinal and time lag changes in memory and cognition in older adults. *Psychology and Aging, 12*, 503–513.

Zelinski, E. M., & Gilewski, M. J. (1988). Memory for prose and aging: A meta-analysis. In M. L. Howe & C. Brainerd (Eds.), *Cognitive development in adulthood: Progress in cognitive development research* (pp. 133–158). New York: Springer-Verlag.

Zelinski, E. M., Gilewski, M. J., & Schaie, K. W. (1993). Individual differences in cross-sectional and 3-year longitudinal memory performance across the adult life span. *Psychology and Aging, 8*, 176–186.

Zelinski, E. M., & Stewart, S. T. (1998). Individual differences in 16-year memory changes. *Psychology and Aging, 13*, 622–630.

Zwaan, R. A. (1999). Situation models: The mental leap into imagined worlds. *Current Directions in Psychological Science, 8*, 15–18.

Zwaan, R. A., Langston, M. C., & Graesser, A. C. (1995). The construction of situation models in narrative comprehension: An event-indexing model. *Psychological Science, 6*, 292–297.

Zwaan, R. A., Magliano, J. P., & Graesser, A. C. (1995). Dimensions of situation model construction in narrative comprehension. *Journal of Experimental Psychology, 21*, 386–397.

Twelve

Language Comprehension and Production in Normal Aging

Robert Thornton and Leah L. Light

Since Cohen introduced the term "gerolinguistics" in 1979, there has been accelerating interest in understanding the nature of language in old age. Searching PsychINFO using the key words "language and aging" generated 9 citations for the decade from 1970 to 1979, 80 for 1980 to 1989, 270 for 1990 to 1999, and 171 for the 5-year period from 2000 to 2004. This surge in interest in language and aging is not surprising. Language is a complex domain that involves the integration of multiple sources of information, including sound, vision, meaning, and intention. Both comprehension and production of language require integration of current inputs and prior knowledge in evolving mental representations. As such, language deals with very high-level constraint integration and thus can serve as a testing ground for theories of language, as well as theories of cognitive aging (see reviews by Burke, MacKay, & James, 2000; Kemper & Mitzner, 2001; Light, 1988, 1990, 2000; MacKay & Abrams, 1996; Schneider & Pichora-Fuller, 2000; Wingfield & Stine-Morrow, 2000). Moreover, older adults rate many aspects of their own receptive and expressive language abilities less highly than young adults, and both young and older adults believe that aging is associated with poorer performance in both areas (Ryan et al., 1992). Declines in language processing can impede effective communication, with negative effects on older adults' social interactions and psychological well-being (Hummert et al., 2004; Kemper & Lacal, 2004; Tesch-Romer, 1997).

This chapter is divided into three major sections that deal with age-related constancy and change in word, sentence, and discourse level processes. Within each section we consider issues related to language perception or comprehension and to language production. This is a structure that is convenient for organizing the material to be covered, but because language is highly interactive, it is not always possible to adhere strictly to this classificatory scheme. Our deviations from it are apparent when they occur. Because our focus is on work that has contributed to framing or resolving theoretical debates about the nature of cognitive aging, we begin with a brief outline of the major cognitive aging perspectives that have been used to interpret findings on language in normal aging. Our review deals almost exclusively with findings at a behavioral level. Although there is increasing interest in the cognitive neuroscience of aging, work on the brain bases of high-level language processing across the life span has lagged behind that in such domains as memory and attention, as suggested by the absence of a chapter on language in a recent volume (Cabeza, Nyberg, & Park, 2004).

Generally speaking, hypotheses about the nature of age-related change and stability in cognition have been couched within broad organizing frameworks rather than systematically developed and computationally implemented theories (for discussions of this issue, see Burke, 1997, Light, 1991; MacKay & James, 2001a). Five such approaches have been prominent over the last two decades. Three attribute age-related deficits in cognition to cognitive slowing (e.g., Salthouse, 1996), problems in working memory that affect storage and manipulation of information (e.g., Carpenter, Miyake, & Just, 1994), or to weakening of inhibitory processes so that older adults are less able to suppress information irrelevant to ongoing goals than are younger adults (Hasher & Zacks, 1988; Zacks & Hasher, 1997). A fourth approach, the transmission deficit account, hypothesizes that many age-related changes in cognition stem from weakened connections among memory representations that reduce the transmission of excitation (e.g., Burke et al., 2000). As elaborated later, this account postulates not only cognitive processes, but also a cognitive architecture that increases its explanatory power. A fifth view targets the possibility that sensory deficits are causally related to reductions in diverse aspects of cognition (e.g., Baltes & Lindenberger, 1997; Lindenberger & Baltes, 1994). In the context of language processing, this question has been raised

most explicitly with respect to speech perception and comprehension (e.g., CHABA, 1988; Frisina & Frisina, 1997; Light, 1988; Schneider & Pichora-Fuller, 2000; Wingfield & Tun, 2001).

Current models usually assume interactions across sensory, phonological or orthographic, lexical, syntactic, and semantic levels of processing, with an interplay between top–down (conceptually driven) and bottom–up (data driven) processing (e.g., Burke et al., 2000; Dell, Burger, & Svec, 1997). The possibility that aging is accompanied by an increase in the effect of top–down processes permeates recent literature on language in old age. An additional theme that has emerged is the possibility that redefined goals, increases in expertise, or changes in processing strategies to compensate for reductions in processing efficacy affect language function as well as cognitive functioning, more generally, in older adults (Adams et al., 1997; Carstensen, Isaacowitz, & Charles, 1999; Hasher & Zacks, 1988; Radvansky et al., 2001; Wingfield & Stine-Morrow, 2000).

I. Lexical Processing

A. Word Recognition

Although changes in vision have consequences for visual language processing (MacKay, Taylor, & Marian, 2005; Scialfa, 2002; Speranza, Daneman, & Schneider, 2000), the role of sensory deficits in auditory language processing has been investigated more extensively (Schneider & Pichora-Fuller, 2000). Presbycusis, or pure-tone hearing loss, especially at higher frequencies represented in speech, constitutes a major sensory decrement in old age and can contribute to poorer identification of single words even in quiet listening situations (e.g., Humes, 1996). Aging is also associated with other changes in the auditory system, including temporal processing of speech (e.g., Pichora-Fuller, 2003). For instance, older adults have difficulty in differentiating voiced from voiceless consonants (e.g., /b/ and /p/), a discrimination that requires detection of the presence or absence of a voice onset time gap of 20–40 ms in duration (Tremblay, Piskosz, & Souza, 2002). The impact of changes in the auditory system may be exacerbated by the fact that sounds in conversational speech are often lost or modified when combined with each other (e.g., *Great Britain* may be rendered as *Grape Britain*). There is also considerable variation in acoustic realizations of speech sounds by different speakers. Listeners maintain perceptual constancy in the face of this variability by a process known as perceptual normalization (Pisoni, 1993). Older adults have poorer perceptual normalization abilities than young adults, i.e., their word identification performance suffers more when words are presented by many talkers rather than by a single speaker (Yonan & Sommers, 2000).

Even older adults with good audiometric profiles show greater impairment than young adults when speech perception is measured under adverse listening conditions, such as when speech is presented in noise (e.g., Frisina & Frisina, 1997; Pichora-Fuller, Schneider, & Daneman, 1995; Tun, 1998; Tun & Wingfield, 1999). Adjusting signal/noise ratios so that identification of easy words (those phonetically similar to few other low-frequency words) is equated across age does not eliminate age differences in identifying hard words that are phonetically similar to many other high-frequency words (Sommers, 1996). Young adults' recall of spoken sentences is not impacted by a single competing speaker talking at a low level of conversational noise, but older adults recall is impaired at low as well as high levels of conversational noise (Tun & Wingfield,

1999). Difficulties in attention needed to segregate the speech of multiple speakers are implicated here.

Both young and older adults identify words in noise better when these are presented in highly predictive sentence contexts (*The witness took a solemn oath*) rather than nonpredictive ones (e.g., *John hadn't discussed the oath*), with older adults often benefiting more (Frisina & Frisina, 1997; Pichora-Fuller et al., 1995; Yonan & Sommers, 2000). In a systematic investigation of this phenomenon, Pichora-Fuller et al. (1995) varied the signal-to-noise ratio of sentences heard in multitalker babble over a wide range to examine the effect of semantic context. Older adults had a greater maximum benefit from sentence predictability than young adults, arguing for a greater top–down benefit for this group.

Older adults are also affected more adversely when speech is time compressed by periodic deletions of small segments, although again such effects are moderated by the presence of semantic or syntactic constraints (e.g., Gordon-Salant & Fitzgibbons, 2001; Tun, 1998; Wingfield et al., 1985). The interaction of processes at various levels is also clear in studies of time-compressed speech in young and older adults. For instance, prefamiliarization of voices improves speech perception in noise for older adults more than for young adults when there are multiple speakers, especially in identifying high probability words in sentence endings (Yonan & Sommers, 2000). When discrimination of consonants is made difficult by artificially varying speech stimuli along continua so that it is hard to decide whether one is hearing *digress* or *tigress*, the perceived boundary between categories is sensitive to the placement of syllabic stress; this effect is stronger in old than in young adults, to the extent that metrical structure may override voice onset time as a cue for phonemic boundaries (Baum, 2003). Older adults also need more information, i.e., greater word onset duration (or *gate*), than young adults to recognize spoken words, but word recognition is facilitated to the same extent across age by adding prosodic information indicating number of syllables and syllabic stress (Wingfield, Lindfield, & Goodglass, 2000). Rapid auditory presentation of sentences with list intonation rather than normal prosody produces repetition deafness, namely failure to report repeated words (contrast *I live at one two two four Canyon Street* with *I live at one five two four Canyon Street*). Older adults are more prone to repetition deafness when sentences are presented as aprosodic lists (MacKay & Miller, 1996); however, normal prosody eliminates repetition deafness for both young and older adults. These are all cases in which higher level cues (e.g., prosody) are constraining lower level speech perception.

There are, nonetheless, limits on the usefulness of linguistic context. Wingfield, Alexander, and Cavigelli (1994) edited words from connected speech and played them in isolation, with context added before the critical word, after the critical word, or both before and after the target. Both young and older adults benefited from context that preceded the target, but context that followed the target was less effective for older adults, suggesting that they were less able to maintain information from unclear stimuli in working memory.

B. Lexical Retrieval

One often-cited example of a positive age-related change in cognitive abilities is the fact that vocabulary continues to grow with age, such that older adults have larger vocabularies than younger ones for a large meta-analysis, (see Verhaeghen, 2003). Despite this positive change, there is a large body of research demonstrating problems older adults have with retrieving lexical information from memory (for a review, see Griffin and Spieler, in press). For example, Connor and colleagues (2004) presented longitudinal data from the Boston naming test and found that performance declined an average of 2% per decade. Research in this area has been particularly fruitful for theory, as some of the most explicit models of language and aging have been developed to explain changes in lexical retrieval.

Two major theories have been invoked to explain age-related changes in lexical processing, above and beyond accounts of general slowing. The inhibition deficit hypothesis proposes that aging weakens inhibitory processes so that older adults are less able to suppress irrelevant information than younger adults (Hasher & Zacks, 1988; Zacks & Hasher, 1997). An alternative theory, the transmission deficit account, hypothesizes that many age-related changes in linguistic processes stem from weakened connections among memory representations that reduce the transmission of excitation, resulting in weakened patterns of activation (Burke et al., 1991; James & Burke, 2000; MacKay, Abrams, & Pedroza, 1999; MacKay & James, 2004).

One of the most studied aspects of lexical retrieval problems in aging is the tip-of-the-tongue (TOT) state, in which a person temporarily cannot recall a well-known word. The frequency of TOT states seems to increase with age, a finding that has been demonstrated both with experimental techniques (e.g., James & Burke, 2000; Maylor, 1990; White & Abrams, 2002) and in natural production (e.g., Burke et al., 1991; Heine, Ober, & Shenaut, 1999).

It is important to note that this age-related change may not affect all words equally. A number of studies have focused on how aging affects the retrieval of proper names (e.g., Burke et al., 2004;

James, 2004), finding that older adults have more retrieval problems than young adults. For example, James (2004) found that older adults had more retrieval failures for proper names than younger adults, but this was not true for remembering someone's occupation (for similar findings, see Barresi, Obler, & Goodglass, 1998 and Evrard, 2002). Instead of suggesting a specific impairment for proper names, these data have been interpreted as resulting from the nature of the semantic representation for words. In the transmission deficit model, proper names have a sparser semantic representation, i.e., fewer interconnections with other concepts in memory, whereas common names are more interconnected. Thus, weakened connections in semantic memory differentially impact the representations for proper names. The James (2004) study is striking in this regard in that she used proper names that could also be occupation titles (e.g., *Mr. Farmer* versus *farmer*) and found that TOT rates were higher for a given word when it was presented as a proper name than as an occupation. Maylor (1997) argued that the perception of greater age-related problems in this area may arise because common objects can have more than one acceptable name and retrieval failures for people's names may have social consequences.

One intuitive explanation for TOTs is that the underlying cause of the TOT state is that a persistent alternative word is competing for activation, thereby blocking activation of the intended word, which would be expected by an inhibition deficit. Interestingly, several lines of research argue against this intuition (e.g., Abrams & Rodriguez, in press; Abrams, White, & Eitel, 2003; Cross & Burke, 2004; James & Burke, 2000; White & Abrams, 2002, 2004). First, if a failure to inhibit alternatives were the cause of TOTs, one would expect to see older adults with more persistent alternatives

than young adults, but the opposite is true (e.g., Burke et al., 1991). Second, older adults have less partial information available about TOTs than young adults (e.g., Burke et al., 1991). Third, providing phonological primes improves retrieval and helps with the resolution of TOTs rather than blocking resolution. For example, James and Burke (2000) found that when TOTs were elicited for a word such as *abdicate*, having been primed by words that shared phonological structure, such as *ab*stract, in*di*gent, and lo*cate*, helped with retrieval rather than blocking it. This finding argues against a blocking or inhibition-deficit account of TOTs and supports the transmission deficit model, under the assumption that the phonological primes helped strengthen age-weakened activation in the phonological system.

Another factor that has been shown to affect TOTs and word retrieval more generally is the number of phonologically similar words and their related frequencies. The term *neighborhood* refers to the set of words that differ from the target by changing exactly one phoneme. Under this definition, the word *cat*'s neighbors would include *bat*, *sat*, *cut*, and *car*, among a large number of other words. The term *neighborhood density* refers to the total number of neighbors a word has, whereas the term *neighborhood frequency* refers to how frequently those neighbors are used. Both neighborhood density and frequency have been shown to affect word recognition (e.g., Vitevitch & Luce, 1998). Older adults report more TOTs for words with low neighborhood frequency (Vitevitch & Sommers, 2003). This finding is consistent with the transmission deficit model because words with high neighborhood frequencies would receive supporting activation from their neighbors, resulting in fewer TOTs. However, because words with low neighborhood frequency would receive little support from neighbors, the observed age-related increase in TOTs is expected. Age-related neighborhood effects show up in other tasks as well. For example, Sommers (1996) found that older adults have greater difficulty identifying relatively low frequency words from dense neighborhoods than young adults. Sommers (1996) interpreted this finding in terms of an inhibition deficit in that low frequency words in high density neighborhoods would be difficult to isolate from higher frequency, phonologically similar competitors. As such, an age-related inhibition deficit would explain the effect in that older adults would be less able to inhibit the competitors, resulting in greater processing difficulty. Sommers and Danielson (1999) further examined the nature of neighborhood effects by examining the effect of context on word identification. They found that the age-related neighborhood effect, that older adults had great difficulty with the "hard" neighborhood words (low frequency, dense neighborhood), was attenuated by context: with highly constraining sentence contexts, no age differences were found. This finding again highlights the beneficial effect that top–down semantic information has in offsetting lower level age-related cognitive problems.

Spieler and Balota (2000) also examined how neighborhood variables affect word recognition in aging. To assess how simple word naming changes with age, they examined three factors known to influence word naming: word frequency, word length, and neighborhood density. They performed a large-scale regression analysis on the naming times of both young and older adults for over 2800 words. They found that all three factors accounted for significant variance in both age groups, but that frequency had a larger influence for the older adults and that length and neighborhood density had less of an influence, contrary to earlier studies that found similar frequency

effects across age groups (e.g., Allen et al., 1993; Stine, 1990). Spieler and Balota (2000) suggested that this effect was observed because older adults typically have more reading experience than younger adults, so their lexical representations have become more unitized, resulting in larger lexical effects (frequency) and smaller sublexical effects (length and neighborhood density). Their data are complicated by a neuroimaging study by Whiting et al. (2003) who found that in a lexical decision task, the regression coefficients for word frequency were similar for young and older adults, whereas word length had a great influence for older than young adults, the opposite of Spieler and Balota's finding. Thus, how the influence of these lexical variables changes with age is still not clear and some of these differences may stem from the task being used (e.g., naming, lexical decision) as well as whether the target words are presented in context (e.g., Stine, 1990) or in isolation (e.g., Spieler & Balota, 2000). Another issue that has not been addressed in detail is the role of visual acuity in age differences in visual word recognition. Although most studies control for basic acuity, some research suggested that even small differences in acuity can have a surprising effect in cognitive aging research (MacKay et al., 2005).

Another finding relevant to the inhibition deficit account comes from work by Hartman and Hasher (1991). When asked to read sentences that have high probability endings that were not actually presented, older adults were more likely to subsequently produce these in a sentence completion task. Hartman (1995), however, reported that older adults were not more likely than young adults to use expected but disconfirmed study words as completions if the to-be-selected words were clearly indicated at study. Also, when the unexpected ending that is to be remembered is followed by a sentence that embeds the to-be-selected target in an elaborated context, age differences in completion rates for no-longer-relevant words are abolished (Hasher, Quig, & May, 1997). Both findings are consonant with the view that older adults have difficulty tracking contextual information about which words are to be remembered and which are to be forgotten, but that this problem can be mitigated under some circumstances (see also May et al., 1999).

Given these well-documented problems older adults have with lexical retrieval, an open question is how these problems affect higher level processing more generally. For instance, Federmeier et al. (2003) found delays on general sensory components of word processing in older adults, as seen in evoked potential responses, but not on associative priming. Also, if older adults are slower and less accurate in lexical processing, then we might expect to see language production in older adults slow down even more as utterances get longer, as a backlog of words to be produced would build. However, this does not seem to be the case. Although older adults might speak a bit more slowly or be slightly less fluent than younger adults (e.g., Bortfeld et al., 2001), we do not observe a lexical traffic jam in their production. A suggestion about how older adults achieve fluency despite retrieval problems is offered by Spieler and Griffin (in press) who presented evidence from a constrained sentence production task that older adults tend to speak more slowly and to plan ahead further so that production is fluent and error free—when they are not under time pressure. However, under time pressure to respond, older adults cannot plan as far ahead and consequently are less fluent, as they are not able to retrieve words to be produced as quickly.

C. Asymmetries in Processing

One problem in applying general theories of cognitive aging, e.g., general slowing, working memory, or inhibition deficits, to linguistic phenomena is that they are indeed general and consequently lack machinery to account for asymmetries in the effects of age on processing. One such asymmetry is between comprehension and production, at least for single words, with observable production deficits for older adults who do not seem to have comparable comprehension deficits. For example, MacKay et al. (1999) examined age-related differences in comprehending (perceiving) and producing spelling. In their comprehension task, participants were presented with a word and pressed a button to indicate whether or not it was spelled correctly. No differences between older and younger adults in detection accuracy were observed. However, older adults were less accurate on the production task, in which participants had to write out the words they had seen, because they misspelled words they had correctly rejected in the comprehension task [also see MacKay and Abrams (1998) MacKay and James (2004) and Stuart-Hamilton and Rabbitt (1997) for similar studies of age-related changes in spelling, as well as Abrams and Stanley (2004), for evidence that even spelling comprehension is impaired in very old adults]. This production-comprehension asymmetry has been demonstrated across a variety of tasks (Burke & MacKay, 1997).

A second age-related asymmetry has been observed for processing of semantic and phonological information. Although older adults demonstrate deficits in a number of areas, several studies have shown only very minor, if any, differences in semantic processing (e.g., Federmeier et al., 2003; Madden, Pierce, & Allen, 1993; Mayr & Kliegl, 2000; Radvansky et al., 2001), with some finding even larger semantic effects for older adults (e.g., Laver & Burke, 1993; Madden, 1988). Several studies have examined the differential impact aging has on phonological and semantic processing in the same individuals. For example, Taylor and Burke (2002) had participants name pictures while ignoring auditory word distractors. They found no age-related differences in interference from the phonologically related distractors, whereas older adults showed more interference from the semantically related distractors. Semantic interference in the picture-naming task arises from priming of semantic connections linking conceptually related nodes and is expected under the transmission deficit hypothesis to be greater in older adults for the same reasons that semantic priming effects are larger—greater richness of semantic connections in old age leading to greater convergence of priming at a lexical node. Another finding that supports the view that older adults tend to rely more on semantics and less on phonology than young adults is reported in Cortese et al. (2003). They examined age-related spelling differences for homophonic words (e.g., *plane* vs *plain*) and found that young adults tended to rely on phonological information, choosing the most regular spelling, whereas older adults tended to rely more on semantics, choosing the orthography consistent with the dominant meaning. The overall pattern of results indicates that the pattern of semantic and phonological effects is different across age (Burke & MacKay, 1997) and is theoretically significant because although predicted by the transmission deficit hypothesis, it runs contrary to the inhibition deficit hypothesis. Inhibitory processes are not specific to semantic or phonological information, so no asymmetry is predicted.

Several accounts have been offered of the preservation and, in some cases,

apparent increases in semantic processing in older adults (Light, 1992). For example, Madden (1988) examined semantic priming from a sentence context to a target word and found that older adults showed a greater effect of context when the target word was degraded. He suggested that this effect resulted because of age-related slowing in the bottom–up processing of the target word, resulting in a compensatory increase in top–down semantic processing, presumably because it has more time to have an effect and support recognition. A second account for the relative sparing of semantic processing with a concomitant decrease in phonological processing comes from the transmission deficit account. In this model, normal aging weakens memory connections. However, semantic representations have more redundant connections, whereas phonological representations are more sparse. Thus, given the same amount of connection weakening, semantic memory will be relatively preserved because of the redundancy of connectivity. This relative sparing of semantics, along with problems with phonology and sensory deficits, explains why we see greater top–down context effects in older adults.

II. Sentence Processing

In order to understand a sentence, comprehenders must encode orthography or phonology to identify and access the meanings of words (word level processes). They must instantiate concepts, assign thematic roles (e.g., identify predicates and their arguments), and form propositions (commonly called idea units). New concepts must be processed when they appear and maintained in memory for later integration with other concepts within and across sentences. Processing times increase at major syntactic boundaries within sentences and at sentence ends, reflecting so-called "wrap-up" or integrative processing of concepts as well as ambiguity resolution. As discussed in more detail later, readers also go beyond what is stated directly to create a mental representation of the situation model of what is described by the text (Gernsbacher, 1990; Kintsch, 1998; Zwaan & Radvansky, 1998). Despite the importance of discourse level processes in sentence comprehension, a great deal of research has been carried out using single sentences in unconnected discourse. The motivation for doing so is to study sentence-level processes independent of discourse. As we will see in our review, however, it can be difficult to disentangle these levels of processing.

A. Sentence Comprehension

It has been widely argued that individual differences in language processing, including age differences, are associated with individual differences in working memory capacity as measured on standard working memory tasks (e.g., Just & Carpenter, 1992). Given well-established declines in working memory with age, it is easy to see why research on language and aging has intensively examined how age-related deficits in memory, especially working memory, affect language, rather than searching for possible age-related deficits in linguistic processes *per se* (e.g., Burke & Light, 1981; Light, 1988, 1990, 2000). As a result, much of this work is "off-line" in that the experimental material is presented some time before the experimental task. Because of this interval between presentation and task, performance on the task depends not only on how the stimuli were processed originally, but how they have been encoded and stored in memory. Waters and Caplan (e.g., Caplan & Waters, 1999; Waters & Caplan, 1996, 2001, 2005) have failed to find a relationship between on-line syntactic processing

and traditional measures of working memory. They have argued that rather than a single resource theory of the relationship between working memory and language, a separate sentence interpretation resource theory is needed. On this view, interpretive processes that assign meaning to sentences are largely unconscious and obligatory and should be resistant to aging, whereas post interpretive processes that involve retaining and referring to sentence meaning and form may be related to traditional working memory measures and should be sensitive to age.

Interpretive processing is studied in on-line comprehension tasks that tap processes that unfold as words are recognized and integrated into the developing syntactic and semantic representation. In auditory or visual moving window paradigms, participants pace themselves through the material, which is presented word by word or in small segments, and the amount of time spent on each word or segment is recorded. In eye-tracking studies, both first pass and regressive eye movements to earlier text provide clues to processing. An assumption is that complex syntactic constructions (e.g., temporary syntactic ambiguities in garden path sentences such as *The experienced soldiers warned about the dangers conducted the midnight raid*) cause interpretive difficulties that result in processing slow-downs at predictable points. Single resource capacity theories predict that older adults should be disproportionately slowed at such points, whereas the Waters and Caplan theory predicts no differential slowing.

Contrary to single resource theory, reading and listening times for isolated sentences in young and older adults have been found to be affected in very similar ways by syntactic manipulations, although older adults are sometimes (but, contra general-slowing views, not always) slower and sometimes perform more poorly on off-line measures collected in the same studies (e.g., Kemper, Crow, & Kemtes, 2004; Stine-Morrow, Loveless, & Soederberg, 1996; Waters & Caplan, 2001). Using structural equation modeling, DeDe et al. (2004) found that verbal working memory measures mediated age-related differences in off-line sentence and text comprehension tasks, but did not predict performance on on-line listening measures. However, outcomes less supportive of separate sentence interpretation resource notions have also been observed (DeDe et al., 2004; Kemper, Crow, & Kemtes, 2004; Kemtes & Kemper, 1997; Stine-Morrow, Ryan, & Leonard, 2000; Waters & Caplan, 2005). For instance, older adults may make more regressive eye movements in reading sentences containing ambiguities, contrary to separate resource views, even when first pass fixations do not show age effects (Kemper, Crow, & Kemtes, 2004; Liu, Kemper, & Herman, 2004). In general, Waters and Caplan have maintained their separate working memory account by suggesting that the evidence that does not support their theory reflects postinterpretative rather than early (i.e., interpretive) syntactic processes (e.g., DeDe et al., 2004), but the way that different types of working memory cooperate in their account has not been elaborated systematically to date (see commentary following Caplan and Waters, 1999).

Stine-Morrow and colleagues have carried out an extensive program of research comparing young and older readers using the visual moving window technique and carrying out regression analyses to determine the contributions of word level, text base level, and situation model variables to reading times, typically at the word level. These studies have found (not surprisingly) that older adults are slower overall than young adults, but that reading times of both groups are responsive to manipulation of variables at the word, textbase, and situation model levels. One area in which differences in resource allocation may differ across age is in sentence wrap-up effects, with young adults showing larger end of sentence wrap-up effects (Stine, 1990; Stine, Cheung, & Henderson, 1995), whereas older adults have shown larger effects of attention to conceptualization within a sentence (Miller & Stine-Morrow, 1998). This suggests that older adults may be breaking up the discourse into small processing units, a strategy to possibly offset age-related working memory problems. Nonetheless, this pattern of differences in wrap-up processes is not observed universally. For instance, in different studies, there have been no age differences in wrap-up times at clausal boundaries coupled with greater sentence boundary wrap-up effects for older adults (Smiler, Gagne, & Stine-Morrow, 2003) and larger wrap-up effects for older adults at both intrasentence and between sentence boundaries (Miller, Stine-Morrow, Kirkorian, & Conroy, 2004; Stine-Morrow et al., 2001). Interestingly, and consistent with the separate sentence interpretation resource hypothesis, resource allocation parameters for wrap-up apparently do not correlate with working memory as assessed by span measures (Smiler et al., 2003; Stine-Morrow, Milinder et al., 2001).

B. Sentence Production

Kemper et al. (2001a) analyzed both cross-sectional and longitudinal language samples and found that syntactic complexity (e.g., the number of propositions or clauses in a sentence, types of syntactic structure used) declines gradually across the life span. These data have been collected from diaries (Kemper, 1990), written language samples in response to elicitation questions (e.g., Kemper et al.,

1989; Kemper, Thompson, & Marquis, 2001), stories told in writing (Kemper et al., 1990), and autobiographies of nuns (Kemper et al., 2001; Snowdon et al., 1996). Consistent with hypotheses that working memory is critical in sentence production, age-related changes in complexity correlate with a number of measures of working memory (Kemper et al., 1989; Kemper, Thompson, & Marquis, 2001b).

Although naturalistic language samples provide important data, the studies are not experimental and variables expected to influence syntactic complexity cannot be manipulated directly. A number of factors beyond working memory limitations could lead to the production of simpler syntactic constructions by older adults, including possible differences in frequency of exposure to complex sentences that can lead to priming of simpler sentences (Altmann et al., 2004) and age differences in pragmatic choices about how to package information for listeners (Kemper, Herman, & Liu, 2004).

Constrained sentence production tasks that avoid these interpretive pitfalls have been used only recently to compare young and older adults. Davidson, Zacks, and Ferreira (2003) gave participants a subject pronoun and a verb followed by additional words and asked them to produce a well-formed sentence using these words. They found that when producing sentences that had two acceptable grammatical orderings (e.g., *he gave the book to the library* versus *he gave the library the book*), both age groups were faster than for sentences that had only one acceptable grammatical ordering (e.g., *he donated the book to the library* as in most dialects of English *he donated the library the book* is unacceptable). Crucially, older adults were just as fast and accurate as younger adults and both groups showed a similar effect of grammatical choice. This study has

interesting theoretical implications. Under at least some conceptions of the task, both working memory and inhibition deficits would have predicted age differences in that it should be harder to keep both alternatives in mind or inhibit the irrelevant grammatical option. Additionally, the findings by Davidson et al. (2003) are interesting because they provide some evidence that the production deficit found at the lexical level does not replicate for sentence production. Another area where we see syntactic preservation in old age is for subject–verb agreement. Thornton, Skovbroten, and Burke (2004) found that overall older adults produced more agreement errors than young adults, but that age did not interact with syntactic variables known to affect agreement (i.e., number). Although age-related memory problems might affect overall error rate, syntactic processing appears to be constant across age here.

Still, on-line sentence production studies that have used more demanding tasks have observed age differences consistent with greater working memory limitations in older adults. Kemper, Herman, and Liu (2004) gave both young and older participants sentence fragments to memorize that varied in syntactic complexity. Participants then had to produce a complete sentence using the fragment. The length, complexity, and propositional content of the young participants' responses were all affected by the complexity manipulation, whereas this was not the case for the older participants' responses. One explanation of this finding is that the difficulty for older adults lies in the comprehension of the material to be retained for elaboration. Also, young adults produce more syntactically complex sentences than older adults when the verb provided takes a complement (Kemper, Herman, & Lian, 2003). Thus, this line of research provides evidence consistent with more naturalistic studies that working memory limitations constrain language production in older adults.

The kind of working memory assumed in accounts of age differences in interpretive processes in sentence production has received little attention. In a novel approach to constrained sentence production, Spieler and Griffin (in press) asked young and older participants to describe pictures containing two objects above a third one and analyzed duration of gazes to pictures, picture name production latencies, and speech disfluencies. They found very similar rates of speech although older adults were slower to initiate speech, similar gaze patterns, and similar delays associated with the difficulty of retrieving words. Moreover, there was evidence that both groups uttered object names shortly after retrieving them, with little buffering of object names while names of other objects to be produced later were accessed. However, when later objects were less codable (had two or more acceptable and presumably competing names) and when phonological encoding was slowed by low frequency names, older adults were considerably more disfluent. Spieler and Griffin (2005) noted that such results are beyond the explanatory power of general slowing theories, which have no detailed way to explain both those aspects of older adults' speech that slowed and the fact of disfluencies in the face of lexical competition. They suggested that the transmission deficit hypothesis can account for their results because the activation of competing lexical names for an object could lead to convergence of semantic priming on more than one lexical node.

We should note that interpretation of constrained sentence processing tasks is not altogether straightforward. These tasks all require comprehension of the material to be produced. Also, one important aspect of production is repair of errors, a topic that is little studied by

cognitive aging researchers (for an exception, see MacKay & James, 2004) but has been the object of study in the production literature more generally (Hartsuiker & Kolk, 2001; Levelt, 1989). Many accounts of monitoring for errors posit that speech is fed back through the comprehension system. Predictions about monitoring differences across age might vary depending on whether comprehension processes during production are thought to tap a separate sentence interpretation resource or some more general resource.

III. Discourse Processes

A. Hearing Loss and Listening Comprehension

Schneider, Daneman, and Pichora-Fuller (2002) have argued that many age-related changes in comprehension of spoken language are due to lower level auditory declines instead of actual high-level changes in linguistic processing. Schneider et al. (2000) investigated age differences in spoken discourse by having both young and older adults listen to passages read in either a quiet or a noisy background. Despite the fact that older adults had good hearing, they answered fewer questions about the passages correctly than young adults. Schneider et al. (2000) hypothesized that the difference might be due to subclinical auditory problems in older adults. To test this hypothesis, they equated the signal-to-noise ratio on a participant-by-participant basis. When the signal-to-noise ratio was equated, no age differences in comprehension were found. Interestingly, adding a secondary task to divide attention had negative effects on comprehension for both young and old, but older adults were not differentially impaired, suggesting that distraction may not have more deleterious consequences for older adults when perceptual stress is equated.

Thus, this study provides good evidence that even subclinical age-related auditory declines can have significant effects on higher level language comprehension. Results from Federmeier et al. (2003) are interesting in this context. As noted earlier, they reported slowing of evoked potential responses at the sensory level in older adults and age differences at the discourse level, but interestingly, no differences at the lexical-semantic level.

One explanation of such effects is that older adults who have poorer processing of acoustic details of speech reallocate cognitive resources to determine the meanings of words from context with the result that higher level processes needed for integration of information (including working memory) suffer (Pichora-Fuller et al., 1995; see also Rabbitt, 1968, 1991). Evidence supporting this proposition comes from a study by McCoy et al. (2005). Older adults with good hearing and older adults with mild–moderate hearing loss were tested in a running memory span task that required recall of the last three words in speech that varied in approximation to English. Even though the hearing loss group could remember the most recent word as well as the good hearing group and though both groups could recall the first two words of a string quite well when approximation to English was high, performance for both groups, especially for the hearing loss group, was poorer when sequential constraints were low. The assumption here is that recall of the final words is proof that all words were perceived correctly by both groups (because the list could be stopped at any point), but that speech perception required extra resources in the hearing loss group that could otherwise have been devoted to maintenance of information in working memory (see also Murphy et al., 2000). As these results suggest, and consistent with the findings of Federmeier et al. (2003),

the effects of sensory deficits are complex and may appear at different levels in different paradigms.

B. Situation Models and Discourse Comprehension

Updating a situation model involves tracking new people and objects that are introduced by the text, causal sequences, temporal and spatial shifts, and changes in the goals and emotional responses of characters. Inferences must often be generated to maintain discourse coherence, although the extent and timing of such inferences have been debated (Kintsch, 1998; McKoon & Ratcliff, 1992). A hypothesis that has garnered considerable recent attention is the possibility that older adults differ from young adults in lower (especially textbase) but not higher (situation model) levels of discourse comprehension.

There is clear evidence from both on-line and off-line paradigms for similar sensitivity to variables that influence situation model or discourse representations across age and, sometimes, for greater dedication of resources (i.e., reading time) to these variables on the part of older adults (Radvansky et al., 2001). For instance, young and older adults are equally responsive to changes in the goal status of characters in a narrative (Radvansky & Curiel, 1998), to shifts in the location of characters and objects within a spatial layout (Radvansky et al., 2003a; Stine-Morrow et al., 2004; Stine-Morrow, Morrow, & Leno, 2002), to the importance of functional spatial locations such as the consequences of standing under a street lamp or a bridge to avoid rain (Radvansky, Copeland, & Zwaan, 2003), to relative shifts in time requiring updating (Radvansky et al., 2003a), to incongruities of emotional responses of characters to situations (Soederberg & Stine, 1995), to discrepancies in the appearance of objects in pictures and information in a text (Dijkstra et al., 2004), to causal relationships between sentences (Hess, 1995; Radvansky et al., 1990; Valencia-Laver & Light, 2000), and to topic shifts (Miller et al., 2004). Allocation of resources to textbase and situation model features can also vary with whether the text is being read initially or is being reread, and allocation strategies appear to depend on age and, within individuals, on text genre (Stine-Morrow et al., 2004). A noteworthy finding is that for both expository and narrative prose, older adults allocated more attention to situation model features on first but not second reading. Generally speaking, across studies in Stine-Morrow's work, young and older adults perform at similarly high levels on off-line tasks, with young and older adults' different in resource allocation strategies both promoting good performance.

With minor exceptions, young and old readers are similarly influenced by story structure variables in terms of reading times (Stine-Morrow, Miller, & Leno, 2001). People generally read faster as they proceed through a text so that less time is spent on sentences later in a passage. Following Gernsbacher (1990), this variable is sometimes treated as evidence that more resource investment (time) is needed early in passage reading to establish the basic form of the situation model, but this interpretation is not universal (e.g., Radvansky et al., 2001). Nonetheless, we note that older adults generally show at least as great an effect of serial position as young adults (e.g., Stine-Morrow et al., 1996).

C. Discourse Production

Processes involved in drawing anaphoric (and other) inferences also appear to be well preserved in old age unless working memory is taxed or specific bits of

recently presented information must be retrieved actively over delays (Light & Albertson, 1988; Light & Capps, 1986; Light et al., 1994; Morrow, Leirer, & Altieri, 1992; Zelinski, 1988) or unless the inference requires understanding unfamiliar words (McGinnis & Zelinski, 2000, 2003) or eponyms (Zelinski & Hyde, 1996). One result that bears note here is the finding by Hamm and Hasher (1992) that when reading garden path passages, in which a plausible interpretation of an event is later shown to be incorrect, older adults are more likely to maintain both correct and incorrect inferences than young adults, consistent with a problem in inhibition. This finding is at odds with the fact that young and older adults are equally able to background completed goals. Radvansky and Curiel (1998) suggested that older adults may have difficulty in relinquishing incorrect inferences when these are both wrong and strong, which was not the case in the goals study. This hypothesis has not, to our knowledge, been submitted to empirical test as yet. Also, there is reason to believe that young adults do not invariably give up incorrect interpretations of sentences readily, so that the Hamm and Hasher (1992) findings may be the exception rather than the rule (Christianson et al., 2001).

As noted earlier, Kemper and colleagues observed a marked reduction in syntactic complexity in older adults in both longitudinal and cross-sectional studies. At the same time, there is evidence for increased skill in situation model level aspects of discourse. Older adults' written diaries and oral stories are more structurally complex than those of young adults in that they include multiple episodes, embedded episodes, and codas that draw a moral lesson from events being narrated (Kemper, 1990; Kemper et al., 1989, 1990; Pratt et al., 1989; Pratt & Robins, 1991). In addition, discourse produced by older adults is rated at least as highly (and sometimes more highly) as that of young adults for story quality, interest, clarity, and informativeness (James et al., 1999; Kemper, 1990; Kemper et al., 1989, 1990; Pratt et al., 1989; Pratt & Robins, 1991). When asked to interpret stories they have read, older adults are more likely to generate elaborated, integrative, symbolically rich responses than young adults, although older adults may recall less of the literal propositional content when asked to do so (Adams et al., 1997).

The conjunction of reduced syntactic complexity and increased narrative quality or focus on discourse level has been interpreted variously as an accommodation to decreases in processing resources or to growing expertise in the communicative nature of discourse (Adams et al., 1997; Kemper, 1990; Kemper et al., 1990), as well as to differences across age in the interpretation of what it means to tell a story or recall a narrative (Adams et al., 2002). This pattern of reduced grammatical complexity, increased structural complexity, and greater elaboration does not, however, mean that all aspects of discourse become more reader or listener friendly in old age. Decreased cohesiveness and greater likelihood of ambiguous reference have also been reported (e.g., Cohen, 1979; Glosser & Deser, 1992; Kemper, 1990; Kemper et al., 1990; Pratt et al., 1989).

D. Off-Target Verbosity

One area in which discourse production of older adults has been said to deteriorate is the ability to remain on topic during conversations. Although older adults do not give off-topic responses with greater frequency than young adults in speech production tasks that do not involve discourse (Burke, 1997), there have been reports of decreased global coherence associated with less good topical organization (Glosser & Deser, 1992) in older

adults. When asked to answer questions about their lives or to narrate personal experiences, older adults do generate longer (more verbose) responses than young adults. In samples of adults over 60 years of age, extreme off-target verbosity may occur in as much as 20% of individuals (Arbuckle & Pushkar Gold, 1993; Gold et al., 1988; Pushkar Gold & Arbuckle, 1995) and has been associated with lower performance on some cognitive tasks that are purported markers of ability to inhibit irrelevant stimuli, less good management of instrumental activities of daily life, and psychosocial variables such as diminished satisfaction with social support. Off-target verbosity may limit the quality of social interactions by making interpersonal communication less satisfying for conversational partners (Pushkar Gold et al., 2000). Indeed, when compared to speakers who are verbose but not off-topic and to on-target speakers, off-target speakers are rated more negatively on dimensions such as intellectual competence, speed of learning, and forgetfulness (Ruscher & Hurley, 2000), and other studies suggest that off-target speakers may be less sensitive to the communicative needs of their partners (Arbuckle, Nohara-LeClair, & Pushkar, 2000).

The generality of off-target verbosity as a characteristic of the discourse of older adults has nevertheless been questioned. For instance, Vandeputte et al. (1999) found no age differences in topic continuations in the get-acquainted conversations of same and mixed-age dyads of younger and older adults. Off-target utterances, when they occur, may be specific to situations in which personal information or experience is transmitted. Comparing young and older adults (aged 60–80) on both descriptions of pictures and narrations of personal topics dealing with family, education, and vacations, James et al. (1999) found that the total number of words elicited for personal topics, but not picture descriptions, was greater for older adults, and the effect for personal topics persisted when only on-topic speech was considered. In addition, instances of off-topic speech were more frequent for older than young adults only for personal topics. Young and older raters judged older speakers as more talkative than younger speakers and young speakers thought the older speakers were less focused on topics. However, older speakers were rated as higher on interest, informativeness, and story quality. James et al. (1999) argued that this pattern of results is inconsistent with inhibitory deficit accounts of off-target speech that have no principled way of accounting for differences across categories of topics and predicted that off-target verbosity should lead to low communicative efficiency, with poorer evaluations of story quality. Instead they suggested that older adults have differences in pragmatic aspects of discourse, placing greater value on meaningful interpretation of past events rather than concise factual descriptions (e.g., Boden & Bielby, 1983; Coupland & Coupland, 1995).

E. Language Addressed to Older Adults: Elderspeak

Negative assumptions about the communicative skills of older adults may lead to inappropriate overaccommodation by young adults who use a specialized speech register resembling baby talk in addressing older adults (Caporael, Lukaszewski, & Culbertson, 1983; Hummert et al., 2004; Ryan et al., 1986). This speech register, usually referred to as *elderspeak*, differs from speech addressed to young adults in information content and packaging. Kemper (1994) reported that speech addressed to older audiences (rather than younger ones) was characterized by fewer clauses per

utterance, shorter utterances, fewer left-branching or self-embedded clauses, more lexical fillers (e.g., you know), more sentence fragments, fewer cohesive ties, fewer words of three or more syllables, more repetitions, slower speech rate, and longer pauses. In addition, the use of diminutives was more frequent in addressing dementing than nondementing older adults in this study, but this may be context specific, inasmuch as young speakers in mixed-age dyads rarely use diminutives in referential communication tasks (Kemper et al., 1995, 1998c). Evaluations of elderspeak may be moderated by context (e.g. institutional vs community settings), characteristics of the listener (e.g., degree of cognitive impairment), and relationship of speaker and listener (e.g., relative vs unfamiliar service provider), but such speech is generally judged to be both inappropriate and patronizing (Hummert & Mazloff, 2001; Kemper et al., 1998a; LaTourette & Meeks, 2000; O'Connor & St. Pierre, 2004; Ryan et al., 2000).

To some extent, use of elderspeak is driven by stereotypical expectations rather than by the actual characteristics of conversational partners. For instance, speech addressed to dementing and nondementing older adults varied very little (Kemper, 1994). Young speakers do not vary speech to older partners in a referential communication task very much regardless of whether the listeners are allowed to interrupt by asking questions or requesting clarification or to provide other feedback (Kemper et al., 1995, 1996). However, repeated practice on the same task (Kemper et al., 1998c), listener speech suggesting cognitive impairment (Kemper et al., 1998b), and simulation of speech to adults experiencing cognitive problems rather than living healthy, independent lives in the community (Kemper et al., 1998a) do lead to exaggerated forms of elderspeak in a referential communication task, suggestive of responsiveness to the communicative needs of partners in this task. Older adults also receive more patronizing messages in a simulated persuasion task, especially if targets are described negatively (Hummert et al., 1998).

Although often viewed as stigmatizing speech, some elements of elderspeak may benefit performance in older adults (Cohen & Faulkner, 1986; McGuire et al., 2000). Performance in a referential communication task is better when older adults receive instruction from young speakers (e.g., Kemper et al., 1995, 1996), but at a cost—older adults also report more expressive and receptive communication problems when interacting with young speakers. This conjunction of improved performance, together with negative self-evaluation, has led to a search for versions of elderspeak that impart performance benefits without being patronizing or insulting (Ryan et al., 1995; Williams, Kemper, & Hummert, 2003). Kemper and Harden (1999), in a careful dissection of the properties of elderspeak, found that increasing semantic elaborations and reducing use of subordinate and embedded clauses improved performance on a referential communication task, but that reduced sentence length, slower speech rate, and higher pitch did not; the latter trio of properties also increased complaints of communication problems.

According to the communicative predicament of aging model (Ryan et al., 1986; see Coupland et al., 1988), recognition of old-age cues triggers stereotyped expectations about aging that give rise to overaccommodative speech to older adults. Recipients of elderspeak may experience diminished self-esteem, reduced communication efficacy, dissatisfaction with communication, and, ultimately, diminished social interaction and loss of control. A revised and elaborated version of this model, the age stereotypes in the interaction model, accounts for both positive and negative effects of stereotypes in communication and includes a feedback mechanism that permits revision of the assessment of the communicative competency of conversational partners (Hummert et al., 2004). In line with this model, older targets that evoke positive rather than negative stereotypes of aging are judged higher in communicative competence (Hummert, Garstka, & Shaner, 1995), instructions to competent older targets contain less patronizing speech (Thimm, Rademacher, Kruse, 1998), and humorous responses by older adults to patronizing speech appear to permit assertiveness without loss of appearance of competence and politeness (Hummert & Mazloff, 2001; Ryan et al., 2000).

Thus far, we have discussed only research on language in intergenerational dyads that has focused on overaccommodative speech by young adults. Interestingly, in referential communication tasks, older adults vary little in the ways in which they convey route information to young and older targets (Kemper et al., 1995, 1996). This does not appear to reflect an inability to change register as a result of working memory or other global age-related deficits—older adults do accommodate when speaking to cognitively impaired partners (Gould & Shaleen, 1999; Kemper et al., 1994) and in retelling stories to children (Adams et al., 2002). There are heated debates in the psycholinguistic literature about issues of common ground—the extent to which speakers take into account the specific conversational needs of their audience (Horton & Keysar, 1996; Lockridge & Brennan, 2002). An important but understudied question is whether there are age differences in the ability to take common ground into consideration. A related issue is the role of gesture, body language, and facial expression in communication by and to older adults. Although these topics have attracted interest in the wider research community (Goldin-Meadow, Alibali, & Church, 1993; McNeil, 1992), they represent terra almost incognita in the language and aging literature (for some exceptions, see Cohen & Borsoi, 1996; Feyereisen & Havard, 1999; Montepare et al., 1999).

IV. A Concluding Word

Many of the broad models of cognitive aging are simply too general to account for the diverse range of data. General slowing cannot readily account for processing asymmetries in lexical processing or for differences in outcomes within single tasks [e.g., different distributions of speech errors across age found by MacKay and James, (2004)]. In some instances, theoretical constructs are in flux or not sufficiently unpacked to be useful in explaining particular patterns of results. Inhibition deficit theory has been criticized for insufficient specificity of its theoretical constructs in particular paradigms [Burke (1997), but see Sommers (1996) for a more specific inhibition account of neighborhood effects]. Although single resource working memory hypotheses have been pitted against multiple resource hypotheses in the context of aging research, some psycholinguistic theorists have argued that there is no working memory resource separate from general processing (MacDonald & Christiansen, 2002). As crucial constructs shift in interpretation, our understanding of the relationships among these constructs, language, and aging will perforce change too.

Unlike the transmission deficit model, the general slowing, working memory, and inhibition deficit hypotheses all lack specific cognitive architectures within which processes might act. This is not a necessary feature of such approaches.

For example, one could imagine embedding an account of inhibition deficits within a specific architecture, such as that of the transmission deficit model, which might allow it to make principled predictions about paradigms to which it has been applied. Even models that do have specific cognitive architectures may lack mechanisms for carrying out particular kinds of language processes. As a case in point, the transmission deficit model does not have a fully developed syntactic processor. Extensions to syntactic processing are possible within the general framework of the transmission deficit model (MacKay & James, 2001b) and it would be interesting to see how it accounts for classic syntactic phenomena.

As emphasized throughout this chapter, understanding the effects of normal aging on language processing requires attention to a complex interaction of processes, from low-level sensory deficits that can affect high-level discourse processes and vice versa. Current models of cognitive aging have typically been applied to only a subset of the phenomena we have discussed at word, sentence, and discourse levels of language comprehension and production. For example, the transmission deficit hypothesis has been applied primarily to lexical processing, whereas working memory accounts of various types have been developed almost exclusively in the realms of sentence and discourse processing. Moreover, the influence of lower level sensory deficits, which can have substantial effects on working memory and higher level comprehension, has generally not played a large role in theory development. To give one example, one could imagine a more explicit model of sensory deficits that would explain some of the phenomena accounted for by inhibition deficits or transmission deficits, perhaps as a result of weakened activation in the system. One could also ask how a separate sentence interpretation resource model might expect interpretive processes to operate on and repair low-quality sensory inputs and how top–down information might offset those degraded representations. Similarly, Waters and Caplan's working memory accounts have been applied for the most part to the syntactic comprehension of single sentences, whereas existing data suggest that working memory can strongly influence the production of language and such models have been much less applied to language processing in connected discourse. Thus, one obvious direction for future research on language and aging is greater theoretical integration across levels of processing in comprehension and production. Incorporating pragmatic aspects of language use such as common ground and accommodation into these approaches serves as a further challenge for cognitive aging researchers.

Acknowledgment

The authors would like to thank Susan Kemper and Patricia Tun for comments on an earlier version of this chapter.

References

Abrams, L., & Rodriguez, E. L. (in press). Syntactic class influences phonological priming of tip-of-the-tongue resolution. *Psychonomic Bulletin & Review*.

Abrams, L., & Stanley, J. H. (2004). The detection and retrieval of spelling in older adults. In S. P. Shohov (Ed.), *Advances in psychology research* (Vol. 33). Hauppauge, NY: Nova Science.

Abrams, L., White, K. K., & Eitel, S. L. (2003). Isolating phonological components that increase tip-of-the-tongue resolution. *Memory & Cognition, 31,* 1153–1162.

Adams, C., Smith, M. C., Nyquist, L., & Perlmutter, M. (1997). Adult age-group differences in recall for the literal and interpretive meanings of narrative text. *Journal of Gerontology: Psychological Sciences, 52B,* 187–195.

Adams, C., Smith, M. C., Pasupathi, M., & Vitolo, L. (2002). Social context effects on story recall in older and younger women: Does the listener make a difference? *Journal of Gerontology: Psychological Sciences, 57B,* 28–40.

Allen, P. A., Madden, D. J., Weber, T. A., & Groth, K. E. (1993). Influence of age and processing stage on visual word recognition. *Psychology and Aging, 8,* 274–282.

Altmann, L. J. P., Kemper, S., Mullin, D. A., & Mathews, A. (2004). *Syntactic priming in older adults*. Poster session presented at the Tenth Cognitive Aging Conference, Atlanta, GA.

Arbuckle, T. Y., Nohara-LeClair, M., & Pushkar, D. (2000). Effect of off-target verbosity on communication efficiency in a referential communication task. *Psychology and Aging, 15,* 65–77.

Arbuckle, T. Y., & Pushkar Gold, D. (1993). Aging, inhibition, and verbosity. *Journal of Gerontology: Psychological Sciences, 48,* 225–232.

Baltes, P. B., & Lindenberger, U. (1997). Emergence of a powerful connection between sensory and cognitive functions across the adult life span: A new window to the study of cognitive aging? *Psychology and Aging, 12,* 12–21.

Barresi, B. A., Obler, L. K., & Goodglass, H. (1998). Dissociation between proper name and common noun learning. *Brain and Cognition, 37,* 21–23.

Baum, S. R. (2003). Age differences in the influence of metrical structure on phonetic identification. *Speech Communication, 39,* 231–242.

Boden, D., & Bielby, D. (1983). The past as resource: A conversational analysis of elderly talk. *Human Development, 26,* 308–319.

Bortfeld, H., Leon, S., Bloom, J., Schober, M., & Brennan, S. (2001). Disfluency rates in conversation: Effects of age, relationship, topic, role, and gender. *Language and Speech, 44,* 123–147.

Burke, D. M. (1997). Language, aging, and inhibitory deficits: Evaluation of a theory. *Journal of Gerontology: Psychological Sciences, 52B,* 254–264.

Burke, D. M., & Light, L. L. (1981). Memory and aging: The role of retrieval processes. *Psychological Bulletin, 90,* 513–546.

Burke, D. M., Locantore, J., Austin, A., & Chae, B. (2004). Cherry pit primes Brad Pitt: Homophone priming effects on young and older adults' production of proper names. *Psychological Science, 15,* 164–170.

Burke, D. M., & MacKay, D. G. (1997). Memory, language, and aging. *Philosophical Transactions of the Royal Society, Biological Sciences, 352,* 1845–1856.

Burke, D. M., MacKay, D. G., & James, L. E. (2000). Theoretical approaches to language and aging. In T. Perfect & E. Maylor (Eds.), *Models of cognitive aging* (pp. 204–237). Oxford, UK: Oxford University Press.

Burke, D. M., MacKay, D.G, Worthley, J. S., & Wade, E. (1991). On the tip of the tongue: What causes word finding failures in young and older adults? *Journal of Memory and Language, 30,* 542–579.

Cabeza, R., Nyberg, L., & Park, D. (Eds.) (2004). *Cognitive neuroscience of aging: Linking cognitive and cerebral aging.* New York: Oxford University Press.

Caplan, D., & Waters, G. S. (1999). Verbal working memory and sentence comprehension. *Behavioral and Brain Sciences, 22,* 77–94.

Caporael, L. R., Lukaszewski, M. P., & Culbertson, G. H. (1983). Secondary baby talk: Judgments by institutionalized elderly and their caregivers. *Journal of Personality and Social Psychology, 44,* 746–754.

Carpenter, P. A., Miyake, A., & Just, M. A. (1994). Working memory constraints in comprehension: Evidence from individual differences, aphasia, and aging. In M. A. Gernsbacher, (Ed.) *The handbook of psycholinguistics.* San Diego: Academic Press.

Carstensen, L. L., Isaacowitz, D., & Charles, S. T. (1999). Taking time seriously: A theory of socioemotional selectivity. *American Psychologist, 54,* 165–181.

Christianson, K., Hollingworth, A., Halliwell, J., & Ferreira, F. (2001). Thematic roles assigned along the garden path linger. *Cognitive Psychology, 42,* 368–407.

Cohen, G. (1979). Language comprehension in old age. *Cognitive Psychology, 11,* 412–429.

Cohen, G., & Faulkner, D. (1986). Does "elderspeak" work? The effect of intonation and stress on comprehension and recall of spoken discourse in old age. *Language & Communication, 6,* 99–112.

Cohen, R., & Borsoi, D. (1996). The role of gestures in description-communication: A cross-sectional study of aging. *Journal of Nonverbal Behavior, 20,* 45–63.

Committee on Hearing, Bioacoustics and Biomechanics (CHABA) (1988). Speech understanding and aging. *Journal of the Acoustical Society of America, 83,* 859–895.

Connor, L. T., Spiro, A., Obler, L. K., & Albert, M. L. (2004). Change in object naming ability during adulthood. *Journal of Gerontology: Psychological Sciences, 59,* P203–P209.

Cortese, M. J., Balota, D. A., Sergent-Marshall, S. D., & Buckner, R. L. (2003). Sublexical, lexical, and semantic influences in spelling: Exploring the effects of age, Alzheimer's disease and primary semantic impairment. *Neuropsychologia, 41,* 952–967.

Coupland, J., Coupland, N., Giles, H., & Henwood, K. (1988). Accommodating the elderly: Invoking and extending a theory. *Ageing and Society, 11,* 189–208.

Coupland, N., & Coupland, J. (1995). Discourse, identity, and aging. In J. F. Nussbaum & J. Coupland (Eds) *Handbook of communication and aging research* (pp. 79–103). Hillsdale, NJ: Lawrence Erlbaum.

Cross, E. S., & Burke, D. M. (2004). Do alternative names block young and older adults' retrieval of proper names? *Brain and Language, 89,* 174–181.

Davidson, D. J., Zacks, R. T., & Ferreira, F. (2003). Age preservation of the syntactic processor in production. *Journal of Psycholinguistic Research, 32,* 541–566.

DeDe, G., Caplan, D., Kemtes, K., & Waters, G. S. (2004). The relationship between age, verbal working memory, and language comprehension. *Psychology and Aging, 19,* 601–616.

Dell, G. S., Burger, L. K., & Svec, W. R. (1997). Language production and serial order: A functional analysis and a model. *Psychological Review, 104,* 123–147.

Dijkstra, K., Yaxley, R. H., Madden, C. J., & Zwaan, R. A. (2004). The role of age and perceptual symbols in language comprehension. *Psychology and Aging, 19*, 352–356.

Evrard, M. (2002). Ageing and lexical access to common and proper names in picture naming. *Brain and Language, 81*, 174–179.

Federmeier, K. D., Van Petten, C., Schwartz, T. J., & Kutas, M. (2003). Sounds, words, sentences: Age-related changes across levels of language processing. *Psychology and Aging, 18*, 858–872.

Feyereisen, P., & Havard, I. (1999). Mental imagery and production of hand gestures while speaking in younger and older adults. *Journal of Nonverbal Behavior, 23*, 153–171.

Frisina, D. R., & Frisina, R. D. (1997). Speech recognition in noise and presbycusis: Relations to possible neural mechanisms. *Hearing Research, 106*, 95–104.

Gernsbacher, M. A. (1990). *Language comprehension as structure building.* Hillsdale, NJ: Lawrence Erlbaum.

Glosser, G., & Deser, T. (1992). A comparison of changes in macrolinguistic and microlinguistic aspects of discourse production in normal aging. *Journal of Gerontology: Psychological Sciences, 47*, 266–272.

Gold, D., Andres, S. D., Arbuckle, T., & Schwartzman, A. (1988). Measurement and correlates of verbosity in elderly people. *Journal of Gerontology: Psychological Sciences, 43*, 27–34.

Goldin-Meadow, S., Alibali, M. W., & Church, R. B. (1993). Transitions in concept-acquisition: Using the hand to read the mind. *Psychological Review, 100*, 279–297.

Gordon-Salant, S., & Fitzgibbons, P. J. (2001). Sources of age-related recognition difficulty for time-compressed speech. *Journal of Speech, Language, & Hearing Research, 44*, 709–719.

Gould, O. N., & Shaleen, L. (1999). Collaboration with diverse partners: How older women adapt their speech. *Journal of Language and Social Psychology, 18*, 395–418.

Griffin, Z. M., & Spieler, D. H. (in press). Observing the what and when of language production for different age groups by monitoring speakers' eye movements. *Brain and Language.*

Hamm, V. P., & Hasher, L. (1992). Age and the availability of inferences. *Psychology and Aging, 7*, 56–64.

Hartman, M. (1995). Aging and interference: Evidence from indirect memory tests. *Psychology and Aging, 10*, 659–669.

Hartman, M., & Hasher, L. (1991). Aging and suppression: Memory for previously relevant information. *Psychology and Aging, 6*, 587–594.

Hartsuiker, R. J., & Kolk, H. H. J. (2001). Error monitoring in speech production: A computational test of the perceptual loop theory. *Cognitive Psychology, 42*, 113–157.

Hasher, L., Quig, M. B., & May, C. P. (1997). Inhibitory control over no longer relevant information. *Memory & Cognition, 25*, 286–295.

Hasher, L., & Zacks, R. T. (1988). Working memory, comprehension and aging: A review and a new view. *The Psychology of Learning and Motivation, 22*, 193–225.

Heine, M. K., Ober, B. A., & Shenaut, G. K. (1999). Naturally occurring and experimentally induced tip-of-the-tongue experiences in three adult age groups. *Psychology and Aging, 14*, 445–457.

Hess, T. M. (1995). Aging and the impact of causal connections on text comprehension and memory. *Aging and Cognition, 2*, 216–230.

Horton, W. S., & Keysar, B. (1996). When do speakers take into account common ground? *Cognition, 59*, 91–117.

Humes, L. E. (1996). Speech understanding in the elderly. *Journal of the American Academy of Audiology, 7*, 161–167.

Hummert, M. L., Garstka, T. A., Ryan, E. B., & Bonnesen, J. L. (2004). The role of age stereotypes in interpersonal communication. In J. F. Nussbaum & J. Coupland (Eds.), *Handbook of communication and aging research* (2nd edition, pp. 91–114). Mahwah, NJ: Lawrence Erlbaum.

Hummert, M. L., Garstka, T. A., & Shaner, J. L. (1995). Beliefs about language performance: Adults' perceptions about self and elderly targets. *Journal of Language and Social Psychology, 14*, 235–259.

Hummert, M. L., & Mazloff, D. C. (2001). Older adults' responses to patronizing advice: Balancing politeness and identity in context. *Journal of Language and Social Psychology, 20*, 168–196.

Hummert, M. L., Shaner, J. L., Garstka, T. A., & Henry, C. (1998). Communication with older adults: The influence of age stereotypes, content, and communicator age. *Human Communication Research, 81*, 774–788.

James, L. E. (2004). Meeting Mr. Farmer versus meeting a farmer: Specific effects of aging on learning proper names. *Psychology and Aging, 19*, 515–522.

James, L. E., & Burke, D. M. (2000). Phonological priming effects on word retrieval and tip-of-the-tongue experiences in young and older adults. *Journal of Experimental Psychology: Learning, Memory, and Cognition, 26*, 1378–1391.

James, L. E., Burke, D. M., Austin, A., & Hulme, E. (1999). Production and perception of "verbosity" in younger and older adults. *Psychology and Aging, 13*, 355–367.

Just, M. A., & Carpenter, P. A. (1992). A capacity theory of comprehension: Individual differences in working memory. *Psychological Review, 98*, 122–149.

Kemper, S. (1990). Adults' diaries: Changes to written narratives across the life span. *Discourse Processes, 13*, 207–223.

Kemper, S. (1994). Elderspeak: Speech accommodations to older adults. *Aging and Cognition, 1*, 17–28.

Kemper, S., Anagnopoulos, C., Lyons, K., & Heberlein, W. (1994). Speech accommodations to dementia. *Journal of Gerontology: Psychological Sciences, 49*, P223–P230.

Kemper, S., Crow, A., & Kemtes, K. (2004). Eye-fixation patterns of high- and low-span young and older adults: Down the garden path and back again. *Psychology and Aging, 19*, 157–170.

Kemper, S., Ferrell, P., Harden, T., Finter-Urczyk, & Billington, C. (1998a). Use of elderspeak by young and older adults to impaired and unimpaired listeners. *Aging, Neuropsychology, and Cognition, 5*, 43–55.

Kemper, S., Finter-Urczyk, A., Ferrell, P., Harden, T., & Billington, C. (1998b). Using elderspeak with older adults. *Discourse Processes, 25*, 55–73.

Kemper, S., Greiner, L. H., Marquis, J. G., Prenovost, K., & Mitzner, T. (2001a). Language decline across the life span: Findings from the Nun study. *Psychology and Aging, 16*, 227–239.

Kemper, S., & Harden, T. (1999). Experimentally disentangling what's beneficial about elderspeak from what's not. *Psychology and Aging, 14*, 656–670.

Kemper, S., Herman, R., & Lian, C. H. T. (2003). Age differences in sentence production. *Journal of Gerontology: Psychological Sciences, 58B*, P260–P268.

Kemper, S., Herman, R. E., & Liu, C.-J. (2004). Sentence production by young and older adults in controlled contexts. *Journal of Gerontology: Psychological Sciences, 59B*, P220–P224.

Kemper, S., Kynette, D., Rash, S., O'Brien, K., & Sprott, R. (1989). Life-span changes to adults' language: Effects of memory and genre. *Applied Psycholinguistics, 10*, 49–66.

Kemper, S., & Lacal, J. C. (2004). Addressing the communication needs of an aging society. R. W. Pew & S. B. Van Hemel (Eds.), *Technology for adaptive aging* (pp. 129–149). Washington, DC: The National Academies Press.

Kemper, S., & Mitzner, T. L. (2001). Production and comprehension. In J. E. Birren & K. W. Schaie (Eds.), *Handbook of the psychology of aging* (5th edition). San Diego: Academic Press.

Kemper, S., Othick, M., Gerhing, H., Gubarchuk, J., & Billington, C. (1998c). The effects of practicing speech accommodations to older adults. *Applied Psycholinguistics, 19*, 175–192.

Kemper, S., Othick, M., Warren, J., Gubarchuk, J., & Gerhing, H. (1996). Facilitating older adults' performance on a referential communication task through speech accommodations. *Aging, Neuropsychology, and Cognition, 3*, 37–55.

Kemper, S., Rash, S., Kynette, D., & Norman, S. (1990). Telling stories: The structure of adults' narratives. *European Journal of Cognitive Psychology, 2*, 205–228.

Kemper, S., Thompson, M., & Marquis, J. (2001b). Longitudinal change in language production: Effects of aging and dementia on grammatical complexity and propositional content. *Psychology and Aging, 16*, 600–614.

Kemper S, Vandeputte, D., Rice, K., Cheung, H., & Gubarchuk, J. (1995).

Speech adjustments to aging during a referential communication task. *Journal of Language and Social Psychology, 14,* 40–59.

Kemtes, K. A., & Kemper, S. (1997). Younger and older adults' on-line processing of syntactically ambiguous sentences. *Psychology and Aging, 12,* 362–371.

Kintsch, W. (1998). *Comprehension: A paradigm for cognition.* New York: Cambridge University Press.

La Tourette, T. R., & Meeks, S. (2000). Perceptions of patronizing speech by older women in nursing homes and in the community: Impact of cognitive ability and place of residence. *Journal of Language and Social Psychology, 19,* 463–473.

Laver, G. D., & Burke, D. M. (1993). Why do semantic priming effects increase in old age? A meta-analysis. *Psychology and Aging, 8,* 34–43.

Levelt, W. J. M. (1989). *Speaking: From intention to articulation.* Cambridge, MA: MIT Press.

Light, L. L. (1988). Language and aging: Competence versus performance. In J. E. Birren & V. L. Bengston (Eds.), *Emergent theories of aging* (pp. 177–213). New York: Springer.

Light, L. L. (1990). Interactions between language and memory in old age. In J. E. Birren & K. W. Schaie (Eds.), *Handbook of the psychology of aging* (3rd edition). New York: Academic Press.

Light, L. L. (1991). Memory and aging: Four hypothesis in search of data. *Annual Review of Psychology, 42,* 333–376.

Light, L. L. (1992). The organization of memory in old age. In F. I. M. Craik & T. A. Salthouse (Eds.), *The handbook of aging and cognition* (pp. 111–165). Hillsdale, NJ: LEA.

Light, L. L. (2000). Memory changes in adulthood. In S. H. Qualls and N. Abeles (Eds.), *Psychology and the aging revolution: How we adapt to longer life* (pp. 73–97). Washington, DC: APA.

Light, L. L., & Albertson, S. A. (1988). Comprehension of pragmatic implications in young and older adults. In L. L. Light and D. M. Burke (Eds.), *Language, memory, and aging* (pp. 133–153). New York: Cambridge University Press.

Light, L. L., & Capps, J. L. (1986). Comprehension of pronouns in young and older adults. *Developmental Psychology, 22,* 580–585.

Light, L. L., Capps, J. L., Singh, A., & Albertson Owens, S. A. (1994). Comprehension and use of anaphoric devices in young and older adults. *Discourse Processes, 18,* 77–103.

Lindenberger, U., Baltes, P. B. (1994). Sensory functioning and intelligence in old age: A strong connection. *Psychology and Aging, 9,* 339–355.

Liu, C. J., Kemper, S., & Herman, R. (2004). *Eye movements of young and older adults in sentence reading.* Poster session presented at the Tenth Cognitive Aging Conference, Atlanta, GA.

Lockridge, C. B., & Brennan, S. E. (2002). Addressees' needs influence speakers' early syntactic choices. *Psychonomic Bulletin & Review, 9,* 550–557.

MacDonald, M. C., & Christiansen, M. H. (2002). Reassessing working memory: A comment on Just & Carpenter (1992) and Waters & Caplan (1996). *Psychological Review, 109,* 35–54.

MacKay, D. G., & Abrams, L. (1996). Language, memory, and aging: Distributed deficits and the structure of new-versus-old connections. In J. E. Birren & K. W. Schaie (Eds.), *Handbook of the psychology of aging* (4th edition, pp. 251–265). San Diego: Academic Press.

MacKay, D. G., & Abrams, L. (1998). Age-linked declines in retrieving orthographic knowledge: Empirical, practical, and theoretical implications. *Psychology and Aging, 13,* 647–662.

MacKay, D. G., Abrams, L., & Pedroza, M. J. (1999). Aging on the input versus output side: Theoretical implications of age-linked asymmetries between detecting versus retrieving orthographic information. *Psychology and Aging, 14,* 3–17.

MacKay, D. G., & James, L. E. (2001a). Is cognitive aging all downhill? Current theory versus reality. *Human Development, 44,* 288–295.

MacKay, D. G., & James, L. E. (2001b). The binding problem for syntax, semantics, and prosody: H. M.'s selective sentence reading deficits under the theoretical–syndrome approach. *Language and Cognitive Processes, 16,* 419–460.

MacKay, D. G., & James, L. E. (2004). Sequencing, speech production, and selective effects of aging on phonological and morphological speech errors. *Psychology and Aging, 19,* 93–107.

MacKay, D. G., & Miller, M. D. (1996). Can cognitive aging contribute to fundamental psychological theory? Repetition deafness as a test case. *Aging, Neuropsychology, and Cognition, 3,* 169–186.

MacKay, D. G., Taylor, J. K., & Marian, D. E. (2005). Unsuspected age-linked acuity deficits and research on reading: Practical and empirical implications. Submitted for publication.

Madden, D. J. (1988). Adult age differences in the effects of sentence context and stimulus degradation during visual word recognition. *Psychology and Aging, 3,* 167–172.

Madden, D. J., Pierce, T. W., & Allen, P. A. (1993). Age-related slowing and the time-course of semantic priming in visual word identification. *Psychology and Aging, 8,* 490–507.

May, C. P., Zacks, R. T., Hasher, L., & Multhaup, K. S. (1999). Inhibition in the processing of garden-path sentences. *Psychology and Aging, 14,* 304–313.

Maylor, E. A. (1990). Recognizing and naming faces: Aging, memory retrieval, and the tip of the tongue state. *Journal of Gerontology, 45,* P215–P226.

Maylor, E. A. (1997). Proper name retrieval in old age: Converging evidence against disproportionate impairment. *Aging, Neuropsychology, and Cognition, 4,* 211–226.

Mayr, U., & Kliegl, R. (2000). Complex semantic processing in old age: Does it stay or does it go? *Psychology and Aging, 15,* 29–43.

McCoy, S. L., Tun, P. A., Cox, L. C., Colangelo, M., Stewart, R. A., & Wingfield, A. (2005). Hearing loss and perceptual effort: Downstream effects on older adults' memory for speech. *Quarterly Journal of Experimental Psychology, 58A,* 22–33.

McGinnis, D., & Zelinski, E. M. (2000). Understanding unfamiliar words: The influence of processing resources, vocabulary knowledge, and age. *Psychology and Aging, 15,* 335–350.

McGinnis, D., & Zelinski, E. M. (2003). Understanding unfamiliar words in young, young-old, and old-old adults: Inferential processing and the abstraction-deficit hypothesis. *Psychology and Aging, 18,* 497–509.

McGuire, L. C., Morian, A., Codding, R., & Smyer, M. A. (2000). Older adults' memory for medical information: Influence of elderspeak and note taking. *International Journal of Rehabilitation and Health, 5,* 117–128.

McKoon, G., & Ratcliff, R. (1992). Inference during reading. *Psychological Review, 99,* 440–466.

McNeil, D. (1992). *Hand and mind.* Chicago: University of Chicago Press.

Miller, L. M. S., & Stine-Morrow, E. A. L. (1998). Aging and the effects of knowledge on on-line reading strategies. *Journal of Gerontology: Psychological Sciences, 53,* P223-P233.

Miller, L. M. S., Stine-Morrow, E. A. L., Kirkorian, H., & Conroy, M. (2004). Adult age differences in knowledge-driven reading. *Journal of Educational Psychology, 96,* 811–821.

Montepare, J., Koff, E., Zaitchik, D., & Albert, M. (1999). The use of body movements and gestures as cues to emotions in younger and older adults. *Journal of Nonverbal Behavior, 23,* 133–152.

Morrow, D. G., Leirer, V. O., & Altieri, P. A. (1992). Aging, expertise, and narrative processing. *Psychology and Aging, 7,* 376–388.

Murphy, D. R., Craik, F. I. M., Li, K., & Schneider, B. A (2000). Comparing the effects of aging and background noise on short-term memory performance. *Psychology and Aging, 15,* 323–334.

O'Connor, B. P., & St. Pierre, E. S. (2004). Older persons' perceptions of the frequency and meaning of elderspeak from family, friends, and service workers. *International Journal of Aging and Human Development, 58,* 197–221.

Pichora-Fuller, M. K. (2003). Processing speed and timing in aging adults: Psychoacoustics, speech perception, and comprehension. *International Journal of Audiology, 42,* S59–S67.

Pichora-Fuller, M. K., Schneider, B. A., & Daneman, M. (1995). How young and old adults listen to and remember speech in noise. *Journal of the Acoustical Society of America, 97*, 593–608.

Pisoni, D. B. (1993). Long-term-memory in speech-perception: Some new findings on talker variability, speaking rate and perceptual-learning. *Speech Communication, 13*, 109–125.

Pratt, M. W., Boyes, C., Robins, S., & Manchester, J. (1989). Telling tales: Aging, working memory, and the narrative cohesion of story retellings. *Developmental Psychology, 25*, 628–635.

Pratt, M. W., & Robins, S. L. (1991). That's the way it was: Age differences in the structure and quality of adults' personal narratives. *Discourse Processes, 14*, 73–85.

Pushkar Gold, D., & Arbuckle, T. Y. (1995). A longitudinal study of off-target verbosity: *Journal of Gerontology: Psychological Sciences, 50B*, 307–315.

Pushkar Gold, D., Basevitz, P., Arbuckle, T., Nohara-LeClair, M., Lapidus, S., & Peled, M. (2000). Social behavior and off-target verbosity in elderly people. *Psychology and Aging, 15*, 361–374.

Rabbitt, P. M. A. (1968). Channel-capacity, intelligibility and immediate memory. *Quarterly Journal of Experimental Psychology, 20*, 241–248.

Rabbitt, P. (1991). Mild hearing loss can cause apparent memory failures which increase with age and reduce with IQ. *Acta Otolaryngolica, 476*, S167–S176.

Radvansky, G. A., Copeland, D. E., Berish, D. E., & Dijkstra, K. (2003a). Aging and situation model updating. *Aging, Neuropsychology, and Cognition, 10*, 158–166.

Radvansky, G. A., Copeland, D. E., & Zwaan, R. A. (2003a). Aging and functional spatial relations in comprehension and memory. *Psychology and Aging, 18*, 161–165.

Radvansky, G. A., & Curiel, J. M. (1998). Narrative comprehension and aging: The fate of completed goal information. *Psychology and Aging, 13*, 69–79.

Radvansky, G. A., Gerard, L. D., Zacks, R. T., & Hasher, L. (1990). Younger and older adults' use of mental models as representations for text materials. *Psychology and Aging, 5*, 209–214.

Radvansky, G. A., Zwaan, R. A., Curiel, J. M., & Copeland, D. E. (2001). Situation models

and aging. *Psychology and Aging, 16*, 145–160.

Ruscher, J. B., & Hurley, M. M. (2000). Off-target verbosity evokes negative stereotypes of older adults. *Journal of Language and Social Psychology, 19*, 141–149.

Ryan, E. B., Giles, H., Bartolucci, G., & Henwood, K. (1986). Psycholinguistic and social psychological components of communication by and with the elderly. *Language & Communication, 6*, 1–24.

Ryan, E. B., Kennaley, D. E., Pratt, M. W., & Shumovich, M. A. (2000). Evaluations by staff, residents, and community seniors of patronizing speech in the nursing home: Impact of passive, assertive, or humorous responses. *Psychology and Aging, 15*, 272–285.

Ryan, E. B., Kwong See, S., Meneer, W. B., & Trovato, D. (1992). Age-based perceptions of language performance among young and older adults. *Communication Research, 19*, 423–443.

Ryan, E. B., Meredith, S. D., MacLean, M. J., & Orange, J. B. (1995). Changing the way we talk with elders: Promoting health using the communication enhancement model. *International Journal of Aging and Human Development, 41*, 89–107.

Salthouse, T. A. (1996). Constraints on theories of cognitive aging. *Psychology and Aging, 3*, 287–299.

Schneider, B. A., Daneman, M., Murphy, D. R., & Kwong See, S. (2000). Listening to discourse in distracting settings: The effects of aging. *Psychology and Aging, 15*, 110–125.

Schneider, B. A., Daneman, M., & Pichora-Fuller, M. K. (2002). Listening in aging adults: From discourse comprehension to psychoacoustics. *Canadian Journal of Experimental Psychology, 56*, 139–152.

Schneider, B. A., & Pichora-Fuller, M. K. (2000). Implications of sensory deficits for cognitive aging. In F. I. M. Craik & T. Salthouse (Eds.), *The handbook of aging and cognition* (2nd edition, pp. 155–219). Mahwah, NJ: Lawrence Erlbaum.

Scialfa, C. T. (2002). The role of sensory factors in cognitive aging research. *Canadian Journal of Experimental Psychology, 56*, 153–163.

Smiler, A. P., Gagne, D. D., & Stine-Morrow, E. A. L. (2003). Aging, memory load, and resource allocation during reading. *Psychology and Aging, 18*, 203–209.

Snowdon, D. A., Kemper, S., Mortimer, J. A., Greiner, L. H., Wekstein, D. R., & Markesbery, W. R. (1996). Cognitive ability in early life and cognitive function and Alzheimer's disease in late life: Findings from the Nun study. *Journal of the American Medical Association, 275*, 528–532.

Soederberg, L. M., & Stine, E. A. L. (1995). Activation of emotion information in text among young and older adults. *Journal of Adult Development, 2*, 23–36.

Sommers, M. S. (1996). The structural organization of the mental lexicon and its contributions to age-related declines in spoken word recognition. *Psychology and Aging, 11*, 333–341.

Sommers, M. S., & Danielson, S. M. (1999). Inhibitory processes and spoken word recognition in young and older adults: The interaction of lexical competition and semantic context. *Psychology and Aging, 14*, 458–472.

Speranza, F., Daneman, M., & Schneider, B. A. (2000). How aging affects the reading of words in noisy backgrounds. *Psychology and Aging, 15*, 253–258.

Spieler, D. H., & Balota, D. A. (2000). Factors influencing word naming in younger and older adults. *Psychology and Aging, 15*, 225–231.

Spieler, D. H., & Griffin, Z. M. (in press). The influence of age on the time course of word preparation in multiword utterances. *Language and Cognitive Processes.*

Stine, E. A. L. (1990). Online processing of written text by younger and older adults. *Psychology and Aging, 5*, 68–78.

Stine, E. A. L., Cheung, H., & Henderson, D. (1995). Adult age-differences in the online processing of new concepts in discourse. *Aging and Cognition, 2*, 1–18.

Stine-Morrow, E. A. L., Gagne, D. D., Morrow, D. G., & DeWall, B. H. (2004). Age differences in rereading. *Memory & Cognition, 32*, 696–710.

Stine-Morrow, E. A. L., Loveless, M. K., & Soederberg, L. M. (1996). Resource allocation in on-line reading by younger and older adults. *Psychology and Aging, 11*, 475–486.

Stine-Morrow, E. A. L., Milinder, L. A., Pullara, O., & Herman, B. (2001). Patterns of resource allocation are reliable among younger and older readers. *Psychology and Aging, 16*, 69–84.

Stine-Morrow, E. A. L., Miller, L. M. S., & Leno, R., III (2001). Aging and resource allocation to narrative text. *Aging, Neuropsychology, and Cognition, 8*, 36–53.

Stine-Morrow, E. A. L., Morrow, D. G., & Leno, R., III (2002). Aging and the representation of spatial situations in narrative understanding. *Journal of Gerontology: Psychological Sciences, 57B*, 91–97.

Stine-Morrow, E. A. L., Ryan, S., & Leonard, J. S. (2000). Age differences in on-line syntactic processing. *Experimental Aging Research, 26*, 315–322.

Stuart-Hamilton, I., & Rabbitt, P. (1997). Age-related decline in spelling ability: A link with fluid intelligence? *Educational Gerontology, 23*, 437–441.

Taylor, J. K., & Burke, D. M. (2002). Asymmetric aging effects on semantic and phonological processes: Naming in the picture-word interference task. *Psychology and Aging, 17*, 662–676.

Tesch-Romer, C. (1997). Psychological effects of hearing aid use in older adults. *Journal of Gerontology: Psychological Sciences, 52*, P127–P138.

Thimm, C., Rademacher, U., & Kruse, L. (1998). Age stereotypes and patronizing messages: Features of age-adapted speech in technical instructions to the elderly. *Journal of Applied Communication Research, 26*, 66–82.

Thornton, R., Skovbroten, K., & Burke, D. M. (2004). *Grammatical agreement processes in young and older adults.* Presented at the Forty-Fifth Annual Meeting of the Psychonomic Society, Minneapolis, MN.

Tremblay, K. L., Piskosz, M., & Souza, P. (2002). Aging alters the neural representation of speech cues. *NeuroReport, 13*, 1865–1870.

Tun, P. A. (1998). Fast noisy speech: Age differences in processing rapid speech with background noise. *Psychology and Aging, 13*, 424–434.

Tun, P. A., & Wingfield A. (1999). One voice too many: Adult age differences in language processing with different types of distracting sounds. *Journal of Gerontology: Psychological Sciences, 54B*, 317–327.

Valencia-Laver, D. L., & Light, L. L. (2000). The occurrence of causal bridging and predictive inferences in young and older adults. *Discourse Processes, 30*, 27–56.

Vandeputte, D. D., Kemper, S., Hummert, M. L., Kemtes, K. A., Shaner, J., & Segrin, C. (1999). Social skills of older people: Conversations in same and mixed age dyads. *Discourse Processes, 27*, 55–76.

Verhaeghen, P. (2003). Aging and vocabulary scores: A meta-analysis. *Psychology and Aging, 18*, 332–339.

Vitevitch, M. S., & Luce, P. A. (1998). When words compete: Levels of processing in perception of spoken words. *Psychological Science, 9*, 325–329.

Vitevitch, M. S., & Sommers, M. S. (2003). The facilitative influence of phonological similarity and neighborhood frequency in speech production in younger and older adults. *Memory & Cognition, 31*, 491–504.

Waters, G. S., & Caplan, D. (1996). The capacity theory of sentence comprehension: Critique of Just and Carpenter (1992). *Psychological Review, 103*, 761–772.

Waters, G. S. & Caplan, D. (2001). Age, working memory and on-line syntactic processing in sentence comprehension. *Psychology and Aging, 16*, 128–144.

Waters, G. S., & Caplan, D. (2005). The relationship between age, processing speed, working memory capacity, and language comprehension. *Memory, 13*, 403–413.

White, K. K., & Abrams, L. (2002). Does priming specific syllables during tip-of-the-tongue states facilitate word retrieval in older adults? *Psychology and Aging, 17*, 226–235.

White, K. K., & Abrams, L. (2004). Phonologically mediated priming of preexisting and new associations in young and older adults. *Journal of Experimental Psychology: Learning, Memory, and Cognition, 30*, 645–655.

Whiting, W. L., Madden, D. J., Langley, L. K., Denny, L. L., Turkington, T. G., Provenzale, J. M., Hawk, T. C., & Coleman, R. E. (2003). Lexical and sublexical components of age-related changes in neural activation during visual word identification. *Journal of Cognitive Neuroscience, 15*, 475–487.

Williams, K., Kemper, S., & Hummert, M. L. (2003). Improving nursing home communication: An intervention to reduce elderspeak. *The Gerontologist, 43*, 242–247.

Wingfield, A., Alexander, A. H., & Cavigelli, S. (1994). Does memory constrain utilization of top–down information in spoken word recognition? Evidence from normal aging. *Language and Speech, 37*, 221–235.

Wingfield, A., Lindfield, K. C., & Goodglass, H. (2000). Effects of age and hearing sensitivity on the use of prosodic information in spoken word recognition. *Journal of Speech, Language, and Hearing Research, 43*, 915–925.

Wingfield, A., Poon, L. W., Lombardi, L., & Lowe, D. (1985). Speed of processing in normal aging: Effects of speech rate, linguistic structure, and processing time. *Journal of Gerontology, 40*, 579–585.

Wingfield, A., & Stine-Morrow, E. A. L. (2000). Language and speech. In F. I. M. Craik & T. A. Salthouse (Eds). *Handbook of Aging and Cognition* (2nd edition, pp. 359–416). Mahwah, NJ: Erlbaum.

Wingfield, A., & Tun, P. A. (2001). Spoken language comprehension in older adults: Interactions between sensory and cognitive change in normal aging. *Seminars in Hearing, 22*, 287–301.

Yonan, C. A., & Sommers, M. S. (2000). The effects of talker familiarity on spoken word identification in younger and older listeners. *Psychology and Aging, 15*, 88–99.

Zacks, R. T., & Hasher, L. (1997). Cognitive gerontology and attentional inhibition: A reply to Burke and McDowd. *Journal of Gerontology: Psychological Sciences, 52B*, 274–283.

Zelinski, E. M. (1988). Integrating information from discourse: Do older adults show deficits? In L. L. Light & D. M. Burke (Eds.), *Language, memory, and aging* (pp. 117–132). Cambridge: Cambridge University Press.

Zelinski, E. M., & Hyde, J. C. (1996). Old words, new meanings: Aging and sense creation. *Journal of Memory and Language, 35*, 689–707.

Zwaan, R. A., & Radvansky, G. A. (1998). Situation models in language comprehension and memory. *Psychological Bulletin, 123*, 162–185.

Thirteen

Selection, Optimization, and Compensation as Developmental Mechanisms of Adaptive Resource Allocation: Review and Preview

Michaela Riediger, Shu-Chen Li and Ulman Lindenberger

I. Introduction

Developmental psychology has investigated a multitude of developmental phenomena in different phases of the life span and in multiple domains of functioning. However, the resulting knowledge about human development in general and aging in particular continues to be fragmented, with relatively little connection across disparate strands of research and different research traditions (Baltes, Lindenberger, Staudinger, in press; Magnusson, 1996). Informed by work of others (e.g., Baltes, 1997; Freund & Baltes, 2000; Marsiske et al., 1995), a central objective of this chapter is to use the conceptual framework of selection, optimization, and compensation (SOC; Baltes & Baltes, 1990) as a tool for integrating research on adaptive resource allocation in life span development. In addition, we propose that the SOC framework helps open up promising research directions, especially if attempts are made to study the interplay of SOC mechanisms from a dynamic systems perspective.

In line with the scope of the SOC framework, the general approach taken in this chapter is inherently life span developmental (e.g., Baltes et al., in press). Our specific focus, however, is on later adulthood and old age. We start by introducing prominent contemporary conceptual frameworks of developmental regulation. In this context, we comment on the benefits and limitations of the resource metaphor for studying developmental regulation, given that resource-allocation mechanisms play a prominent role in all considered frameworks. Then we describe the SOC framework in more detail and conclude that this framework may serve as a heuristic tool for arriving at a more integrated picture of human development and aging. We elaborate this claim in two major ways. First, we make use of SOC to integrate evidence of a great variety of different resource allocation processes. Here, we selectively review conceptual approaches and recent empirical findings in two research domains: (a) motivational–volitional processes and (b) cognitive–sensorimotor functioning.

Handbook of the Psychology of Aging

Second, we illustrate the fecundity of the SOC framework for conceptualizing new research avenues. Here we emphasize the need for age-comparative assessments of SOC-related processes in single-person and multiple-person systems and on multiple levels of analyses (e.g., neuronal, behavioral, interpersonal). In conclusion, we advocate the use of formal models to further enhance the testability and predictive power of SOC mechanisms for describing, explaining, and modifying life span differences in the adaptive dynamics of resource allocation.

To avoid misunderstandings, the conceptual status and scope of SOC are clarified at the outset of this chapter. As a conceptual framework, SOC helps to synthesize existing and instigate novel strands of empirical research on developmental regulation. Thus, as is typical for conceptual cores of empirical research programs (e.g., Lakatos, 1970), the SOC framework is not amenable to direct testing (falsification) but serves to organize and guide an empirical research. However, as shown in the course of this chapter, the SOC framework leads to explicit and testable (falsifiable) predictions when it is brought to bear upon specific research questions and developmental domains, such as life span differences in selection mechanisms of cognitive processing. Furthermore, the conceptual scope of SOC is broader than represented in this chapter. Most importantly, SOC encompasses both mechanisms of resource *generation* and mechanisms of resource *allocation* (e.g., Krampe & Baltes, 2003), whereas this chapter is restricted to the latter.

II. Resource-Allocation Processes in Life Span Development

During all phases of life, human development unfolds within the range of opportunities and constraints that

biological, psychological, and contextual characteristics provide. Such opportunities and constraints for development can be subsumed under the general notion of *resources*. Resources are as diverse as the life domains and situations in which development takes place (for resource taxonomies illustrating this diversity, see Hobfoll, 1998; Read & Miller, 1989; Wilensky, 1983). Individuals differ in their access to resources. Moreover, for the same individual, the availability and efficiency of resources undergo fundamental changes throughout life. Adult development is characterized by a shift in directions of lesser resource gains and more resource losses (e.g., Baltes, 1987). Although individuals might gain, for example, in social status, material belongings, knowledge, and professional expertise, other resources such as physical fitness, health, sensory acuity, multitasking ability, or functional brain efficacy decrease throughout adulthood.

The decreasing gain–loss ratio of resources across the adult life span does not inevitably compromise adaptive functioning. This is perhaps best illustrated by the finding of an age-related increase of heterogeneity in functional status, with a good proportion of individuals aging successfully by various subjective and objective criteria, at biological, cognitive, and social levels. Hence, an intriguing task, also at the heart of research on successful aging (for an overview, see Freund & Riediger, 2003), is to better understand *how* individuals manage to reach and maintain desirable levels of functioning in a life phase that is characterized by a wealth of objective and subjective resource losses.

In line with Navon (1984), we regard it as helpful to distinguish two classes of resources: *commodities* and *alterants* (Freund & Riediger, 2001; Li & Freund, 2005). The central characteristic of commodities is their finitude. Many important resources, such as time, physical energy, and neurocognitive capacity, are only available in limited amounts. In contrast, alterants, are not finite in themselves but influence the efficiency of using finite commodities. In the context of cognitive aging research, for instance, processing speed, working memory, and attention as well as their neural correlates are assumed, with varying degrees of explanatory power depending on theoretical preferences, as finite, depleting resources. Lifelong experiences in specific domains (expertise) and various forms of contextual support (e.g., from social networks to technologically engineered environmental support for older people), however, can be considered as alterants that improve the efficiency of applying depleting cognitive resources.

Various current conceptual frameworks in life span development emphasize the interaction between life span changes in the availability of limited resources (commodities) and ways in which individuals utilize these resources for successful development (alterants). Next, we briefly discuss the central propositions of four such current frameworks: socioemotional selectivity theory (Carstensen, Isaacowitz, & Charles, 1999); dual-process model of assimilative and accommodative coping (Brandtstädter & Renner, 1990), optimization in primary and secondary control (Heckhausen & Schulz, 1995), and selection, optimization, and compensation (Baltes & Baltes, 1990). We then focus specifically on the latter framework and demonstrate its utility for integrating findings on diverse developmental phenomena and for conceptualizing new lines of research.

III. Four Current Approaches to Adaptive Regulation of Life Span Development

This section introduces four current approaches to adaptive regulation of life span development. All four frameworks converge on the assumption that the adaptive regulation of life span development requires suitable mechanisms for the allocation of limited resources. They vary, however, in their particular focus (e.g., on social motivation, coping, or control), in the particular characteristics of the proposed resource-allocation mechanisms, and in their postulated generality.

A. Socioemotional Selectivity Theory

Focusing on social relationships, Carstensen and colleagues postulated socioemotional selectivity as a mechanism regulating age-associated changes in future time perspective (e.g., Carstensen, 1993, 1998; Carstensen et al., 1999). The authors propose two primary motivations for social interaction, emotion regulation and knowledge acquisition. Perceived future time perspective is assumed to determine the relative importance of these motivational objectives. An *extended* future time perspective tends to be related to knowledge-related goals. A *limited* future time perspective, in contrast, tends to be related to emotion-related goals.

The authors further postulate that knowledge- and emotion-related goals are more likely to be achieved by interactions with different social partners. Emotion regulation is enhanced with familiar and close interaction partners. Knowledge acquisition, in contrast, often requires interacting with people who are emotionally not very close, but who can give access to desired information. Based on these considerations, the authors argue that the well-documented reduction in social contacts in later adulthood largely results from a selective pruning process that older adults intentionally initiate in accordance with their social–interactional priorities. Because of their limited future time extension, older adults are assumed to be more motivated to regulate emotions than to acquire knowledge. Older adults are therefore predicted to discard emotionally less important relationships in order to selectively invest time and effort into the maintenance of intensive relations to emotionally close interaction partners.

The basic predictions of socioemotional selectivity theory have received empirical support in a variety of studies (for an overview, see Carstensen, Fung, & Charles, 2003). Empirical evidence also indicates that socioemotional selectivity is not exclusive to old age. Rather, and in line with the theory, it appears to operate whenever future time perspective is perceived as limited, such as in the case of severe illness (e.g., Fredrickson & Carstensen, 1990; Fung, Carstensen, & Lutz, 1999).

B. Dual-Process Model of Assimilative and Accommodative Coping

Whereas the socioemotional selectivity theory focuses on social–motivational phenomena, the dual-process model proposed by Brandtstädter and colleagues (e.g., Brandtstädter & Greve, 1994; Brandtstädter & Renner, 1990) addresses coping strategies for maintaining a sense of continuity and efficacy in the face of resource losses. According to this framework, people use two complementary forms of coping to reestablish congruence between desired and actual states when faced with difficulties. *Assimilation* (e.g., tenacious goal pursuit) involves active and intentional efforts to change *life circumstances* such that the discrepancy between actual and desired states reduces or disappears. *Accommodation* (e.g., flexible goal adjustment), in contrast, denotes discrepancy reduction through the automatic (i.e., unintentional)

adjustment of *preferences and goals* to situational constraints.

The authors posit that people usually first employ assimilative coping efforts to actively overcome obstacles that block their goals. If these attempts turn out unsuccessful, a gradual shift to accommodative processes of automatic goal adjustment is postulated, which is modulated by personal and situational factors (e.g., goal importance, success probability, Brandtstädter & Wentura, 1995).

Empirical evidence demonstrates a general shift from assimilative to accommodative coping and an increasing adaptiveness of the latter in later adulthood when losses become more widespread and resources necessary for tenacious goal pursuit in the face of obstacles decline (Brandtstädter & Renner, 1990; Brandtstädter, Rothermund, & Schmitz, 1997; Brandtstädter, Wentura, & Greve, 1993).

C. Optimization in Primary and Secondary Control

The model of optimization in primary and secondary control proposed by Heckhausen and Schulz (1995) assumes that humans have a basic need for control. The primary way to achieve control is by modifying the environment according to one's goals. If such primary control efforts are not available or fail, a secondary way to achieve control (i.e., to protect oneself in the face of difficulties and setbacks) is to modify one's goals and standards or to engage in self-protective attributions and social comparisons. At first glance, this bipartite partitioning of control needs resembles the dual-process model proffered by Brandtstädter and colleagues. However, whereas Heckhausen and Schulz (1995) posit a developmental ordering of control mechanisms as primary and secondary, the dual-process model does not assign a developmental or conceptual priority to assimilation or accommodation but emphasizes their interplay through all phases of life (e.g., Brandtstädter & Rothermund, 2002; cf. Piaget, 1980).

Heckhausen and Schulz (1995) further proposed that selectivity and failure compensation are two basic requirements for adaptive developmental regulation. Integrating these two basic requirements of human functioning and the two fundamental types of control, these authors postulated four developmental regulatory mechanisms. *Selective primary control* denotes the focused investment of resources (e.g., time, effort) into the pursuit of a chosen goal. *Compensatory primary control* involves the recruitment of external help or technical aids for the attainment of a chosen goal. *Selective secondary control* subsumes metavolitional strategies to keep oneself focused on the pursuit of selected goals, e.g., by avoiding distractions. Finally, *compensatory secondary control* serves to buffer negative effects of failure experiences. It involves, for instance, such strategies as disengagement from unattainable goals, downward social comparisons, or external causal attributions.

According to the authors, none of these four strategies is functional per se. Rather, a higher order *optimization* process is postulated that coordinates control strivings such that the potential for primary control is maximized across the life span. Consistent with this proposition is empirical evidence indicating that self-protective compensatory strategies (compensatory secondary control) become more prevalent and more adaptive in later adulthood and when opportunity structures for goal attainment are unfavorable (Wrosch & Heckhausen, 1999), whereas continued involvement in primary control efforts may be maladaptive in such situations (Chipperfield, Perry, & Menec,

1999; Heckhausen, Wrosch, & Fleeson, 2001).

D. The Meta-Model of Selection, Optimization, and Compensation

From the outset (e.g., Baltes & Baltes, 1990), the model of selection, optimization, and Compensation was proposed as a *general framework of adaptive development* that is apt to represent the dynamics between developmental gains and losses across various periods of the life span (e.g., childhood, adolescence, adulthood, old age), at different levels of analyses (e.g., neuronal, behavioral, societal), and within and across domains of functioning (e.g., cognitive development, affect regulation).

Within the SOC framework, adaptive development is defined as a tendency toward simultaneous minimization of losses that impair effective functioning and maximization of gains that promote growth and maintenance. It proposes that adaptive development results from the interaction of three general mechanisms for generating, releasing, and allocating resources: *selection, optimization, and compensation*. As a meta-theory, the SOC framework does not designate any specific content to these mechanisms, which are proposed to have a multitude of possible phenotypic realizations that may vary along dimensions, such as active–passive, internal–external, and intentional–unintentional. Specific implementations depend on the situation, the relevant domain of functioning, the sociocultural context, individual resources, and personal preferences (Baltes, 1997).

Because pursuing all potentially possible developmental pathways typically exceeds available resources, SOC theory posits that *selection* from the pool of available alternatives is one of the main mechanisms of developmental regulation (Waddington, 1975). The model distinguishes two forms of selection that serve different regulatory functions in life span development: *Elective selection* occurs in response to new demands or tasks, whereas *loss-based selection* occurs as a consequence of actual or anticipated loss of resources. Focused investment of resources gives development its direction and is a precondition for developmental specialization and the achievement of higher levels of functioning. *Optimization* reflects the gain aspect of development, defined as the acquisition, refinement, and coordinated application of resources directed at the achievement of higher functional levels. Finally, *compensation* addresses the regulation of loss in development. It involves efforts to maintain a given level of functioning despite decline in, or loss of, previously available resources. It thus represents an alternative to loss-based selection, which implies a reorganization of life and functioning around the loss.

IV. The Utility of SOC as an Integrative Framework: Selective Review of Empirical Findings

So far, we have introduced four different conceptual frameworks that seek to identify developmental processes that regulate the allocation of limited resources to various life domains and life tasks. Next, we review empirical evidence of resource allocation in adulthood and old age, drawing primarily, but not exclusively, on research motivated by the SOC framework. This section focuses on two research domains in which research on SOC mechanisms has been most active: motivational–volitional processes and sensorimotor–cognitive functioning.

A. Motivation and Volition: Mechanisms of Active Life Management

To date, the SOC framework has been most influential in stimulating research on *active life management* (cf. Freund & Baltes, 2000) or *intentional self-development* (cf. Brandtstädter, 1999). Both notions emphasize the assumption that individuals themselves actively influence the course of their lives through goal-directed action.

Freund and Baltes (2000) elaborated that, in the domain of active life management, SOC mechanisms become evident in motivational and volitional processes. For instance, the selection mechanism unfolds in the process of goal selection. Goals are "desired states that people seek to obtain, maintain, or avoid" (Emmons, 1996, p. 314). *Elective selection* here denotes committing oneself to goals directed at the achievement of higher levels of functioning. In contrast, *loss-based selection*, involves changing goals or the goal system in response to losses in previously available goal-relevant resources. It is proposed to represent an adaptive strategy for focusing or redirecting resources when compensatory efforts (see later) to maintain one's goal(s) in the face of resource loss are either not possible or would be invested at the expense of other, more promising goals. In contrast, *optimization* and *compensation* are reflected in behaviors involved in goal pursuit. The distinguishing characteristic is the absence or presence of loss in previously available goal-relevant resources. Compensation, in contrast to optimization, aims at counteracting or avoiding losses rather than achieving higher levels of functioning.

Freund and Baltes (2002a) used proverbs to assess people's intuitive knowledge about the effectiveness of these life-management strategies. Proverbs contain historically accumulated cultural experience and provide guidelines of how one should act in certain situations or contexts. The authors identified a large range of proverbs that reflect instantiations of selection (e.g., "Those who follow every path never reach any destination."), optimization (e.g., "Practice makes perfect."), and compensation (e.g., "When there's no wind, grab the oars."). In a series of studies, the authors then paired these proverbs with proverbs representing alternative, non-SOC-relevant life management strategies (e.g., "Good things come to those who wait"). Proverbs in each pair were matched with regard to familiarity, comprehensibility, and perceived meaningfulness. Younger and older participants typically chose SOC-related proverbs as giving better general advice and as matching general life decision situations better than proverbs representing alternative life management strategies. However, when the task was to decide which proverb matches better in situations that focus on relaxation, such as during a vacation, participants typically preferred the alternative to the SOC-related proverbs. The authors concluded that cultural as well as individual knowledge about the pragmatics of life includes representations of selection, optimization, and compensation and that this knowledge is well elaborated and context specific.

Other research indicates that people not only know about but also engage in SOC strategies and that this is associated positively with indicators of adaptive development in various life domains. Such research has employed different measures of SOC. The so far most frequently used instrument is a self-report questionnaire (SOC questionnaire, Baltes et al., 1999; Freund & Baltes, 2002b). Other indicators have been derived, for example, from minute-to-minute reconstructions of the sequence, duration, geographical, and social context of everyday activities

(Baltes & Lang, 1997; Lang, Rieckmann, & Baltes, 2002), from content analyses of strategies employed to cope with disability (Bouchard Ryan et al., 2003; Gignac, Cott, & Badley, 2000, 2002), or from patterns of self-reported resource investment in various domains of life (e.g., Staudinger & Freund, 1998; Staudinger et al., 1999; Wiese, 2000; Wiese & Freund, 2000).

These measures of engagement in SOC strategies have been linked to various general and domain-specific indicators of adaptive development. *General* criteria involved, for example, facets of positive psychological functioning, emotional well-being, or life/aging satisfaction (e.g., Chou & Chi, 2002; Freund & Baltes, 1998, 2002b; Jopp, 2002; Staudinger & Freund, 1998; Staudinger et al., 1999). *Domain-specific* indicators have so far been obtained primarily in the partnership/family and work/study domains. Examples are partnership and job satisfaction (e.g., Wiese, Freund, & Baltes, 2000, 2002), workplace performance (Abraham & Hansson, 1995; Bajor & Baltes, 2003), experience of work-related stressors, family-related stressors, and work–family conflict (Baltes & Heydens-Gahir, 2003), or learning quantity and learning quality in university students (Wiese & Schmitz, 2002). Without exception, these studies demonstrated that higher engagement in SOC-relevant life management strategies is predictive of concurrent as well as future developmental success (for examples of prospective study designs, see Jopp, 2002; Wiese et al., 2002). This predictive value of SOC has been shown in samples of healthy adults in different age groups, namely younger adults (e.g., Wiese, 2000; Wiese & Freund, 2000; Wiese et al., 2000, 2002; Wiese & Schmitz, 2002), middle-aged adults (e.g., Bajor & Baltes, 2003), old and very old adults (e.g., Chou & Chi, 2002; Freund & Baltes, 1998), and in a sample covering the adult life span (Freund

& Baltes, 2002b). In all, these findings of positive (rather than negative or no) associations between SOC-relevant strategies and indicators of adaptive development are consistent with the proposition that engagement in SOC-relevant strategies fosters adaptive regulation of life span development.

In the Freund and Baltes (2002b) study, adults of various age groups differed in their self-reported engagement in SOC (assessed with the SOC questionnaire; Baltes et al., 1999). Middle-aged adults reported stronger engagement than younger and older adults in loss-based selection, optimization, and compensation. Elective selection showed a linear increase from younger, to middle-aged, and older adulthood. Using a qualitative approach to the assessment of SOC, Gignac et al. (2002) observed a similar pattern in a sample of older patients. These authors content-coded patients' descriptions of behavioral adaptations to osteoarthritis along dimensions of selection (not distinguishing between elective and loss-based selection), optimization, and compensation. In this sample (patients older than 55 years), engagement in all three SOC strategies was slightly negatively associated with age.

Freund and Baltes (2002b) offered the following interpretation of these cross-sectional age gradients. In younger adulthood, individuals may still need to explore different developmental pathways to find their way in life, and also have the necessary resources for such explorations (e.g., time to live, energy). As individuals move into middle adulthood, they acquire and refine resource-efficient life management strategies (SOC). Engagement in SOC, however, is itself resource intensive. In older adulthood, therefore, engagement in SOC strategies may again decrease because their implementation is more effortful than alternative behaviors and actions, such as immediately giving up goals

in the face of difficulties without attempting to compensate or to select alternative goals. An aging-associated decline in goal-relevant resources therefore limits the expression of optimizing goal pursuit and counteracting goal-related losses in later adulthood. For the same reason, elective selection may become more pronounced with age because the necessity to focus the remaining resources efficiently on selected goals increases.

In support of the assumption that engagement in SOC strategies is resource intensive, studies have shown that resource-rich individuals tend to exhibit higher levels of engagement in SOC strategies than resource-poor individuals (Baltes & Lang, 1997; Jopp, 2002; Lang et al., 2002). Furthermore, there is accumulating evidence that engagement in SOC-related life management strategies is particularly effective when resources are limited (Abraham & Hansson, 1995; Chou & Chi, 2002; Jopp, 2002; Staudinger & Freund, 1998; Staudinger et al., 1999). In such situations, engagement in SOC strategies has been shown to buffer the negative effect of scarce resources on indicators of adaptive development. Chou and Chi (2002), for example, showed that engagement in selection and optimization, as assessed with the SOC questionnaire, moderated the negative association between financial strain and life satisfaction among elderly Chinese. Elderly participants experiencing high financial strain reported less impaired life satisfaction when they were highly engaged in these strategies and more impaired life satisfaction when they were not.

In summary, in the domain of active life management, SOC-related processes become evident in the selection of personal goals, optimization of goal pursuit, and compensation of goal-relevant resource losses. Empirical evidence demonstrates that people have intuitive knowledge about the effectiveness of these life management strategies and that engagement in these strategies is related positively to a diversity of indicators of developmental success, particularly so in increasingly resource-constraining life conditions, such as older adulthood.

We propose that future research on motivational and volitional aspects of developmental regulation would benefit from using the SOC framework to identify specific aspects of goal selection and goal pursuit behaviors that foster adaptive development in adulthood and old age. Various authors have argued that not all expressions of goal selection and pursuit (SOC) are equally adaptive (Freund & Baltes, 2000; Freund, Li, & Baltes, 1999; Marsiske et al., 1995). Selecting too early or too few goals, for example, might impair one's flexibility, a characteristic necessary for continued growth and development (Heckhausen, 1999). Similarly, optimization and compensation can take inappropriate forms and have negative consequences (e.g., Bäckman & Dixon, 1992). Not investing enough resources, investing resources that do not have the desired effect, or overinvesting resources at the expenses of other goals or one's own health and well-being would be examples for SOC-related actions with potentially maladaptive consequences. These examples underscore that SOC mechanisms need to be tuned to the developmental task and orchestrated among each other in order to be adaptive (e.g., equilibrated; cf. Piaget, 1985). For more effective separation of adaptive from less adaptive forms of goal selection and pursuit in a particular developmental situation, person and context characteristics as well as dynamics among SOC mechanisms need to be taken into account (for examples, see Riediger & Freund, 2004; Riediger, Freund, & Baltes, 2005). From an applied perspective, such knowledge would provide an empirical foundation for intervention programs aimed at fostering successful development and aging in particular target groups (for similar propositions, see Cerrato & Fernanández de Trocóniz, 1998; Chou & Chi, 2002; Vondracek & Porfeli, 2002).

B. Cognitive and Sensorimotor Dual Tasking: Adaptive Cross-Domain Resource Allocation

A salient and ecologically valid component of active life management consists in the simultaneous management of cognitive and sensorimotor aspects of behavior. Cognitive and sensorimotor requirements frequently have to be mastered simultaneously, for example, when conducting a conversation while walking. Therefore, life span changes in coordinating simultaneous demands on sensorimotor and cognitive functions provide a fertile ground for exploring SOC mechanisms.

The resource metaphor has a long tradition in cognitive psychology (e.g., Miller, 1956). Defined as a set of functions or structures relevant to perform a task (Heuer, 1996), it captures processing constraints during single and multi-tasking at a molar level of analysis, i.e., above the level of specific task-relevant processes. A good example is the unitary resource theory proposed by Kahneman (1973). This framework assumes that different tasks require different amounts of a general mental resource (referred to as attention, capacity, or effort), which is limited, although the limit is variable, and divisible between tasks (cf. Kinsbourne & Hicks, 1978). Thus, cognitive resources considering as a finite commodity that can be allocated in a highly flexible manner and theorizing at the level of cognitive resources allow researchers to make and test predictions about life span changes in adaptive resource allocation.[1]

Research on cognitive–sensorimotor couplings in adulthood has provided ample evidence for three interrelated assumptions. First, both cognitive and sensorimotor tasks draw upon attentional resources, with much variability among tasks in both domains of functioning (e.g., Woollacott, 2000). Second, the overall capacity of available attentional resources decreases with advancing adult age (e.g., Craik & Byrd, 1982). Third, due to increasing frailty, sensory impairments, and less reliable sensory coordination processes, older adults need to invest more cognitive resources, in both absolute and relative terms, into the regulation of sensorimotor behavior than younger adults (e.g., Brown & Woollacott, 1998). This increasing need for a decreasing resource constitutes a quandary of behavioral aging (Lindenberger, Marsiske, & Baltes, 2000).

Supportive evidence for these claims is typically based on dual-task experiments, in which participants perform a single cognitive task (e.g., memorize a word list), a single sensorimotor task (e.g., walk a narrow track), and both tasks simultaneously. Dual-task costs are then determined as the relative decrement in performance in dual-task as compared to single-task conditions.

[1]Various process accounts of resource restrictions have been proposed. For instance, it has been proposed (a) that some mental process needed for one task must wait as long as the person engages in another task (single-channel hypothesis, e.g., K. J. W. Craik, 1948); (b) that processes of stimulus identification and interpretation are inherently limited, which forces people to work on one task at a time only (perceptual bottleneck hypothesis, e.g., Broadbent, 1958); or (c) that individuals can only select responses for one task at a time (response-selection bottleneck hypothesis, e.g., Pashler, 1984). The purpose of this chapter is not to discriminate among these accounts, but to provide a more general overview of life span dynamics in sensorimotor–cognitive couplings from a SOC perspective.

Various studies using different cognitive and sensorimotor tasks demonstrated that aging is associated with increasing dual-task costs (for overviews, see Li, Krampe, & Bondar, in press; Woollacott & Shumway-Cook, 2002). Li and colleagues (2001) extended the dual-task paradigm by varying task difficulty levels. Younger adults' cognitive dual-task costs were independent of the difficulty of the sensorimotor task. Older adults' cognitive performance, however, was significantly more impaired when simultaneously performing a difficult rather than an easy sensorimotor task. These results are consistent with the view that sensorimotor functioning in older adulthood draws increasingly on attentional resources.

SOC provides a suitable framework for investigating adaptive resource allocation processes in dual-task situations involving cognitive and sensorimotor functioning. The framework suggests that selection (i.e., prioritization of more important situational demands at the cost of less important ones) and compensation (i.e., utilization of compensatory means to counteract losses in prioritized aspects of the situation) should be effective mechanisms to cope with age-related declines in cognitive and sensorimotor capacity. Because declining physical capacity in older adulthood results in a higher vulnerability to falls and, in the case of falling, in aggravated risk of serious injuries with debilitating long-term health outcomes, securing one's sensorimotor functioning (e.g., walking safely, keeping one's balance) should have a higher immediate relevance for adaptive functioning in older than in younger adulthood. Older adults should therefore be inclined to protect their sensorimotor functioning (e.g., to walk safely or keep their balance) even at the cost of cognitive performance. This prediction has received initial, but not unequivocal, empirical support by recent experimental studies.

Several studies found that older participants tend more to prioritize sensorimotor functioning (e.g., postural control) over cognitive performance than younger adults (e.g., Brown et al., 2002; Lajoie et al., 1996; Teasdale et al., 1992, 1993). For instance, Lövdén et al. (in press) found that older adults profited more than young adults when they were allowed to hold onto a handrail while walking on a treadmill and performing a spatial navigation task. Li et al. (2001) found that younger and older adults did not differ in dual-task costs of *walking* performance when simultaneously memorizing word lists, but that older adults showed higher dual-task *memory* costs. Other researchers, e.g., Lindenberger et al. (2000), however, did not observe this pattern, perhaps because the difficulty level of the sensorimotor task was not sufficiently high to induce older adults to protect their bodies at the expense of cognitive performance.

Further findings on the selective use of external aids are of particular interest from a SOC perspective. Li et al. (2001) provided memory and walking aids that participants could use in a self-paced manner in conditions with increased task difficulty. The memory aid delayed the presentation of to-be-remembered words to enhance encoding. The walking aid consisted of a handrail that participants could use to stabilize their balance. Older participants not only preferred but also benefited more from using external aids to optimize their walking performance than younger adults. In contrast, younger adults preferred and benefited more from aid use to optimize their memory performance (for another example of age group differences in compensatory strategies in dual-task situations of a different nature, see Kemper, Herman, & Lian, 2003).

These findings on age differential resource allocation in cognitive–sensorimotor dual-task settings open up a

difficult question: To what extent does the observed prioritization of sensorimotor over intellectual dimensions of behavior among older adults result from the flexible and deliberate use of resource allocation strategies (e.g., SOC at the level of deliberate action), as opposed to an automatic mechanism protecting bodily integrity (e.g., SOC at the level of behavioral regulation)? One way to investigate this question is to employ different task-emphasis instructions in dual-task designs. Although some studies show age-related deficits in deliberate resource allocations (Anderson, Craik, & Naveh-Benjamin, 1998; Tsang & Shaner, 1998), the majority of available studies show that older adults are as able as younger adults to deliberately emphasize either one (e.g., motor) or the other (e.g., cognitive) component task when instructed to do so (Crossley & Hiscock, 1992; Salthouse, Rogan, & Prill, 1984; Somberg & Salthouse, 1982). For example, Bondar, Krampe, and Baltes (2005) found that older adults were equally or better able than younger adults to follow instructions of varying task emphasis under dual-task conditions, i.e., to prioritize either sensorimotor or cognitive aspects of performance. The authors concluded that older adults' selective prioritization of sensorimotor aspects in multiple-task situations resulted from their ability to flexibly and deliberately withdraw cognitive resources from a cognitive component in order to secure the more survival-relevant sensorimotor functioning. Such deliberate strategic choices may be operating on top of more automated protection mechanisms.

In summary, research on resource allocation processes in multitask situations involving cognitive and sensorimotor tasks has demonstrated an aging-associated increase in loss-based selection and selective compensation. Older adults tend to prioritize safe sensorimotor functioning (e.g., walking, keeping balance) at the cost of simultaneous cognitive demands. To some degree at least, this form of selective optimization appears to result from older adults' maintained ability to flexibly allocate attentional resources. Given the increased susceptibility to, and aggravated consequences of falling, prioritization of sensorimotor functioning can tentatively be classified as an adaptive strategy of older adults. Future research would benefit from further investigation of the adaptive values of resource allocation processes in sensorimotor–cognitive dual task settings. For example, are there interindividual differences among older adults in the ability to flexibly allocate attentional resources to protect sensorimotor functioning? Are older adults who tend to be less selective in this respect more susceptible to falls, as clinical observations would suggest (Sattin, 1992; Tinetti, 1995)? From an applied perspective, responses to these questions might help conceptualizing prevention programs targeting older adults at high risk of falling.

V. Research on SOC: Future Directions

Thus far, we have used the SOC framework to organize and integrate evidence on resource allocation processes across age periods, levels of analysis, and content domains. Resource allocation processes in domains as diverse as motivation/volition and cognitive–sensorimotor functioning can be phrased and interpreted in terms of selection, optimization, and compensation mechanisms. In this manner, the SOC framework may contribute to a more coherent and holistic picture of human development and aging. Moreover, the SOC framework also has the potential to inspire new research questions and paradigms. This section

illustrates this claim with select research examples, again drawn from the domains of active life management and cognition. Finally, we propose formal modeling to further develop the predictive potential of the SOC framework.

A. Social Embedding of Active Life Management: SOC in Multiple-Person Systems

There is clear agreement among current developmental psychologists that an individual's development is fundamentally shaped and constrained by his or her environment. It is also generally acknowledged that such contextual forces are manifold, including normative age-graded, normative history-graded, and nonnormative influences (see Baltes, 1987), and that many of these influences involve social aspects and processes. Despite this general acknowledgement of the importance of social contexts (Baltes & Staudinger, 1996), the majority of studies in developmental psychology, including those reviewed earlier, have taken a person-centered route. We propose that the SOC framework may serve as an organizing framework for surpassing this incongruence between theory and methods. Research on active life management may serve as an example to illustrate this claim.

Active life management refers to the fact that people themselves influence their development within the range of available opportunities. In this regard, SOC mechanisms have been proposed to unfold in the *selection* of personal goals, *optimization* of goal pursuit, and *compensation* of losses in goal-relevant resources (Freund & Baltes, 2000; Freund et al., 1999). We propose that future research should investigate the social foundations of these processes. We regard two research perspectives as particularly promising.

From a *social-interactive perspective*, motivational and volitional processes within individuals can be viewed both as a source and as a target of social influence. This approach can yield important information on other people's influence on the content and pursuit of an individual's goals, on the impact of an individual's goal selection and pursuit on his or her social environment, and especially on the development of such social-interactive components and their associations with successful life management in various phases of the life span, such as older adulthood.

From a social-interactive perspective, the focus is on the individual as embedded in social contexts. From a *collective perspective*, the focus is on social systems (e.g., dyad, family, work group) as a whole. According to the SOC framework, selection, optimization, and compensation also operate at this level of analysis (e.g., Baltes & Carstensen, 1998). In terms of life management, then, social systems can be seen as selecting goals and as striving toward goal attainment (see also von Cranach, Ochsenbein, & Valach, 1986). This perspective can yield important information on processes fostering successful development of social units, such as partnerships or intergenerational relations.

In our view, SOC is apt to synthesize both perspectives, social interactive and collective, within the same theoretical framework. This has two advantages. First, it allows relating formerly disconnected evidence from the social-interactive perspective (e.g., finding of a dependence support script that undermines older adults' striving for independence, Baltes, 1996), on the one hand, and the collective perspective (e.g., finding that collective goal setting improves work group performance, Wegge, 2000), on the other. Second, it stimulates empirical research efforts that combine both perspectives. Such research might address, for example, interrelations among individual and collective goal processes, antecedents and consequences of collective goal processes on the individual and collective level, or life span trajectories of competencies involved in individual and collective goal processes.

B. Life Span Development of Selection Mechanisms

According to the SOC framework, selection is particularly important when processing resources are scarce. Everyday cognitive functioning is a continuous stream of simultaneous and sequential multitasking (e.g., finding one's way through a mall while memorizing a shopping list, watching one's purse, and talking to a friend), thus requiring flexible resource allocation across functions and task domains on the part of the individual. Resource allocation is in turn supported by selection mechanisms that are either primarily more resource based or more process based, as discussed here.

1. Resource-Based Selection

Conceptually, scarcity in processing resources refers to cases where total demands required by multiple tasks exceed the total available resources. An example is reading a text while taking care of a small child. Overlap in resources, however, refers to situations where multiple tasks overlap substantially in the resources they require, such as when taking care of several small children. Although resource scarcity and resource overlap may be independent of each other, most daily cognition involves carrying out multiple tasks with overlapping requirements on limited resources, simultaneously, sequentially, or both.

2. Process-Based Selection

Other than resource-based selection, a less noted aspect of selection refers to processing conflict, such as a mismatch between current task requirement and already well-established behavioral or neurocognitive processing patterns. Such processing conflicts between old habits and new task demands occur regularly in everyday life, for example, when there is change in contexts (e.g., a move to a new apartment), in contact persons (e.g., new neighbors), or in properties of daily devices (e.g., a new personal computer). Such changes necessitate selecting between competing processes, which we refer to as process-based selection (see also Miller & Cohen, 2001). Throughout life, experiential selection generates habits that could either facilitate or hamper goal or process selection in specific life or task contexts. Experiential selection not only operates at the behavioral level to shape the individual's specific behavioral and cognitive characteristics, it also operates at the neuronal level. Both the selective stabilization theory of neuronal epigenesis (Changeux, 1985) and the neuronal group selection theory (Edelman, 1987) postulate that during early brain development selective experiential influences shape the details of structural and functional organization. Similarly, the neural constructivist view stresses that experiences can selectively strengthen the synaptic efficacy of frequently activated neural assemblies to construct cortical circuits for different specialization (e.g., Johnson, 2001; Quartz & Senjowski, 2000).

In our view, resource- and process-based selection are not independent of each other and should both be emphasized conjointly in future behavioral and cognitive neuroscience research on life span age differences in selection regulation. The following sections propose (a) how life span age differences in resource-based selection can be studied in the context of multitasking paradigms and (b) how life span age differences in process-based selection can be investigated using differential training and context shift paradigms. In both cases, implementing specific aspects of SOC concepts, such as selection mechanisms, leads to empirically testable predictions.

C. Age Differences in Resource-Based Selection: The Concept of Selection Margins

Informed by early work of Brim (1992), we propose that the concept of *selection margins* may help extend our knowledge of the development of adaptive resource allocation processes in multiple-task situations. We define selection margins as the discrepancy between the number of multiple tasks an individual could maximally manage given the available processing resources and the number of tasks he or she actually selects to work on. Selection margins have three central characteristics: their (a) width, (b) direction, and (c) function for adaptive development (see Figure 13.1).

The *width* of selection margins refers to the extent of the deviation between self-selected and maximally manageable number of simultaneous tasks. We assume that this width is influenced by the accuracy of people's estimates of the number of tasks they can maximally manage, which in turn should be a function of performance variability and the accuracy of performance and error monitoring. During childhood and aging, when cognitive resources and their underlying neurobiological substrates undergo growth and decline respectively (Li et al., 2004), individuals' performance variability has been shown to be larger and their monitoring operations to be less precise than during late adolescence and adulthood when resources are more

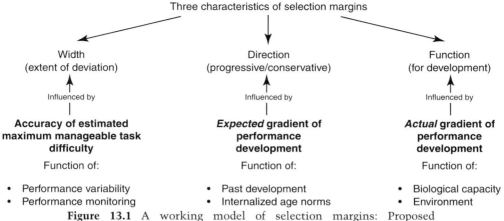

Three characteristics of selection margins

Width (extent of deviation)	Direction (progressive/conservative)	Function (for development)
Influenced by	Influenced by	Influenced by
Accuracy of estimated maximum manageable task difficulty	***Expected* gradient of performance development**	***Actual* gradient of performance development**
Function of:	Function of:	Function of:
• Performance variability • Performance monitoring	• Past development • Internalized age norms	• Biological capacity • Environment

Figure 13.1 A working model of selection margins: Proposed characteristics and antecedents.

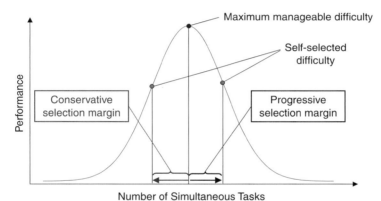

Figure 13.2 The concept of selection margins defined as discrepancy between the number of subtasks an individual could maximally manage given the available processing resources and the number of tasks he or she actually selects to work on.

stable (e.g., Davies, Segalowitz, & Gavin, 2004; Li et al., 2004; Nieuwenhuis et al., 2002). It can therefore be expected that older adults and children show wider selection margins in cognitive tasks than young adults.

The *direction* of selection margins is characterized by whether individuals choose task numbers or task difficulties in excess of or below their current ability levels. If an individual chooses to work with a number of subtasks that is smaller than his or her maximum manageable difficulty, the selection margin is *conservative*. Conversely, if the individual selects to work with a number of subtasks that is greater than his or her maximum manageable difficulty, the selection margin is *progressive* (see Figure 13.2). We assume that the direction of selection margins is influenced by people's expectations of the future development of their performance. Progressive selection margins should result from expected improvement, and conservative selection margins from expected decline. We further assume that such expectations are, to some extent, a function of past experiences of improvement or decline in abilities, and of age-normative expectations. Therefore, older adults may be more likely to adopt conservative selection margins, whereas children are expected to prefer progressive selection margins.

Finally, we assume that the *function* or adaptivity of selection margins depends on the actual gradient of performance development, which is a function of biological capacity and contextual opportunities and constraints. As a general rule, progressive selection margins may, on average, be more adaptive in childhood, when cognitive abilities are on a growth trajectory and when working on a number of tasks that exceeds the child's current resources should stimulate the full utilization of the developmental potential, thus accelerating the improvement of functioning. Progressive selection margins of moderate width might be most adaptive in this regard. Working on a number of tasks that substantially exceeds the child's current ability level may eventually undermine the task-relevant motivation.

In turn, whenever progressive selection margins are unlikely to result in accelerated enhancement of behavioral competence, neutral or conservative selection margins may be more adaptive. Therefore, we assume that older adults are more likely to adopt conservative selection margins in functional domains that are characterized by normative age-related decline such as memory and perceptual speed. In SOC terminology, conservative selection margins would function as a mechanism of anticipatory loss-based selection in this case. We assume that conservative selection margins of small width might be most adaptive because they keep individuals safely away from their limits without severely constraining the utilization of the available capacity.

D. Age Differences in Process-Based Selection: Habituation and Context-Shifting Paradigms

Adult age differences in maintenance of and reliance on context information for memory processes have been well established. Memory for context is particularly vulnerable in old age (Spencer & Raz, 1995). At the same time, older adults are also more dependent on the match between encoding and retrieval contexts (e.g., Braver et al., 2001; Castel & Craik, 2003). Older adults are also less able to inhibit a potent habitual process or behavior and are more susceptible to interference (e.g., Nieuwenhuis et al., 2002). Generalizing from these findings, experimental paradigms that involve a first phase of habituation training for strengthening a particular selection option and a second phase of context match that systematically varies the degree of match between current task context and the habituated context may be a fruitful approach to study life span age differences in process-based selection. On the one hand, if the current task context is particularly similar to the training context, habituation should facilitate the required selection in the current task. On the other hand, if the requirement of the current task context is quite different from the already established habit, processing conflict may result and hamper selection (see Figure 13.3). Thus for old adults, a habituated selection mechanism may be particularly detrimental for selecting the appropriate processes when inference between the habitual context and the current task demand is high.

It has been proposed that the anterior cingulate cortex (ACC) plays an important role in monitoring processing conflict. According to one account, activities in ACC send signals of conflict in processing pathways to the prefrontal

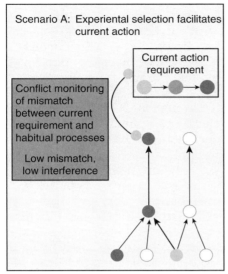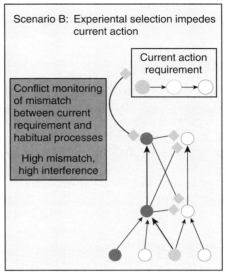

Figure 13.3 Schematic diagram of two scenarios of possible interactions between experiential selection and current actions: Habituated (experientially selected) processes are linked with thick dark lines. When the conflict between current action requirements and experientially selected processes is low, experiential selection facilitates current action (scenario A). In contrast, when conflict between current action requirements and experientially selected processes is high, experiential selection hampers current action (scenario B).

cortex (PFC) in order to generate stronger PFC representations to support (direct) processing in the task-relevant pathways (e.g., Cohen, Aston-Jones, & Gilzenrat, 2004). Given that aging-related declines implicate both brain regions and the neuromodulatory mechanisms therein (Bäckman & Farde, 2005; Ohnishi et al., 2001), older adults can be expected to be less efficient at monitoring process conflicts between habituated behavioral patterns and new task demands.

E. Toward Formalization of the SOC Framework

During the last decade, theoretical implications of the SOC framework have been developed and elaborated with widespread success, but, for the most part, without recourse to formal modeling (e.g., Baltes & Baltes, 1990; Baltes, 1997; Freund & Baltes, 2000; Marsiske et al., 1995; see, however, Chow & Nesselroade, 2004). In our view, formalizing the SOC framework through mathematical or computational models carries the advantage of making the dynamics of SOC mechanisms more explicit and empirically testable. Two specific modeling approaches, nonlinear dynamical systems and neural network models, are used to illustrate this claim.[2]

[2]As a third class of models, agent-based approaches may be particularly suitable for formal analyses of age differences in resource-based selection as observed in multitasking situations (Sy-Miin Chow and Paul B. Baltes, personal communication, 2005).

Dynamic Modeling of Age Differences in Resource Competition and Task Prioritization

Dynamic systems models characterize changes according to functional relations and parameters that determine their current state according to previous ones. Developmental psychologists have used dynamic systems notions both as conceptual theories and in various formal mathematical treatments (e.g., connectionist models and catastrophe theories) of developmental changes (for a review, see Smith and Thelen, 2003).

Predator–prey models, a subclass of dynamical models, have been applied successfully to study adult age differences in dual-task resource competition (Chow & Nesselroade, 2004). In these models, the performance of the two tasks can be specified as a set of two interrelated differential equations to predict learning rates, as well as the intratask and intertask dynamics of adaptive resource allocation. Specifically, age differences in intra- and intertask resource competition can be expressed as differences in the parameters of the differential equation system. We suggest extending these models by including parameters that capture age differences in task prioritization (e.g., emphasizing task domains that have more salient functional significance) in order to formally examine age differences in resource competition as a function of task selection.

Dynamic Neural Network Modeling of Age Differences in Experiential Selection

A second class of dynamic process models that has been commonly applied in studying developmental changes during childhood is neural networks (for a review, see Munakata & McClelland, 2003). We suggest that the dynamic adaptive properties of neural networks, with internal representations depending jointly on network parameters, input–output mapping, and training history, provide suitable frameworks for studying age differences in process-based selection.

Throughout life, experiences help shape the individual's habits and preferences. Such habits and preferences could, in turn, affect goal and task selection, either intentionally or unintentionally. In cases where past experiences match well with current situations, habits help the deliberation of selecting a particular goal or process. In other cases, habits may introduce conflict between current task requirement and old patterns of behavior or processes (see Figure 13.3). Neural network models have been applied to study the phenomenon of habitual word processing, leading to a color naming disadvantage in the traditional Stroop interference task (Cohen, Dunbar, & McClelland, 1990), habituation processes in infant cognition (for a review, see Sirois & Mareschal, 2004), and aging effects on context processing, susceptibility to inference, and conflict monitoring between targeted performance and error (Braver et al., 2001; Li, Lindenberger, & Sikström, 2001; Nieuwenhuis et al., 2002). Building on this past work, we propose that neural network simulations are a suitable means for studying interactions between aging-related decline in cognitive resources and process-based selection in situations that require conflict monitoring between current task requirement and well-established habits.

VI. Summary and Outlook

In our view, the SOC framework, originally developed by Baltes and Baltes (1990), is a valuable meta-theoretical tool for integrating research on life span development across functional domains, life periods, and levels of analysis (cf. Baltes et al., in press). Its explicit focus on selection, optimization, and compensation as three key mechanisms of developmental resource generation and allocation effectively counteracts the fragmentation of knowledge that characterizes much of the work in child development and aging.

The first part of this chapter reviewed empirical findings on adaptive resource allocation in adulthood and old age, primarily from a SOC perspective. Special emphasis was given to two research domains: motivation–volition, and cognitive–sensorimotor functioning. We illustrated how the development, expression, and function of diverse developmental phenomena such as goal selection and pursuit and performance in cognitive–sensorimotor dual tasks can be regarded as specific implementations of the component processes of selection, optimization, or compensation. We also noted how future research might strengthen the predictive power of the SOC framework.

The second part of this chapter delineated new research directions within the SOC framework. Our choice of suggested research topics was neither exhaustive nor representative. Rather, we opted for a selection of particularly promising and divergent themes to illustrate the range of applicability of the SOC framework. In the social domain, we suggested that future research would benefit from the investigation of age differences in characteristics of resource allocation mechanisms in single- and multiple-person systems. In the motivational domain, we explored how SOC theorizing can be used for deriving research questions that explicitly address the social foundation of active life management. In the cognitive domain, we introduced the concept of selection margins and discussed conflict monitoring between habitual processing and novel task demands. Finally, we argued that formal modeling provides a promising methodological tool for investigating the dynamics of adaptive resource allocation processes in life span development and for formalizing the dynamic properties of SOC theory.

This present chapter focused on the suitability of the SOC framework for understanding regulatory processes of adaptive resources allocation. Such processes play a central role in all functional domains and at all levels of analysis (e.g., interpersonal, behavioral, neuronal), especially when resource limitations become more pronounced, as is the case in old age. We reiterate, however, that the scope of the SOC framework extends beyond resource *allocation* to resource *generation*, i.e., it also speaks to the ontogeny of behavioral repertoires and action propensities. In our view, future research would profit from increased attention to the resource generation facet of SOC theory. Such increased attention would also result in a broader appreciation of the optimization mechanism, which presumably plays a key role in resource generation.

Acknowledgement

We thank Paul B. Baltes and Alexandra M. Freund for many insightful comments and stimulating discussions on SOC theory.

References

Abraham, J. D., & Hansson, R. O. (1995). Successful aging at work: An applied study of selection, optimization, and compensation through impression management. *Journal of Gerontology: Psychological Sciences, 50B,* P94–P103.

Anderson, N. D., Craik, F. I. M., & Naveh-Benjamin, M. (1998). The attentional demands of encoding and retrieval in younger and older adults. 1. Evidence from divided attention costs. *Psychology and Aging, 13,* 405–423.

Bäckman, L., & Dixon, R. A. (1992). Psychological compensation: A theoretical framework. *Psychological Bulletin, 112,* 259–283.

Bäckman, L., & Farde, L. (2005). The role of dopamine systems in cognitive aging. In R. Cabeza, L. Nyberg, & D. Park (Eds.), *Cognitive neuroscience of aging* (pp. 58–84). New York: Oxford University Press.

Bajor, J. K., & Baltes, B. B. (2003). The relationship between selection optimization with compensation, conscientiousness, motivation, and performance. *Journal of Vocational Behaviour, 63,* 347–367.

Baltes, B. B., & Heydens-Gahir, H. A. (2003). Reduction of work-family conflict through the use of selection, optimization, and compensation behaviors. *Journal of Applied Psychology, 88,* 1005–1018.

Baltes, M. M. (1996). *The many faces of dependency in old age.* New York: Cambridge University Press.

Baltes, M. M., & Carstensen, L. L. (1998). Social psychological theories and their applications to aging: From individual to collective. In V. L. Bengtson & K. W. Schaie (Eds.), *Handbook of theories of aging* (pp. 209–226). New York: Springer.

Baltes, M. M., & Lang, F. R. (1997). Everyday functioning and successful aging: The impact of resources. *Psychology and aging, 12,* 433–443.

Baltes, P. B. (1987). Theoretical propositions of life-span developmental psychology: On the dynamics between growth and decline. *Developmental Psychology, 23,* 611–626.

Baltes, P. B. (1997). On the incomplete architecture of human ontogeny: Selection, optimization, and compensation as foundation of developmental theory. *American Psychologist, 52,* 366–380.

Baltes, P. B., & Baltes, M. M. (1990). Psychological perspectives on successful aging: The model of selective optimization with compensation. In P. B. Baltes & M. M. Baltes (Eds.), *Successful aging: Perspectives from the behavioral sciences* (pp. 1–34). New York: Cambridge University Press.

Baltes, P. B., Baltes, M. M., Freund, A. M., & Lang, F. R. (1999). *The measurement of selection, optimization, and compensation (SOC) by self-report: Technical report 1999.*

Berlin: Max Planck Institute for Human Development.

Baltes, P. B., Lindenberger, U., & Staudinger, U. M. (in press). Life span theory in developmental psychology. In W. Damon (Series Ed.) & R. M. Lerner (Vol. Ed.), *Handbook of child psychology* (6th edition, vol.1). New York: Wiley.

Baltes, P. B., & Staudinger, U. M. (1996). Interactive minds in a life-span perspective: Prologue. In P. B. Baltes & U. M. Staudinger (Eds.), *Interactive minds* (pp. 1–32). New York: Cambridge University Press.

Bondar, A., Krampe, R. T., & Baltes, P. B. (2005). *The dynamics between balance and cognition in young and old adults: Older adults maintain adaptive flexibility of resource allocation despite higher dual-task costs.* Unpublished manuscript.

Bouchard Ryan, E., Anas, A. P., Beamer, M., & Bajorek, S. (2003). Coping with age-related vision loss in everyday reading activities. *Educational Gerontology, 29,* 37–54.

Brandtstädter, J. (1999). The self in action and development. Cultural, biosocial, and ontogenetic bases of intentional self-development. In J. Brandtstädter & R. M. Lerner (Eds.), *Action and self-development: Theory and research through the life span* (pp. 37–65). Thousand Oaks, CA: Sage.

Brandtstädter, J., & Greve, W. (1994). The aging self: Stabilizing and protective processes. *Developmental Review, 14,* 52–80.

Brandtstädter, J., & Renner, G. (1990). Tenacious goal pursuit and flexible goal adjustment: Explication and age-related analysis of assimilative and accommodative strategies of coping. *Psychology and Aging, 5,* 58–67.

Brandtstädter, J., Rothermund, K., & Schmitz, U. (1997). Coping resources in later life. *European Review of Applied Psychology, 47,* 107–114.

Brandtstädter, J., & Rothermund, K. (2002). The life-course dynamics of goal pursuit and goal adjustment: A two-process framework. *Developmental Review, 22,* 117–150.

Brandtstädter, J., & Wentura, D. (1995). Adjustment to shifting possibility frontiers in later life: Complementary adaptive modes. In R. A. Dixon & L. Bäckman

(Eds.), *Compensating for psychological deficits and declines: Managing losses and promoting gains* (pp. 83–106). Hilldale, NJ: Erlbaum.

Brandtstädter, J., Wentura, D., & Greve, W. (1993). Adaptive resources of the aging self: Outlines of an emergent perspective. *Journal of Behavioral Development, 16,* 323–349.

Braver, T. S., et al. (2001). Context processing in older adults: Evidence for a theory relating cognitive control to neurobiology in healthy aging. *Journal of Experimental Psychology: General, 130,* 746–763.

Brim, G. (1992). *Ambition: How we manage success and failure throughout our lives.* New York: Basic Books.

Broadbent, D. E. (1958). *Perception and communication.* New York: Pergamon Press.

Brown, L. A., Sleik, R. J., Polych, M. A., & Gage, W. H. (2002). Is the prioritization of postural control altered in conditions of postural threat in younger and older adults? *Journal of Gerontology: Medical Sciences, 57A,* M785–M792.

Brown, L. A., & Woollacott, M. H. (1998). The effects of aging on the control of posture and locomotion in healthy older adults: An emphasis on cognition. *Psychologische Beiträge, 40,* 27–43.

Carstensen, L. L. (1993). Motivation for social contact across the life span: A theory of socioemotional selectivity. In J. E. Jacobs (Ed.), *Nebraska Symposium on Motivation, 1992: Developmental perspectives on motivation. Current theory and research in motivation* (Vol. 40, pp. 209–254). Lincoln, NE: University of Nebraska Press.

Carstensen, L. L. (1998). A life-span approach to social motivation. In J. Heckhausen (Ed.), *Motivation and self-regulation across the life span* (pp. 341–363). New York: Cambridge University Press.

Carstensen, L. L., Fung, H. H., & Charles, S. T. (2003). Socioemotional selectivity theory and the regulation of emotion in the second half of life. *Motivation and Emotion, 27,* 103–123.

Carstensen, L. L., Isaacowitz, D. M., & Charles, S. T. (1999). Taking time seriously: A theory of socioemotional selectivity. *American Psychologist, 54,* 165–181.

Castel, A. D., & F. I. M. Craik (2003). The effects of aging and divided attention on memory for item and associative information. *Psychology & Aging, 18,* 873–885.

Cerrato, I. M., & Fernanández de Trocóniz, M. I. (1998). Successful aging. But, why don't the elderly get more depressed? *Psychology in Spain, 2,* 27–42.

Changeux, J.-P. (1985). *Neuronal man.* New York: Oxford University Press.

Chipperfield, J. G., Perry, R. P., & Menec, V. H. (1999). Primary and secondary control-enhancing strategies: Implications for health in later life. *Journal of Aging and Health, 11,* 517–539.

Chou, K.-L., & Chi, I. (2002). Financial strain and life satisfaction in Hong Kong elderly Chinese: Moderating effect of life management strategies including selection, optimization, and compensation. *Aging and Mental Health, 6,* 172–177.

Chow, S. M., & Nesselroade, J. R. (2004). General slowing or decreased inhibition? Mathematical models of age differences in cognitive functioning. *Journals of Gerontology Series B: Psychological Sciences, 59,* P101–P109.

Cohen, J. D., Aston-Jones, G., & Gilzenrat, M. S. (2004). A system level theory of attention and cognitive control. In M. I. Posner (Eds.) *Cognitive neuroscience of attention,* (pp. 71–90). New York: Guilford Press.

Cohen, J. D., Dunbar, K., & McClelland, J. L. (1990). On the control of automatic processes: A parallel distributed-processing account of the Stroop effect. *Psychological Review, 97,* 332–361.

Craik, F. I. M., & Byrd, M. (1982). Aging and cognitive deficits: The role of attentional resources. In F. I. M. Craik & S. Trehub (Eds.), *Aging and cognitive processes* (pp. 191–211). New York: Plenum.

Craik, K. J. W. (1948). Theory of the human operator in control systems. II. Man as an element in a control system. *British Journal of Psychology, 38,* 142–148.

Crossley, M., & Hiscock, M. (1992). Age-related differences in concurrent-task performance in normal adults: Evidence for a decline in processing resources. *Psychology and Aging, 7,* 499–506.

Davies, P. L., Segalowitz, S. J., & Gavin, W. J. (2004). Development of response-monitoring ERPs in 7-to-25 year-olds. *Developmental Neuropsychology, 25,* 355–376.

Edelman, G. M. (1987). *Neural Darwinism: The theory of neuronal group selection.* New York: Basic Books.

Emmons, R. A. (1996). Striving and feeling: Personal goals and subjective well-being. In P. M. Gollwitzer & J. A. Bargh (Eds.), *The psychology of action: Linking cognition and motivation to behavior* (pp. 313–337). New York: Guilford Press.

Fredrickson, B. L., & Carstensen, L. L. (1990). Choosing social partners: How old age and anticipated endings make people more selective. *Psychology and Aging, 5,* 335–347.

Freund, A. M., & Baltes, P. B. (1998). Selection, optimization, and compensation as strategies of life management: Correlations with subjective indicators of successful aging. *Psychology and Aging, 13,* 531–543.

Freund, A. M., & Baltes, P. B. (2000). The orchestration of selection, optimization and compensation: An action-theoretical conceptualization of a theory of developmental regulation. In W. J. Perrig & A. Grob (Eds.), *Control of human behavior, mental processes, and consciousness: Essays in honor of the 60th birthday of August Flammer* (pp. 35–58). Mahwah, NJ: Lawrence Erlbaum.

Freund, A. M., & Baltes, P. B. (2002a). The adaptiveness of selection, optimization, and compensation as strategies of life management: Evidence from a preference study on proverbs. *Journal of Gerontology: Psychological Sciences, 57B,* P426–P434.

Freund, A. M., & Baltes, P. B. (2002b). Life-management strategies of selection, optimization, and compensation: Measurement by self-report and construct validity. *Journal of Personality and Social Psychology, 82,* 642–662.

Freund, A. M., Li, K. Z. H., & Baltes, P. B. (1999). Successful development and aging: The role of selection, optimization, and compensation. In J. Brandtstädter & R. M. Lerner (Eds.), *Action and self-development: Theory and research through the life span* (pp. 401–434). Thousand Oaks, CA: Sage.

Freund, A. M., & Riediger, M. (2001). What I have and what I do: The role of resource loss and gain throughout life. *Applied Psychology: An International Review, 50,* 370–380.

Freund, A. M., & Riediger, M. (2003). Successful aging. In R. M. Lerner, M. A. Easterbrooks & J. Mistry (Eds.), *Handbook of psychology:* (vol. 6, pp. 601–628). New York: Wiley.

Fung, H. H., Carstensen, L. L., & Lutz, A. M. (1999). Influence of time on social preference: Implications for life-span development. *Psychology and Aging, 14,* 595–604.

Gignac, M. A. M., Cott, C., & Badley, E. M. (2000). Adaptation to chronic illness and disability and its relationship to perceptions of independence and dependence. *Journal of Gerontology: Psychological Sciences, 55B,* P362–P372.

Gignac, M. A. M., Cott, C., & Badley, E. M. (2002). Adaptation to disability: Applying selective optimization with compensation to behaviors of older adults with osteoarthritis. *Psychology and Aging, 17,* 520–524.

Heckhausen, J. (1999). *Developmental regulation in adulthood: Age-normative and sociostructural constraints as adaptive challenges.* New York: Cambridge University Press.

Heckhausen, J., & Schulz, R. (1995). A life-span theory of control. *Psychological Review, 102,* 284–304.

Heckhausen, J., Wrosch, C., & Fleeson, W. (2001). Developmental regulation before and after a developmental deadline: The sample case of "biological clock" for childbearing. *Psychology and Aging, 16,* 400–413.

Heuer, H. (1996). Dual-task performance. In O. Neumann & A. F. Sanders (Eds.), *Handbook of perception and action* (Vol. 3, pp. 113–153). London: Academic Press.

Hobfoll, S. E. (1998). *Stress, culture, and community: The psychology and philosophy of stress.* New York: Plenum Press.

Johnson, M. H. (2001). Functional brain development in humans. *Nature Review Neuroscience, 2,* 475–483.

Jopp, D. (2002). *Successful aging: On the functional interplay between personal resources and adaptive strategies of life management.* Doctoral dissertation, Free

University Berlin. Retrieved October 10, 2004, from http://www.diss.fu-berlin.de/2003/50/

Kahneman, D. (1973). *Attention and effort.* Englewood Cliffs, NJ: Prentice-Hall.

Kemper, S., Herman, R. E., & Lian, C. H. T. (2003). The costs of doing two things at once for younger and older adults: Talking while walking, finger tapping, and ignoring speech or noise. *Psychology and Aging, 18,* 181–192.

Kinsbourne, M., & Hicks, R. E. (1978). Functional cerebral space: A model for overflow, transfer and interference effects in human performance: A tutorial review. In J. Requin (Ed.), *Attention and performance VII* (pp. 345–362). Hillsdale, NJ: Lawrence Erlbaum.

Krampe, R. T., & Baltes, P. B. (2003). Intelligence as adaptive resource development and resource allocation: A new look through the lenses of SOC and expertise. In R. J. Sternberg & E. L. Grigorenko (Eds.), *Perspectives on the psychology of abilities, competencies, and expertise* (pp. 31–69). New York: Cambridge University Press.

Lajoie, Y., Teasdale, N., Bard, C., & Fleury, M. (1996). Attentional demands for walking: Age-related changes. In A.-M. Ferrandez & N. Teasdale (Eds.), *Changes in sensory motor behavior in aging* (pp. 235–256). Amsterdam: Elsevier Science.

Lakatos, I. (1970). Falsification and the methodology of scientific research programmes. In I. Lakatos & A. Musgrave (Eds.), *Criticisms and the growth of knowledge* (pp. 91–196). Cambridge, England: Cambridge University Press.

Lang, F. B., Rieckmann, N., & Baltes, M. M. (2002). Adapting to aging losses: Do resources facilitate strategies of selection, compensation, and optimization in everyday functioning. *Journal of Gerontology: Psychological Sciences, 57B,* P501–P509.

Li, K. Z. H., Krampe, R. T., & Bondar, A. (in press). An ecological approach to studying aging and dual-task performance. In R. W. Engle, G. Sedek, U. von Hecker, & D. N. McIntosh (Eds.), *Cognitive limitations in aging and psychopathology.* New York: Cambridge University Press.

Li, K. Z. H., Lindenberger, U., Freund, A. M., & Baltes, P. B. (2001). Walking while memorizing: Age-related differences in compensatory behavior. *Psychological Science, 12,* 230–237.

Li, S.-C., & Freund, A. M. (2005). Advances in lifespan psychology: A focus on biocultural and personal influences. *Research in Human Development, 2,* 1–23.

Li, S.-C., Lindenberger, U., Hommel, B., Aschersleben, G., Prinz, W., & Baltes, P. B. (2004). Lifespan transformations in the couplings of mental abilities and underlying cognitive processes. *Psychological Science, 15,* 155–163.

Li, S.-C., Lindenberger, U., & Sikström, S. (2001). Aging cognition: From neuromodulation to representation. *Trends in Cognitive Sciences, 5,* 479–486.

Lindenberger, U., Marsiske, M., & Baltes, P. B. (2000). Memorizing while walking: Increase in dual-task costs from young adulthood to old age. *Psychology and Aging, 15,* 417–436.

Lövdén, M., Schellenbach, M., Grossmann-Hutter, B., Krüger, A., & Lindenberger, U. (in press). Environmental topography and postural control demands shape aging-associated decrements in spatial navigation performance. *Psychology and Aging.*

Magnusson, D. (Ed.) (1996). *The life span development of individuals: Behavioral, neurobiological, and psychosocial perspectives: A synthesis.* Cambridge, UK: Cambridge University Press.

Marsiske, M., Lang, F. B., Baltes, P. B., & Baltes, M. M. (1995). Selective optimization with compensation: Life-span perspectives on successful human development. In R. A. Dixon & L. Baeckman (Eds.), *Compensating for psychological deficits and declines: Managing losses and promoting gains* (pp. 35–79). Mahwah, NJ: Lawrence Erlbaum.

Miller, E. K., & J. D. Cohen (2001). An integrative theory of prefontal cortex function. *Annual Review of Neuroscience, 24,* 167–202.

Miller, G. A. (1956). The magical number seven, plus or minus two: Some limits on our capacity for processing information. *Psychological Review, 63,* 81–97.

Munakata, Y., & McClelland, J. L. (2003). Connectionist models of development. *Developmental Sciences, 6,* 413–429.

Navon, D. (1984). Resources: A theoretical soup stone? *Psychological Review, 91,* 216–234.

Nieuwenhuis, S., Ridderinkhof, K. R., Talsma, D., Coles, M. G. H., Holroyd, C. B., Kpk, A., & Van der Molen, M. W. (2002). A computational account of altered error processing in older age: Dopamine and error-related processing. *Cognitive, Affective, and Behavioral Neuroscience, 2,* 19–36.

Ohnishi, T., Matsuda, H., Tabira, T., Asada, T., & Uno, M. (2001). Changes in brain morphology in Alzheimer disease and normal aging: Is Alzheimer disease an exaggerated aging process? *American Journal of Neuroradiology, 22,* 1680–1685.

Pashler, H. (1984). Processing stages in overlapping tasks: Evidence for a central bottleneck. *Journal of Experimental Psychology: Human Perception and Performance, 10,* 358–377.

Piaget, J. (1980). *Les formes élémentaires de la dialectique.* Paris: Gallimard.

Piaget, J. (1985). *The equilibrium of cognitive structures: The central problem of intellectual development.* Chicago: University of Chicago Press.

Quartz, S., & Sejnowski, T. (2000). Constraining constructivism: cortical and subcortical constraints on learning in development. *Behavioral and Brain Sciences, 23,* 785–792.

Read, S. J., & Miller, L. C. (1989). Inter-Personalism: Toward a goal-based theory of persons in relationships. In L. A. Pervin (Ed.), *Goal concepts in personality and social psychology* (pp. 413–472). Hillsdale, NJ: Lawrence Erlbaum.

Riediger, M., & Freund, A. M. (2004). Interference and facilitation among personal goals: Differential associations with subjective well-being and persistent goal pursuit. *Personality and Social Psychology Bulletin, 30,* 1511–1523.

Riediger, M., Freund, A. M., & Baltes, P. B. (2005). Managing life through personal goals: Intergoal facilitation and intensity of goal pursuit in younger and older adulthood. *Journal of Gerontology: Psychological Sciences, 60B,* P84–P91.

Salthouse, T. A., Rogan, J. D., & Prill, K. A. (1984). Division of attention: Age differences on a visually presented memory task. *Memory and cognition, 12,* 613–620.

Sattin, R. W. (1992). Falls among older persons: A public health perspective. *Annual Reviews in Public Health, 13,* 489–508.

Sirois, S., & Mareschal, D. (2004). An interacting system model of infant habituation. *Journal of Cognitive Neuroscience, 16,* 1352–1362.

Smith, L. B., & Thelen, E. (2003). development as a dynamic system. *Trends in Cognitive Sciences, 7,* 343–348.

Somberg, B. L., & Salthouse, T. A. (1982). Divided attention abilities in young and old adults. *Journal of Experimental Psychology: Human Perception and Performance, 8,* 651–663.

Spencer, W. D., & Raz, N. (1995). Differential effects of aging on memory for content and context: A meta-analysis. *Psychology and Aging, 10,* 527–539.

Staudinger, U. M., & Freund, A. M. (1998). Sick and "poor" in old age and still in good spirits? A study of psychological resilience. *Zeitschrift für Klinische Psychologie, Forschung und Praxis, 27,* 78–85.

Staudinger, U. M., Freund, A. M., Linden, M., & Maas, I. (1999). Self, personality, and life regulation: Facets of psychological resilience in old age. In P. B. Baltes & K. U. Mayer (Eds.), *The Berlin Aging Study: Aging from 70 to 100* (pp. 302–328). New York: Cambridge University Press.

Teasdale, N., Bard, C., Dadouchi, F., Fleury, M., LaRue, J., & Stelmach, G. E. (1992). Posture and elderly persons: Evidence for deficits in the central integrative mechanisms. In G. E. Stelmach & J. Requin (Eds.), *Tutorials in motor behavior II* (pp. 917–931). Amsterdam: Elsevier Science.

Teasdale, N., Bard, C., LaRue, J., & Fleury, M. (1993). On the cognitive penetrability of posture control. *Experimental Aging Research, 19,* 1–13.

Tinetti, M. E. (1995). Falls. In W. R. Hazzard, E. L. Bierman, J. P. Blass, W. H. Ettinger, & J. B. Halter (Eds.), *Principles of Geriatric Medicine and Gerontology* (3rd edition). New York: McGraw-Hill.

Tsang, P. S., & Shaner, T. L. (1998). Age, attention, expertise, and time-sharing performance. *Psychology and Aging, 13,* 323–347.

von Cranach, M., Ochsenbein, G., & Valach, L. (1986). The group as a self-active system: Outline of a theory of group action. *European Journal of Social Psychology, 16,* 193–229.

Vondracek, F. W., & Porfeli, E. J. (2002). Life-span developmental perspectives on adult career development: Recent advances. In S. G. Niles (Ed.), *Adult career development: Concepts, issues and practices* (3rd edition, pp. 20–38). Columbus, OH: National Career Development Association.

Waddington, C. H. (1975). *The evolution of an evolutionist.* Edinburgh: Edinburgh University Press.

Wegge, J. (2000). Participation in group goal setting: Some novel findings and a comprehensive model as a new ending to an old story. *Applied Psychology: An International Review, 49,* 498–516.

Wiese, B. S. (2000). *On the dynamics of goal structures in the domains of work and partnership.* Münster, Germany: Waxmann.

Wiese, B. S., & Freund, A. M. (2000). The interplay of work and family in young and middle adulthood. In J. Heckhausen (Ed.), *Motivational psychology of human development: Developing motivation and motivating development* (pp. 233–250). Amsterdam, Netherlands: Elsevier.

Wiese, B. S., Freund, A. M., & Baltes, P. B. (2000). Selection, optimization, and compensation: An action-related approach to work and partnership. *Journal of Vocational Behaviour, 57,* 273–300.

Wiese, B. S., Freund, A. M., & Baltes, P. B. (2002). Subjective career success and emotional well-being: Longitudinal predictive power of selection, optimization, and compensation. *Journal of Vocational Behaviour, 60,* 321–335.

Wiese, B. S., & Schmitz, B. (2002). Study-related action in the context of a developmental-psychological meta-model. *Zeitschrift für Entwicklungspsychologie und Pädagogische Psychologie, 34,* 80–94.

Wilensky, R. (1983). *Planning and Understanding.* Reading, MA: Addison-Wesley.

Woollacott, M. H. (2000). Systems contributing to balance disorders in older adults. *Journal of Gerontology: Medical Sciences, 55A,* M424–M428.

Woollacott, M. H., & Shumway-Cook, A. (2002). Attention and the control of posture and gait: A review of an emerging area of research. *Gait and Posture, 16,* 1–14.

Wrosch, C., & Heckhausen, J. (1999). Control processes before and after passing a developmental deadline: Activation and deactivation of intimate relationship goals. *Journal of Personality and Social Psychology, 77,* 415–427.

Fourteen

Everyday Problem Solving and Decision Making

Michael Marsiske and Jennifer A. Margrett

I. Introduction

Three main questions guide the study of everyday problem solving and decision making. First, in contrast to many academic and laboratory measures of cognition, does real world problem solving show the benefits of experience and is it protected against age-related declines? Second, what is the relationship between basic or laboratory cognitive measures, which were originally designed to predict academic performance, and everyday problem solving? Third, if measures of everyday problem solving capture some aspect of individuals' behavior in the everyday world, are they useful predictors of how people actually manage their daily affairs? This chapter reviews evidence for each of these three questions and builds on previous *Handbook of the Psychology of Aging* reviews by Rabbitt (1977), Reese and Rodeheaver (1985), Salthouse (1990), and Willis (1996c). We will argue that there are now fairly clear answers to the first two questions, but that insufficient attention has been paid to the third.

The first section of this chapter considers definitional, theoretical, and operational (i.e., task characteristics) issues that have influenced current knowledge about everyday problem solving and decision making. The second section considers evidence for the three major questions (relatedness of everyday problem solving to age, cognition, and everyday function). The chapter closes by considering some emerging issues, including the clinical and practical value of everyday problem-solving assessment, as well as intervention and enhancement approaches.

A. Definitional Issues

The field of everyday problem solving has been characterized as heterogeneous or disordered (Allaire & Marsiske, 1999; Berg, 2005; Sinnott, 1989a; Marsiske & Willis, 1995), largely due to the diversity of problem types and scoring approaches used. Even nomenclature has varied, including practical problem solving (Denney, 1989), everyday cognition (Poon, Rubin, & Wilson, 1989), pragmatics of intelligence (Baltes, 1987), and practical intelligence (Sternberg & Wagner, 1986). One reason for these discrepancies likely stems from the varied theoretical roots from which everyday problem solving and decision-making research has emerged. Following the recommendations of Thornton and Dumke (2005) and Berg (2005), this chapter employs "everyday problem solving" as the most general label.

Problem solving and *decision making* both refer to goal-directed cognition, in which an individual constructs plans and/or formulates behavioral responses aimed at resolving a discrepancy between an initial state and a desired end state. Problem solving originated from cognitive psychology, and research in this tradition has focused more on the outcomes of problem solving and the effectiveness of solutions generated (Reitman, 1965; Simon, 1973). In addition, studies from this orientation have tended to focus on more instrumental tasks (i.e., solutions involving manipulation of data or objects in the service of self- and home-maintenance goals) and have tended to be well structured (i.e., initial state, available means/information, and desired end state are all provided to the problem solver; e.g., Allaire & Marsiske, 2002).

A second tradition of problem-solving research, from clinical psychology, is more related to studies of coping and is concerned both with how individuals appraise or represent problems (e.g., causal attributions, self-efficacy expectations, coping orientation) and their problem-solving skills (problem definition and formulation, solution generation and monitoring; e.g., D'Zurilla et al., 1998). Research in this tradition has focused more on the strategies and coping styles used by individuals, and the problems studied have tended to be relatively interpersonal (i.e., dilemmas involving conflict and cohesion with friends, families, and co-workers) and ill-structured (i.e., some information about initial state and/or available solution means and/or desired end state is not provided; e.g., Berg & Klaczynksi, 1996).

Decision-making studies are closely allied with problem-solving research, but such studies have focused more on the process of problem solving, particularly on how individuals evaluate multiple alternatives and choices. It has been common in decision-making studies to examine how much information individuals use to solve highly structured choice problems, as well as the time spent and the information search strategies employed (Peters et al., 2000; Sanfrey & Hastie, 2000).

A critical issue for this chapter concerns how a problem or decision earns the "everyday" modifier. The core idea seems to be that everyday problems are contextualized, i.e., (a) they resemble challenges or dilemmas that individuals might actually confront in their lives, (b) they seem important and relevant, (c) their effective solution relies on accumulated experience, and (d) the means and ends of the problem exist and are common or familiar (Baddeley, 1989; Bahrick, 1989). These ideas are revisited in our consideration of ecological validity in a later section.

B. Theoretical Issues

Four major theoretical ideas have guided research on adult everyday problem solving. *Contextualism* (Berg & Sternberg, 1985) or neofunctionalism (Dixon & Baltes, 1986) addresses the idea that individuals develop in specific life circumstances and niches. This implies that to truly measure an individual's effectiveness with managing daily life challenges, we must identify those particular tasks that occur with high frequency and that might have high survival value for the individual (Frederiksen, 1986; Schaie, 1978; Willis & Schaie, 1986).

Experientialism (Berg & Sternberg, 1985) is related to contextualism in that individuals are expected to have had high levels of practice and experience with highly relevant and personally important problems. Through practice, substantial bodies of procedural and declarative knowledge are built (e.g., Ackerman, 2005; Baltes; 1987, 1993; Baltes, Staudinger, & Lindenberger, 1999; Beier & Ackerman, 2005; Cattell, 1987; Denney, 1989; Ericsson & Charness, 1994; Rybash, Hoyer, & Roodin, 1986). Such knowledge seems to remain relatively preserved into old age (e.g., Charness, 2005). Decision-making researchers encompass this idea in the notion of *heuristics*, which refer to stored scripts, schemas, preferences, and routines. Heuristics constitute mental shortcuts, which permit individuals to generate consistent responses in new situations (Chasseigne et al., 1999; Peters et al., 2000). Reliance on heuristics can reduce the processing demands of complex problems (by reliance on the products of past processing) and increase the speed and efficiency of decision making ("fast and frugal" problem solving; Marsh, Todd, & Gigerenzer, 2004). However, overreliance on heuristics may lead to biased and inappropriate responding when past situations are not isomorphic with current problems (Peters et al., 2000).

Componentialism (Berg & Sternberg, 1985) reflects the role of the broader cognitive system when acquired knowledge and heuristics are not adequate for problem solving, as in novel or unfamiliar situations. When individuals deal with novelty, they must increasingly rely upon adaptive abilities and skills, such as attention, speed of response, working memory, reasoning skills, and executive functioning. However, it is precisely these aspects of cognitive functioning that are affected most negatively by age in both cross-sectional and longitudinal studies (Schaie, 2005; Lövdén, Ghisletta, & Lindenberger, 2004). Willis and Schaie (1986, 1993) have argued, therefore, that we can best understand everyday problem solving from a "hierarchical" perspective (see also Marsiske & Willis, 1998; Willis & Marsiske, 1991). In this view, everyday problem solving is a higher order ("compiled"; Salthouse, 1990) skill, dependent for performance on many constituent abilities (domain-specific knowledge, as well as basic cognitive abilities).

Postformalism has also been an influential perspective. Developed as an extension of Piagetian theory, the core contribution of this line of thought is the recognition that adult problem solving is not always strictly *rational*. In the real world, when pondering life dilemmas, individuals also consider their own preferences, values, and feelings as well as those of their social partners and cultural context, in addition to purely cognitive considerations (Kramer & Woodruff, 1986; Labouvie-Vief, 1985, 1992; Sinnott, 1989b). Thus, scoring adult problem solutions on strictly rational grounds may reveal age *differences*; however, such differences may not necessarily imply age *deficits* because they could instead reflect qualitative changes in problem solving (see also Berg et al., 1994; Reese & Rodeheaver, 1985).

C. Operational Issues

There has been wide variability across laboratories in the conceptualization and measurement of everyday problem solving. Table 14.1 summarizes five major dimensions along which everyday problems have varied and also highlights the challenge when trying to make generalizations about everyday problem solving in later life. Thus, differences

Table 14.1
Sources of Heterogeneity across Studies of Everyday Problem Solving

Dimension	Exemplar	Example studies
Structure	Well-structured: Problems present individuals with specific stimuli (e.g., compare nutrition label) and ask them to answer questions about them (e.g., which product has the least salt?).	Allaire & Marsiske, 1999, Diehl et al., 2005; Meyer et al., 1995; Willis, 1996b
	Ill-structured: Brief narrative vignettes are presented describing dilemmas or situations where available means or solution goals may not be explicit (e.g., "A couple moves to a new town; how should they continue to associate with people?").	Artistico, Cervone, & Pezzuti, 2003; Berg et al., 1998; Blanchard-Fields, Stein, & Watson, 2004; Denney & Pearce, 1989
Breadth of domains	Single-domain studies: All problems fall within a single category or domain (e.g., medication use, financial decisions, selecting a car).	Capon, Kuhn, & Carretero, 1989; Finucane et al., 2005; Hershey & Walsh, 2000–2001; Johnson & Drungle, 2000
	Multiple-domain studies: The set of problems is varied and includes multiple instrumental (e.g., nutrition, medication use, finance) and/or interpersonal (e.g., dealing with co-workers, friends, family members) domains within a single instrument.	Allaire & Marsiske, 1999; Cornelius & Caspi, 1987; Denney, 1989; Diehl, Willis, & Schaie, 1995; Hartley, 1989; Willis & Marsiske, 1993
Content	Instrumental: Problems involve the manipulation of implements or data, usually in the service of a larger goal, such as maintaining health or well-being.	Chen & Sun, 2003; Hershey & Farrell, 1999; Diehl et al., 2005
	Social: management of personal relationships, collaboration, coping with conflicts.	Berg et al., 1998; Blanchard-Fields, 1986; Crawford & Channon, 2002
Type	Performance-based, paper and pencil: Participants actually solve the problem for the investigator (e.g., compare two brands) and record their answer.	Allaire & Marsiske, 2002; Whitfield et al., 1999
	Performance-based, behavioral observation: Participants solve the problem behaviorally for the experimenter (e.g., look up and dial a long-distance number; make change).	Diehl, Willis, & Schaie, 1995; Owsley, Sloane, McGwin, & Ball, 2001
	Performance-based, computer-administered: Problems are studied on-screen, and individuals must select the order and amount of information to review and make a decision.	Johnson, 1990; Finucane et al., 2005; Patrick, 1995
	Problem vignettes with strategy selection: After a dilemma is presented, participants are given one or more potential solution strategies and are asked to rate their likelihood of using each strategy.	Cornelius & Caspi, 1987; D'Zurilla et al., 1998; Haught et al., 2000

Scoring		
	Problem vignettes with open-ended responses: Participants "think aloud" or write narrative essays about how they might deal with the challenge.	Artistico et al., 2003
	Accuracy/correctness: Participants' solutions are scored as correct/incorrect or effective/ineffective.	Allaire & Marsiske, 2002; Willis & Marsiske, 1993
	Fluency: The number of solutions is counted; may be combined with accuracy (i.e., the number of *effective* solutions).	Artistico et al., 2003; Allaire & Marsiske, 2002; Denney & Pearce, 1989
	Coping-style strategies: Participant-described solutions are coded for type (e.g., problem-focused, interpersonal/dependent, cognitive/analytic, avoidant).	Berg et al., 1998; Blanchard-Fields et al., 1995
	Decisional criteria: Parameters such as study time, number of pieces of information viewed and re-viewed, systematicity of information review, consistency of responding are recorded.	Finucane et al., 2002; Johnson, 1990; Patrick, 1995

in findings between studies may reflect variation in task features or scoring approaches, a situation that is compounded by the clustering of several task and sample properties across investigations. For example, investigators studying well-structured problems also mostly focus on instrumental activities using accuracy/effectiveness coding. Moreover, these studies typically have included only adults aged 50 and older. Thus, it is somewhat difficult to disentangle the unique effects of these various dimensions, although Thornton and Dumke (2005) have made an important initial attempt at this in a meta-analysis.

II. Evaluating Age, Cognition, and Function Relatedness

The introduction to this chapter argued that the three main questions motivating research on everyday problem solving have been whether (a) there is maintenance of performance with age; (b) whether everyday problem solving is related to, or independent of, traditionally measured cognition; and (c) everyday problem solving is a useful predictor of real world functioning and adaptation. The next sections evaluate evidence regarding these questions.

A. Age

The focus on age effects in the everyday problem-solving literature has been dominant. As is true for much cognitive aging research, most work has been cross-sectional, meaning that maturational and generational effects tend to be confounded (Schaie, 1965; Baltes, 1968). Age ranges studied have varied substantially; the extreme age group design (i.e., comparison of "younger" participants, usually undergraduates in their twenties, and "older" participants, typically 65 years

of age and older) is modal. A smaller number of studies also includes a middle-aged group or sample continuously across the adult age range. Because of the substantial number of studies examining age effects, we summarize the literature separately for problem-solving and decision-making studies.

1. Problem Solving

There is some consistency to the age-relationship findings when we divide studies into four major areas: (a) studies that emphasize accuracy or effectiveness of problem solving, (b) studies that measure the number of solutions (fluency), (c) other studies (mostly relying on participant ratings), and (d) studies that have focused on the strategies employed rather than the effectiveness of solutions.

a. Accuracy/Effectiveness Studies
Table 14.2 summarizes some of the major instruments used across a variety of studies, as well as the age ranges covered in these studies, and the reported age effects, mostly in samples aged sixty and older. As shown, most of the measures in this grouping have examined participant performance on domains drawn from the instrumental activities of daily living (IADL; food preparation, medication use, financial management, housekeeping, laundry, shopping, transportation; Lawton & Brody, 1969); some have used paper-and-pencil tests, whereas others have used behavioral observations.

The focus on older adults only is likely a manifestation of contextualism: Problems designed to be relevant for older adults are presumed to be relatively meaningless to examine in broad age ranges. In the young-old to old-old age range studied, there have been near-universal negative cross-sectional effects of age. While most of the studies have emphasized European American samples,

Table 14.2

Problem-Solving Instruments with Accuracy/Effectiveness Scoring: Examples of Measures, Age Ranges, and Cross-Sectional Associations with Age in Unimpaired Samples

Instrument	Summary	Example studies	Age range (years)	Association with age
Accuracy/effectiveness scores: Paper-and-pencil Test of Basic Skills (TBS; Educational Testing Service, 1977)	Participants study everyday printed stimuli (directions, charts, forms) and answer questions about them	Willis & Schaie, 1986	60-88	—[a]
Everyday Problems Test (EPT; Willis & Marsiske, 1993)	Similar to TBS, but all stimuli designed to be old-age appropriate in domains of food preparation, medication use, financial management, etc.	Marsiske & Willis, 1995 Whitfield et al., 1999	68-94 50-90	$r=-0.41$ $r=-0.34$
Everyday Cognition Battery (ECB)	Subtasks include reasoning, declarative memory, knowledge, and working memory; items cover nutrition, medication use, finance	Allaire & Marsiske, 1999	60-92	$r=-0.23$ to -0.37
Practical reasoning/practical knowledge	German adaptations of TBS and WAIS Information/similarities, respectively	Lindenberger et al., 1993	70-103	$r=-0.45$[b]
Accuracy/effectiveness scores: Behavioral Observed Tasks of Daily Living (OTDL)	Participants are observed enacting requested behaviors (e.g., looking up and dialing a phone number; paying a bill by mail) in areas such as food preparation, telephone use, finance, and medication use	Diehl, Willis, & Schaie, 1995 Diehl et al., 2005 Goverover, 2004 Goverover & Hinojosa, 2002 Goverover & Josman, 2004	66-87 65-90	$r=-0.42$ $r=-0.24$ —[a] —[a] —[a]
Timed Instrumental Activities of Daily Living Test (TIADL)	Both accuracy and speed of everyday visual search behaviors (e.g., looking up a number in a phone directory, counting change, finding items on a pantry shelf) are recorded	Owsley et al., 2001	66-87	$r=0.29$[c]

[a]Not reported.

[b]Correlation reflects association between age and a reasoning composite on which the practical reasoning task had a standardized factor loading of 0.83.

[c]Positive direction reflects coding of variable; age was associated with increases in time needed to complete visual searches accurately.

studies by Allaire and Marsiske (1999), Diehl et al. (2005), and Whitfield et al. (1999) indicate that these problem-solving measures have similar psycho-metric properties and age trends in African-American samples.

There have been two exceptions to the dominance of cross-sectional studies, one using the Test of Basic Skills (TBS; Willis et al., 1992; see also Willis & Marsiske, 1991) and one using the Every-day Problems Test (EPT; Willis, 1996b). Participants in these studies (adults who at baseline ranged in age from the sixties to the nineties) showed a reliable but modest decline over a 7-year period, with the magnitude of decline larger at higher ages. In the Willis et al. (1992) study, intraindividual change analyses revealed that the majority of participants (57%) showed no reliable intraindividual decline (defined as changes of less than one standard error of measurement) over 7 years.

b. Fluency studies Table 14.3 summarizes a number of the studies that have used some version of fluency rating. In these studies, fluency is operationalized as the number of safe and effective solutions generated by participants for open-ended vignettes. The rationale for fluency scoring relates to the difficulty of scoring responses to open-ended, ill-structured vignettes (i.e., what constitutes a "correct" answer?). Drawing on the example problem in Table 14.3, if one's refrigerator breaks down in the middle of the night, is checking the fuse panel (for a blown fuse) more correct than calling an adult child for help? Moreover, individuals often spontaneously generate more than one possible solution, particularly when the problems are not constrained regarding means or goals.

In several cross-sectional studies reported by Denney and colleagues, including persons covering the full adult age range, there was a curvilinear age trend with a "midlife peak," favoring those in midlife (e.g., Denney & Palmer, 1981; Denney & Pearce, 1989; Denney, Pearce, & Palmer, 1982; Denney, Tozier, & Schlotthauer, 1992). An exception to this pattern was reported by Denney et al. (1982), who found that younger adults performed best on "age-matched" problems. Artistico, Cervone, and Pezzuti (2003) have reported a similar "age-match" effect using their own open-ended vignettes: in that study, younger and older adults demonstrated the best performance and had the highest self-efficacy for problems identified as relevant to their age group.

While most studies have focused on age effects across adulthood, a few studies have examined the young-old to old-old differences, as in the accuracy/effectiveness studies. In the Georgia Centenarian Study, which included parti-cipants in their sixties, eighties, and hundreds, age was strongly negatively associated with fluency in two studies (Poon et al., 1992; Holtsberg et al., 2002), although Holtsberg et al. (2002) reported that age differences were actually confined to the best educated participants (perhaps because well-educated 60 year olds were more like Denney's middle-aged subjects and had not yet experienced declines). Findings similar to those of Holtsberg et al.'s less educated adults were reported by Marsiske and Willis (1995). The latter study found no relationship between age and fluency ($r = -.08$) on the Denney and Pearce (1989) task.

Berg, Meegan, and Klaczynski (1999) presented younger and older adults with open-ended problems about physician visits and attending a dinner party. Participants were asked to describe every-thing they would do between first making the decision to attend and later leaving the office/party. Participants described both preferred strategies and

Table 14.3

Problem-Solving Instruments with Fluency Scoring: Examples of Measures, Age Ranges, and Cross-Sectional Associations with Age in Unimpaired Samples

Instrument	Summary	Example studies	Age range
Denney practical problems (PP)	Problems varied from study to study, but all took the form of vignettes (e.g., "an older woman's refrigerator breaks down in the middle of the night; what should she do?") to which participants are encouraged to generate as many safe and effective solutions as possible.	Denney & Palmer, 1981	20–79
		Denney & Pearce, 1989	20–79
		Denney et al., 1982	20–79
		Denney et al., 1992	20–79
		Heidrich & Denney, 1994	18–81
		Poon et al., 1992	60–69, 80–89, 100+
		Holtsberg et al., 2002	60–69, 80–89, 100+
		Marsiske & Willis, 1995	68–94
Other vignette-based tasks	Tasks designed to be age appropriate.	Artistico et al., 2003	20–29, 65–75
		Berg et al., 1999	$M = 21$ and $M = 73^{a}$

[a]Age ranges not reported; cross-sectional associations with age are not shown because most of these studies relied on analysis of variance comparisons of adults of different ages and did not report effect sizes.

information needed to deal with the problem. Both age groups reported similar amounts of experience with the tasks, and script reports were similarly detailed across groups. Younger adults reported more strategies and requested more information in their problem solving, although the investigators were mindful that these differences might not reflect aging deficits, but rather greater goal and task focus in older participants. Indeed, the authors proposed that age differences in strategies might be characterized as "exhaustive/youthful style" versus "selective/older style," a theme that also emerges in the decision-making research (discussed later).

In one of the few studies to examine both solution effectiveness and solution fluency, Crawford and Channon (2002) examined responses to social dilemmas. The investigators reported that, relative to younger adults, older adults generated slightly fewer solutions. Interestingly, their work hinted at a possible compensatory process in older adults, trading quality for quantity (i.e., "older style"). The solutions of the older adults were rated as higher in effectiveness than those of younger participants, even though they were fewer in number.

c. Meta-analysis Thornton and Dumke (2005) conducted a meta-analysis of 33 age-difference studies of everyday problem solving and decision making. Many of the studies included in their review used experimenter ratings of solution quality (e.g., attempts to code the quality of participant-generated solutions). Other reviewed studies employed participant self-ratings of the likelihood of using particular experimenter-provided solutions or participant's confidence self-ratings about the effectiveness of self-generated solutions. To be included in the meta-analysis, studies had to include at least one age comparison (e.g., young vs old,

middle-aged vs old, young vs middle-aged). Across studies, older adults tended to perform more poorly than either middle-aged/younger adults, with a medium effect size (Cohen's $d = 0.48$, which translates roughly to an average correlation of $r = |0.29|$, according to Cohen, 1988). Estimates of average everyday problem solving were equivalent in young and middle-aged adults, in contrast to Denney's (1989) "midlife peak."

As shown in Table 14.1, problem-solving studies varied substantially in the method of response and scoring. Thus, Thornton and Dumke (2005) contrasted age differences in those studies where experimenters rated participant performance with studies using one of two forms of participant self-ratings (likelihood ratings or confidence ratings). Both experimenter ratings and participant confidence ratings showed similar negative age effects, favoring younger and middle-aged adults. Participants' likelihood self-ratings, in contrast, favored older adults. Thornton and Dumke (2005) also contrasted instrumental versus social problems. They found negative age effects for both problem types, but age differences were significantly smaller for the social problems. This is consistent with an analysis conducted by Marsiske and Willis (1995), who administered two social problem-solving measures (i.e., Cornelius & Caspi, 1987; Denney & Pearce, 1989) and one instrumental measure (Willis & Marsiske, 1995) in a single sample of older adults. Marsiske and Willis (1995) found no relationship between social problems and age, but a negative age relationship with the instrumental task.

d. Problem Strategy Studies Sinnott (1989b), among others, has suggested that qualitative aspects of everyday problem solving require at least as much attention as actual performance. Two research groups (Blanchard-Fields and Berg) have done the most work in this area. Several general findings have emerged.

First, on interpersonal and emotionally salient problems, older adults were more likely than younger adults to use both *emotional* coping strategies (i.e., managing their feelings) and *problem-focused action* (i.e., independent behavioral initiatives to solve the problem). This integration of emotional and rational styles is consistent with postformalist theories (Watson & Blanchard-Fields, 1998).

Second, evidence shows that older adults used more passive-dependent and avoidant-withdrawal solutions with interpersonal dilemmas than younger and middle-aged adults. This was true regardless of whether problems are self-generated or other-generated (e.g., Blanchard-Fields, Camp, & Jahnke, 1995).

Third, just as Artistico et al. (2003) reported that individuals had the poorest performance on problems for which they had the lowest self-efficacy, avoidant-denial solutions occurred disproportionately with problems for which individuals had the least confidence in their abilities (Blanchard-Fields, Chen, & Norris, 1997).

Fourth, even when middle-aged and older adults were compared in their use of emotional coping, there were qualitative differences in the type of coping. Middle-aged persons demonstrated more active (e.g., seeking out social support, confronting negative emotions directly) emotional coping, whereas older adults used more passive (e.g., denial, suppressing emotion, accepting the situation) emotion-focused strategies (Blanchard-Fields, Stein, & Watson, 2004).

Fifth, there may be a Denney-style midlife peak in interpersonal problem solving; D'Zurilla, Maydeu-Olivares, and Kant (1998) compared adults aged 17–80 and reported that middle-aged

participants obtained the highest scores on positive problem orientation and rational problem solving and the lowest scores on negative problem orientation, impulsivity and carelessness, and avoidance. Individuals at midlife were also most likely to identify interpersonal elements as the most salient features of everyday problems they encountered (Strough, Berg, & Sansone, 1996).

There may be some domain specificity in strategy use based on studies comparing instrumental versus social everyday problems. Blanchard-Fields, Chen, and Norris (1997), for example, showed that older adults were more likely to be problem focused with instrumental dilemmas, but emotion focused with interpersonal dilemmas. Sperling (2003) examined coping responses of adults aged 43 to 63 in one social and three instrumental life domains (marriage/partnership, health care system, housing, finances) and also found evidence for domain specificity. For example, with a social problem (marriage dilemmas), individuals were more likely to prefer interpersonal coping strategies, whereas for a health care problem, individuals were more likely to employ strategies utilizing formal institutional assistance.

Berg and colleagues (1998) found a similar match between problem domain (interpersonal or instrumental) and chosen strategies, but there were no age differences in this "domain match" of strategies to problems. Age differences in strategies were observed only for "free choice" self-generated problems (i.e., participants could name any problem they wanted to). Here, older adults reported using more problem-focused action and less cognitive regulation than younger age groups.

2. Decision Making

As with the everyday problem-solving research, it is possible to examine age effects both on decision-making performance (e.g., quality or suitability of choice made) and in the strategies used (e.g., amount of information studied, time spent, organization of feature searches). Table 14.4 offers a summary of several representative studies that suggested, relative to younger adults, older participants tended to use less information and reviewed fewer bits of information regarding the use of information and exhaustiveness of search (Finucane et al., 2005; Johnson, 1990; Johnson & Drungle, 2000; Meyer, Russo, & Talbot, 1995; Patrick, 1995). This tendency of older adults to be less exhaustive reflects, in part, the use of "noncompensatory" decision rules (e.g. ranking attributes in terms of importance and only comparing products/services on a subset of attributes that are judged as "important"; Johnson, 1990; Patrick, 1995; Finucane et al., 2002; Finucane et al., 2005) and is consistent with the "older/selective" problem-solving style described by Berg et al. (1999). Such noncompensatory strategies are assumed to be reducing cognitive processing demands by excluding some dimensions from consideration, thereby reducing task complexity and working memory load.

Second, while increased age has been associated with poorer decision-making performance, there seems to be substantial task specificity in findings. While the Thornton and Dumke (2005) meta-analysis suggested a negative relationship between age and solution quality (see also Finucane et al., 2002, 2005), other studies have found age invariance in solution quality. Patrick (1995) failed to find age differences in solution quality in a highly structured car-shopping task, as did Walker et al. (1997) in a driving decisions task and Meyer et al. (1995) in a breast cancer decision-making task. In the driving study, older adults tended to vary their decisions more (i.e., greater inconsistency) and have less confidence

about their decisions, but the overall quality of younger and older adults' route decisions was similar (Walker et al., 1997). Kim and Hasher (2005) actually found a performance advantage for older adults relative to undergraduates. In decision-making tasks in two domains (earning extra credit in a course and grocery shopping), undergraduates were actually more prone to an erroneous heuristic bias (the "attraction effect" or a preference for previously seen solutions, even if they are no longer optimal) than older adults on the grocery task. The investigators speculated that lack of interest/motivation by the younger adults for the grocery problem might have explained why they paid less attention to this task. Affect and motivation have been implicated as strong predictors of decision making in several studies (Finucane, Peters, & Slovic, 2003; Peters et al., 2000).

Third, while increased task complexity (i.e., having to evaluate a larger number of alternatives or features) is associated with greater error and more inconsistency, it does not appear to put older adults at a disproportionate disadvantage. Age-by-complexity interactions seldom reach significance (e.g., Finucane et al., 2005).

Fourth, prior experience and expertise with a task leads to better decisions, although this factor also does not appear to interact with age. In her car-shopping task, Patrick (1995) found that experts (salespeople) used as much time as other participants (average and novice car shoppers) to make their decisions, but the quality of their decisions was better. Similarly, in a study comparing younger, middle-aged, and older pilots and non-pilots on their memory and comprehension of navigational air traffic control messages, Morrow et al. (2001) found significantly poorer performance in older participants. Pilots outperformed nonpilots,

Table 14.4
Everyday Decision-Making Tasks: Examples

Task	Study	Description	IADL domain(s) assessed
Instrumental/interpersonal situations	Berg et al. (1999)	"Tell me everything that happens, from the time you make decision to go until the time you leave, at a _____"; options were "dinner party" and "physician visit"	n/a
Choices among health plans, food items, and banks	Finucane et al. (2005)	Included health plan choices similar to Finucane et al. (2002), as well as similarly presented choice tasks in the domains of food item comparison and financial institution comparisons	Medication, finance, and food preparation
Health care plan choices	Finucane et al. (2002)	Individuals were either provided with multiple pieces of information about a single HMO or with a table that compared multiple HMOs on several dimensions and were asked to find the best plans for certain scenarios	Medication/finance
Car shopping	Johnson (1990)	Make purchasing decisions about several vehicles, comparing them on multiple features	Shopping
Airplane navigation decisions	Morrow et al. (2001)	Younger, middle-aged, and older pilots and nonpilots on their memory and comprehension of navigational air traffic control messages	Transportation
Car shopping	Patrick (1995)	Make purchasing decisions about several vehicles, arrayed in an 8 (car) × 8 (feature) matrix	Shopping
Driving decisions task	Walker et al. (1997)	Evaluate information about traffic density and speed limits of main and secondary routes to minimize the time needed to traverse between two points	Transportation

but expertise status did not moderate negative age effects.

Fifth, it appears that older adults require more time with decision-making tasks to produce solutions of equal quality as younger adults (Walker et al., 1997), although they may choose to spend less (Johnson, 1990; Johnson & Drungle, 2000; Meyer et al., 1995) or equivalent (Patrick, 1995) amounts of time.

B. Relationship to Cognition and Intelligence

Sternberg and Wagner (1986) coined the phrase "practical intelligence" to reflect the idea that cognition in everyday contexts was something emergent in adulthood, distinct from what they labeled "academic intelligence." The underlying argument was that there should be little relationship between everyday problem solving and traditional measures of intelligence and cognition. In research with older adults, study findings have generally not supported the idea of distinct "academic" and "practical" intelligences, particularly with well-structured instrumental everyday problems tasks.

A number of studies have shown strong relationships between accuracy/effectiveness of problem solving and measures of intelligence and cognition. Table 14.5 summarizes some of these investigations and demonstrates several key findings. First, consistent with the predictions of Chapman (1993), well-structured problem-solving tasks have substantial overlap with traditional measures of intelligence and cognition. Indeed, in most studies, between 50 and 80% of the individual differences in problem solving were associated with traditional cognitive and intellectual measures. Second, in a number of studies, fluid and crystallized intelligence appeared to be the most important correlates

of problem solving. Often, the relative regression weights of fluid and crystallized intelligence were roughly equal, suggesting that both prior knowledge and current reasoning have similar importance in predicting problem-solving performance (e.g., Allaire & Marsiske, 1999; Diehl, Willis, & Schaie, 1995; Willis et al., 1992; Willis & Schaie, 1986). It is likely that these strong relationships with basic measures of intelligence, particularly age-sensitive fluid measures, help explain why the dominant cross-sectional pattern for everyday problem solving has been negative.

The importance of fluid and crystallized intelligence may be a function of the kinds of problems that are typically presented. For example, for the Timed Instrumental Activities of Daily Living (TIADL; Owsley et al., 2001), which measured speed of correct responding to a variety of everyday visual search activities (e.g., finding items on a pantry shelf, looking up a phone number), a measure of visual processing speed was the most important unique regression predictor of this measure.

Relatively few decision-making studies have included cognitive correlates of performance. Finucane et al. (2005) reported that their measures of information comprehension and decision-making consistency in the domains of nutrition, health, and finance were significantly associated (range: $r = .19$ to .39) with measures of vocabulary, number span, and perceptual speed.

The bottom half of Table 14.5 shows cognitive correlations with social/interpersonal problems. Consistent with postformal perspectives, which argue that such problems are less rational and performance should be less related to cognitive functioning, social problem solving does appear to be less strongly related to intellectual abilities. It is important to note, however,

Table 14.5

Relationship between Cognition/Intelligence and Everyday Problem Solving; Well-Structured Accuracy/Effectiveness Measures

Study	Problem-solving measure	Cognitive domains/measures assessed	Summary of relationships observed
Instrumental problems			
Allaire & Marsiske (1999)	Everyday Cognition Battery (ECB)	Fluid reasoning, verbal knowledge, list memory, working memory	Strong positive correlations (range: $r = .42$ to $r = .86$) between all intellectual abilities and problem solving
Hartley (1989)	Medicare choice task, automobile choice task, advice giving task	Memory, embedded figures tasks, reading task	Cognitive measures were related positively to all problem-solving tasks and explained about 40% of the variance in each
Diehl, Willis, & Schaie (1995)	Observed Tasks of Daily Living (OTDL)	Fluid reasoning, crystallized verbal knowledge, memory span, perceptual speed	All abilities were strong correlates (range: $r = .37$ to $r = .59$); in a path model, fluid and crystallized measures mediated memory- and speed-related variance
Goverover (2004); Goverover & Hinojosa (2002)	OTDL	Categorization ability, deductive reasoning, awareness of deficit	In acute neurology patients, all cognitive measures were significantly related to OTDL performance
Willis & Schaie (1986)	Test of Basic Skills (TBS)	Fluid and crystallized intelligence, memory span, perceptual speed	Marker tests of fluid and crystallized intelligence accounted for 80% of the variance in the total basic skills measure
Willis et al. (1992)	TBS	Fluid and crystallized intelligence, memory span, perceptual speed	After controlling for autoregression, fluid reasoning at baseline was the best predictor of performance 7 years later
Owsley et al. (2001)	Timed Instrumental Activities of Daily Living Test (TIADL)	Inductive reasoning, list and prose memory, visual processing speed	All abilities were associated with TIADL, although there was a significant unique association with visual processing speed
Social/interpersonal problems			
Camp et al. (1989)	Denney's Practical Problems (PP)	WAIS similarities and information tests; Raven's progressive matrices	Correlations ranged from $r = .29$ to $r = .40$

(continued)

Table 14.5
Continued

Study	Problem-solving measure	Cognitive domains/measures assessed	Summary of relationships observed
Cornelius & Caspi (1987)	Everyday Problem-Solving Inventory (EPSI; participant scored higher if they selected solutions that were congruent with an optimal judge-rated pattern)	Inductive reasoning (letter sets) and verbal ability (vocabulary)	Correlations with EPSI were 0.29 (letter sets) and 0.27 (verbal ability)
Crawford & Channon (2002)	Fluency-based scores of individuals' responses to social dilemmas	Executive skills (neuropsychological) measures	Older adults were slightly less fluent and slightly more effective than younger adults in their problem solutions, but younger adults outperformed older adults significantly in executive functioning, suggesting a decoupling of problem solving from executive functions
Heidrich & Denney (1994)	Denney's PP (divided into social and interpersonal subscores)	WAIS vocabulary and Raven's progressive matrices	Correlation between WAIS vocabulary and social problems was $r = 0.36$; correlation between Raven's matrices and practical problems was $r = .36$.

that there is a nonzero relationship in most studies, suggesting that there is not complete independence of between cognitive performance and social problem solving.

C. Relationship to Everyday Function

As discussed in the introduction to this chapter, everyday problem-solving work is premised on an ecological validity assumption. If everyday problems are closer to the "real world," then they should be strongly related to real world outcomes. One difficulty in establishing ecological validity is that of identifying an appropriate validation criterion. Willis (e.g., 1996c) has made a strong case for validating everyday problems by examining the extent to which they might explain individual differences in IADL (Lawton & Brody, 1969) competence. IADL domains (e.g., food preparation, medication use, financial management) have been widely studied in gerontological research and geriatric practice and are related to the ability to live independently and in good health (e.g., Branch & Jette, 1982; Fried et al., 2001).

IADLs are problematic as validation criteria, however, because they are frequently assessed via caregiver or self-reports, which have the potential for substantial reporting bias (e.g., Rubenstein et al., 1984). In addition to a reluctance to admit one's frailties, for those with cognitive impairment, anosognosia (lack of awareness of deficits) may further work to diminish the accuracy of ratings.

Even if self-ratings are valid, there is an implied ceiling effect in the IADLs of most community-dwelling elders. It is only after the onset of major losses (e.g., mobility impairments due to falls or stroke; cognitive impairment due to dementia) that individuals would expect to experience substantial IADL impairments. Thus, in community-dwelling elders, traditionally measured IADLs will typically have a restricted range and therefore cannot be expected to show substantial associations with other variables. Despite these caveats, Diehl et al. (1995) reported a correlation of $r = .50$ between IADL ratings and performance on the Observed Tasks of Daily Living.

One difficulty with such bivariate correlations is that they fail to capture the *unique* association between measures when other variables are controlled. Here, the critical question is whether measures of everyday problem solving are any more useful in predicting real world functioning than traditional cognitive measures. Because everyday problem-solving tests take substantial effort to develop, it would seem to be important that such new tests demonstrate some kind of "value added" above and beyond existing cognitive measures.

The additional value of everyday tasks could take several forms. First, and most desirably, everyday problem-solving measures should predict individual differences in outcomes, such as IADLs, better than traditional cognitive and intellectual measures (Fillenbaum, 1985; 1988). Second, because everyday problem-solving measures tend to be related to multiple cognitive domains, they may offer an efficiency advantage (i.e., one relatively brief everyday problem-solving measure might efficiently capture variance that would typically require a longer battery of multiple cognitive or neuropsychological measures). A third possible area of added value is motivational; if everyday problems tasks seem relevant and familiar, they may encourage greater self-efficacy (e.g., Artistico et al., 2003) and willingness to agree to testing (Cornelius, 1984).

Allaire and Marsiske (2002) investigated the first form of "added value," examining whether several measures of everyday problem solving could predict everyday function (IADL and advanced IADLs) as well as, or better, than a traditional cognitive battery. Two measures, the Everyday Cognition Battery (ECB, a well-structured test of instrumental problem solving) and a solution fluency measure (for problems of food preparation, medication use, and financial management), explained more than 50% of the reliable variance in reported everyday function. After allowing ECB and solution fluency to predict IADL scores, there was no residual relationship between IADL and traditional measures of cognition (reasoning, memory, vocabulary, working memory); indeed, the everyday problem-solving measures explained unique variance in the IADL score above and beyond basic cognitive measures. Thus, this study suggested that measures of everyday problem solving could show ecological validity (relationship to everyday function) and, moreover, could pass the "value added" test; replication and extension of these findings with other everyday problem-solving and cognition measures are necessary.

It should also be noted that the predominant focus on IADL functioning as the outcome of everyday problem solving may ignore the other important potential consequences of effective everyday problem solving (Berg, 2005; Willis, 1991). In particular, well-being, life satisfaction, and the absence of depression seem particularly relevant as outcomes of social and interpersonal problem solving. Indeed, clinical studies of problem solving often view depression remediation and effective coping as key outcome measures (D'Zurilla et al., 1998). The validation of late life everyday problem-solving measures in terms of their relationship to affective and well-being outcomes represents virtually unexplored territory.

III. Unanswered Questions and Future Directions

This final section considers two lines of inquiry that are nascent, but that seem to have substantial potential for advancing the practical, clinical, and scientific contributions of everyday problem-solving research. First, we consider the possible role of everyday problem solving in the detection of functional and cognitive impairment in later life. Second, we discuss three approaches to intervening with, or supporting, everyday cognitive performance.

A. Integrating Everyday Problem Solving with Evaluation of Functional and Cognitive Decline

Cross-sectional evidence suggests that late life is a period of decline for most types of everyday problem solving and decision making, which is supported by the few available longitudinal investigations. It is intriguing to know whether everyday problem-solving measures might also offer a window into the prodromal functional impairments that individuals experience prior to the onset of cognitive decline. More importantly, might subtle patterns of decline on everyday problem-solving measures serve as useful "early warning" indicators of incipient cognitive decline and functional impairment? From a clinical perspective, it has been generally assumed that everyday functioning remains "intact" in later life, even in the early stages of preclinical cognitive impairment (Peterson, 2003). Impairments in IADLs and more basic activities of daily living (ADLs, e.g., Katz et al., 1963) are not expected until individuals progress to later stages of dementia.

This all-or-none view of functional impairment may be too simplistic.

Nygard (2003) suggested that it could be useful to develop better evidence regarding the subtle clinical signs of cognitive IADL impairment that might signal incipient dementia-related changes. Indeed, a growing corpus of literature suggests that various measures of everyday problem solving might be useful in identifying cognitive impairment. For example, Baird et al. (2001) reported that a performance-based measure of everyday cognition in IADL domains, the *Independent Living Scales* (Loeb, 1996), was strongly associated with the Dementia Rating Scale and the Boston Naming Test, two commonly used tools for dementia assessment. Similarly, a version of the Everyday Problems Test that was adapted for use with demented populations, the Everyday Problems Test for Cognitively Challenged Elderly (EPCCE), discriminated persons at different levels of diagnosed dementia and was well correlated with other neuropsychological measures sensitive to cognitive impairment (especially executive function measures). Self- and caregiver ratings of functional impairment were also related to EPCCE (Bertrand & Willis, 1999; Willis, 1996a; Willis et al., 1998). Good discrimination between demented and nondemented elders was also reported using the Test of Problem Solving (Bowers et al., 1996), which was originally designed as a measure of real world critical thinking and problem-solving fluency (Ripich, Fritsch, & Ziol, 2002). Goverover and Josman (2004) reported that while the Observed Tasks of Daily Living (Diehl et al., 1995) were useful in discriminating adults with schizophrenia from unimpaired elders, they were not useful in separately discriminating older adults with cognitive impairment, although statistical power in that study was quite low.

The ability to use everyday problem-solving measures to identify subtle preclinical changes (e.g., early cognitive losses, as in mild cognitive impairment;

Peterson, 2000, 2003), as opposed to later stages of dementia, is one issue that needs further study. Allaire and Willis (in press) have reported one of the few investigations that explored everyday problem solving in a prospective study of dementia and found that EPCCE scores differentiated among cognitively impaired, "possibly impaired," and unimpaired older adults, although the contrast between the first two groups disappeared after controlling for age, gender, and education. Participants were also examined longitudinally; nonimpaired individuals declined on the EPCCE at a slower rate than impaired participants.

Another potential use of everyday problem solving and decision-making assessment with cognitive impairment relates to competency loss or, more precisely, identification of the point at which individuals can no longer make sound health care, financial, or other consent-related decisions (Barbas & Wilde, 2001). Marson and colleagues, for example, have developed model-based instruments of financial capacity that present individuals with financial tasks graded in difficulty (from basic money counting tasks through more complex financial decision making); such instruments may be useful in characterizing individuals' competence to continue making independent financial decisions (Marson et al., 2000; Marson, 2001a, b, 2002). The decision-making tasks of Finucane et al. (2005) offer another promising avenue for assessing such competence in multiple critical domains (health care, nutrition, finance).

B. Approaches for Improving Performance

Related to the identification of impairment, a question that emerges is whether everyday problem-solving measures, if they are in fact ecologically valid and reflect real world competencies, can be modified or improved. Strategies to enhance performance, in public health parlance, might constitute primary and secondary prevention strategies to minimize age-associated losses and maximize everyday independence. We briefly consider two possible approaches to intervening with everyday problem solving.

One approach to be considered is formal cognitive interventions, or training. Given the consistent finding of significant relations between basic measures of cognition and intelligence, and measures of everyday problem solving, it seems reasonable that interventions to improve basic abilities may also improve everyday problem solving. One difficulty with devising formal interventions to improve everyday cognition, however, is the long-standing finding that training effects tend to be highly specific and do not transfer easily to even closely related untrained tasks (e.g., Detterman & Sternberg, 1993; Salomon & Perkins, 1989). One study, Advanced Cognitive Training for Independent and Vital Elderly (ACTIVE; Ball et al., 2002; Jobe et al., 2001), was designed to investigate just this question. The purpose of ACTIVE was to evaluate the efficacy and subsequent transfer to everyday functioning of three established interventions focusing on inductive reasoning, memory, and speed of processing, all of which had been shown to be strongly related to various measures of everyday problem solving. Initial findings from this study showed that while the training programs had large, significant, and durable (2-year maintenance) effects, there was no evidence of concurrent improvement in three related everyday problem-solving measures (Everyday Problems Test,

Observed Tasks of Daily Living, and the Timed Instrumental Activities of Daily Living). Planned long-term follow-ups (5 years posttraining) will examine whether there are any emergent differences in the decline trajectories of trained and untrained participants. The difficulty of achieving training transfer has led some investigators to intervene, successfully, with everyday cognitive tasks such as automatic teller machines (e.g., Jamieson & Rogers, 2000; Mead & Fisk, 1998) and blood glucose meters (Mykityshyn, Fisk, & Rogers, 2002). Thus, further investigation is needed to determine whether there might be any general cognitive interventions that could enhance or postpone decline in a broad set of everyday problem domains.

A second possible approach for enhancing everyday problem solving is by encouraging collaboration. This relates directly to contextualist arguments: an ongoing criticism of cognitive aging research in general, including everyday problem solving, concerns the reliance on the "individual problem solving" approach. In truth, in the everyday world, many older individuals conduct many of their daily activities with social partners (e.g., M. Baltes, Wahl, & Schmid-Furstoss, 1990); thus, it is meaningful to consider how social partners might help or harm such problem solving (Meegan & Berg, 2002; Strough & Margrett, 2002). There is now consistent evidence that colloboration among older adults may yield performance improvements for older adults on a variety of basic and everyday cognitive tasks, including "transactive" memory (Andersson & Rönnberg, 1995, 1996), prose recall (e.g., Dixon & Gould, 1996), inductive reasoning (Margrett & Willis, in press), integrative and everyday tasks (i.e., route planning: Cheng & Strough, 2004) errand planning and comprehension of printed materials (Margrett & Marsiske, 2002) referential tasks (Gould et al., 2002), and social problem solving (Margrett & Marsiske, 2002; Staudinger & Baltes, 1996), as well as more complex everyday tasks, such as coping with prostate cancer and managing diabetes (Palmer et al., 2004; Wiebe et al., 2005). In general, collaboration appears to be beneficial to performance, particularly when it is with a familiar partner, such as a spouse (e.g., Gould, Trevithick, & Dixon, 1991; Gould, Kurzman, & Dixon, 1994; Margrett and Marsiske, 2002; for an exception, see Gould et al., 2002).

There may also be costs to collaboration; for example, Margrett and Marsiske (2002) reported that older women experienced collaboration with an unfamiliar male more negatively compared to their male partners. Gould and colleagues (1991, 1994) found that when collaborating with strangers, time on task could actually be reduced due to the distraction of needing to spend time on getting to know one's partner. Nonetheless, particularly with familiar dyads, the lion's share of evidence suggests that there are benefits to working with a partner. Further research is needed to identify the most important interactive elements of successful collaborations (although research on small group collaborations in industry or earlier in the life span may be useful starting points) and how to train or facilitate such interactions in older adults. In advanced old age, as individuals are increasingly likely to live alone, it may be more difficult to identify partners for collaboration, even if it is useful.

IV. Conclusions

In conclusion, research on everyday problem-solving continues to evolve.

There seem to be fairly clear answers to two of the three questions that have motivated this field. With regard to age differences and age changes, the picture from at least midlife through old-old age appears to be one of negative effects; these effects seem to be stronger in instrumental, well-structured tasks than in interpersonal, ill-structured tasks. It is also important to note that these negative age effects may not always reflect "deficits." Reduced fluency in social problem-solving tasks, for example, may reflect greater focus or a qualitatively different style of processing.

There also seems to be converging evidence that everyday problem solving and traditional measures of intelligence and cognition are related. As with the age difference patterns, there seems to be a dissociation between instrumental and interpersonal problems, with the former more strongly related to intellectual abilities, particularly fluid and crystallized intelligence.

The third question to motivate this line of research, which concerned the putative ecological validity of everyday problems and their presumed enhanced ability to predict real world outcomes, has received much less attention. Relatively few studies have tried to validate everyday problem solving against any criterion (the two most common to date have been IADL ratings and cognitive status). Moreover, few investigators have begun to think about what other meaningful validation criteria might be or how they could best be measured. This is an important next step to further demonstrate the practical utility of this line of research. Given the substantial progress that has already been made, there is room for optimism that researchers can now successfully tackle this next set of questions.

References

Ackerman, P. L. (2005). Ability determinants of individual differences in skilled performance. In R. J. Sternberg & J. E. Pretz (Eds.), *Cognition and intelligence: Identifying the mechanisms of the mind* (pp. 142–159). New York: Cambridge University Press.

Allaire, J. C., & Marsiske, M. (1999). Everyday cognition: Age and intellectual ability correlates. *Psychology and Aging, 14,* 627–644.

Allaire, J. C., & Marsiske, M. (2002). Well- and ill-defined measures of everyday cognition relationship to older adults' intellectual ability and functional status. *Psychology and Aging, 17,* 101–115.

Allaire, J. C., & Willis, S. L. (in press). Everyday activities as a predictor of cognitive risk and mortality. *Aging, Neuropsychology and Cognition.*

Andersson, J., & Rönnberg, J. (1995). Recall suffers from collaboration: Joint recall effects of friendship and task complexity. *Applied Cognitive Psychology, 9,* 199–211.

Andersson, J., & Rönnberg, J. (1996). Collaboration and memory: Effects of dyadic retrieval on different memory tasks. *Applied Cognitive Psychology, 10,* 171–181.

Artistico, D., Cervone, D., & Pezzuti, L. (2003). Perceived self-efficacy and everyday problem solving among young and older adults. *Psychology & Aging, 18,* 68–79.

Baddeley, A. (1989). Finding the bloody horse. In L. W. Poon, D. C. Rubin, & B. A. Wilson (Eds.), *Everyday cognition in adulthood and late life* (pp. 104–115). New York: Cambridge University Press.

Bahrick, H. P. (1989). The laboratory and ecology: Supplementary sources of data for memory research. In L. W. Poon, D. C. Rubin, & B. A. Wilson (Eds.), *Everyday cognition in adulthood and late life* (pp. 73–83). New York: Cambridge University Press.

Baird, A., Podell, K., Lovell, M., & McGinty, S. B. (2001). Complex real-world functioning and neuropsychological test performance in older adults. *Clinical Neuropsychologist, 15,* 369–379.

Ball, K., Berch, D. B., Helmers, K. F., Jobe, J. B., Leveck, M. D., Marsiske, M., Morris, J. N., Rebok, G. W., Smith, D. M., Tennstedt, S. L., Unverzagt, F. W., & Willis, S. L. (2002). *Journal of the American Medical Association, 288*(18), 2271–2281.

Baltes, M. M., Wahl, H.-W., & Schmid-Furstoss, U. (1990). The daily life of elderly Germans: Activity patterns, personal control, and functional health. *Journal of Gerontology: Psychological Sciences, 45,* P173–P179.

Baltes, P. B. (1968). Longitudinal and cross-sectional sequences in the study of age and generation effects. *Human Development, 11,* 145–171.

Baltes, P. B. (1987). Theoretical propositions of life span developmental psychology: On the dynamics between growth and decline. *Developmental Psychology, 23,* 611–626.

Baltes, P. B. (1993). The aging mind: Potentials and limits. *Gerontologist, 33,* 580–594.

Baltes, P. B., Staudinger, U. M., & Lindenberger, U. (1999). Lifespan psychology: Theory and application to intellectual functioning. *Annual Review Of Psychology, 50,* 471–507.

Barbas, N. R., & Wilde, E. A. (2001). Competency issues in dementia: Medical decision making, driving, and independent living. *Journal of Geriatric Psychiatry And Neurology, 14,* 199–212.

Beier, M. E., & Ackerman, P. L. (2005). Age, ability, and the role of prior knowledge on the acquisition of new domain knowledge: Promising results in a real-world learning environment. *Psychology and Aging, 20,* 341–355.

Berg, C. A. (2005, May) The future of everyday problem solving: Linking everyday problem solving to real-world indicators of successful aging. Paper presented at the International Conference on the Future of Cognitive Aging Research, Pennsylvania State University, State College, PA.

Berg, C. A., Calderone, K. S., Sansone, C., Strough, J., & Weir, C. (1998). The role of problem definitions in understanding age and context effects on strategies for solving everyday problems. *Psychology and Aging, 13,* 29–44.

Berg, C. A., & Klaczynski, P. A. (1996). Practical intelligence and problem solving: Searching for perspectives. In F. Blanchard-Fields & T. M. Hess (Eds.), *Perspectives on cognitive change in adulthood and aging* (pp. 323–357). Boston: McGraw-Hill.

Berg, C. A., Klaczynski, P. A., Calderone, K. S., & Strough, J. (1994). Adult age differences in cognitive strategies: Adaptive or deficient? In J. D. Sinnott (Ed.), *Interdisciplinary handbook of adult lifespan learning* (pp. 371–388). Westport, CT: Greenwood Press/Greenwood Publish Group, Inc.

Berg, C. A., Meegan, S. P., & Klaczynski, P. (1999). Age and experiential differences in strategy generation and information requests for solving everyday problems. *International Journal of Behavioral Development, 23*, 615–639.

Berg, C. A., & Sternberg, R. J. (1985). A triarchic theory of intellectual development during adulthood. *Developmental Review, 5*, 334–370.

Bertrand, R. M., & Willis, S. L. (1999). Everyday problem solving in Alzheimer's patients: A comparison of subjective and objective assessments. *Aging & Mental Health, 3*, 281–293.

Blanchard-Fields, F. (1986). Reasoning on social dilemmas varying in emotional saliency: An adult developmental perspective. *Psychology & Aging, 1*(4), 325–333.

Blanchard-Fields, F., Camp, C., & Jahnke, H. C. (1995). Age differences in problem-solving style: The role of emotional salience. *Psychology and Aging, 10*, 173–180.

Blanchard-Fields, F., Chen, Y., & Norris, L. (1997). Everyday problem solving across the adult life span: Influence of domain specificity and cognitive appraisal. *Psychology and Aging, 12*, 684–693.

Blanchard-Fields, F., Stein, R., & Watson, T. L. (2004). Age differences in emotion-regulation strategies in handling everyday problems. *Journals of Gerontology Series B Psychological Sciences and Social Sciences, 59*, P261–P269.

Bowers, L., Huisingh, R., Barrett, M., Orman, J., & LoGiudice, C. (1996). *Test of Problem Solving - Elementary, Revised* (TOPS-E, revised). East Moline, IL: LinguiSystems.

Branch, L. G., & Jette, A. M. (1982). A prospective study of long-term care institutionalization among the aged. *American Journal of Public Health, 72*, 1373–1379.

Camp, C. J., Doherty, K., & Moody-Thomas, S. (1989). Practical problem solving in adults: A comparison of problem types and scoring methods. In J. Sinnott (Ed.), *Everyday problem solving: Theory and applications* (pp. 211–228). New York: Praeger.

Capon, N., Kuhn, D., & Carretero, M. (1989). Consumer reasoning. In J. D. Sinnott (Ed.), *Everyday problem solving: Theory and applications* (pp. 153–174). New York: Praeger.

Cattell, R. B. (1987). *Intelligence: Its structure, growth, and action.* New York: Elsevier Science.

Chapman, M. (1993). Everyday reasoning and the revision of belief. In J. M. Puckett & H. W. Reese (Eds.), *Mechanisms of everyday cognition* (pp. 93–113). Hillsdale, NJ: Erlbaum.

Charness, N. (2005, May). Expertise and knowledge. Paper presented at the International Conference on the Future of Cognitive Aging Research, Pennsylvania State University, State College, PA.

Chasseigne, G., Grau, S., Mullet, E., & Cama, V. (1999). How well do elderly people cope with uncertainty in a learning task? *Acta Psychologica, 103*, 229–238.

Chen, Y., & Sun, Y. (2003). Age differences in financial decision-making: Using simple heuristics. *Educational Gerontology, 29*, 627–635.

Cheng, S., & Strough, J. (2004). A comparison of collaborative and individual everyday problem solving in younger and older adults. *International Journal of Aging and Human Development, 58*(3), 167–195.

Cohen, J. (1988). *Statistical power analysis for the behavioral sciences* (2nd Edition). Hillsdale, NJ: Lawrence Erlbaum.

Cornelius, S. W. (1984). Classic pattern of intellectual aging: Test familiarity, difficulty, and performance. *Journal of Gerontology, 39*, 201–206.

Cornelius, S. W., & Caspi, A. (1987). Everyday problem solving in adulthood and old age. *Psychology and Aging, 2*, 144–153.

Crawford, S., & Channon, S. (2002). Dissociation between performance on abstract tests of executive function and problem solving in real-life-type situations in normal aging. *Aging and Mental Health, 6*, 12–21.

Denney, N. W. (1989). Everyday problem solving: Methodological issues, research findings, and a model. In L. W. Poon,

D. C. Rubin, & B. A. Wilson (Eds.), *Everyday cognition in adulthood and late life* (pp. 330–351). New York: Cambridge University Press.

Denney, N. W., & Palmer, A. M. (1981). Adult age differences on traditional and practical problem-solving measures. *Journal of Gerontology, 36,* 323–328.

Denney, N. W., & Pearce, K. A. (1989). A developmental study of practical problem solving in adults. *Psychology and Aging, 4,* 438–442.

Denney, N. W., Pearce, K. A., & Palmer, A. M. (1982). A developmental study of adults' performance on traditional and practical problem-solving tasks. *Experimental Aging Research, 8*(2), 115–118.

Denney, N. W., Tozier, T. L., & Schlotthauer, C. A. (1992). The effect of instructions on age differences in practical problem solving. *Journal of Gerontology, 47,* 142–145.

Detterman, D. K., & Sternberg, R. J. (Eds.) (1993). *Transfer on trial: Intelligence, cognition, and instruction.* Norwood, NJ: Ablex Publishing Corporation.

Diehl, M, Marsiske, M., Horgas, A. L., Rosenberg A., Saczynski, J. S., & Willis, S. L. (2005). The revised observed tasks of daily living: A performance-based assessment of everyday problem solving in older adults. *Journal of Applied Gerontology, 24,* 211–230.

Diehl, M., Willis, S. L., & Schaie, K. W. (1995). Everyday problem solving in older adults: Observational assessment and cognitive correlates. *Psychology and Aging, 10,* 478–491.

Dixon, R. A., & Baltes, P. B. (1986). Toward life-span research on the functions and pragmatics of intelligence. In R. J. Sternberg & R. K. Wagner (Eds.), *Practical intelligence: Nature and origins of competence in the everyday world* (pp. 203–235). New York: Cambridge University Press.

Dixon, R. A., & Gould, O. N. (1996). Adults telling and retelling stories collaboratively. In P. B. Baltes & U. M. Staudinger (Eds.), *Interactive minds: Life-span perspective on the social foundation of cognition* (pp. 221–241). New York: University Press.

D'Zurilla, T. J., Chang, E. C., Nottingham, E. J., & Faccini, L. (1998). Social problem-solving deficits and hopelessness, depression, and suicidal risk in college students and psychiatric inpatients. *Journal of Clinical Psychology, 54,* 1091–1107.

D'Zurilla, T. J., Maydeu-Olivares, A., & Kant, G. L. (1998). Age and gender differences in social problem-solving ability. *Personal and Individual Differences, 25,* 241–252.

Educational Testing Service (1977). *Test of basic skills.* Princeton, NJ: Educational Testing Service.

Ericsson, K. A., & Charness, N. (1994). Expert performance: Its structure and acquisition. *American Psychologist, 49,* 725–747.

Fillenbaum, G. G. (1985). Screening the elderly: A brief instrumental activities of daily living measure. *Journal of the American Geriatrics Society, 33,* 698–706.

Fillenbaum, G. G. (1988). *Multidimensional functional assessment of older adults: The Duke Older Americans Resources and Services Procedures.* Hillsdale, NJ: Lawrence Erlbaum.

Finucane, M. L., Mertz, C. K., Slovic, P., & Schmidt, E. S. (2005). Task complexity and older adults' decision-making competence. *Psychology And Aging, 20,* 71–84.

Finucane, M. L., Peters, E., & Slovic, P. (2003). Judgment and decision making: The dance of affect and reason. In S. L. Schneider & J. Shanteau (Eds.), *Emerging perspectives on judgment and decision research* (pp. 327–364). New York: Cambridge University Press.

Finucane, M. L., Slovic, P., Hibbard, J. H., Peters, E., Mertz, D. K., & McGregor, D. G. (2002). Aging and decision-making competence: An analysis of comprehension and consistency skills in older versus younger adults. *Journal of Behavioural Decision Making, 15,* 141–164.

Frederiksen, N. (1986). Toward a broader conception of human intelligence. In R. J. Sternberg & R. K. Wagner (Eds.), *Practical intelligence: Nature and origins of competence in the everyday world* (pp. 84–116). New York: Cambridge University Press.

Fried, T. R., Bradley, E. H., Williams, C. S., & Tinetti, M. E. (2001). Functional disability and health care expenditures for older persons. *Archives of Internal Medicine, 161,* 2602–2607.

Gould, O., Kurzman, D., & Dixon, R. A. (1994). Communication during prose recall conversations by young and old dyads. *Discourse Processes, 17,* 149–165.

Gould, O. N., Osborn, C., Krein, H., & Mortenson, M. (2002). Collaborative recall in married and unacquainted dyads. *International Journal of Behavioral Development, 26*(1), 36–44.

Gould, O. N., Trevithick, L., & Dixon, R. A. (1991). Adult age differences in elaborations produced during prose recall. *Psychology & Aging, 6*(1), 93–99.

Goverover, Y. (2004). Categorization, deductive reasoning, and self-awareness: Association with everyday competence in persons with acute brain injury. *Journal Of Clinical And Experimental Neuropsychology, 26,* 737–749.

Goverover, Y., & Hinojosa, J. (2002). Categorization and deductive reasoning: Predictors of instrumental activities of daily living performance in adults with brain injury. *American Journal Of Occupational Therapy, 56,* 509–516.

Goverover, Y., & Josman, N. (2004). Everyday problem solving among four groups of individuals with cognitive impairments: Examination of the discriminant validity of the observed tasks of daily living-revised. *OTJR-Occupation Participation and Health, 24,* 103–112.

Hartley, A. A. (1989). The cognitive ecology of problem solving. In L. W. Poon, D. C. Rubin, & B. A. Wilson (Eds.), *Everyday cognition in adulthood and late life* (pp. 300–329). New York: Cambridge University Press.

Haught, P. A., Hill, L. A., Nardi, A. H., & Walls, R. T. (2000). Perceived ability and level of education as predictors of traditional and practical adult problem solving. *Experimental Aging Research, 26,* 89–101.

Heidrich, S. M., & Denney, N. W. (1994). Does social problem solving differ from other types of problem solving during the adult years? *Experimental Aging Research, 20*(2), 105–126.

Hershey, D. A., & Farrell, A. H. (1999). Age differences on a procedurally oriented test of practical problem solving. *Journal of Adult Development, 6,* 87–104.

Hershey, D. A., & Walsh, D. A. (2000–2001). Knowledge versus experience in financial problem solving performance. *Current Psychology: Developmental, Learning, Personality, Social, 19,* 261–291.

Holtsberg, P. A., Poon, L. W., Noble, C. A., & Mapstone-Johnson, M. (2002). Everyday problem-solving in community-dwelling cognitively intact centenarians. *Hallym International Journal of Aging, 4,* 83–97.

Jamieson, B. A., & Rogers, W. A. (2000). Age-related effects of blocked and random practice schedules on learning a new technology. *Journals of Gerontology: Series B: Psychological Sciences & Social Sciences, 55,* P343–P353.

Jobe, J. B., Smith, D. M., Ball, K., Tennstedt, S. L., Marsiske, M., Rebok, G. W., Morris, J. N., Willis, S. L., Helmers, K., Leveck, M. D., and Kleinman, K. (2001). ACTIVE: A cognitive intervention trial to promote independence in older adults. *Controlled Clinical Trials, 22*(4), 453–479.

Johnson, M. M. (1990). Age differences in decision making: A process methodology for examining strategic information processing. *Journal of Gerontology: Psychological Sciences, 45,* P75–P78.

Johnson, M. M. S., & Drungle, S. C. (2000). Purchasing OTC medications: The influence of age and familiarity. *Experimental Aging Research, 26,* 245–261.

Katz, S., Ford, A. B., Moskowitz, R. W., Jackson, B. A., & Jaffee, M. W. (1963). Studies of illness in the aged. The index of ADL: A standardized measure of biological and psychological function. *Journal of the American Medical Association, 185,* 94–101.

Kim, S., & Hasher, L. (2005). The attraction effect in decision making: Superior performance by older adults. *Quarterly Journal of Experimental Psychology Section A-Human Experimental Psychology, 58*(1), 120–133.

Klumb, P. L., & Baltes, M. M. (1999). Validity of retrospective time-use reports in old age. *Applied Cognitive Psychology, 13,* 527–539.

Kramer, D., & Woodruff, D. (1986). Relativistic and dialectical thought in three adult age groups. *Human Development, 29,* 280–290.

Labouvie-Vief, G. (1985). Intelligence and cognition. In J. E. Birren & K. W. Schaie (Eds.), *Handbook of the psychology of aging* (2nd edition, pp. 500–530). New York: Van Nostrand Reinhold.

Labouvie-Vief, G. (1992). A neo-Piagetian perspective on adult cognitive development. In R. J. Sternberg & C. A. Berg (Eds.), *Intellectual development* (pp. 239–252). New York: Cambridge University Press.

Lawton, M. P., & Brody, E. M. (1969). Assessment of older people: Self-maintaining and instrumental activities of daily living. *The Gerontologist, 9,* 179–185.

Lindenberger, U., Mayr, U., & Kliegl, R. (1993). Speed and intelligence in old age. *Psychology and Aging, 8,* 207–220.

Loeb, P. A. (1996). *The independent living scales.* New York: Psychological Corporation.

Lövdén, M., Ghisletta, P., & Lindenberger, U. (2004). Cognition in the Berlin Aging Study (BASE): The first 10 years. *Aging, Neuropsychology, & Cognition, 11,* 104–133.

Margrett, J. A., & Marsiske, M. (2002). Gender differences in older adults' everyday cognitive collaboration. *International Journal of Behavioral Development, 26,* 45–59.

Margrett, J. A., & Willis, S. L. (In press). In-home cognitive training with older married couples: Individual versus collaborative learning. *Aging, Neuropsychology, and Cognition.*

Marsh, B., Todd, P. M., & Gigerenzer, G. (2004). Cognitive heuristics: Reasoning the fast and frugal way. In J. P. Leighton (Ed.) *Nature of reasoning* (pp. 273–287). New York: Cambridge University Press.

Marsiske, M., & Willis, S. L. (1995). Dimensionality of everyday problem solving in older adults. *Psychology and Aging, 10,* 269–283.

Marsiske, M., & Willis, S. L. (1998). Practical creativity in older adults' everyday problem solving: Life-span perspectives. In C. E. Adams-Price (Ed.), *Creativity and aging: Theoretical and empirical approaches* (pp. 73–113). New York: Springer.

Marson, D. C. (2001a). Loss of competency in Alzheimer's disease: Conceptual and

psychometric approaches. *International Journal Of Law And Psychiatry, 24,* 267–283.

Marson, D. C. (2001b). Loss of financial competency in dementia: Conceptual and empirical approaches. *Aging Neuropsychology and Cognition, 8,* 164–181.

Marson, D. (2002). Competency assessment and research in an aging society. *Generations-Journal of the American Society on Aging, 26,* 99–103.

Marson, D. C., Sawrie, S. M., Snyder, S., McInturff, B., Stalvey, T., Boothe, A., Aldridge, T., Chatterjee, A., & Harrell, L. E. (2000). Assessing financial capacity in patients with Alzheimer disease: A conceptual model and prototype instrument. *Archives of Neurology, 57,* 877–884.

Mead, S., & Fisk, A. D. (1998). Measuring skill acquisition and retention with an ATM simulator: The need for age-specific training. *Human Factors, 40,* 516–523.

Meegan, S. P., & Berg, C. A. (2002). Contexts, functions, forms, and processes of collaborative everyday problem solving in older adulthood. *International Journal of Behavioral Development, 26,* 6–15.

Meyer, B. J. F., Russo, C., & Talbot, A. (1995). Discourse comprehension and problem solving: Decisions about the treatment of breast cancer by women across the life span. *Psychology and Aging, 10,* 84–103.

Morrow, D. G., Menard, W. E., Stine-Morrow, E. A. L., Teller, T., & Bryant, D. (2001). The influence of expertise and task factors on age differences in pilot communication. *Psychology and Aging, 16,* 31–46.

Mykityshyn, A. L., Fisk, A. D., & Rogers, W. A. (2002). Learning to use a home medical device: Mediating age-related differences with training. *Human Factors, 44,* 354–364.

Nygard, L. (2003). Instrumental activities of daily living: A stepping-stone towards Alzheimer's disease diagnosis in subjects with mild cognitive impairment? *Acta Neurologica Scandinavica, 107,* 42–46.

Owsley, C., Sloane, M. E., McGwin, G. J., & Ball, K. (2001). Timed instrumental activities of daily living tasks: Relationship to cognitive function and everyday performance assessments in older adults. *Gerontology, 48,* 254–265.

Palmer, D. L., Berg, C. A., Wiebe, D. J., Beveridge, R. M., Korbel, C. D., Upchurch, R., Swinyard, M. T., Lindsay, R., & Donaldson, D. L. (2004). The role of autonomy and pubertal status in understanding age differences in maternal involvement in diabetes responsibility across adolescence. *Journal of Pediatric Psychology, 29,* 35–46.

Patrick, J. M. H. (1995). Age and expertise effects on decision making processes and outcomes. *Dissertation Abstracts International: Section B The Sciences and Engineering, 56,* 4607.

Peters, E., Finucane, M. L., MacGregor, D., & Slovic, P. (2000). The bearable lightness of aging: Judgment and decision processes in older adults. In National Research Council, P. C. Stern, & L. L. Carstensen (Eds.), *The aging mind: Opportunities in cognitive research* (pp. 144–165). Washington, DC: National Academy.

Peterson, R. C. (2000). Aging, mild cognitive impairment, and Alzheimer's disease. *Neurologic Clinics, 18,* 789–806.

Peterson, R. C. (2003). *Mild cognitive impairment: Aging to Alzheimer's disease.* New York: Oxford University Press.

Poon, L. W., Rubin, D. C., & Wilson, B. A. (1989). *Everyday cognition in adulthood and late life.* New York: Cambridge University Press.

Poon, L. W., Messner, S., Martin, P., Noble, C. A., Clayton, G. M., & Johnson, M. A. (1992). The influences of cognitive resources on adaptation and old age. *International Journal of Aging and Human Development, 34,* 31–46.

Rabbitt, P. (1977). Changes in problem solving ability in old age. In J. E. Birren & K. W. Schaie (Eds.), *Handbook of the psychology of aging* (pp. 606–625). New York: Van Nostrand Reinhold.

Reese, H. W., & Rodeheaver, D. (1985). Problem solving and complex decision making. In K. W. Schaie (Ed.), *Handbook of the psychology of aging* (2nd edition, pp. 474–499). New York: Academic Press.

Reitman, W. R. (1965). *Cognition and thought: An information processing approach.* Oxford, UK: Wiley.

Ripich, D. N., Fritsch, T., & Ziol, E. (2002). Everyday problem solving in African Americans and European Americans with Alzheimer's disease: An exploratory study. *International Psychogeriatrics, 14,* 83–95.

Rubenstein, L. Z., Schairer, C., Wieland, G. D., & Kane, R. (1984). Systematic biases in functional status assessment of elderly adults: Effects of different data sources. *Journal of Gerontology, 39,* 686–691.

Rybash, I. M., Hoyer, W. J., &. Roodin, P. A. (1986). *Adult cognition and aging: Developmental changes in processing, knowing, and thinking.* New York: Pergamon.

Salthouse, T. A. (1990). Cognitive competence and expertise in aging. In J. E. Birren & K. W. Schaie (Eds.), *Handbook of the psychology of aging* (3rd edition, pp. 310–319). San Diego: Academic Press.

Salomon, G., & Perkins, D. N. (1989). Rocky roads to transfer: Rethinking mechanisms of a neglected phenomenon. *Educational Psychologist, 24,* 113–142.

Sanfrey, A. G., & Hastie, R. (2000). Judgment and decision making across the adult life span: A tutorial review of psychological research. In D. C. Park & N. Schwarz (Eds.), *Cognitive aging: A primer* (pp. 253–273). New York: Psychology Press.

Schaie, K. W. (1965). A general model for the study of developmental problems. *Psychological Bulletin, 64,* 92–107.

Schaie, K. W. (1978). External validity in the assessment of intellectual development in adulthood. *Journal of Gerontology, 33,* 695–701.

Schaie, K. W. (2005). *Developmental influences on adult intelligence: The Seattle Longitudinal Study.* London: Oxford University Press.

Simon, H. A. (1973). The structure of ill-structured problems. *Artificial Intelligence, 4,* 181–201.

Sinnott, J. D. (Ed.) (1989a). *Everyday problem solving: Theory and applications.* New York: Praeger.

Sinnott, J. D. (1989b). A model for solution of ill-structured problems: Implications for every-day and abstract problem solving. In J. D. Sinnott (Ed.), *Everyday problem solving: Theory and applications* (pp. 72–99). New York: Praeger.

Sperling, U. (2003). Responses to the demands of everyday life: Domain-specific or general coping? *Journal of Adult Development, 10,* 189–201.

Staudinger, U. M., & Baltes, P. B. (1996). Interactive minds: A facilitative setting for wisdom-related performance? *Journal of Personality and Social Psychology, 71,* 746–762.

Sternberg, R. J., & Wagner, R. K. (1986). *Practical intelligence: Nature and origins of competence in the everyday world.* Cambridge: Cambridge University Press.

Strough, J., Berg, C. A., & Sansone, C. (1996). Goals for solving everyday problems across the life span: Age and gender differences in the salience of interpersonal concerns. *Developmental Psychology, 32,* 1106–1115.

Strough, J., & Margrett, J. A. (2002). Introduction: Collaboration in later life. *International Journal of Behavior Development, 26,* 2–5.

Thornton, W. J. L., & Dumke, H. A. (2005). Age differences in everyday problem-solving and decision-making effectiveness: A meta-analytic review. *Psychology and Aging, 20,* 85–99.

Walker, N., Fain, W. B., Fisk, A. D., & McGuire, C. L. (1997). Aging and decision making: Driving-related problem-solving. *Human Factors, 39,* 438–444.

Watson, T. L., & Blanchard-Fields, F. (1998). Thinking with your head and your heart: Age differences in everyday problem-solving strategy preferences. *Aging Neuropsychology And Cognition, 5,* 225–240.

Whitfield, K. E., Baker-Thomas, T., Heyward, K., Gatto, M., & Williams, Y. (1999). Evaluating a measure of everyday problem solving for use in African Americans. *Experimental Aging Research, 25,* 209–221.

Wiebe, D. J., Berg, C. A., Korbel, C., Palmer, D. L., Beveridge, R. M., Upchurch, R., Lindsay, R., Swinyard, M. T., & Donaldson, D. L. (2005). Children's appraisals of maternal involvement in coping with diabetes: Enhancing our understanding of adherence, metabolic control, and quality of life across adolescence. *Journal of Pediatric Psychology, 30,* 167–178.

Willis, S. L. (1991). Cognition and everyday competence. In K. W. Schaie (Ed.), *Annual review of gerontology and geriatrics* (Vol. 11, pp. 80–109). New York: Springer.

Willis, S. L. (1996a). Assessing everyday competence in the cognitively challenged elderly. In M. A. Smyer (Ed.), *Older adults' decision-making and the law* (pp. 87–127). New York: Springer.

Willis, S. L. (1996b). Everyday cognitive competence in elderly persons: Conceptual issues and empirical findings. *Gerontologist, 51,* 11–17.

Willis, S. L. (1996c). Everyday problem solving. In J. E. Birren & K. W. Schaie (Eds.), *Handbook of the psychology of aging* (4th edition, pp. 287–307). New York: Academic Press.

Willis, S. L., Allen-Burge, R., Dolan, M. M., Bertrand, R. M., Yesavage, J., & Taylor, J. L. (1998). Everyday problem solving among individuals with Alzheimer's disease. *The Gerontologist, 38,* 569–577.

Willis, S. L., Jay, G. M., Diehl, M., & Marsiske, M. (1992). Longitudinal change and prediction of everyday task competence in the elderly. *Research on Aging, 14,* 68–91.

Willis, S. L., & Marsiske, M. (1991). Life span perspective on practical intelligence. In T. E. Tupper & K. D. Cicerone (Eds.), *The neuropsychology of everyday life: Issues in development and rehabilitation* (pp. 183–197). Boston: Kluwer.

Willis, S. L., & Marsiske, M. (1993). *Manual for the everyday problems test.* University Park, PA: Department of Human Development and Family Studies, Pennsylvania State University.

Willis, S. L., & Schaie, K. W. (1986). Practical intelligence in later adulthood. In R. J. Sternberg & R. K. Wagner (Eds.), *Practical intelligence: Nature and origins of competence in the everyday world* (pp. 236–268). New York: Cambridge University Press.

Willis, S. L., & Schaie, K. W. (1993). Everyday cognition: Taxonomic and methodological considerations. In J. M. Puckett & H. W. Reese (Eds.), *Mechanisms of everyday cognition* (pp. 33–54). Hillsdale, NJ: Lawrence Erlbaum.

Fifteen

Aging and the Intersection of Cognition, Motivation, and Emotion

Laura L. Carstensen, Joseph A. Mikels, and Mara Mather

As in the mainstream of psychology, the field of psychology and aging has been parsed into subareas according to topical focus. Cognitive psychology concerns processing capacity, memory, and knowledge. Social and personality psychology address socioemotional aspects of aging, such as well-being and self-regulation. Historically, these subareas have operated relatively independently of one another. Admittedly, cognitive psychologists have often included measures of personality or mood in their studies, usually to ensure that age groups are comparable along these dimensions, and social psychologists have included gross measures of cognitive function in their studies in order to be sure that their findings are not simply artifacts of impaired intellectual functioning. However, until very recently, there has been little serious consideration of the interactions among cognition, emotion, and motivation. We maintain that a sea change is underway. Empirical findings from a number of laboratories are beginning to converge to suggest that the interplay of cognitive, emotional, and motivational processes may offer important insights into the aging mind and, in doing so, point to ways to improve functioning.

The chapter is organized into multiple sections. The first two sections, respectively, provide broad overviews of cognitive and socioemotional aging, noting opposing aging trajectories. Next, we offer socioemotional selectivity theory—a life span model of motivation—as one conceptual framework within which to generate hypotheses about interactions between these functional domains. Finally, we review recent empirical evidence that memory and attention operate, in part, in the service of emotion regulation. We maintain that such age-related patterns are systematic and robust and conclude that consideration of the interplay of cognition, motivation, and emotion can provide a more complete and more nuanced understanding of the psychology of aging.

I. Cognitive Aging

The cognitive lives of older adults are characterized by stability, decline, and improvement; however, at the aggregate,

Handbook of the Psychology of Aging

deterioration generally characterizes cognitive aging. In attempts to explain cognitive aging, much attention in the field has been paid to developing theories that postulate underlying basic mechanisms. Sensory function (Baltes & Lindenberger, 1997; Lindenberger & Baltes, 1994) and speed of processing (Salthouse, 1991, 1996) have been theorized to account for the myriad declines in cognitive ability. Equally compelling are theories positing that fundamental deficits in processing resources (Craik & Byrd, 1982), inhibitory control (Hasher & Zacks, 1988), or the ability to refresh recently activated information (Johnson et al., 2002) underlie the declines in cognitive performance. It is becoming increasingly clear that these theories are not necessarily mutually exclusive. Rather each mechanism appears to play a fundamental role in cognitive decline (Park, 2000).

Decades of research in cognitive aging have documented systematic deterioration in effortful cognitive functions, such as verbal and visuospatial working memory (Park et al., 2002; Park et al., 1996), free- and cued-recall long-term memory (Park et al., 1996, 2002), selective attention (Plude & Doussard-Roosevelt, 1989), divided attention (Madden, 1986; McDowd & Craik, 1988), mental imagery (Dror & Kosslyn, 1994), verbal fluency (Mathuranath et al., 2003; Phillips, 1999), reasoning and problem solving (Salthouse, 1996), language comprehension (for a review, see Carpenter, Miyake, & Just, 1995), and language production (Burke & Shafto, 2004; MacKay & James, 2004).

Decline is most pronounced in effortful and resource-intensive processing. Less decline is observed in relatively automatic processing, which requires fewer processing resources and does not require extensive deliberative processing (Craik & Salthouse, 2000; Hedden & Gabrieli, 2004; Johnson & Raye, 2000;

Park & Schwarz, 2000). For instance, implicit and procedural memory (Fleischman et al., 2004; Jacoby, 1991; Laver & Burke, 1993; Light & La Voie, 1993; Light & Singh, 1987; Mitchell, Brown, & Murphy, 1990; Park & Shaw, 1992) as well as picture recognition (Park, Puglisi, & Smith, 1986) are well maintained in old age.

In addition to the relative maintenance of performance on tasks involving automatic processing, general world knowledge and specified knowledge in areas of expertise increase across adulthood (Schaie, 2005). Such expertise can even offset cognitive decline (Mireles & Charness, 2002). Performance on tasks tapping expertise in matters of everyday life (e.g., wisdom and life management) remains stable (Baltes & Staudinger, 2000; Staudinger, 1999), whereas on tasks that require solving interpersonal problems, older people show greater flexibility than younger people, especially when problems are emotionally charged (Blanchard-Fields, Jahnke, & Camp, 1995).

Moreover, even in areas that show reliable performance deficits, such as memory, there is considerable evidence for plasticity in performance. In a now classic study, reported by Baltes and Kliegl (1992; see also Kliegl & Baltes, 1991), older peoples' performance on a memory task benefited from practice so much so that after relatively few practice sessions, older people performed as well as younger people who had not practiced. Younger people also improved with practice such that younger people at all points in the study outperformed older people. Thus, the study elegantly demonstrated evidence for benefits of practice at the same time it demonstrated limits of such practice. More recently, Logan and colleagues (2002) have shown that the observed underrecruitment of frontal lobe regions can be eliminated when older adults are explicitly provided strategies to use on a memory task.

In light of acknowledged malleability or plasticity of cognitive performance, researchers began to turn their attention to questions about social conditions that may enhance or impede performance. Rahhal, Hasher, and Colcombe (2001) documented performance differences as a function of experimental instructions. They reasoned that because there are widespread beliefs in the culture that memory declines with age, tests that explicitly feature memory may invoke performance deficits in older people. They compared memory performance under two conditions. In one condition, experimental instructions stressed that memory was being tested, with the experimenter stating repeatedly that participants should "remember" as many statements from a list as they could. In the other condition, experimental instructions were identical except that emphasis was placed instead on learning, i.e., participants were instructed to "learn" as many statements as they could. In this study, rather dramatic effects were obtained. Age differences were found when memory was emphasized, but were eliminated when learning was emphasized.

Hess and colleagues (2003) also documented deficits in performance when aging decline was emphasized to participants before the experiment. In their study, older participants read one of three simulated newspaper articles prior to completing a memory task. One article reaffirmed memory decline and stated that older people should rely on others to help them. Another article described research findings suggesting that memory may improve in some ways with age. The third article was memory neutral. In Hess's study, younger people outperformed older people in each condition, but the age difference was reduced significantly in participants who read the positive account of memory. Most important, Hess's team identified a potential mediator of these performance differences. Participants had been required to write down as many words as they could remember. Those who had read the positive account about memory were more likely to use an effective memory strategy, called semantic clustering, in which similar words are grouped together. Thus, it appeared that strategic efforts were not recruited as skillfully in those participants who were reminded of age deficits.

Findings such as these begin to speak to the potential influence of emotion and motivation on cognitive performance. Interest in social and emotional influences on cognitive performance is all the more interesting in light of emerging evidence that socioemotional functioning is well maintained or even improved with age. The next section overviews key findings from this area and then offers socioemotional selectivity theory as one conceptual model that may help to inform interactions among motivation, cognition, and emotion.

II. Socioemotional Aging

The literature on socioemotional aging paints a very different picture than the literature on cognitive aging. Whereas emotional aging was initially characterized as a period of ubiquitous deterioration (Banham, 1951), it is becoming increasingly clear that this is not the case. Emotion regulation and emotional experience in old age are as good if not better than they are in younger years. Laboratory studies of emotional experience reveal that the emotional lives of older adults are very similar to those of younger adults or differ in ways that indicate improved emotion regulation (Carstensen, Fung, & Charles, 2003).

The basic components of emotion, namely subjective experience, expression and physiological responsivity, change little with age. Older adults do not differ from younger adults in their self-reports of emotional intensity (Carstensen et al., 2000; Levenson et al., 1991; Malatesta et al., 1987; Mikels et al., 2005; Tsai, Levenson, & Carstensen, 2000), in emotion-specific patterns of physiological reactivity (Levenson et al., 1991; Levenson, Carstensen, & Gottman, 1994), or in the spontaneous production of emotional facial expressions, as well as other emotional expressive behavior [Levenson et al., 1991; Tsai et al., 2000; note, however, that Malatesta-Magai et al. (1992) found old adults to be more expressive]. Despite the lack of change in these aspects of emotional experience and expression, there are a few aspects of emotional experience in which there is decline. Older adults relative to their younger counterparts show overall decreases in the magnitude of their physiological reactions (Levenson et al., 1991, 1994; Tsai et al., 2000) and report fewer negative emotional experiences (Carstensen et al., 2000; Gross et al., 1997; Mroczek & Kolarz, 1998), especially reductions in anger (Lawton, Kleban, & Dean, 1993; Magai, 1999). Finally, in addition to the sustained and diminished aspects of emotional experience and expression in old age, there also appear to be gains in regulation. Older adults relative to younger adults report greater emotional control (Gross et al., 1997; Lawton et al., 1992), an increase in positive affect (Mroczek & Kolarz, 1998) or, at minimum, sustained levels of positive affect (Carstensen et al., 2000), and more complex emotional experiences, namely greater poignancy or the cooccurrence of positive and negative affect (Carstensen et al., 2000).

The pattern described above is also reflected at the evaluative level. Satisfaction with life increases or at least is well maintained across adulthood (Diener & Lucas, 1999; Diener & Suh, 1997; however, see Mroczek & Spiro, 2005). Older adults report a greater sense of environmental mastery relative to their younger counterparts (Ryff, 1991; Ryff & Keyes, 1995). Relationships with family are described more positively by older adults (Fingerman, 2000). Even rates of depression and anxiety disorders are lower among older adults than their younger counterparts (George et al., 1988). Rather than heighten risk, advanced age appears to protect against psychopathology (Gatz et al., 1993).

Importantly, this patchwork pattern of sustained, diminished, and increased aspects of emotional experience and expression coalesce to indicate an overall pattern that suggests that age benefits emotion regulation (Carstensen et al., 2003). The sustained aspects of older adults' emotional lives make evident that the emotion system is as functional as it is in younger adults. The decreases in negative affect and increase in positive affect and emotional control indicate that the emotional lives of older adults are more pleasant and manageable relative to their younger counterparts. Thus, although distinct components of emotional processing show different trajectories, i.e., remaining the same, declining, or improving across the life span, at the aggregate emotional experience is enhanced.

III. Socioemotional Selectivity Theory

The juxtaposition of decline in cognitive and physical aging and the maintenance or improvement of well-being has been referred to as "the paradox of aging." How can it be that people suffer significant loss with age but experience life more positively? Socioemotional selectivity theory offers an explanation based on motivation (Carstensen, 1993, 1995; Carstensen, Isaacowitz, & Charles, 1999). The theory is distinguished from other life span theories in that its principal focus concerns the motivational consequences of perceived time left in life. Instead of relying on the more traditional yardstick of age, namely time since birth (or chronological age), socioemotional selectivity theory considers the effects of a continually changing temporal horizon on human development. The theory holds that when time is perceived as open ended, as it typically is in youth, people are strongly motivated to pursue information. They attempt to expand their horizons, gain knowledge, and pursue relationships. Information is gathered relentlessly. In the face of a long and nebulous future, even information that is not immediately relevant may become so somewhere down the line.

In contrast, when time is perceived as constrained, as it typically is in later life, people are motivated to pursue emotional satisfaction. They invest in sure things, deepen existing relationships, and savor life. Under these conditions, people are less interested in banking information and instead invest resources in the regulation of emotion. In this way, socioemotional selectivity theory specifies the direction of the age-related motivational shift and offers hypotheses about social preferences and goals as well as the types of material that people of different ages are most likely to attend to and remember. To be clear, the theory does not speak against experience-based change. Rather it postulates that some of the age differences long thought to reflect intractable, unidirectional change instead reflect changes in motivation, and as such the theory contributes to a more nuanced interpretation of age differences.

The theory leads to a number of postulates (for review, see Carstensen et al., 1999). Among them is the assertion that heightened attention to emotion should lead to the allocation of more cognitive resources to emotional tasks. In other words, if greater priority is placed on the regulation of emotion states and emotional aspects of life, this motivational shift should have consequences for cognitive processing. Adding to the potential for such theoretical reasoning is the observation of different aging trajectories for effortful and automatic — also called deliberative and intuitive — processes. Although at times emotion regulation is effortful, much emotion regulation has become automatic. Thus, two factors may contribute to changes in cognitive processes: Priorities may change with age and/or temporal horizons such that more resources are allocated to emotion regulation; and to the extent that regulation has become relatively automatic it may be easier to engage such strategies than effortful strategies involving acquiring new information.

IV. Emotion–Cognition Interactions with Age

From socioemotional selectivity theory, we can derive two postulates about how motivation might affect attention and memory. The first is that, as people age, they allocate a larger proportion of their cognitive resources to all types of emotionally relevant information, as both negative and positive emotional information is relevant for emotion regulation. The second is that selective cognitive processing is a component of effective emotion regulation, and therefore older adults are likely to devote their attention and memory capacity to information that will enhance their current mood. A growing body of research supports this second postulate. Whereas younger people tend to favor negative material in information processing, increasingly older groups favor positive material. We refer to the developmental trend as the positivity effect (see Carstensen & Mikels, 2005; Mather & Carstensen, 2005).

V. Memory for Emotion in General

Most of the initial research investigating emotion–cognition interactions and aging did not distinguish between negative and positive information. A number of these studies support the idea that with age, people allocate more of their cognitive resources to emotional information. As part of this, they seem to focus on their own internal thoughts and feelings more than younger adults. For example, in one study, younger and older adults participated in a series of "mini-events" in which they followed a script to complete actions such as packing a picnic basket or to imagine completing such actions (Hashtroudi, Johnson, & Chrosniak, 1990). When participants returned a day later and assessed the amount of perceptual and contextual detail and thoughts and feelings associated with their memories, older adults gave higher ratings for their thoughts and feelings than younger adults. In their recall of the events, younger adults recalled more spatial and contextual detail than older adults, whereas older adults recalled more associated thoughts and feelings than younger adults. Older adults not only were more likely to allocate their memory resources to thoughts and feelings, but they also seemed to base their confidence in their memories more on the strength of their associated thoughts and feelings than younger adults, as indicated by higher correlations between ratings of thoughts and feelings and memory confidence judgments than seen among younger adults (Johnson & Multhaup, 1992). Similar findings were seen in a study of

memory for pictures in which participants were asked to list reasons why they indicated certain memories were vivid (Comblain et al., 2004). Older adults were more likely than younger adults to say that the memories seemed vivid because they recollected their emotional reactions.

This increased focus on internal emotional states with age seems to be one reason that older adults' memories tend to be more influenced by schemas than those of younger adults (for a review, see Mather, 2004). Focusing on one's own feelings enhances memory for semantic content but impairs memory for contextual details (Johnson, Nolde, & De Leonardis, 1996; Mather, Johnson, & De Leonardis, 1999), which may lead people to rely more on their general semantic knowledge about the event when reconstructing it later. Instructing younger adults to focus on their internal emotional states as they experience or review an event leads their memories to be more consistent with their schemas or general knowledge (Mather & Johnson, 2000, 2003). In fact, younger adults in emotion-focus conditions show the same biases in memory as older adults in control conditions, who presumably are more likely to focus on their feelings without being prompted to do so (Kennedy, Mather, & Carstensen, 2004; Mather & Johnson, 2000, 2003).

A few studies also suggest that, compared with younger adults, older adults allocate more resources to emotional information in the external world than to neutral information. One study had participants from four different age groups spanning from 20 to 83 years of age read and then recall a narrative that contained about the same amount of emotional and neutral information (Carstensen & Turk-Charles, 1994). The proportion of information recalled that was emotional increased linearly with age. Similar findings were found in a study examining the recall of slogans and brand names from advertisements that were presented with a slogan that evoked either an emotionally meaningful goal (e.g., "Take flight … your loved ones await" for an airline ad) or an information-seeking goal (e.g., "Take flight … expand your horizons") (Fung & Carstensen, 2003). Older adults preferred the emotional versions of the ads and remembered the slogans and brand names better than in the knowledge-related versions, even though the two versions of the ads only differed in their slogans.

Older adults also remember the source of information better when the sources are framed in emotional terms than when they are framed in nonemotional terms (Rahhal, May, & Hasher, 2002). In one such experiment, older adults listened to a tape of a female and a male speaker each saying some trivia statements. The experimenters told them that all of the statements made by the female were true and all of the statements made by the male were false (or vice versa). After a delay, they were given a source memory test consisting of a list of the statements they had heard. In the emotional source task condition, participants were asked whether each statement was true or false. In the perceptual source task condition, participants were asked whether each statement was said by the male or by the female. As found in many previous studies, older adults were worse than younger adults at identifying who said each statement. However, there were no age differences in memory for which statements were true or false, even though that affective information was originally indicated by which speaker said the statement. Hess, Rosenberg, and Waters (2001) reported similar findings on an impression formation task. When the task was made personally relevant (e.g., participants were told that they would share their impressions with another person), older adults were more

likely to remember inconsistencies in the behavior of the target they were asked to describe.

Thus, these studies suggest that older adults allocate relatively more resources to encoding and retrieving relevant information. We go one step further and argue that "relevance" is systematic. Information that is related to older peoples' own internal emotional states or represents emotional aspects of the external environment assumes greater relevance. Given that experimental instructions reliably elicit and diminish such effects, we contend that motivation appears to be the key factor in creating these age differences. We note, however, that relatively well-maintained brain regions associated with emotional processing among older adults (Mather, 2004) may be an important precondition allowing older adults to effectively focus on and manage emotional information and reactions.

Because the studies reviewed earlier do not distinguish between negative and positive emotional information, they do not indicate whether older adults use attention and memory as an emotion regulation tool by focusing on the information that should make them feel best or whether they are especially attuned to all emotional information.

VI. Positivity Effects in Memory

Studies that distinguish positive and negative information reveal a positivity effect in older adults' memories that manifests itself in a number of different contexts and testing paradigms. We define the positivity effect as a developmental pattern in which a disproportionate preference for negative material in youth shifts across adulthood to disproportionate preference for positive information in later life. Operationally, the positivity effect is the age difference in the ratio of positive to negative material in information processing. For example, older adults show positivity effects in both recall and recognition of pictures (Charles, Mather, & Carstensen, 2003). Charles et al. (2003) asked 48 younger (18–29 years), 48 middle-aged (41–53 years), and 48 older (65–80 years) adults to watch a slide show consisting of positive, negative, and neutral pictures and to complete a 15-min filler task before recalling as many pictures as they could. Following the recall test, participants also completed a recognition test. Across each successive age group, memory recall increasingly consisted of positive pictures. Recognition also showed a shift in emotional memory, but on this measure, younger adults were most accurate for negative pictures, an advantage that disappeared in middle and old age.

Charles et al. (2003) controlled for a number of possible influencing variables. Half of the pictures from each emotional category depicted people and half did not. The numbers of men and women, white- and blue-collar workers, and European and African Americans were the same across each age group. None of these factors moderated the age by valence interactions. In addition, in a second study, including mood ratings as a covariate did not eliminate the age differences. Thus, the increase with age in the relative advantage of positive information over negative information in memory occurs across socioeconomic status, gender, and race and is not driven by age differences in mood.

Not only is the positivity effect present in long-term memory, but also in working memory. Mikels and colleagues (2005) examined working memory for visual and emotional information in older and younger adults. As expected from the pervasive declines in working memory described earlier, an age deficit in working memory for visual information emerged in that older adults performed significantly worse than younger adults. However, no age deficit emerged in working memory for emotional information; older and younger adults performed equivalently. Further, whereas younger adults showed superior working memory for negative relative to positive emotional stimuli, older adults exhibited superior working memory for positive relative to negative emotional stimuli. Thus, even within a fundamental component of the information processing system, a positivity effect is evident.

When remembering choices, older adults also remember in a way that is more emotionally gratifying than younger adults. They are more accurate at recognizing positive features (e.g., "spacious kitchen" for an apartment) than negative features (e.g., "low ceilings") from choices in contexts in which younger adults are about equally accurate for both types of features (Mather, Knight, & McCaffrey, 2005). In addition, when asked "which choice option was this feature associated with?" older adults are more likely than younger adults to attribute features from choices in a way that supports the option they chose (Mather & Johnson, 2000), attributing more positive features to chosen options and more negative features to rejected options than younger adults. Older adults show a stronger choice-supportive bias even when their overall source-monitoring accuracy is equated with that of younger adults. Supporting the idea that older adults remember in a more choice-supportive way than younger adults because of age differences in motivation is an additional condition in which younger adults were asked to think about how they felt about their choices after they made them. In this condition, younger adults were as choice supportive as older adults in the control condition, indicating that when emotional goals are made more salient for them, they are as likely as older adults to remember in ways that are emotionally gratifying.

Positivity effects are also seen more among older adults than younger adults in autobiographical memory (see Chapter 21). For example, when interviewed repeatedly throughout their lifetime, participants in a longitudinal study reported their childhood as being happier the older they were (Field, 1981). When recalling the 1992 election, older supporters of Ross Perot were more likely to underestimate how sad they had been than younger supporters (Levine & Bluck, 1997). This age difference was only present among those supporters who still wished Perot had been elected. Presumably, among those supporters who no longer wished he had been elected, memory for emotions when he withdrew from the race did not have as much relevance for current emotion regulation. In another study, nuns were asked to recall personal information from 14 years earlier when they had filled out a questionnaire about their health and personal habits (Kennedy et al., 2004). In the control condition in which participants simply filled out the questionnaire with questions about themselves 14 years ago, the oldest nuns distorted their memories in a positive direction more than the youngest nuns did. However, the youngest nuns had as strong a positivity bias as the oldest nuns in an emotion-focus condition in which they were asked to complete a brief emotion rating scale every so often during the questionnaire. Thus, this study, like Mather and Johnson (2000), demonstrates that age differences can be eliminated by making emotional goals more salient for younger adults.

In addition, the nuns in the Kennedy et al. (2004) study completed mood rating scales both before and after completing the memory questionnaire. Both the oldest nuns in the control condition and the nuns in the emotion-focus condition were in better moods after completing the memory questionnaire than when they started, an indication that the positivity biases in their memories helped improve their moods. In contrast, the youngest nuns and the nuns in an accuracy-focus condition did not show this improvement in mood, consistent with their lack of positivity bias in memory. The idea that older adults use memory as an emotion regulation tool is consistent with a study that examined emotions during various everyday activities (Pasupathi & Carstensen, 2003). Age was correlated with improved emotional experience only during episodes of reminiscing; no effects of age on mood were seen during other daily activities.

VII. Positivity Effects in Initial Attention

Initial indications of older adults' positivity biases can be seen in the way they first process information. When two faces appear on a computer screen side by side for 1 sec. followed by a dot in the same location as one of the faces, older adults are slower to indicate which side of the screen the dot is on if it appeared behind a negative face than a neutral or a positive face (Mather & Carstensen, 2003). Thus, older adults appeared to have detected the negative face and then avoided attending to it.

The ability to downregulate initial responses to negative stimuli was also found in a study that monitored participants' brain activity using functional magnetic resonance imaging (fMRI) while they viewed emotional pictures (Mather et al., 2004). The study focused on the amygdala, a region of the brain that has been found to enhance memory for emotionally arousing information (e.g., Cahill et al., 1996; Canli et al., 2000;

Phelps et al., 1998). Both older and younger adults showed greater amygdala activation while viewing emotional pictures than while viewing neutral pictures, but for older adults the amygdala activity was greater for the positive than the negative pictures, whereas this was not the case for younger adults. Thus, when left to their own devices, older adults are more likely than younger adults to downregulate responses to negative stimuli. Interestingly, younger adults also show decreased amygdala activation in response to negative pictures when given an explicit regulatory goal by experimenters (Ochsner et al., 2004).

In addition, studies examining age difference in information search during choices reveal differences in attention allocation. When allowed to search through a comparison chart about different cars available to purchase, older adults spend a larger proportion of their time looking at the positive features (e.g., a good safety rating feature) than the negative features (e.g., a bad safety rating feature) than younger adults (Mather et al., 2005). A study examining information search during health-related decisions found that, as in memory retrieval contexts (Kennedy et al., 2004; Mather & Johnson, 2000), this age difference in the positivity effect can be eliminated by explicitly focusing both younger and older adults on the details of the situation (Löckenhoff & Carstensen, 2004).

In contrast with the studies reviewed earlier, several studies have found no evidence for age-related positivity effects in memory (Comblain et al., 2004; Kensinger et al., 2002) or have found only marginally significant positivity effects (Denburg et al., 2003). One potential reason for the failure of these studies to replicate the positivity effect may be a lack of statistical power. The positivity effect is typically manifested in age by valence interactions with medium effect sizes (e.g., Charles et al., 2003; Mather & Knight, 2005). According to Cohen (1988), an N of 20 in each group, as used in Comblain et al. (2004) and Kensinger et al. (2002), only provides 34% power to detect a medium effect size. Another important and potentially meaningful methodological difference is that Charles et al. (2003) and Mather and Knight (2005) showed participants the picture slide shows without any encoding task; participants were simply asked to watch a slide show. In contrast, studies that have found no positivity effects have had participants either make valence/arousal ratings or asked them to try to feel the emotion being depicted in each picture. Including specific encoding instructions may equate performance across subgroups by limiting the implementation of more typical strategies. Another potential difference between the studies that do find a positivity effect and those that do not may be the cognitive abilities of the older participants. Higher executive functioning appears to be related to greater positivity, a point to which we return later.

VIII. Mechanisms Underlying the Positivity Effect

Given what we know about the numerous declines seen with age in various types of memory, one obvious possible explanation for the positivity effect is that it results from some sort of declining ability. As mentioned previously, older adults show diminished physiological responses to emotional stimuli (Levenson et al., 1991, 1994; Tsai et al., 2000). This diminished level of physiological responding occurs despite the lack of age differences in subjective emotional experience in the same studies, thus it is not clear how they might be associated with memory. Many studies with younger adults indicate that memory is enhanced for emotionally arousing elements of a scene but impaired for peripheral details of arousing scenes (for reviews, see Cahill & McGaugh, 1998; McGaugh, 2000; Reisberg & Heuer, 2004). Highly arousing stimuli are more likely to be negative (Lang, 1995), thus if arousal no longer affects memory as much for older adults, they may show less vivid memories for negative stimuli.

However, there is growing evidence that older adults gain the same benefits and suffer the same costs of emotional arousal as younger adults. Like younger adults, they recall the gist of emotionally arousing pictures better than neutral pictures (Denburg et al., 2003), but recognize the details of emotionally arousing scenes less well than details from neutral scenes (Denburg et al., 2003; Kensinger et al., 2005). The maintained effect of arousal among older adults is consistent with neurological evidence that the amygdala shows relatively little decline with age (for a review, see Mather, 2004). Thus, older adults' bias to forget negative information more quickly than positive information does not seem to be the result of declines in the influence of emotional arousal on memory.

As reviewed earlier, one of the most consistent themes in cognitive aging research is the decline in effortful and resource-intensive processes versus the stability of more automatic processes. From this perspective, one likely account of the positivity effect is that it some-how results from declines in the ability to engage in more resource-intensive processes. However, it has been shown that positivity effects rely on resource-intensive executive processes (Mather & Knight, 2005). In one experiment in this study, older and younger adults were shown a slide show of emotional pictures, like the ones seen in

Charles et al. (2003), and were asked to remember them 20 min later. In addition, they completed several tasks associated with executive function and were split into low and high groups based on their performance on these tasks. Older adults who performed well on the ability to ignore goal-irrelevant information while performing a task (Fan et al., 2002) or well on the ability to refresh just-activated information in memory (Johnson et al., 2002) had larger positivity biases in memory than older adults who performed poorly on these tasks. In contrast, performing well on the executive tasks had little relation with the positivity of younger adults' memories.

In another experiment, distracting older adults while they viewed the picture slide show eliminated their positivity effect in a later memory test, whereas it had no effect on the positivity of younger adults' memories. In fact, distracting older adults during encoding not only eliminated but reversed their positivity effect, such that they showed a negativity effect, with most of their recall consisting of negative pictures. These findings indicate that older adults automatically detect negative information in the environment (see also Mather & Knight, 2003), even when they are distracted. In fact, when older adults' attention is divided, they seem to be even more susceptible to the influence of negative and highly arousing stimuli (Mather & Knight, 2005; Wurm et al., 2004).

However, when they have the available cognitive resources, they act quickly to diminish their response to the negative information. This goal-directed stage of the process is more likely to be engaged in by older adults than by younger adults because emotion regulation becomes a more salient goal as people approach the end of life (Carstensen & Charles, 1998; Carstensen et al., 1999).

Supporting the role of time perspective in older adults' positivity effects, controlling for the amount of time participants felt they had left in life can eliminate age differences in the positivity effect (Löckenhoff & Carstensen, 2004).

IX. Future Directions

Until recently, the ways that motivation and cognition might interact were rarely considered by researchers, investigating the effects of aging. However, increasingly research suggests that neither age-related cognitive nor emotional processes can be understood fully in isolation. Age-related stereotype threat, for example, worsens performance (Hess et al., 1999), whereas emotional content that appeals strongly to the emotion regulatory goals of older individuals appears to improve performance (Carstensen et al., 2003).

We have interpreted the changes in emotion regulation with age in motivational terms and argue that experimental evidence for flexibility in performance based on instructional conditions that direct motivation is compelling (Hess, Waters, & Bolstad, 2000; Kennedy et al., 2004; Rahhal et al., 2002). Still other factors may contribute to the pattern of age differences emerging in the literature. Differential changes in the neural substrates underlying cognitive and emotional processes could explain some of the behavioral patterns reviewed previously. From functional neuroimaging we now know that on tasks that place a large demand on controlled and deliberative processes, such as working memory, older adults evidence bilateral prefrontal activation. Importantly, this bilateral prefrontal activation has been observed in the dorsolateral prefrontal cortex, the area critical to the executive and deliberative processes involved in working memory tasks

(Smith & Jonides, 1999). This overactivation has been interpreted as compensation for the neural degradation present with increasing age (Park et al., 2001; Reuter-Lorenz, 2002). As such, it reflects previously unsuspected neural plasticity across the life span even into old age. This compensatory model has been driven by the assumption that degeneration of the adult brain is responsible for losses in domains such as working memory and executive function (Park et al., 2001; Reuter-Lorenz, 2002).

Consistent with this degenerative process explanation, the documented improvements in emotion regulation and experience with age may merely be the result of neural change associated with aging. For instance, the finding of disproportionately greater atrophy of the dorsolateral prefrontal cortex relative to the orbital frontal cortex (Duara et al., 1983; Haug et al., 1983; Salat, Kaye, & Janowsky, 2001; however, see Raz et al., 1997) may help support preserved emotion regulation in the face of declines in cognitive deliberative processes and executive processing of nonemotional information. Teasing apart these alternative explanations and scenarios represents an exciting frontier in explorations of the aging mind and brain.

With socioemotional selectivity theory, we interpret the findings reviewed earlier in motivational terms. There are, however, other developmental models within which to consider emotion–cognition interactions. For example, Labouvie-Vief (2003) distinguished between affective experience and cognitive-affect complexity, the former referring to emotions experienced in everyday life and the latter referring to a conceptual understanding of emotional experience. Labouvie-Vief (2003) argued that these two aspects of emotional aging are separable and further that they show different aging trajectories with experience improving but emotional understanding declining as people move from middle to old age. Her group maintains that less sophisticated understanding may actually contribute to a more positive experience because of its relatively simple structure and that older adults are increasingly likely to use emotion regulation strategies that are automated and do not rely on cognitive resources. Thus, she suggested that "negative affect—but not positive affect—is related to cognitive functioning, perhaps because processing negative experience is more cognitively demanding" (Labouvie-Vief, 2003, p. 202). Labouvie-Vief argued that in contrast to the cognitive demands of integrating negative affect into one's experience, "optimization is automatic and relatively effortless" (Labouvie-Vief, 2003, p. 202). Mather and Knight's (2005) study provides a counterexample to this idea, as older people who reported the most positive memories scored highest on cognitive tests and reducing cognitive resources eliminated older adults' positivity effects. Thus, Labouvie-Vief's theory also predicts that emotional and cognitive trajectories are interrelated but in a quite different form. Future research is needed to better understand the relationship between cognitive functioning and affect among older adults.

Most life span theories view selection as a key component of development. As Hess et al. (2001) observed, most view selection as motivated by age-related loss and the subsequent need to husband resources toward increasingly circumscribed domains of life (Baltes & Baltes, 1990; Brandtstädter & Greve, 1994; Heckhausen & Schulz, 1995). Socioemotional selectivity theory asserts a different type of selection, not motivated by individualized goals and strivings but by broadly generalizable shifts in motivation that result from changes in temporal horizons. Such motivational shifts result in a favoring of positive over negative information in the processing of information.

There is, of course, much to learn. One important line of inquiry concerns the ways in which emotional material draws attention away from material highly relevant to the task. Consedine, Magai, and King (2004) pointed out that we are only beginning to understand the role of discrete emotions and their interactions with cognition. Although well-being may benefit from changes described earlier, there may be problems in other areas. In keeping with life span theory, development entails gains and losses. Research attention to such issues is likely to be fruitful in the future.

X. Summary

This chapter sought to integrate the disparate domains of cognitive aging and socioemotional aging from the perspective of a motivational theory of life span development. In order to accomplish this endeavor, we reviewed the dominant findings in cognitive and socioemotional aging, introduced socioemotional selectivity theory as one potential integrative perspective, and then demonstrated how changes in emotion–cognition interactions serve the emotion regulatory goals of older adults. The research presented in this final section suggests that a thorough understanding of how the human mind adapts ontogenetically requires an integrative perspective of cognition, emotion, and motivation.

The aging mind is generally characterized by divergent trajectories. Research in cognitive aging indicates that old age is marked by deterioration; most mental processes, especially those that are effortful and deliberative, decline ubiquitously while a few automatic processes and well-learned expertise-related functions remain unscathed. Importantly, evidence also indicates that even in old age there is remarkable plasticity of function. Not only can practice improve the performance of older adults, but instructional frames that portray a positive account of aging and memory can also improve performance. Such malleability suggests that motivation and emotion may play critical roles in the cognitive lives of older individuals. Thus, the nature of changes in the emotional lives of older adults should figure prominently in accounts of cognitive aging. In stark contrast to cognitive deterioration, emotional experience and emotion regulation emerge enhanced across the life span. Most emotional processes remain intact, and any changes, such as decreases in negative affect or increases in emotional control, indicate enhancements in the emotional lives of older adults. Understanding the intersection of cognitive decline and emotional enhancement appears to be critical to understanding the aging mind.

Socioemotional selectivity theory offers a motivational explanation for these changes in suggesting that due to an expanded time perspective, younger adults seek information, whereas due to a limited time perspective, older adults seek emotional satisfaction. The theory also generates hypotheses about emotion–cognition interactions in that the postulated emotion focus of older adults could direct attention and memory in line with emotional goals. The research reviewed in this chapter supports this postulate. Not only do older adults prefer, attend to, and show superior memory for emotional relative to nonemotional stimuli, but this emotion effect is disproportionate for positively relative to negatively valenced stimuli. This positivity effect associated with age appears to rely on resource-intensive processing, further suggesting that information processing changes in older adults are goal directed (Mather & Carstensen, 2005).

It appears that the long-standing independence of socioemotional and cognitive research arenas may have led to the inadvertent exclusion of important aspects of the psychology of aging. Whereas motivation has been a central focus in the area of *social* cognition, it has received relatively little attention in studies of basic mechanisms involved in information processing. This likely reflects a tacit assumption that social motives and social context affect social processes but not the basic elements of attention, memory, and other aspects of information processing. Research reviewed herein suggests that a more complete understanding demands consideration of the interplay of emotion, motivation, and cognition.

References

Baltes, P. B., & Baltes, M. M. (1990). Psychological perspectives on successful aging: The model of selective optimization with compensation. In P. B. Baltes & M. M. Baltes (Eds.), *Successful aging: Perspectives from the behavioral sciences* (pp. 1–34). New York: Cambridge University Press.

Baltes, P. B., & Kliegl, R. (1992). Further testing of limits of plasticity: Negative age differences in a mnemonic skill are robust. *Developmental Psychology, 28*(1), 121–125.

Baltes, P. B., & Lindenberger, U. (1997). Emergence of a powerful connection between sensory and cognitive functions across the adult life span: A new window at the study of cognitive aging? *Psychology of Aging, 12*, 12–21.

Baltes, P. B., & Staudinger, U. M. (2000). Wisdom: A metaheuristic (pragmatic) to orchestrate mind and virtue toward excellence. *American Psychologist, 55*(1), 122–136.

Banham, K. M. (1951). Senescence and the emotions: A genetic study. *Journal of Genetic Psychology, 78*, 175–183.

Birren, J. E., & Schroots, J. J. F. (2005). Autobiographical memory and the narrative self over the life span. In J. E. Birren & K. W. Schaie (Eds.), *Handbook of the psychology of aging* (6 ed.). San Diego, CA: Academic Press.

Blanchard-Fields, F., Jahnke, H. C., & Camp, C. (1995). Age differences in problem-solving style: The role of emotional salience. *Psychology & Aging, 10*(2), 173–180.

Brandtstädter, J., & Greve, W. (1994). The aging self: Stabilizing and protective processes. *Developmental Review, 14*(1), 52–80.

Burke, D. M., & Shafto, M. A. (2004). Aging and language production. *Current Directions in Psychological Science, 13*(1), 21.

Cahill, L., Haier, R. J., Fallon, J., Alkire, M. T., Tang, C., Keator, D., et al. (1996). Amygdala activity at encoding correlated with long-term, free recall of emotional information. *Proceedings of the National Academy of Sciences of the United States of America, 93*(15), 8016–8021.

Cahill, L., & McGaugh, J. L. (1998). Mechanisms of emotional arousal and lasting declarative memory. *Trends in Neurosciences, 21*(7), 294–299.

Canli, T., Zhao, Z., Brewer, J. B., Gabrieli, J. D. E., & Cahill, L. (2000). Event-related activation in the human amygdala associates with later memory for individual emotional response. *Journal of Neuroscience, 20*(19), RC99.

Carpenter, P. A., Miyake, A., & Just, M. A. (1995). Language comprehension: Sentence and discourse processing. *Annual Review of Psychology, 46*, 91–120.

Carstensen, L. L. (1993). Perspective on research with older families: Contributions of older adults to families and to family theory. In P. A. Cowan & D. Field (Eds.), *Family, self, and society: Toward a new agenda for family research* (pp. 353–360). Hillsdale, NJ: Lawrence Erlbaum.

Carstensen, L. L. (1995). Evidence for a life span theory of socioemotional selectivity. *Current Directions in Psychological Science, 4*(5), 151–156.

Carstensen, L. L., & Charles, S. T. (1998). Emotion in the second half of life. *Current Directions in Psychological Science, 7*, 144–149.

Carstensen, L. L., Fung, H. H., & Charles, S. T. (2003). Socioemotional selectivity theory and the regulation of emotion in the second half of life. *Motivation & Emotion, 27*(2), 103–123.

Carstensen, L. L., Isaacowitz, D. M., & Charles, S. T. (1999). Taking time seriously: A theory of socioemotional selectivity. *American Psychologist, 54*(3), 165–181.

Carstensen, L. L., & Mikels, J. A. (2005). At the intersection of emotion and cognition: aging and the positivity effect. *Current Directions in Psychological Science, 14*(3), 117–121.

Carstensen, L. L., Pasupathi, M., Mayr, U., & Nesselroade, J. R. (2000). Emotional experience in everyday life across the adult life span. *Journal of Personality & Social Psychology, 79*(4), 644–655.

Carstensen, L. L., & Turk-Charles, S. (1994). The salience of emotion across the adult life course. *Psychology and Aging, 9*, 259–264.

Charles, S. T., Mather, M., & Carstensen, L. L. (2003). Aging and emotional memory: The forgettable nature of negative images for older adults. *Journal of Experimental Psychology: General, 132*(2), 310–324.

Comblain, C., D'Argembeau, A., Van der Linden, M., & Aldenhoff, L. (2004). Impact of ageing on the recollection of emotional and neutral pictures. *Memory, 12*, 673–684.

Considine, N. S., Magai, C., & King, A. R. (2004). Deconstructing positive affect in later life: A differential functionalist analysis of joy and interest. *International Journal of Aging & Human Development, 58*(1), 49–68.

Craik, F. I. M., & Byrd, M. (1982). Aging and cognitive deficits: The role of attentional resources. In F. I. M. Craik & S. Trehub (Eds.), *Aging and cognitive processes* (pp. 191–211). New York: Plenum Press.

Craik, F. I. M., & Salthouse, T. A. (Eds.) (2000). *The handbook of aging and cognition* (2nd ed.). Mahwah, NJ: Lawrence Erlbaum.

Denburg, N. L., Buchanan, D., Tranel, D., & Adolphs, R. (2003). Evidence for preserved emotional memory in normal elderly persons. *Emotion, 3*, 239–254.

Diener, E., & Lucas, R. E. (1999). Personality and subjective well-being. In D. Kahneman, E. Diener, & N. Schwarz (Eds.), *Well-being: The foundations of hedonic psychology* (pp. 213–229). New York: Russell Sage Foundation.

Diener, E., & Suh, E. (1997). Measuring quality of life: Economic, social, and subjective indicators. *Social Indicators Research, 40*(1–2), 189–216.

Dror, I. E., & Kosslyn, S. M. (1994). Mental imagery and aging. *Psychology & Aging, 9*(1), 90–102.

Duara, R., Margolin, R. A., Robertson-Tchabo, E. A., London, E. D., Schwartz, M., Renfrew, J. W., et al. (1983). Cerebral glucose utilization, as measured with positron emission tomography in 21 resting healthy men between the ages of 21 and 83 years. *Brain*(106), 761–775.

Fan, J., McCandliss, B. D., Sommer, T., Raz, A., & Posner, M. I. (2002). Testing the efficiency and independence of attentional networks. *Journal of Cognitive Neuroscience, 14*(3), 340–347.

Field, D. (1981). Retrospective reports by healthy intelligent elderly people of personal events of their adult lives. *International Journal of Behavioral Development, 4,* 77–97.

Fingerman, K. L. (2000). "We had a nice little chat": Age and generational differences in mothers' and daughters' descriptions of enjoyable visits. *Journals of Gerontology: Psychological Sciences, 55,* P95–P106.

Fleischman, D. A., Wilson, R. S., Gabrieli, J. D. E., Bienias, J. L., & Bennett, D. A. (2004). A longitudinal study of implicit and explicit memory in old persons. *Psychology & Aging, 19*(4), 617–625.

Fung, H. H., & Carstensen, L. L. (2003). Sending memorable messages to the old: Age differences in preferences and memory for advertisements. *Journal of Personality and Social Psychology, 85*(1), 163–178.

Gatz, M., Johansson, B., Pedersen, N., Berg, S., & Reynolds, C. (1993). A cross-national self-report measure of depressive symptomatology. *International Psychogeriatrics, 5,* 14–156.

George, L. K., Blazer, D. F., Winfield-Laird, I., Leaf, P. J., & Fischback, R. L. (1988). Psychiatric disorders and mental health service use in later life: Evidence from the Epidemiologic Catchment Area Program. In J. Brody & G. Maddox (Eds.), *Epidemiology and aging* (pp. 189–219). New York: Springer.

Gross, J. J., Carstensen, L. L., Pasupathi, M., Tsai, J. L., Goetestam Skorpen, C., & Hsu, A. Y. C. (1997). Emotion and aging: Experience, expression, and control. *Psychology & Aging, 12*(4), 590–599.

Hasher, L., & Zacks, R. T. (1988). Working memory, comprehension, and aging: A review and a new view. In *The psychology of learning and motivation: Advances in research and theory* (Vol. 22, pp. 193–225). San Diego: Academic Press.

Hashtroudi, S., Johnson, M. K., & Chrosniak, L. D. (1990). Aging and qualitative characteristics of memories for perceived and imagined complex events. *Psychology and Aging, 5,* 119–126.

Haug, H., Barmwater, U., Eggers, R., Fischer, D., Kuhl, S., & Sass, N. L. (1983). Anatomical changes in aging brain: Morphometric analysis of the human prosencephalon. In J. Cervos-Navarro & H. I. Sarkander (Eds.), *Brain aging: Neuropathology and neuropharmacology* (pp. 1–12). New York: Raven Press.

Heckhausen, J., & Schulz, R. (1995). A life span theory of control. *Psychological Review, 102*(2), 284–304.

Hedden, T., & Gabrieli, J. D. E. (2004). Insights into the ageing mind: A view from cognitive neuroscience. *Nature Reviews Neuroscience, 5*(2), 87–U12.

Hess, T. M., Auman, C., Colcombe, S. J., & Rahhal, T. A. (2003). The impact of stereotype threat on age differences in memory performance. *Journals of Gerontology: Series B: Psychological Sciences & Social Sciences, 58B*(1), 3–11.

Hess, T. M., Bolstad, C. A., Woodburn, S. M., & Auman, C. (1999). Trait diagnosticity versus behavioral consistency as determinants of impression change in adulthood. *Psychology & Aging, 14*(1), 77–89.

Hess, T. M., Rosenberg, D. C., & Waters, S. J. (2001). Motivation and representational processes in adulthood: The effects of social accountability and information relevance. *Psychology and Aging, 16*(4), 629–642.

Hess, T. M., Waters, S. J., & Bolstad, C. A. (2000). Motivational and cognitive influences on affective priming in adulthood. *Journals of Gerontology: Series B: Psychological Sciences & Social Sciences, 55B*(4), 193–204.

Jacoby, L. L. (1991). A process dissociation framework: Separating automatic from intentional uses of memory. *Journal of Memory & Language, 30*(5), 513–541.

Johnson, M. K., & Multhaup, K. S. (1992). Emotion and MEM. In S.-A. Christianson (Ed.), *The handbook of emotion and memory: Current research and theory* (pp. 33–66). Hillsdale, NJ: Lawrence Erlbaum.

Johnson, M. K., Nolde, S. F., & De Leonardis, D. M. (1996). Emotional focus and source monitoring. *Journal of Memory and Language, 35*, 135–156.

Johnson, M. K., & Raye, C. L. (2000). Cognitive and brain mechanisms of false memories and beliefs. In D. L. Schacter & E. Scarry (Eds.), *Memory, brain, and belief* (pp. 25–86). Cambridge, MA: Harvard University Press.

Johnson, M. K., Reeder, J. A., Raye, C. L., & Mitchell, K. J. (2002). Second thoughts versus second looks: An age-related deficit in reflectively refreshing just-activated information. *Psychological Science, 13*(1), 64–67.

Kennedy, Q., Mather, M., & Carstensen, L. L. (2004). The role of motivation in the age-related positivity effect in autobiographical memory. *Psychological Science, 15*, 208–214.

Kensinger, E. A., Brierley, B., Medford, N., Growdon, J. H., & Corkin, S. (2002). Effects of normal aging and Alzheimer's disease on emotional memory. *Emotion, 2*(2), 118–134.

Kensinger, E. A., Piguet, O., Krendl, A. C., & Corkin, S. (2005). Memory for contextual details: Effects of emotion and aging. *Psychology and Aging, 20*, 241–250.

Kliegl, R., & Baltes, P. B. (1991). Testing-the-Limits kognitiver Entwicklungskapazität in einer Gedächtnisleistung. *Zeitschrift für Psychologie, Supplement 11*, 84–92.

Labouvie-Vief, G. (2003). Dynamic integration: Affect, cognition, and the self in adulthood. *Current Directions in Psychological Science, 12*(6), 201–206.

Lang, P. J. (1995). The emotion probe: Studies of motivation and attention. *American Psychologist, 50*, 372–385.

Laver, G. D., & Burke, D. M. (1993). Why do semantic priming effects increase in old age? A meta-analysis. *Psychology & Aging, 8*(1), 34–43.

Lawton, M. P., Kleban, M. H., & Dean, J. (1993). Affect and age: Cross-sectional comparisons of structure and prevalence. *Psychology & Aging, 8*(2), 165–175.

Lawton, M. P., Kleban, M. H., Rajagopal, D., & Dean, J. (1992). Dimensions of affective experience in three age groups. *Psychology & Aging, 7*(2), 171–184.

Levenson, R. W., Carstensen, L. L., Friesen, W. V., & Ekman, P. (1991). Emotion, physiology, and expression in old age. *Psychology & Aging, 6*(1), 28–35.

Levenson, R. W., Carstensen, L. L., & Gottman, J. M. (1994). Influence of age and gender on affect, physiology, and their interrelations: A study of long-term marriages. *Journal of Personality & Social Psychology, 67*(1), 56–68.

Levenson, R. W., Friesen, W. V., Ekman, P., & Carstensen, L. L. (1991). Emotion, physiology, and expression in old age. *Psychology and Aging, 6*(1), 28–35.

Levine, L. J., & Bluck, S. (1997). Experienced and remembered emotional intensity in older adults. *Psychology and Aging, 12*(3), 514–523.

Light, L. L., & La Voie, D. (1993). Direct and indirect measures of memory in old age. In P. Graf & M. E. J. Masson (Eds.), *Implicit memory: New directions in cognition, development, and neuropsychology* (pp. 207–230). Hillsdale, NJ: Lawrence Erlbaum.

Light, L. L., & Singh, A. (1987). Implicit and explicit memory in young and older adults. *Journal of Experimental Psychology: Learning, Memory, & Cognition, 13*(4), 531–541.

Lindenberger, U., & Baltes, P. B. (1994). Sensory functioning and intelligence in old age: A strong connection. *Psychology & Aging, 9*(3), 339–355.

Löckenhoff, C. E., & Carstensen, L. L. (2004). Socioemotional selectivity theory, aging, and health: The increasingly delicate balance between regulating emotions and making tough choices. *Journal of Personality, 72*, 1395–1424.

Logan, J. M., Sanders, A. L., Snyder, A. Z., Morris, J. C. & Buckner, R. L. (2002). Underrecruitment and non-selective recruitment: Dissociable neural mechanisms associated with aging. *Neuron, 33*, 827–840.

MacKay, D. G., & James, L. E. (2004). Sequencing, speech production, and selective effects of aging on phonological and morphological speech errors. *Psychology and Aging, 19*(1), 93–107.

Madden, D. J. (1986). Adult age differences in the attentional capacity demands of visual search. *Cognitive Development, 1*(4), 335–363.

Magai, C. (1999). Affect, imagery, attachment: Working models of interpersonal affect and the socialization of emotion. In J. Cassidy & P. R. Shaver (Eds.), *Handbook of attachment theory and research* (pp. 787–802). New York: Guilford.

Malatesta, C. Z., Izard, C. E., Culver, C., & Nicolich, M. (1987). Emotion communication skills in young, middle-aged, and older women. *Psychology and Aging, 2*, 193–203.

Malatesta-Magai, C., Jonas, R., Shepard, B., & Culver, L. C. (1992). Type A behavior pattern and emotion expression in younger and older adults. *Psychology and Aging, 7*(4), 551–561.

Mather, M. (2004). Aging and emotional memory. In D. Reisberg & P. Hertel (Eds.), *Memory and Emotion* (pp. 272–307). London: Oxford University Press.

Mather, M., Canli, T., English, T., Whitfield, S. L., Wais, P., Ochsner, K. N., et al. (2004). Amygdala responses to emotionally valenced stimuli in older and younger adults. *Psychological Science, 15*, 259–263.

Mather, M., & Carstensen, L. L. (2003). Aging and attentional biases for emotional faces. *Psychological Science, 14*, 409–415.

Mather, M., & Carstensen, L. L. (2005). Aging and motivated cognition: The positivity effect in attention and memory. *Trends in Cognitive Sciences, 9*, 496–502.

Mather, M., & Johnson, M. K. (2000). Choice-supportive source monitoring: Do our decisions seem better to us as we age? *Psychology & Aging, 15*(4), 596–606.

Mather, M., & Johnson, M. K. (2003). Affective review and schema reliance in memory in older and younger adults. *American Journal of Psychology, 116*, 169–189.

Mather, M., Johnson, M. K., & De Leonardis, D. M. (1999). Stereotype reliance in source monitoring: Age differences and neuropsychological test correlates. *Cognitive Neuropsychology, 16*, 437–458.

Mather, M., & Knight, M. (2003). *No age-related impairment in the detection of threatening faces.* Paper presented at the annual meeting of the Cognitive Neuroscience Society, New York.

Mather, M., & Knight, M. (2005). Goal-directed memory: The role of executive processes in older adults' emotional memory. *Psychology and Aging.*

Mather, M., Knight, M., & McCaffrey, M. (2005). The allure of the alignable: False memories of choice features. *Journal of Experimental Psychology: General, 134*, 38–51.

Mathuranath, P. S., George, A., Cherian, P. J., Alexander, A., Sarma, S. G., & Sarma, P. S. (2003). Effects of age, education and gender on verbal fluency. *Journal of Clinical and Experimental Neuropsychology, 25*(8), 1057–1064.

McDowd, J. M., & Craik, F. I. (1988). Effects of aging and task difficulty on divided attention performance. *Journal of Experimental Psychology: Human Perception & Performance, 14*(2), 267–280.

McGaugh, J. L. (2000). Memory: A century of consolidation. *Science, 287*, 248–251.

Mikels, J. A., Larkin, G. R., Reuter-Lorenz, P. A., & Carstensen, L. (2005). Divergent trajectories in the aging mind: Changes in working memory for affective versus visual information with age. *Psychology and Aging.*

Mireles, D. E., & Charness, N. (2002). Computational explorations of the influence of structured knowledge on age-related cognitive decline. *Psychology & Aging, 17*(2), 245–259.

Mitchell, D. B., Brown, A. S., & Murphy, D. R. (1990). Dissociations between procedural and episodic memory: Effects of time and aging. *Psychology and Aging, 5*(2), 264–276.

Mroczek, D. K., & Kolarz, C. M. (1998). The effect of age on positive and negative affect: A developmental perspective on happiness. *Journal of Personality & Social Psychology, 75*(5), 1333–1349.

Mroczek, D. K., & Spiro, A., III (2005). Change in life satisfaction during adulthood: findings from the veterans affairs normative aging study. *Journal of Personality & Social Psychology, 88*(1), 189–202.

Ochsner, K. N., Ray, R. D., Cooper, J. C., Robertson, E. R., Chopra, S., Gabrieli, J. D. E., et al. (2004). For better or for worse: Neural systems supporting the cognitive down- and up-regulation of negative emotion. *Neuroimage, 23*(2), 483–499.

Park, D. C. (2000). The basic mechanisms accounting for age-related decline in cognitive function. In D. C. Park & N. Schwarz (Eds.), *Cognitive aging: A primer*. Philadelphia, PA: Psychology Press/Taylor & Francis.

Park, D. C., Lautenschlager, G., Hedden, T., Davidson, N. S., Smith, A. D., & Smith, P. K. (2002). Models of visuospatial and verbal memory across the adult life span. *Psychology & Aging, 17*(2), 299–320.

Park, D. C., Polk, T. A., Mikels, J. A., Taylor, S. F., & Marshuetz, C. (2001). Cerebral aging: integration of brain and behavioral models of cognitive function. *Dialogues in Clinical Neuroscience, 3*(3), 151–165.

Park, D. C., Puglisi, J. T., & Smith, A. D. (1986). Memory for pictures: Does an age-related decline exist? *Psychology & Aging, 1*(1), 11–17.

Park, D. C., & Schwarz, N. (Eds.) (2000). *Cognitive aging: A primer*. Philadelphia, PA: Psychology Press/Taylor & Francis.

Park, D. C., & Shaw, R. J. (1992). Effect of environmental support on implicit and explicit memory in younger and older adults. *Psychology & Aging, 7*(4), 632–642.

Park, D. C., Smith, A. D., Lautenschlager, G., & Earles, J. L. (1996). Mediators of long-term memory performance across the life span. *Psychology & Aging, 11*(4), 621–637.

Pasupathi, M., & Carstensen, L. L. (2003). Age and emotional experience during mutual reminiscing. *Psychology & Aging, 18*, 430–442.

Phelps, E. A., LaBar, K. S., Anderson, A. K., O'Connor, K. J., Fulbright, R. K., & Spencer, D. D. (1998). Specifying the contributions of the human amygdala to emotional memory: A case study. *Neurocase, 4*(6), 527–540.

Phillips, L. H. (1999). Age and individual differences in letter fluency. *Developmental Neuropsychology, 15*, 249–267.

Plude, D. J., & Doussard-Roosevelt, J. A. (1989). Aging, selective attention, and feature integration. *Psychology & Aging, 4*(1), 98–105.

Rahhal, T. A., Hasher, L., & Colcombe, S. J. (2001). Instructional manipulations and age differences in memory: Now you see them, now you don't. *Psychology & Aging, 16*(4), 697–706.

Rahhal, T. A., May, C. P., & Hasher, L. (2002). Truth and character: Sources that older adults can remember. *Psychological Science, 13*(2), 101–105.

Raz, N., Gunning, F. M., Head, D., Dupuis, J. H., McQuain, J., Briggs, S. D., et al. (1997). Selective aging of the human cerebral cortex observed in vivo: Differential vulnerability of the prefrontal gray matter. *Cerebral Cortex, 7*, 268–282.

Reisberg, D., & Heuer, F. (2004). Memory for emotional events. In D. Reisberg & P. Hertel (Eds.), *Memory and emotion*. New York: Oxford University Press.

Reuter-Lorenz, P. A. (2002). New visions of the aging mind and brain. *Trends in Cognitive Sciences, 6*(9), 394–400.

Ryff, C. D. (1991). Possible selves in adulthood and old age: A tale of shifting horizons. *Psychology & Aging, 6*(2), 286–295.

Ryff, C. D., & Keyes, C. L. M. (1995). The structure of psychological well-being revisited. *Journal of Personality & Social Psychology, 69*(4), 719–727.

Salat, D. H., Kaye , J. A., & Janowsky, J. S. (2001). Selective preservation and degeneration within the prefrontal cortex in aging and Alzheimer disease. *Archives of Neurology, 58*(9), 1403–1408.

Salthouse, T. A. (1991). *Theoretical perspectives on cognitive aging*. Hillsdale, NJ: Lawrence Erlbaum.

Salthouse, T. A. (1996). The processing-speed theory of adult age differences in cognition. *Psychological Review, 103*(3), 403–428.

Schaie, K. W. (2005). *Developmental influences on adult intelligence: The Seattle longitudinal study*. New York: Oxford University Press.

Smith, E. E., & Jonides, J. (1999). Storage and executive processes in the frontal lobes. *Science, 283*(5408), 1657–1661.

Staudinger, U. M. (1999). Older and wiser? Integrating results on the relationship between age and wisdom-related performance. *International Journal of Behavioral Development, 23,* 641–664.

Tsai, J. L., Levenson, R. W., & Carstensen, L. L. (2000). Autonomic, subjective, and expressive responses to emotional films in older and younger Chinese Americans and European Americans. *Psychology & Aging, 15*(4), 684–693.

Wurm, L. H., Labouvie-Vief, G., Aycock, J., Rebucal, K. A., & Koch, H. E. (2004). Performance in auditory and visual emotional Stroop tasks: A comparison of older and younger adults. *Psychology and Aging, 19*(3), 523–535.

Sixteen

Personality and Aging

Daniel K. Mroczek, Avron Spiro III, and Paul W. Griffin

The study of personality and aging is currently in a state of good health. The study of personality characteristics in and of themselves within older adults is flourishing (Hooker & McAdams, 2003; Mroczek & Spiro, 2003a; Small et al., 2003), and scholars are fruitfully using personality variables to predict important outcomes in older adulthood, particularly mortality (Wilson et al., 2004). With respect to the former, intriguing new findings have permitted a deeper and more complex understanding of personality development in older adulthood, which is especially true with respect to stability and change in personality traits over long-term periods (Mroczek et al., 2005). This chapter gives ample attention to the stability-change issue in personality, as well as the organization of personality variables and their utility in predicting mortality among older adults. We believe that conceptual and empirical work by developmentalists in these three areas (personality organization, personality development, and the personality–mortality association) has been particularly interesting since publication of the last volume of this handbook, justifying the selective focus on

these three topics. We start with the issue of organization, then discuss stability and change, followed by a consideration of what may explain why some are stable and others not, and finally conclude with a treatment of the issue of personality and mortality in older adulthood.

I. Personality Organization: The Broadening of Conceptual Models

Through most of the 1980s and 1990s, scholarly work on personality organization focused almost exclusively on the factor structure of traits (Costa & McCrae, 1994; Goldberg, 1993). These research efforts concluded that the five-factor model, informally known as the big five, adequately described the general factorial structure of personality traits, although each of the five (extroversion, agreeableness, conscientiousness, neuroticism, openness) was so broad that many narrow factors comprised each. This program of research was extended to older adults and established that this broad factor structure held within older samples as well as younger ones (Mroczek et al., 1998).

However, even as the big five gained widespread acceptance in the 1990s, skeptics pointed out shortcomings of the model (Block, 1995; McAdams, 1992). By the turn of the century it was clear that although the big five may provide an adequate framework for traits, it left out many other types of personality variables. Nontrait approaches were largely excluded in the big five model. Funder (2001) identified three major approaches to personality psychology: trait, social–cognitive, and psychodynamic approaches. Although not a formal organizational structure, Funder (2000) did describe the frameworks that encompass the vast majority of personality researchers. He additionally indicated that two of these approaches (trait and social–cognitive) were on an integrative course and that the next 10–20 years would witness the fusion of these major areas.

We believe Funder is correct about these two areas integrating, and gerontologists are at the forefront of conceptual efforts that utilize both trait and social–cognitive variables. The burgeoning area of *developmental regulation* is a testament to such integration (Brandtstadter & Renner, 1990; Heckhausen & Schulz, 1995; Martin, 2001; Wrosch, Heckhausen, & Lachman, 2000). Theories of developmental regulation stress the importance of the person (and person-based characteristics) in shaping one's own development and life context throughout the entire life span. Traits and social–cognitive variables are each key components in these frameworks, which themselves are part of the larger conception of *self-regulation*, which maintains that people actively fashion their own behavior (Carver & Scheier, 1982, 1998). However, while theories of developmental and self-regulation utilize both trait and

social–cognitive variables, their purpose is to explain behavior and development, not provide an integrative framework for the field of personality psychology. Yet again, developmentalists in general and gerontologists in particular are at the forefront of efforts to build a broad framework for all personality variables (Diehl, 2005; Lang, Reschke, & Neyer, 2005; Roberts & Wood, 2005).

Hooker and McAdams (2003) combined concepts from the trait and social–cognitive approaches to create a six-foci model for understanding personality and its development. Hooker and McAdams (2003) organized the foci along two dimensions. These are *structure* and *process*. Structure is grounded in concepts from the trait approach, such as extroversion and neuroticism. Process refers to concepts from the social cognitive approach, such as situational variability (e.g., the pattern of a person's behavior across situations). These two concepts can be likened to structural and process elements of an automobile. A car has certain fixed, structural components, such as the chassis and windshield. These elements represent "structure." A car also possesses dynamic elements, such as the process that converts gasoline into energy that powers the engine and moves the vehicle forward. These elements represent "process." Human personality encompasses both structural and process elements, and Hooker and McAdams (2003) used these two concepts to provide a dual backbone of their model. Their three structural aspects of personality are traits, characteristic adaptations, and life stories; their three process aspects are states, self-regulation, and self-narration. The structural dimensions comprise aspects of personality that change slowly, although among the three, some change less slowly than others. In the six-foci model, traits change the least and life stories the most. However, none of the variables that lie within the structural foci are dynamic, i.e., they do not display short-lived, but rather systematic, changes that play out over periods of weeks, days, hours, minutes, or seconds. Personality variables that change very quickly, often in response to a contextual variable (such as stress), and retain the ability to snap back to prior levels are the purview of Hooker and McAdams' process dimension. These variables display change, but the change is temporary and strongly linked to context.

The Hooker–McAdams model is important for the field of personality psychology in general because it provides a broader framework than that of the big five, which is too strongly attached to structure approaches, particularly the trait approach. Every conceivable personality characteristic has a place within the model. However, the Hooker–McAdams model is important for the area of personality and aging in particular because it incorporates issues of development into its very core. Hooker and McAdams (2003) make specific theoretical predictions about which of the six foci should display more long-term change. The development of personality over the life span is not an afterthought in their model. It is part and parcel of its foundation. For these reasons, we expect the Hooker–McAdams model to receive increasing attention in the coming years within personality psychology in general and life span personality development in particular.

II. Personality Development: Individual Differences in Change

The debate over change in personality has quietly transformed over the past several years. The old, simple question of whether personality traits are stable or not has given way to the more subtle and complex perspective that change is an individual differences variable in and of itself. Some people are stable, whereas others are not. This perspective has its origins in the life span developmental concept of *individual differences in intraindividual change* (Alwin, 1994; Baltes & Nesselroade, 1973; Baltes, Reese, & Nesselroade, 1977; Nesselroade, 1988, 1991; Ozer, 1986; Schaie, 1996; Wohlwill, 1973). Since the mid-1970s, personality development researchers have rarely focused on individual differences in personality change, focusing instead on aggregate statistical approaches to the question, such as repeated-measures means and correlation coefficients. These approaches have yielded valuable results, establishing that rank-order stability is high for the big five traits (extroversion, neuroticism, agreeableness, conscientiousness, openness), even into older adulthood (Caspi & Roberts, 2001; Roberts & DelVecchio, 2000; Costa & McCrae, 1988, 1994). These studies have also determined that mean-level stability varies by trait over the course of adulthood (Costa & McCrae, 1994; Roberts & Walton, 2004).

As valuable as these studies are, they have narrowed the focus of research on personality development in adulthood. Scholars became habituated to thinking in terms of change or stability in means or in relative positioning within a distribution (rank orders) or change in group-level means. Much of the important early work on personality stability and change concentrated on one or both of these forms, as summarized in meta-analyses (Roberts & DelVecchio, 2000; Roberts & Walton, 2004). However, they largely conceal individual differences in stability and change (Aldwin et al., 1989; Lamiell, 1981; Mroczek & Spiro, 2003a). As a result of overreliance on these statistics and the preponderance of them in the literature, many researchers have concluded that personality is stable for all or most individuals, without actually evaluating the extent of the individual differences in stability. Do some individuals remain stable and others change? Do some change in one direction, while others change in the opposite direction?

Personality psychology is strongly identified with the science of individual differences, yet it is ironic that it has largely overlooked the possibility of individual differences in stability and change. Another major reason why the notion of individual differences in change remained an obscure and mainly theoretical concept for many years was the lack of adequate statistical models to estimate change accurately. With the development of such models (McArdle, 1991; Meredith & Tisak, 1990; Muthen, 2002; Raudenbush & Bryk, 2002; Rogosa, Brandt, & Zimowski, 1982; Singer & Willett, 2003), investigators have been able to estimate more accurately overall (sample-level) rates of change as well as individual differences in rate of change and in higher order parameters (e.g., curvature). Collectively known as growth curve models (latent growth curves if estimated via structural equation models; McArdle, 1991), this family of techniques has allowed researchers to confirm that the life span principle of individual differences in intraindividual change is an empirical fact and no longer a theoretical conjecture with respect to personality traits.

Studies documenting individual differences in rate of change in personality traits are now numerous (Helson, Jones, & Kwan, 2002; Jones & Meredith, 1996; Jones, Livson, & Peskin, 2003; Mroczek & Spiro, 2003a; Mroczek, Spiro, & Almeida, 2003; Roberts & Chapman, 2001; Small et al., 2003). Together, they have established that a large number of traits show variability across individuals in rate of change, including each of the big five constructs (Small et al., 2003). Jones et al. (2003) termed this

heterogeneous change, meaning that some people change, others do not, and the direction or pattern of change (e.g., linear, quadratic) varies across people. Put more simply, there is a range of change. These studies have also documented overall (sample-level) changes in some traits as people age, most notably declines in neuroticism (Mroczek & Spiro, 2003a; Small et al., 2003) and increases in agreeableness and concientiousness (Helson, Jones, & Kwan, 2002; Small et al., 2003).

Complementing these long-term studies of intraindividual change are shorter term studies that carry out intensive measurements (usually daily assessments) of personality traits. These studies have largely found that there is great day-to-day variation in traits, meaning that sometimes people rate themselves as extroverted but other times as introverted (Jones, Nesselroade, & Birkel, 1991; Nesselroade & Jones, 1991). This kind of change is very different from the long-term (trajectory) change described earlier. In fact, some have argued it should not be called change at all, but rather intraindividual variability or fluctuation (Nesselroade & Featherman, 1991). This shorter term intraindividual variability can coexist with longer term intraindividual change (or stability) because they refer to two different aspects of a longitudinal series of measurement occasions. For a given person, the concept of intraindividual change captures the direction of his or her overall trajectory and its rate of change, whereas the concept of intraindividual variability captures the variation in the measurements around that trajectory for that person.

Fleeson (2001) proposed an elegant framework for understanding the difference between these concepts. He argues that the personality-related behavior over a period of time (usually a few weeks) for a given person is characterized by a density distribution (Fleeson & Jolley, 2005). That distribution will contain behaviors that span the full spectrum for a given personality dimension, e.g., extroversion. Over that period of weeks, one will observe both extroverted and introverted behaviors at various times for that person. Fleeson (2001) demonstrated empirically that the full spectrum of behaviors for a trait is manifested in nearly every person over a period of a few weeks. However, people vary greatly from one another in how many of these behaviors they emit. Some people emit far more extroverted behaviors than others, skewing the mean of their distribution toward the extroverted end. Conversely, others display more introverted behaviors over a multi-week period, skewing their mean toward the introverted end. The concept of density distribution makes it easy to see how a person's typical way of behaving (the mean) is separate from the variability around that mean (the variance, corresponding to Nesselroade's concept of intraindividual variability). The mean can either change or remain stable, depending on the person. This is what growth curve studies of traits have documented (Mroczek & Spiro, 2003a; Small et al., 2003). Similarly, the variance can either change or remain stable, depending on the person. We know of no studies that have tracked this change in variances over long periods of time. Thus, the self-regulation and process constructs in Hooker and McAdams' (2003) model have not been studied by scholars in the long-term manner that traits have. This is a large gap in the literature. It is hoped that by the next edition of this handbook, researchers interested in self-regulation and other "process" personality concepts will have begun some long-term (5–10 years or more) studies of these constructs to correct the imbalance. That said, some interesting studies of

the correlates of shorter term intraindividual variability have been carried out. Most notably, variability in perceived control beliefs over a multi week period predicted mortality 5 years later in a sample of older adults (Eizenman et al., 1997).

III. What Gives Rise to Individual Differences in Intraindividual Personality Change?

Although it is now clear that over long-term periods some people change more than others (and some people do not change at all), it is less clear why some people change and others remain stable. A number of theorists have speculated on the factors that bring about individual differences in personality changes. People differ with respect to the environments to which they are exposed, the genetic makeup they possess, and the active ways they bring about behavioral change in themselves (Caspi & Roberts, 2001; Lerner & Busch-Rossnagel, 1981; Levenson & Crumpler, 1996; Mroczek & Spiro, 2003b; Roberts & Wood, 2005). People actively make decisions regarding aspects of themselves they wish to change, they actively turn to therapy and spirituality, and they rearrange the contexts that surround them. Moreover, these active behaviors surely interact with biological and environmental sources of personality change, and these biological and environmental sources themselves interact with one another (e.g., Caspi et al., 2002). All of these may produce individual differences in the developmental trajectories of personality dimensions.

For example, a number of contextual variables have been shown to influence personality change. For example, Clausen and Jones (1998) found that disorderly careers and divorce may disrupt personality stability and bring about trait change. Additionally, Martin and

Mroczek (2005) indicated that work and family overload in adults at midlife are associated with mean differences in big five traits when compared to younger or older adults. Specifically, agreeableness and extroversion both showed a nadir in midlife. However, work overload explained this effect for extroversion, and family overload explained it for agreeableness. These results indicate a certain sensitivity of personality to contextual events and stressors.

Additionally, history-graded normative influences (perhaps contained within birth cohorts) may influence personality trajectories (Baltes, 1987; Nesselroade & Baltes, 1974). Indeed, evidence suggests that there are birth cohort differences in the level of (Twenge, 2000, 2001) and rate of change in extroversion and neuroticism (Mroczek & Spiro, 2003a). Specifically, older cohorts decline on neuroticism at a slower rate than younger cohorts, and older cohorts decline on extroversion whereas younger cohorts rise or remain stable.

Age-graded life events, especially relationship events, can alter personality trajectories as well. Getting married typically increases conscientiousness and lowers neuroticism (Neyer & Asendorpf, 2001). In older adulthood, death of spouse and remarriage are relationship events that can influence personality trajectories. Neuroticism rose initially, but then declined at a faster rate in the years after a spouse died, and among those who remarried, neuroticism declined at a faster rate (Mroczek & Spiro, 2003a).

Speculatively, age-graded changes in health may also influence personality trajectories. If a person's health deteriorates to the point where they are unable or unwilling to socialize with others, this could create a shift toward less extroversion, greater neuroticism, and perhaps less agreeableness. Moreover, it is possible that changes in physical health may feed on changes in personality, creating a vicious cycle. For example, a decline in health may bring about a decline in extroversion. Declining extroversion may then decrease motivation to stay healthy, in turn contributing to further declines in physical health. Understanding these potential vicious cycles has important implications for the prevention and treatment of disease in older adults and for the ongoing treatment of chronic disorders.

Most of the theorizing and empirical work on what predicts personality change has focused on environmental or contextual explanations. Biological influences have generally been ignored. This is unfortunate because we now have evidence that individual differences in genes (whether a person possesses a particular variant or not) and individual differences in exposure to particular contexts (e.g., whether one was abused as a child or not), as well as their interaction, give rise to individual differences in certain personality outcomes. Specifically, possessing a combination of a particular gene and an abusive environment produced higher levels of antisocial behavior and a higher tendency toward depression 18 years later (Caspi et al., 2002, 2003). This longitudinal study documented a clear gene–environment interaction in producing downstream personality outcomes, in this case, almost two decades later. Speculatively, similar combinations of biological (such as, but not exclusively, genetic predispositions) and environmental factors may predict individual differences in long-term personality trajectories as well.

Explaining variability in personality trajectories in older adulthood, especially in rates of change, is an important task facing personality development researchers. Yet those who have attempted to account for such individual differences in change have often run into difficulties. Frequently, the hypothesized predictors do not predict as expected. One reason for this may be that personality trajectories are more responsive to idiosyncratic factors such as genetic makeup or nonnormative life events than normative or age-graded biological or contextual events (Baltes, 1987; Baltes, Reese, & Nesselroade, 1977). Variability in personality trajectories may reflect, to some degree, very specific circumstances in individual lives. One way around this is to identify people whose trajectories show either great change or stability and determine what environmental or biological factors may have promoted such high stability or change. Another possibility is to incorporate time-varying covariates into personality growth curve models (Singer & Willett, 2003). This refers to variables who values may change over time and which are entered into the growth curve model as a within-person covariate or predictor. Such models have been used in modeling change in well-being over time (Lucas et al., 2003, 2004). Life events or health events are placed in the model when they occur, allowing for more proximal prediction. These kinds of models may eventually prove superior to static-predictor (between-person) models in accounting for individual differences in personality trajectories because they mimic the vicissitudes of life more accurately.

Again, the effects of change in personality and health may work both ways. Change in personality may also have a protective effect on health. People who increase in conscientiousness or decrease in neuroticism may enjoy a concomitant increase in physical health or, more likely, stability in his or her good health trajectory (Aldwin & Levenson, 1994; Aldwin, Sutton, & Lachman, 1996). In this sense, a change in personality may indicate resiliency, protecting a person against disease in older adulthood (Ryff & Singer, 1998).

IV. Personality and Mortality among Older Adults

This final section focuses on a specific issue in personality and aging. This is the question of the influence of personality on mortality in adulthood, especially older adulthood. Earlier we indicated that a change in personality in late life may be a marker of decline in health, but other evidence suggests it may be more than simply a marker. A number of studies over the past decade have reported that certain personality dispositions predict time to mortality. Low levels of conscientiousness and extroversion and high levels of neuroticism and negative affect are associated with earlier mortality (Almada et al., 1991; Christensen et al., 2002; Friedman et al., 1993; Kubzansky et al., 1997; Maruta et al., 2000; Wilson et al., 2003, 2004). Greater variability in day-to-day feelings of personal control over a month-long period also predicted mortality in an institutionalized sample of older adults (Eizenman et al., 1997). Positive outlooks on life, such as that assessed by dispositional optimism (Scheier & Carver, 1985), have been associated with longer life (Levy et al., 2002). Further, people who had high neuroticism and low agreeableness possessed poor health profiles that were associated with higher mortality (Aldwin et al., 2001).

The first study to document the relationship between personality and mortality was investigation using the Terman sample (Friedman et al., 1993). It used personality assessed in childhood to predict time to death, finding that lower conscientiousness (greater impulsivity) was associated with earlier mortality. It was hypothesized that this relationship rested on health behaviors. People who are more planful and conscientious display better health outcomes than those who are less so

(Roberts & Bogg, 2004). However, people low in conscientiousness engage in more risky behaviors (alcohol and drug abuse, risky sex, impulsive behaviors that lead to fatal accidents) that end their lives sooner. This makes sense for young or middle-aged adults, but among older adults, many impulsive individuals would have been removed from the population, thus weakening or rendering nonsignificant the conscientiousness–mortality association. However, Wilson et al. (2004) found that the conscientiousness–mortality relationship held among older adults. Thus, there may be more to this intriguing association. One hypothesis is that people high in conscientiousness engage in good health behaviors, such as eating a healthy diet and exercising, which keeps them alive longer than people who are lower in this trait, but not so low that they would have died young (e.g., people very low in conscientiousness). If so, the protective effects of conscientiousness may last well into older adulthood. More research is needed to verify these hypotheses and further elucidate this interesting association.

The mechanisms underlying the relationship between other traits and mortality are similarly unclear. For example, the association between mortality and neuroticism may have roots in sensitivity to stress. One of the effects of stress is to elevate levels of stress hormones (e.g., cortisol) that can damage arteries (Kiecolt-Glaser & Glaser, 1986). Psychological stress can increase the corticotrophin-releasing hormone, activate the hypothalamic–pituitary–adrenal stress (HPA) axis, and promote secretion of glucocorticoids (e.g., cortisol) into the blood circulation. Persistent elevated levels of cortisol are symptomatic of general poor physical health, especially wear and tear on the HPA axis (Kiecolt-Glaser & Glaser, 1986). Because neuroticism is associated with greater exposure

and reactivity to stress (Bolger & Schilling, 1991), including in older adults (Mroczek & Almeida, 2004), the physical effects of stress may underlie the effect of neuroticism on mortality. Indeed, neuroticism and a prolonged negative affect have been linked to dysregulation of the HPA, and some have suggested that high levels of neuroticism over a lifetime may give rise to dysregulated emotion in older adulthood (Kendler, Thornton, & Gardner, 2001; Wilson et al., 2003, 2004). Studies of stress reactivity and neuroticism in older adults are consistent with this hypothesis. Mroczek and Almeida (2004) found that older adults, especially those high in neuroticism, were much more emotionally reactive to daily stressors than younger or midlife adults. It may be that a lifetime of high neuroticism and its concomitant stress sensitivity (and potentially elevating levels of harmful stress hormones such as cortisol) may cause physical damage to one's arteries and heart, contributing to mortality.

Earlier we discussed the ample documentation of long-term change in personality traits, which gives rise to an interesting question. Is change in personality associated with mortality? If high neuroticism is associated with higher mortality, then what happens when someone increases or decreases this trait? Does risk of dying at a given age rise or fall as the level of neuroticism changes? Change in risk of death may be a consequence of personality change itself. If someone is able to lower his or her level or neuroticism via therapy or by making conscious efforts to defuse feelings of anxiety, then the personality change itself may lead to a better physical well-being and alter one's risk of dying. However, any such effects are likely observable over very long periods of time, in terms of years or decades.

In contrast, there may be forms of change in personality that are associated with mortality, but only in very late life. This is a very different type of association than the one discussed earlier, and is similar to the concept of "terminal decline" (Berg, 1996; Small & Backman, 1997; Small et al., 2003), where considerable drops in cognitive functioning precede death. Terminal decline is speculatively attributed to neurological problems (e.g., ministrokes) that do serious health damage "silently," even while allowing people to maintain a relatively high level of daily physical functioning (Berg, 1996; Small & Backman, 1997). However, reports have shown that terminal decline occurs regardless of cause of death (e.g., cerebrovascular, cardiac, cancer; Small et al., 2003). It thus appears to be a general phenomenon. We do know that changes in personality accompany other forms of slow-moving but debilitating neurological diseases, such as Alzheimer's (Oppenheim, 1994; Wild et al., 1994). Is there a similar type of terminal decline for personality in which change over a short period (a year or two) in these constructs precedes death? Berg (1996) indicated that this may be the case. Similarly, do increases or decreases in life satisfaction and affect, well-being variables that are closely associated with personality, raise or lower one's risk of dying? These interesting questions require answers, but would also help tie together two streams of research on personality and aging. It would bring together studies on stability and change in personality in older adulthood, with the important question of how personality impacts mortality.

V. Future Directions in the Study of Personality and Aging

What are some of the pressing issues for future research based on the theory and empirical investigations reviewed in this chapter? First, researchers have applied growth curve and latent growth models to only a handful of personality dimensions in older adults. Most of these have focused on traits. Among other types of personality variables (e.g., social–cognitive personality dimensions), there have been few long-term studies, let alone studies that apply modern techniques for analyzing change such as growth curve modeling.

Second, there is a need to continue examining potential predictors of change. For some personality dimensions, we will undoubtedly find that change occurs in lockstep, i.e., everyone changes in the same direction and at the same rate. However, these dimensions will likely be in the minority. Most will be governed by the life span principle of individual differences in intraindividual change (Baltes, Reese, & Nesselroade, 1977). On those dimensions that show individual differences in change (some people changing at various rates, some not changing at all), we need to explain such variability across persons. These investigations will require the utilization of both environmental and biological predictors and should utilize time-varying predictors. Undoubtedly, some static and unchanging variables (e.g., gender, ethnicity) will prove to be useful predictors of personality change. These static variables may account for important portions of the individual differences in a personality dimensions pattern of change (e.g., women may rise faster on conscientiousness than men). However, more interesting is the possibility that time-varying covariates shift either the level or the rate of change in personality dimensions. Perhaps the best recent examples of this, using a well-being dimension, are two studies by Lucas and colleagues (2003, 2004). In one (Lucas et al., 2003), marital status, which varies over time as many people slip into marriage and out again (and often back again), was used to predict changes in long-term life satisfaction. In the other (Lucas et al., 2004), employment status, which also can vary over time, was used to predict changes in life satisfaction over a 15-year period. The use of time-varying covariates is an exciting new vista for the analysis of change in personality among older adults. Another exciting new technique is the coupled change growth model (Hertzog & Nesselroade, 2003; MacCallum et al., 1997; Sliwinski, Hofer, & Hall, 2003), which can permit examinations of whether change in one dimension is related to change in another dimension.

Third, personality change may prove a valuable predictor of important outcomes. As noted in several prior studies (Helson et al., 2002; Jones & Meredith, 1996; Jones et al., 2003; Mroczek & Spiro, 2003a; Small et al., 2003), many personality dimensions display individual differences in rate of change. Are these differences in rate of change in and of themselves predictive of certain outcomes? Earlier we discussed the possibility that a change in particular traits (conscientiousness, neuroticism) may predict how long a person will live. Decreases in certain cognitive dimensions are associated with mortality (Small & Backman, 1997). Are there similar effects for decreases or increases in personality dimensions? Does a sharp decline in extroversion signal impending death? Future studies of change in personality should take up these questions, although certain statistical challenges will require solving. These analyses would involve a combination of the growth curve with proportional hazards models. Such a combination would require a less desirable two-step process or some innovative mixing of the two models to allow simultaneous estimation.

This review was selective and omitted many interesting programs of research on personality and aging. The good health of this area is a product not only of the research reviewed here, but also of others that have used personality variables as predictors or outcomes in older adulthood. Perhaps the surest sign of the health of the study of personality and aging are the many studies cited that were conducted by nonpsychologists. Over the past decade, epidemiologists, sociologists, and biomedical scientists working in gerontology have discovered the usefulness of personality dimensions. This is perhaps the clearest testament that the study of personality and aging is doing very well at the outset of the 21st century.

Acknowledgment

This work was supported by grants from the National Institute on Aging (R01-AG018436 and P01-AG020166).

References

Aldwin, C. M., & Levenson, M. R. (1994). Aging and personality assessment. In M. P. Lawton & J. Teresi (Eds.), *Annual review of gerontology/geriatrics* (pp. 182–209). New York: Springer.

Aldwin, C. M., Spiro, A., III, Levenson, M. R., & Cupertino, A. P. (2001). Longitudinal findings from the Normative Aging Study. III. Personality, health trajectories, and mortality. *Psychology and Aging, 16,* 450–465.

Aldwin, C. M., Sutton, K., & Lachman, M. (1996). The development of coping resources in adulthood. *Journal of Personality, 64,* 91–113.

Almada, S. J., Zonderman, A. B., Shekelle, R. B., Dyer, A. R., Daviglus, M. L., Costa, P. T., et al. (1991). Neuroticism, cynicism and risk of death in middle-aged men: The Western Electric Study. *Psychosomatic Medicine, 53,* 165–175.

Alwin, D. F. (1994). Aging, personality, and social change: The stability of individual differences over the adult span. In D. L. Featherman, R. M. Lerner, & M. Perlmutter (Eds.), *Life-span development and behavior* (Vol. 12, pp. 135–185). Hillsdale, NJ: Lawrence Erlbaum.

Baltes, P. B. (1987). Theoretical propositions of life-span developmental psychology: On the dynamics between growth and decline. *Developmental Psychology, 23,* 611–626.

Baltes, P. B., & Nesselroade, J. R. (1973). The developmental analysis of individual differences on multiple measures. In J. R. Nesselroade & H. W. Reese (Eds.), *Life-span developmental psychology: Methodological issues* (pp. 219–251). New York: Academic Press.

Baltes, P. B., Reese, H. W., & Nesselroade, J. R. (1977). *Life span developmental psychology: Introduction to research methods.* Monterey, CA: Brooks Cole.

Berg, B. (1996). Aging, behavior, and terminal decline. In J. E., Birren & K. W. Schaie (Eds.), *The handbook of the psychology of aging* (4th edition, pp. 323–337). San Diego: Academic Press.

Block, J. (1995). A contrarian view of the five-factor approach to personality description, *Psychological Bulletin, 117,* 187–215.

Bolger, N., & Schilling, E. A. (1991). Personality and problems of everyday life: The role of neuroticism in exposure and reactivity to daily stressors. *Journal of Personality, 59,* 356–386.

Brandstadter, J., & Renner, G. (1990). Tenacious goal pursuit and flexible goal adjustment: Explication and age-related analysis of assimilative and accommodative strategies of coping. *Psychology & Aging, 5,* 58–67.

Carver, C. S., & Scheier, M. F. (1982). Control theory: A useful conceptual framework for personality-social, clinical and health psychology. *Psychological Bulletin, 92,* 111–135.

Carver, C. S., & Scheier, M. F. (1998). *On the self-regulation of behavior.* New York: Cambridge University Press.

Caspi, A., McClay, J., Moffitt, T., E., Mill, J., Martin, J., Craig, I. W., Taylor, A., & Poulton, R. (2002). Role of genotype in the cycle of violence in maltreated children. *Science, 297,* 851.

Caspi, A., & Roberts, B. W. (2001). Personality development across the life: The argument for change and continuity. *Psychological Inquiry, 12,* 49–66.

Caspi, A., Sugden, K., Moffitt, T., Taylor, A., Craig, A. S., Harrington, H., McClay, J., Mill, J., Martin, J., Braithwaite, A., & Poulton, R. (2003). Influence of life stress on depression: Moderation by a polymorphism in the 5-HTT gene. *Science, 301,* 386–389.

Christensen, A. J., Ehlers, S. L., Wiebe, J. S., Moran, P. J., Raichle, K., Ferneyhough, K., & Lawton, W. J. (2002). Patient personality and mortality: A 4-year prospective examination of chronic renal insufficiency. *Health Psychology, 21,* 315–320.

Clausen, J. A., & Jones, C. J. (1998). Predicting personality stability across the life span: The role of competence and work and family commitments. *Journal of Adult Development, 5,* 73–83.

Costa, P. T., & McCrae, R. R. (1988). Personality in adulthood: A six-year longitudinal study of self-reports and spouse ratings on the NEO Personality Inventory. *Journal of Personality and Social Psychology, 54,* 853–863.

Costa, P. T., & McCrae, R. R. (1994). Set like plaster? Evidence for the stability of adult personality. In T. F. Heatherton & J. L. Weinberger (Eds.), *Can personality change?* (pp. 21–40). Washington, DC: American Psychological Association.

Diehl, M. (2005). Development of self-representation in adulthood. In D. K. Mroczek & T. D. Little (Eds.), *Handbook of personality development.* Mahwah, NJ: Laurence Erlbaum.

Eizenman, D. R., Nesselroade, J. R., Featherman, D. L. & Rowe, J. W. (1997). Intraindividual variability in perceived control in an older sample: The MacArthur successful aging studies. *Psychology & Aging, 12,* 489–502.

Fleeson, W. (2001). Toward a structure- and process-integrated view of personality: Traits as density distributions of states. *Journal of Personality and Social Psychology, 80,* 1011–1027.

Fleeson, W., & Jolley, S. (2005). The challenge and opportunity of intraindividual variability in trait-relevant behavior: A theory of human flexibility. In D. K. Mroczek & T. D. Little (Eds.), *Handbook of personality development*. Mahwah, NJ: Laurence Erlbaum.

Friedman, H. S., Tucker, J. S., Tomlinson-Keasey, C., Schwartz, J. E., Wingard, D. L., & Criqui, M. H. (1993). Does childhood personality predict longevity? *Journal of Personality and Social Psychology*, 65, 176–185.

Funder, D. (2001). Personality. *Annual Review of Psychology*, 52, 197–231.

Goldberg, L. R. (1993). The structure of phenotypic personality traits. *American Psychologist*, 48, 26–34.

Heckhausen, J., & Schulz, R. (1995). A life-span theory of control. *Psychological Review*, 102, 284–304.

Helson, R., Jones C. J., & Kwan, S. Y. (2002). Personality change over 40 years of adulthood: Hierarchical linear modeling analyses of two longitudinal samples. *Journal of Personality & Social Psychology*, 83, 752–766.

Hertzog, C., & Nesselroade, J. R. (2003). Assessing psychological change in adulthood: An overview of methodological issues. *Psychology & Aging*, 18, 639–657.

Hooker, K., & McAdams, D. P. (2003). Personality reconsidered: A new agenda for aging research. *Journal of Gerontology: Psychological Sciences*, 58, 296–304.

Jones, C. J., Livson, N., & Peskin, H. (2003). Longitudinal hierarchical linear modeling analyses of California Psychological Inventory data from age 33 to 75: An examination of stability and change in adult personality. *Journal of Personality Assessment*, 80, 294–308.

Jones, C. J., & Meredith, W. (1996). Patterns of personality change across the life-span. *Psychology and Aging*, 11, 57–65.

Jones, C. J., Nesselroade, J. R., & Birkel, R. C. (1991). Examination of staffing level effects in the family household: An application of P-technique factor analysis. *Journal of Environmental Psychology*, 11, 59–73.

Kendler, K. S., Thornton, L. M., & Gardner, C. O. (2001). Genetic risk, number of previous depressive episodes, and stressful life events in predicting onset of major depression. *American Journal of Psychiatry*, 158, 582–586.

Kiecolt-Glaser, J. K., & Glaser, R. (1986). Psychological influences on immunity. *Psychosomatics: Journal of Consultation Liaison Psychiatry*, 27, 621–624.

Kubzansky, L. D., Kawachi, I., Spiro, A., Weiss, S. T., Vokonas, P. S., & Sparrow, D. (1997). Is worrying bad for your heart? A prospective study of worry and coronary heart disease in the Normative Aging Study. *Circulation*, 95, 818–824.

Lamiell, J. T. (1981). Toward an idiothethic psychology of personality. *American Psychologist*, 36, 276–289.

Lang, F., Reschke, F., & Neyer, F. J. (2005). Social relationships, transitions and personality development across the life span. In D. K. Mroczek & T. D. Little (Eds.), *Handbook of personality development*. Mahwah, NJ: Lauernce Erlbaum.

Lerner, R. M., & Busch-Rossnagel, N. (1981). *Individuals as producers of their development: A life-span perspective*. New York: Academic Press.

Levenson, M. R., & Crumpler, C. A. (1996). Three models of adult development. *Human Development*, 39, 135–149.

Levy, B. R. et al. (2002). Longevity increased by positive self-perceptions of aging. *Journal of Personality & Social Psychology*, 83, 261–270.

Lucas, R. E., Clark, A. E., Georgellis, Y., & Diener, E. (2003). Reexamining adaptation and the set point model of happiness: Reactions to changes in marital status. *Journal of Personality and Social Psychology*, 84, 527–539.

Lucas, R. E., Clark, A. E., Georgellis, Y., & Diener, E. (2004). Unemployment alters the set point for life satisfaction. *Psychological Science*, 15(1), 8–13.

MacCallum, R. C., Kim, C. Malarkey, W. B., & Kiecolt-Glaser, J. (1997). Studying multivariate change using multilevel models and latent curve models. *Multivariate Behavioral Research*, 32, 215–253.

Martin, M. (2001). *Research on cognitive development as resource-oriented basic research*. Habilitation, University of Heidelberg, Germany.

Martin, M., & Mroczek, D. K. (2005). Are personality traits across the life span sensitive to environmental demands? *Journal of Adult Development*.

Maruta, T., Colligan, R. C., Malinchoc, M., & Offord, K. P. (2000). Optimists vs. pessimists: Survival rate among medical patients over a 30-year period. *Mayo Clinic Proceedings, 75*, 140–143.

McAdams, D. (1992). The five-factor model in personality: A critical appraisal. *Journal of Personality, 60*, 329–361.

McArdle, J. J. (1991). Structural models of development theory in psychology. *Annals of Theoretical Psychology, 7*, 139–159.

Meredith, W., & Tisak, J. (1990). Latent curve analysis. *Psychometrika, 55*, 107–122.

Mroczek, D. K., & Almeida, D. M. (2004). The effects of daily stress, personality, and age on daily negative affect. *Journal of Personality, 72*, 355–378.

Mroczek, D. K., Almeida, D. M. Spiro, A., III, & Pafford, C. (2005). Intraindividual stability and change in personality. In D. K. Mroczek & T. D. Little (Eds.), *Handbook of personality development*. Mahwah, NJ: Laurence Erlbaum.

Mroczek, D. K., Ozer, D. J., Spiro, A., III, & Kaiser, R. T. (1998). Evaluating a measure of the five factor model of personality. *Assessment, 5*, 285–299.

Mroczek, D. K., & Spiro, A, III. (2003a). Modeling intraindividual change in personality traits: Findings from the Normative Aging Study. *Journals of Gerontology: Psychological Sciences, 58B*, 153–165.

Mroczek, D. K., & Spiro, A., III (2003b). Personality structure and process, variance between and within: Integration by means of developmental framework. *Journals of Gerontology: Psychological Sciences, 58B*, 305–306.

Mroczek, D. K., Spiro, A., & Almeida, D. M. (2003). Between- and within-person variation in affect and personality over days and years: How basic and applied approaches can inform one another. *Ageing International, 28*, 260–278.

Muthen, B. O. (2002). Beyond SEM: General latent variable modeling. *Behaviormetrika, 29*, 81–117

Nesselroade, J. R. (1988). Sampling and generalizability: Adult development and aging issues examined within the general methodological framework of selection. In K. W. Schaie, R. T. Campbell, W. M. Meredith, & S. C. Rawlings (Eds.), *Methodological issues in aging research*. New York: Springer.

Nesselroade, J. R. (1991). Interindividual differences in intraindividual change. In L. M. Collins & J. L. Horn (Eds.), *Best methods for the analysis of change* (pp. 92–105). Washington, DC: American Psychological Association.

Nesselroade, J. R., & Baltes, P. B. (1974). Adolescent personality development and historical changes: 1970–1972. *Monographs of the Society for Research in Child Development, 39* (1, Serial No. 154).

Nesselroade, J. R., & Featherman, D. L. (1991). Intraindividual variability in older adults depression scores: Some implications for developmental theory and longitudinal research. In D. Magnusson, R. L. Bergman, G. Rudinger, & B. Torestad (Eds.), *Problems and methods in longitudinal research: Stability and change*. Cambridge: Cambridge University Press.

Nesselroade, J. R., & Jones, C.J (1991). Multi-modal selection effects in the study of adult development: A perspective on multivariate, replicated, single-subject, repeated measures designs. *Experimental Aging Research, 17*, 21–27.

Neyer, F. J., & Asendorpf, J. B. (2001). Personality-relationship transaction in young adulthood. *Journal of Personality and Social Psychology, 81*, 1190–1204.

Oppenheim, G. (1994). The earliest signs of Alzheimer's disease. *Journal of Geriatric Psychiatry and Neurology, 7*, 116–120.

Ozer, D. J. (1986). *Consistency in personality: A methodological framework*. Berlin: Springer.

Raudenbush, S. W., & Bryk, A. S. (2002). *Hierarchical linear models: Applications and data analysis methods (2nd edition)*. Thousand Oaks, CA: Sage.

Roberts, B. W., & Bogg, T. (2004). A longitudinal study of the relationships between conscientiousness and the social-environmental factors and substance-use behaviors that influence health. *Journal of Personality, 72*, 325–353.

Roberts, B. W., & Chapman, C. N. (2001). Change in dispositional well-being and its relations to role quality: A 30-year longitudinal study. *Journal of Research in Personality, 34*, 26–41.

Roberts, B. W., & DelVecchio, W. F. (2000). The rank order consistency of personality traits from childhood to old age: A quantitative review of longitudinal studies. *Psychological Bulletin, 126*, 3–25.

Roberts, B. W., & Walton, K. (2005). *Patterns of mean-level change in personality traits across the life course: A meta-analysis of longitudinal studies.* Unpublished manuscript. University of Illinois, Urbana-Champaign.

Roberts, B. W., & Wood, D. (2005). Personality development in the context of the neo socioanalytic model of personality. In D. K. Mroczek & T. D. Little (Eds.). *Handbook of personality development.* Mahwah, NJ; Laurence Erlbaum.

Rogosa, D. R., Brandt, D., & Zimowski, M. (1982). A growth curve approach to the measurement of change. *Psychological Bulletin, 92*, 726–748.

Ryff, C. D., & Singer, B. (1998). The contours of positive human health. *Psychological Inquiry, 9*, 1–28.

Schaie, K. W. (1996). Intellectual development in adulthood. In J. E. Birren & K. W. Schaie (Eds.), *Handbook of the psychology of aging* (4th edition, pp. 266–286). San Diego: Academic Press.

Scheier, M. F., & Carver, C. S. (1985). Optimism, coping and health: Assessment and implications of generalized outcome expectancies. *Health Psychology, 4*, 219–247.

Singer, J. D., & Willett, J. B. (2003). *Applied longitudinal analysis: Modeling change and event occurrence.* New York: Oxford University Press.

Sliwinski, M. J., Hofer, S. M., & Hall, C. (2003). Correlated and coupled change in older adults with and without preclinical dementia. *Psychology & Aging, 18*, 672–683.

Small, B. J., & Backman, L. (1997). Cognitive correlates of mortality: Evidence from a population-based sample of very old adults. *Psychology & Aging, 12*, 309–313.

Small, B. J., Frantiglioni, L., von Strauss, E., & Backman, L. (2003). Terminal decline and cognitive performance in very old age: Does cause of death matter? *Psychology & Aging, 18*, 193–202.

Small, B. J., Hertzog, C., Hultsch, D. F., & Dixon, R. A. (2003). Stability and change in adult personality over 6 years: Findings from the Victoria Longitudinal Study. *Journals of Gerontology: Psychological Sciences & Social Sciences, 58B*, 166–176.

Twenge, J. M. (2000). The age of anxiety? The birth cohort change in anxiety and neuroticism, 1952–1993. *Journal of Personality and Social Psychology, 79*, 1007–1021.

Twenge, J. M. (2001). Birth cohort changes in extroversion: A cross-temporal meta-analysis, 1966–1993. *Personality and Individual Differences, 30*, 735–748.

Wild, K. V., Kaye, J. A., & Oken, B. S. (1994). Early non-cognitive change in Alzheimer's disease and healthy aging. *Journal of Geriatric Psychiatry and Neurology, 7*, 199–205.

Willett, J. B., & Sayer, A. G. (1994). Using covariance structure analysis to detect correlates and predictors of individual change over time. *Psychological Bulletin, 116*, 363–381.

Wilson, R. S., Bienas, J. L., Mendes de Leon, C. F., Evans, D. A., & Bennett, D. A. (2003). Negative affect and mortality in older persons. *American Journal of Epidemiology, 158*, 827–835.

Wilson, R. S., Evans, D. A., Bienas, J. L., Mendes de Leon, C. F., Schneider, D. F., & Bennett, D. A. (2003). Proneness to psychological distress is associated with risk of Alzheimer's Disease. *Neurology, 61*, 1479–1485.

Wilson, R. S., Mendes de Leon, C. F., Bienas, J. L., Evans, D. A., & Bennett, D. A. (2004). Personality and mortality in old age.

Journal of Gerontology: Psychological Sciences, 59B, 110–116.

Wohlwill, J. F. (1973). *The study of behavioral development*. New York: Academic Press.

Wrosch, C., Heckhausen, J., & Lachman, M. E. (2000). Primary and secondary control strategies for managing health and financial stress across adulthood. *Psychology & Aging, 15*, 387–399.

Seventeen

Attitudes toward Aging and Their Effects on Behavior

Thomas M. Hess

I. Introduction

Attitudes have historically been a central focus of social psychological research due to their assumed importance in directing behavior. At its most basic level, an attitude can be defined as an evaluation of a stimulus as reflected in our affective, cognitive, and behavioral responses to it (Fiske & Taylor, 1991). The evaluation of someone or something and our subsequent response may reflect a relatively conscious process as the individual considers information about the attitude object and then decides on a specific response. Alternatively, the linkage between evaluation and behavior may be relatively automatic in nature due to repeated experiences of particular responses being associated with specific attitude objects (Bargh, 1997). The basis of attitudes is also varied, with evaluation reflecting direct or indirect experiences as well as cognitive constructions that may have a basis in reality. Of importance for the present chapter is the fact that attitudes often have a social basis, reflecting one's past experiences within specific social, cultural, and historical contexts.

A further factor of importance for our understanding of the relationship between attitudes and behavior relates to the fundamental nature of attitudes in the processing of information. Research has suggested that almost everything that we encounter has an evaluative component to it (e.g., Bargh et al., 1992). In addition, this evaluation occurs at a relatively early stage of processing with little demand on cognitive resources (e.g., Bargh et al., 1989). This primacy of evaluation and the fact that it may occur with little awareness on the part of the individual suggest a relatively powerful and potentially insidious influence on behavior.

In the field of gerontology, research has focused on the extent to which attitudes regarding the aging process can be used to understand the social basis of older adults' functioning. A traditional approach in the field has been to focus on societal attitudes regarding the aging process, with studies examining affective reactions, beliefs and knowledge, and specific behavioral responses. A common perspective in such studies is that culturally based attitudes about aging influence social structures and the treatment of older adults, which in turn affect the behavior of older adults, as well as perpetuate these attitudes. In other words, the focus is on understanding how the social environment affects the behavior of older adults. More recently, an emerging emphasis has been on how attitudes possessed by the individual might influence his or her own behavior. In both approaches, a primary assumption is that the social environment influences the behavior of older adults — and the aging process itself — through socially shared attitudes about aging.

An additional emphasis in research is on the distinction between explicit and implicit attitudes (i.e., evaluations available or unavailable to conscious experience). These two types of attitudes are not necessarily consistent with one another and they may operate in qualitatively different ways to influence behavior. For example, implicit attitudes may be contrary to those that are expressed explicitly (e.g., representing general, culturally shared knowledge), but may still exert an important influence on behavior without the individual's awareness. This influence may be especially problematic when the attitudes are associated with negative stereotypes.

In this chapter, the goal is to review research relevant to understanding the impact of aging attitudes on behavior. As a starting point, research on the nature of attitudes about aging in adults of all ages is discussed, as well as moderators of these attitudes. The conditions governing their activation in others and the responses of older adults are then examined. The focus then switches to research examining the impact of one's own attitudes about aging on behavior, including the mechanisms and moderators of such effects. Finally, conclusions regarding the influence of attitudes on the behavior of older adults and the aging process itself are presented.

II. Other's Attitudes about Aging

As noted earlier, attitudes reflect one's valenced evaluation of a stimulus, i.e., how positively or negatively predisposed one is toward a particular attitude object. There is general agreement in the field that these evaluations can have affective, cognitive, and behavioral components associated with them (Petty, Priester, & Wegener, 1994), with the influence being bidirectional. That is, attitudes can influence content in all three components (e.g., one acts in a manner consistent with evaluations of the attitude object) or content can influence attitudes (e.g., evaluation is based on one's response to an attitude object). All three components have received attention in research on aging.

A. Indicators of Attitudes

1. Affective Components

The affective component of aging attitudes is perhaps less clearly delineated in research than are cognitive and behavioral components. An indication of affective responses can be seen, however, in research examining explicit, general attitudes toward younger and older adults. In a meta-analysis of such studies, Kite and Johnson (1988) found a clear bias toward judging older people more negatively than younger people in individuals of all ages. Although not all study effects supported this conclusion, 30 of 43 effect sizes were consistent with this bias and the overall effect size $(d = .39)$ was moderate. The lack of consistency across studies is important, however, and is suggestive of contextual factors that may moderate attitudes.

This negative evaluation of older adults can also be found in specific contexts. For example, research in work settings has indicated that older workers are generally evaluated more negatively than younger workers (see Finkelstein, Burke, & Raju, 1995). What is particularly interesting here is the fact that older workers in most industrial/organizational psychology studies include an age range (55 to 65) that most people would not consider to be old, highlighting the context specificity of many aging-related attitudes. An additional important point to be made here has to do with the fact that these age differences in performance evaluations are inconsistent with findings demonstrating little relationship between age and various aspects of worker performance (for reviews, see McCann & Giles, 2002; Warr, 1994).

Other studies have employed instruments designed to assess implicit attitudes that, by definition, are inaccessible to conscious examination. These investigations rely on associations between age and evaluative categories that are tapped in an indirect fashion through measures of memory and speed of classification. For example, Perdue and Gurtman (1990) found that young adults evaluated positive trait terms more quickly if preceded by the subliminal prime word "young," whereas negative traits were evaluated more quickly if primed with the word "old." Consistent with network theories of memory, the facilitating effect of the word *old* in making judgments about negative traits suggests a strong association between the two.

Chasteen, Schwarz, and Park (2002) noted that the negative words in this study were more reflective of stereotypes of the old, whereas the positive words were more reflective of views of youth, raising concerns that the results reflected stereotype-based associations rather than age-based evaluative differences. Using a lexical decision task in which stereotypicality and valence of the trait terms were disentangled, these researchers actually found relatively positive general attitudes toward older adults for both young and older participants.

Importantly, however, stereotypical associations with negative traits were still in evidence.

Research using the implicit association test (IAT; Greenwald, McGhee, & Schwartz, 1998) has supported the general conclusions of Perdue and Gurtman (1990). This test intermixes two categorization tasks, one involving the contrast of interest (e.g., classifying a person as young vs old) and the other involving an evaluative judgment (e.g., classifying an object as pleasant or unpleasant). Implicit attitudes are then determined by examining the facilitating effect on performance when a particular response (e.g., pressing a computer key with the right hand) is associated with both a specific category and the evaluative judgment assumed to be congruent with that category (e.g., old and unpleasant, young and pleasant) versus when the response is associated with evaluations that are incongruent with the category (e.g., young and unpleasant). In line with research using explicit means of evaluation, studies employing the IAT have found consistent negative evaluations of older adults when compared with young adults (Hummert et al., 2002; Karpinski & Hilton, 2001; Nosek, Banaji, & Greenwald, 2002). As an indication of the strength of these effects, Nosek et al. (2002) noted that the negative implicit attitudes toward older adults obtained in their study were stronger than any of the others assessed, including those associated with race and gender. In addition, the strength of these attitudes does not wane with increasing age: older adults' implicit attitudes are just as strong as those of younger adults. Finally, the strength of these negative implicit attitudes is reduced only slightly following the introduction of specific information designed to activate positive associations with old age.

One final observation about implicit attitudes is that they tend to be weakly associated with explicit attitudes. For example, Hummert et al. (2002) found consistently negative implicit attitudes about older adults across three age groups (18–29, 55–74, 75–93), but explicit judgments revealed more positive evaluations of older adults in the youngest group when compared to the two older groups. Nosek et al. (2002) also demonstrated a dissociation between implicit and explicit attitudes, with negative explicit responses toward old being smaller than those observed with the implicit measure. In contrast to Hummert et al. (2002), however, these researchers found that negative explicit evaluations of older adults declined with increasing age.

2. Cognitive Components

A great deal of research that has focused primarily on the examination of beliefs, stereotypes, and perceptions about older adults and the aging process is relevant to understanding the cognitive component of attitudes. This is due to the fact that the content associated with these constructs is assumed to be evaluative in nature, and thus to reflect attitudes. Studies have been conducted within the context of several research traditions (see Heckhausen, Dixon, & Baltes, 1989). For example, from a sociological perspective, the interest has been in understanding beliefs about aging and their role in structuring the life course through societal institutions and structures guided by age norms. From a more psychological perspective, interest has focused more on examining the nature of aging-related beliefs and stereotypes with an eye toward understanding their role both in determining behaviors directed toward older adults and in guiding one's own behavior through the course of development.

Research examining beliefs has proceeded from a relatively generic position in which the goal was to understand how people view aging to more focused studies in which the goal is to examine beliefs about specific aspects of behavior in order to understand the linkage between such beliefs and functioning. Good examples of the former are studies by Heckhausen and colleagues (Heckhausen & Baltes, 1991; Heckhausen et al., 1989) that investigated subjective conceptions of development as reflected in beliefs about the sensitivity of personal traits to change along with the timing and controllability of such change. Several interesting findings emerged from these investigations. First, adults of all ages expected behavioral losses to dominate over gains with increasing age. Second, the desirability of specific traits was correlated negatively with both the age of onset and the age of cessation of development, such that desirable traits were more likely to emerge and cease development earlier in adulthood than undesirable traits. Finally, desirability was correlated positively with perceived controllability. Although there were certain exceptions, general characterization of the aging process captured in these studies is rather negative in terms of the losses of desirable traits, the advent of undesirable ones, and the perceived inability to control the latter.

Other studies have looked at beliefs tied to specific domains. Traditionally, the most well-investigated domain has to do with cognition and, in particular, memory functioning. The results of these more focused studies are consistent with more general characterizations of aging. For example, Ryan (1992) and Ryan and Kwong See (1993) had a diverse group of participants with respect to age rate the memory ability of typical 25, 45, 65, and 85 year olds. They found that, regardless of type of memory examined, the expectation was that performance would decline in later adulthood, with a significant decline in some cases beginning during the period between 45 and 65. Interestingly, these same researchers found no significant variation in beliefs regarding control over memory across the same age range.

In another series of studies, Lineweaver and Hertzog (1998) and Hertzog, McGuire, and Lineweaver (1998) found strong agreement among young, middle-aged, and older adults concerning the course of memory decline, with all perceiving performance to be relatively stable up to age 30 or 40 and then decreasing thereafter. The type of memory task moderated this trend somewhat, with decline perceived to be less severe for memory for daily schedules and remote events. Importantly, however, belief in decline was pervasive across skills regardless of participant age. Similar results were obtained regarding beliefs about one's control over memory, with control over current and future functioning expected to decline beginning around the fourth decade of life. Consistent findings have been observed in other realms of cognitive functioning (e.g., Camp & Pignatiello, 1988; Ryan et al., 1992).

Research has also demonstrated that not all beliefs regarding aging and cognition are negative, with differences in attitudes being observed as a function of domain. Thus, for example, while old age might be associated with declining physical and cognitive skills, it is also thought to be associated with growth or maintenance of other aspects of functioning, such as those associated with expressive behavior or wisdom (e.g., Heckhausen et al., 1989; Slotterback & Saarnio, 1996).

Another approach to understanding attitudes about aging is through investigations of stereotypes about older adults, which can be thought of as organized knowledge structures that are used to categorize individuals on the basis of age. Similar to the functions of schemas and categories, stereotypes are used both to structure our perceptions of others and to make inferences about them (e.g., causal mechanisms underlying their behavior). Consistent with the foregoing discussion on affective responses, research on stereotypes has emphasized the relatively negative evaluations of older adults that exist in our culture.

Much of the initial work on aging stereotypes employed questionnaires that assessed agreement with statements describing stereotypic characteristics (e.g., Tuckman & Lorge, 1953) or that examined differences in responses associated with older adults versus those associated with people in general (Kogan, 1979). Another common manner of assessing aging stereotypes was — and still is — through the use of semantic differential instruments (e.g., Rosencranz & McNevin, 1969). Although these methodologies proved valuable in highlighting common perceptions about older adults, including the fact that they are not all negative, they are problematic in terms of a more functional approach to the study of stereotypes.

From a social cognitive perspective, stereotypes represent categories that play a critical role in the person perception process (Hummert, 1999). Researchers adopting this perspective have attempted to describe the content of stereotypes as well as their hierarchical nature. These studies have revealed that the superordinate category of "older adult" does not do a good job of characterizing people's cognitive representations, and thus instruments that focus simply on describing attributes of this category do not do justice to the complexity of people's representations. Instead, stereotypes of aging are multifaceted, representing several subcategories that differentiate between subtypes of older adults. Brewer and colleagues (Brewer, Dull, & Lui, 1981; Brewer & Lui, 1984) were among the first to highlight the complex nature of aging stereotypes.

They found that both young and older adults possessed subtypes of older adults and that these subtypes represented both positive and negative views of aging.

This research was extended by others using more complex methods. For example, Schmidt and Boland (1986) and Hummert and colleagues (1990, 1994) employed cluster analyses on trait sortings and found evidence for multiple negative ($n = 7$–8) and positive ($n = 3$–5) stereotypes of older adults. Whereas these findings still highlight the generally negative attitudes toward older adults in our society, they also illustrate the facts that aging stereotypes are multifaceted and that the schemas used for categorizing older adults are not invariably negative.

A qualifying alternative view of this multifacetedness, however, comes from work by Fiske and co-workers (2002) on the nature of stereotypes. These researchers have argued that stereotypes of outgroups can be characterized in terms of their placement along two independent dimensions: competence and warmth. The in-group tends to be perceived as being high on both dimensions. In contrast, out-groups are perceived typically as being higher along one dimension than another, with the specific placement based on perceptions of status and competition relative to the in-group. According to research conducted by Fiske et al. (2002), the general stereotype of older adults is characterized as high in warmth — reflecting low competition — and low in competence — reflecting low perceptions of status. This appears to be consistent with earlier discussed findings relating to beliefs about older adults' cognitive skills.

This same framework, however, suggests that most of the seemingly positive stereotypes identified in research on aging can also be characterized as negative along one of the two content dimensions (Cuddy & Fiske, 2002).

For example, using the seven stereotypes that Hummert (1999) suggested were widely shared across age groups in our culture, only one — the *golden ager* — appears to be high on both warmth and competence. (Interestingly, Hummert notes that *golden ager* only emerges when middle-aged and older adults are included in the sample generating the stereotypes.) Others could be characterized as being low on at least one of the dimensions of competence (*perfect grandparent, severly impaired, recluse*) or warmth (*John Wayne conservative, despondent, shrew/curmudgeon*). Thus, whereas research on stereotypes does indicate that our conceptions of older adults are not all negative, this structural analysis of stereotype content in relationship to the aging stereotypes identified in the literature suggests an underlying negative component to most categories of older adults.

Another fruitful line of research examining cognitive components of attitudes has used a person-perception paradigm that focuses on observers' reactions to the behavior of others. Attitudes are inferred from the different interpretations of and attributions for this behavior as a function of the age of the individual performing the behavior. Much of this work has focused on cognition, with a particular emphasis on memory functioning. In general, responses are consistent with expectations derived from the just-discussed work on beliefs and aging. For example, Erber (1989) found that an identical memory failure was judged as more serious in an older adult than in a younger adult, particularly by younger observers. This age-based double standard was evident in other studies as well, where memory failures were more likely to be attributed to internal stable causes (e.g., ability) in older adults, whereas attributions based in internal, unstable causes (e.g., effort) were more prevalent for younger adults' failures

(Erber, Szuchman, & Rothberg, 1990; Parr & Siegert, 1993). Similarly, observers were more likely to recommend medical evaluations following memory failures in older adults than they were for the same failures in younger adults (Erber & Rothberg, 1991).

Bieman-Copland and Ryan (1998) extended this research by examining responses to both memory successes and failures, with similar results. Specifically, successes were viewed as more typical in younger than in older adults, and failures were seen as more worrisome and diagnostic of mental difficulties in older than in younger adults. In addition, younger adults were perceived as having greater control in general over their memory functioning, and memory failures were more likely to be attributed to ability in older than in younger adults.

Similar findings have been obtained when other aspects of functioning have been examined. For example, Kwong See and Heller (2004) examined perceptions of different-aged adults who exhibited high and low levels of language performance and found that judgments reflected age-based stereotypic expectations (i.e., good performance in young adults, poor performance in older adults). Thus, poor-quality language performance in older adults was judged less negatively than it was in younger adults, whereas high-quality performance was judged relatively more positively. Such findings are consistent with the shifting standards model of stereotype-based judgments (Biernat, 2003).

Related attitudes are operative in specific contexts in which older adults function. For example, several investigations have examined perceptions of older workers, with results suggesting that aging-related biases are conveyed in judgments regarding capabilities. Relative to younger workers, older workers are perceived as less physically capable, less healthy, lower in productivity, inflexible,

resistant to new ideas, and less capable of being trained. These attitudes are reflected in institutional behaviors that result in, for example, older workers being given fewer opportunities for training and learning of new skills (e.g., Capowski, 1994). The disturbing aspect of such findings is that these attitudes typically fly in the face of reality. For example, as noted previously, there is little relationship between age and job productivity, and absenteeism is actually lower in older than in younger workers. What is equally disturbing is that these negative perceptions of older workers occur at an earlier age than commonly associated with more general aging attitudes, suggesting that the time frame typically associated with perceptions regarding the development of negative aging-related characteristics is compressed in the workplace.

Investigators have also examined perceptions in courtroom settings, revealing something of a mixed bag with respect to attitudes regarding older eyewitnesses. Relative to younger eyewitnesses, older adults are perceived as more honest, but less reliable (Kwong See, Hoffman, & Wood, 2001; Yarmey, 1984). Interestingly, research has also demonstrated that witness age has little impact on perceptions of guilt (Brimacombe et al., 1997), suggesting perhaps that these two trends offset each other in jurors' perceptions of witness credibility. A clever study by Kwong See et al. (2001) examined the impact of stereotypic beliefs in a more indirect fashion by testing whether participants would modify their own memory reports based on inaccurate information about the same event provided by either a young or older witness. Consistent with research examining more explicit attitudes, these researchers found that stereotypes were operative in that younger adults were more likely to adjust their memory to be consistent with a young witness perceived to be high in competence than they were to an older witness of similar standing.

3. Behavioral

Attitudes are also reflected in behaviors toward older adults, which have been examined in a number of ways (for a review, see Pasupathi & Löckenhoff, 2002). For example, several investigations have examined the nature of communication with older adults. One finding from this research is that younger adults often use patronizing talk in their conversations with older individuals. Such talk is characterized by attributes such as simplification, superficiality of conversations, demeaning emotional tone, use of clarification strategies (e.g., careful articulation), and, in some cases, controlling or disapproving messages (Hummert & Ryan, 1996). For example, younger adults have been shown to use simpler structures and a more patronizing tone when providing instructions to older adults than they do when communicating with same-aged peers (e.g., Rubin & Brown, 1975; Thimm, Rademacher, & Kruse, 1998). The adaptations to older adults were viewed by participants in these studies as accommodative, but they were also consistent with their stereotypes regarding the competencies of older adults. In its most extreme form, communication takes the form of baby talk by caregivers to institutionalized adults, and such talk has been associated with stereotypical beliefs regarding dependency in older adults (e.g., Caporeal, Lukaszewski, & Culbertson, 1983).

Aging-related attitudes also influence interactions with older adults in a variety of important social contexts. For example, research on doctor–patient interactions has suggested that physicians' patterns of communication vary with the age of the patient. Greene and colleagues (1986) observed that doctors were more respectful, provided more specific information, and were more responsive to younger and middle-aged adults than they were to older adults. They also tend to spend less time with older adults (e.g., Radecki et al., 1988). In addition, physicians may also attribute older individuals' treatable conditions to old age (e.g., Adelman et al., 1990), a situation with potentially grave consequences.

These findings clearly indicate that older adults are often responded to in a manner that is consistent with aging-related stereotypes. In extreme cases, these behaviors might be construed as ageist in nature in that they appear to be primarily in response to an individual's age. In addition to being reflections of negative attitudes about older adults, such ageist behavior can have important consequences in terms of shaping and maintaining these views among members of a culture through such things as language, opportunities for older adults (e.g., receiving new training in the workplace), the creation of social structures (e.g., mandatory retirement ages), and even the design and reporting of psychological research (Schaie, 1988, 1993). These same factors can obviously have profound effects on older adults themselves through beliefs regarding the aging process conveyed in these behaviors and the constraints imposed by age-graded roles and social structures.

Note, however, that not all behavior reflective of negative attitudes about aging should be regarded as ageist. In certain situations, for example, use of elderspeak may actually reflect an adaptive accommodation on the part of the communicator to actual characteristics of the individual. As Pasupathi and Löckenhoff (2002) argued, it is important to consider the type of behavior, the cause of the behavior, and the characteristics of the target in making judgments about whether specific actions toward an older adult are ageist or not.

D. Reactions of Older Adults

Negative attitudes are important to the extent that responses of those holding such attitudes affect older adults. Whereas such influence can occur within the context of everyday interpersonal interactions, it may also be evident at a more macrolevel in terms of institutional and social policies (e.g., age-related opportunities for training in the workplace). For present purposes, however, the focus is on the former type of influence with a specific emphasis on two areas in which there has been a fair amount of systematic research. The first area of investigation focuses on the effects of the previously discussed use of patronizing talk toward older adults, where the communication predicament of aging model (Ryan et al., 1986) has been developed to help understand such effects. This model posits that communications with older adults particularly those who are unknown to the speaker or who are in institutionalized settings are shaped by the speaker's stereotypes of aging. This results in the use of patronizing talk as well as other forms of behavior (e.g., overhelping) that may reinforce stereotyped behaviors and negatively impact older adults in a number of ways, including loss of self-esteem (e.g., O'Connor & Rigby, 1996), lowered motivation and confidence in their ability (Avorn & Langer, 1982), reduced participation in activities, and loss of control (e.g., Rodin & Langer, 1977). These changes toward stereotype-consistent behavior may reinforce the speaker's use of patronizing talk and other sorts of stereotype-based behaviors, conceivably resulting in even greater frequency of use. In support of such conjecture, patronizing speech has been found to have a negative impact on perceptions of the competence

older adult targets of such speech (e.g., Harwood et al., 1997).

A second area of research has focused on behaviors reflecting dependence and independence. Investigations in this realm have suggested that stereotype-based behaviors can serve to foster dependency in older adults. Baltes and Wahl (1992, 1996) have found that older adults are more frequently reinforced—in terms of attention from social partners—for dependent than for independent behavior, and that such reinforcement generalizes across cultures, gender, health status, and settings. Independent behaviors on the part of older adults receive less frequent attention, particularly in institutionalized settings. The implication is that some stereotype-consistent behavior on the part of older adults is prompted by the social environment in order to promote social interaction. This dependence support script, as it is termed by Baltes and Wahl (1996), can be modified through interventions designed to reinforce independent behaviors (e.g., Baltes, Neuman, & Zank, 1994; Rodin & Langer, 1977). Whereas it is clear that aging attitudes shape dependence-related behaviors in older adults, it is also important to note that such behaviors may not always be reactions to the external environment. Instead, they may reflect selective processes designed to foster control and conserve resources (Baltes & Baltes, 1990).

E. Activators and Moderators of Attitudes

The foregoing discussion has painted a rather negative picture of societal perceptions of older adults and the impact on their behavior. Whereas the evidence does suggest a rather pervasive set of negative attitudes, even in those circumstances where more positive attitudes are apparent (e.g., stereotypes), there is also research demonstrating that attitudes toward and treatment of older adults are moderated by particular factors. For example, stereotypes and beliefs regarding the negative aspects of aging are less strong in those who have high levels of knowledge about aging, frequent exposure and interactions with older adults, and are able to assume the perspective of older adults (e.g., Galinsky & Moskowitz, 2000; Hale, 1998; Luszcz & Fitzgerald, 1986). There is also some evidence that attitudes about aging are moderated by one's culture (e.g., Ikels, 1990; Levy & Langer, 1994), although it should be noted that negative attitudes are commonplace in many cultures, including those depicted popularly as having more positive attitudes (for discussions of cross-cultural issues, see Ng, 2002).

Another moderator of attitudes relates to the nature of cues and the presence of counterstereotypic information in specific individuals. Research has demonstrated repeatedly that stereotypes about aging are most likely to influence perceptions of and interactions with older adults when age information and age-related cues are dominant and little individuating information is present. For example, the presence of aging-related physical cues associated with facial characteristics (Hummert, Garstka, & Shaner, 1997), gait (Montepare & Zebrowitz-McArthur, 1988), and verbal behavior (Bieman-Copland & Ryan, 2001) has been shown to increase the probability of stereotypic attributions and inferences.

Similarly, stereotypes are most likely to be activated and applied when specific information about an individual is lacking and age is the most dominant cue. When individuating information is available, especially when it is relevant to the social context in which the older adult is encountered, stereotypes are much less likely to be applied. For example, person-perception studies examining evaluations of memory skills have shown that variations in judgments about older and younger adults disappear when specific information is provided about the capabilities of the individual being judged (e.g., Erber, Etheart, & Szuchman, 1992; Erber et al., 1996). Similarly, perceptions of older workers are less biased when the salience of age is decreased and context-relevant information (e.g., worker's qualification for their job) is presented (Finkelstein, Burke, & Raju, 1995). Such findings are consistent with models of stereotyping that assume their operation in the absence of more specific information about the individual (e.g., Fiske & Neuberg, 1990; Leyens, Yzerbyt, & Schadron, 1994).

Another factor that moderates the severity of aging-related attitudes is the age of the individual. Although the relatively negative attitudes about aging evident in young adulthood are shared by older individuals as well (e.g., Heckhausen et al., 1989; Hummert et al., 1994), there does appear to be a metamorphosis in the nature of these attitudes as a function of one's experience of getting older and the gradual transformation of older adulthood from out-group to in-group status. Research on aging stereotypes has shown that middle-aged and older adults have more positive and more complex representations of old age than younger individuals (e.g., Brewer & Lui, 1984; Hummert et al., 1994; Linville, Fischer, & Salovey, 1989), perhaps reflecting an in-group bias that is commonly reflected in greater complexity of categories to which the perceiver belongs (e.g., Linville, Salovey, & Fischer, 1986). Consistent with this view, Brewer and Lui (1984) found that the differentiation and complexity of aging stereotypes were greatest for the subcategory to which older adults perceived themselves as belonging. This aging-related complexity is also manifested in findings that older adults view the subtypes of older age identified in stereotype research as being less typical than younger adults (Hummert et al., 1994), perhaps reflecting greater perceptions of variability by older adults of individuals within their age group due to greater familiarity (Linville et al., 1989). Older adults also appear to have more complex characterizations of the nature and controllability of development (Heckhausen & Baltes, 1991; Heckhausen et al., 1989). Contradictory evidence in this regard also exists. For example, Lineweaver and Hertzog (1998) found that general memory efficacy beliefs corresponded well with more personal beliefs, with few age differences in the degree of correspondence.

Interestingly, increasing age not only appears to be associated with more positive attitudes about older adults (e.g., Chasteen, 2000), but also with more positive and less prejudicial attitudes toward younger adults (e.g., Chasteen, 2005; Mathesen, Collins, & Kuehne, 2000). This positive attitude toward an out-group by older adults is inconsistent with responses based on social identity theory (e.g., Tajfel, 1981) and may reflect the relatively unique status of age as a marker of group status. Specifically, the fact that older adults were once younger adults may result in greater familiarity with and empathy toward this out-group, which in turn has been shown to be associated with more favorable attitudes (e.g., Batson et al., 2002). Older adults' former status as younger adults might also be seen in the nature of self-referent beliefs. Mueller, Wonderlich, and Dugan (1986) found that older adults were just as likely to ascribe traits associated with young adulthood to themselves and similar-aged others as they were those associated with old age, whereas younger adults exhibited a clear self-referential bias for youthful traits.

These age differences are also reflected in attitudes toward one's own aging. Younger adults tend to have less positive views of their own aging than do older adults, at least up to around age 75 (Chasteen, 2000). Research has suggested that the degree to which one holds negative views of aging is in part related to concerns about one's own aging (e.g., Braithwaite, Lynd-Stevenson, & Pigram, 1993). Relatedly, older adults often have more positive attitudes about themselves than about same-aged peers (e.g., Heckhausen & Brim, 1997; Heckhausen & Krueger, 1997; Luszcz & Fitzgerald, 1986), although this is not always observed (e.g., Ryan & Kwong See, 1993).

Hummert (1999) has further argued that cues associated with older adults' physical appearance and behavior may activate aging stereotypes in others, which in turn influence their behavior toward these same individuals. For example, research has shown that many individuals use patronizing talk with older adults (e.g., Kemper, 1994), even though it is viewed as demeaning and disrespectful (e.g., Ryan, Meredith, & Shantz, 1994). Stereotyped-based treatment by others may heighten older adults' awareness of the aging-related beliefs held by these individuals as well as the fact that they are being viewed as members of the stereotyped group. Such treatment may serve as a mechanism through which stereotypes can influence older adults' memory performance, for example, through the impact of associated affective responses or activated belief systems (e.g., Cavanaugh, Feldman, & Hertzog, 1998).

In conclusion, there is strong evidence for negative attitudes regarding aging within Western culture. These attitudes are reflected in affective, cognitive, and behavioral components of behavior and they are relatively pervasive, both across individuals and across contexts. In addition, evidence suggests that older adults

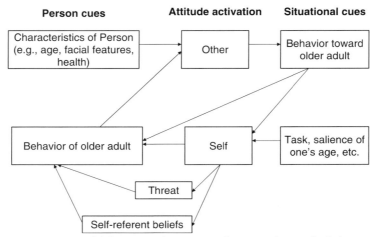

Figure 17.1 Model depicting the reciprocal nature of attitude–behavior relationships.

are aware of these attitudes — and in fact express them in a rather strong manner themselves — and that they are influenced by treatment by others based in these attitudes. On a more positive note, attitudes regarding aging are not all negative, and perceptions about older adults may be relatively positive in certain contexts. There is also good evidence that older adults are most likely to be perceived in terms of negative stereotypes when individuating information is not present and age-based cues are the most obvious characteristics available about the individual. This suggests that negative attitudes about aging, reflected in feelings toward, knowledge about, and responses to older adults are moderated by context. At the same time, the pervasiveness of generally negative attitudes about aging in our culture results in such attitudes serving as the default baseline for judging older individuals, with this influence being strongest in situations involving unfamiliar individuals or under conditions where there is minimal incentive for the perceiver to extensively process information about an older individual.

This section emphasized the general conceptual perspective that emphasizes the degree to which the attitudes held by others shape the behaviors of older adults. A general schematic of this relationship is provided at the top of Figure 17.1. This diagram depicts the flow associated with external sources of influence, as cues associated with the older adult affect the activation of attitudes associated with old age in others, which influence their behaviors (e.g., speech, assistance) toward the older adult. These, in turn, affect the older adults' actual behavior as he or she responds to these behaviors. Note that the modes of external influence can occur at a number of different levels, ranging from individual reactions to older adults in one-on-one situations to the sociocultural level, where responses may take the form of policies and social structures with implications for older adults.

The behaviors of others can be thought of as part of a larger category of situational cues relating to more internal modes of attitude–behavior influence (see lower portion of Figure 17.1). Such cues may serve to activate self-related attitudes, which in turn influence behavior. The next section reviews research that attempts to understand this relationship between the older adult's own aging-related attitudes and their behavior.

III. Self-Related Attitudes

As just described, much research on attitudes about aging has focused on the nature of those attitudes, their impact on the treatment of older adults, and the effects of this treatment on the behavior of older adults. Another important area of research — and a potentially more meaningful one for understanding aging-related change — has examined the relationship of older adults' attitudes about aging to their own behavior. As just documented, even though older adults have more complex and positive representations about aging than younger individuals, they still share many of the same attitudinal components with their younger compatriots. This continuity presumably represents the acquisition of socially shared beliefs regarding old age that they acquired at a younger age (e.g., Levy, 2003), at which time old age was still an out-group and thus susceptible to many of the biases in behavior and perception common to in-group members. The relatively positive view of youth versus old age may also be seen in the fact that research using the IAT has shown that there is greater identity with youth than old age across adulthood (Greenwald et al., 2002; Hummert et al., 2002).

In addition, although older adults are less likely to ascribe the negative characterizations of aging used to describe others in their age group to themselves, their views of their own behavior still reflect beliefs and stereotypes about aging. For example, Luszcz and Fitzgerald (1986) had participants rate the characteristics of adolescents, middle-aged adults, older adults, and themselves. Although older adults exhibited less negative views

of their group than younger individuals, as well as less negative views of themselves than of other older adults, their ratings for self and other older adults were still less positive than their ratings of middle-aged adults. Similarly, Heckhausen and Krueger (1993) found that adults of all ages expected more positive development for self than for others, and this trend was particularly enhanced in older adults. At the same time, however, older adults still described developmental trajectories for themselves that reflected typically documented beliefs of declines in desirable traits and increases in undesirable traits in later life. In a related study, Heckhausen and Brim (1997) found that older adults perceived themselves to have fewer problems relative to peers, but age differences in self-reported problems were consistent with expectations (e.g., more health problems with increasing age).

The traditional approach to investigating relationships between one's attitudes and their behavior is through an examination of self-referent beliefs (e.g., control, self-efficacy), which are presumed to reflect attitudes regarding aging. A more recent approach has been to examine more direct avenues of influence between attitudes and behaviors that do not necessarily rely on the mediating role of beliefs. Research of both types is discussed in the next sections.

A. Beliefs

Much of the research on self-referent beliefs has focused on memory, and that focus is reflected in this review. Note that there are several excellent reviews of this literature (e.g., Berry, 1999; Hertzog & Hultsch, 2000; Miller & Lachman, 1999), and thus the main goal in this section is to use representative findings to illustrate the role of beliefs in determining age differences in memory instead of providing an exhaustive review.

Research on memory-related beliefs in relation to aging has been conducted from a wide range of perspectives, with the primary emphasis being on the examination of expectations about change in one's own ability (e.g., self-efficacy) and the factors that influence performance and change (e.g., control). Whereas the focus of these two types of self-referent beliefs varies, the results of research suggest a common theme that is consistent with the previously reviewed research on aging attitudes; specifically, aging is associated with declining memory skills and reductions in the ability to control memory.

Although older adults tend to have more optimistic views of themselves than of same-aged peers, research has also demonstrated consistently that older adults in general have more negative views about their memory than younger or middle-aged adults. This is true both for self-efficacy (e.g., Berry, West, & Dennehy, 1989; Gilewski, Zelinski, & Schaie, 1990; Hultsch, Hertzog, & Dixon, 1987) and for control beliefs (e.g., Heckhausen & Baltes, 1991; Hertzog, McGuire, & Lineweaver, 1998; Hultsch et al., 1987; Lachman, 1986). Whereas there may be some legitimate basis for these variations in self-efficacy and control beliefs as we age, there is also evidence that our implicit theories about aging may influence perceptions of change in areas where there is little evidence of change (Lineweaver & Hertzog, 1998; McDonald-Miszczak, Hertzog, & Hultsch, 1995; McFarland, Ross, & Giltrow, 1992).

Studies examining the relationship between beliefs and behavior have shown that control and self-efficacy beliefs are associated positively with performance on a variety of memory tasks (e.g., Berry et al., 1989; Hertzog et al., 1998; Lachman, Steinberg, &

Trotter, 1987; Riggs, Lachman, & Wingfield, 1997; Zelinski, Gilewski, & Anthony-Bergstone, 1990). In most cases, the strength of this relationship is relatively modest (see Hertzog & Hultsch, 2000), but increases with increasing task familiarity and experience (e.g., Berry et al., 1989; Cavanaugh & Poon, 1989). Similar relationships between beliefs and memory have also been observed in longitudinal studies (e.g., Johannsson, Allen-Burge, & Zarit, 1997; Lane & Zelinski, 2003; McDonald-Miszczak et al., 1995; Seeman et al., 1996), with higher control/self-efficacy beliefs at initial testing associated with better performance or maintenance of ability at later times of test. In addition, those older adults with higher self-efficacy beliefs have also been found to benefit more from memory training (Rebok & Balcerak, 1989).

Findings that memory-related beliefs decline with age and that beliefs are associated with performance suggest that observed aging-related declines in memory may in part be accounted for by changing belief systems. Unfortunately, few studies have tested this prediction, with most focusing on belief–performance relationships within age groups. Hertzog et al. (1998) did find that age differences in self-efficacy and task-specific control beliefs indirectly influenced memory through strategy use, although a significant amount of age-related variance in recall (about 75%) remained after controlling for beliefs.

The difficulty associated with demonstrating specific causal links between beliefs and performance may have to do with the fact that beliefs not only influence performance, but also change in response to ability, reflecting a relatively complex reciprocal relation between these factors (e.g., Bandura, 1997; Berry, 1999; Lachman, 2000). Consistent with this view, several studies have demonstrated that memory training, either alone or accompanied by a focus on beliefs or goal setting, can result in changes in memory-related beliefs along with improvements in performance (e.g., Lachman et al., 1992; West, Welch, & Thorn, 2001). Poor relationships between performance and beliefs may also reflect the fact that personal beliefs are grounded in cultural stereotypes rather than the individual's own experience (Lineweaver & Hertzog, 1998).

In sum, evidence shows that beliefs about cognitive ability across adulthood reflect stereotypes based in aging-related attitudes. Such beliefs are also related to performance, suggesting that changes in beliefs could, in part, account for changes in cognitive performance. Evidence is somewhat mixed in this regard, with the inconsistency perhaps based in the complexity associated with examining the hypothesized reciprocal relationship between beliefs and performance. The relatively modest relations between these two factors, however, may also suggest problems in the conceptualization of the belief–performance relationship.

B. Attitudes about Aging

An underlying assumption of much of the just-discussed work is that self-relevant memory beliefs are an indirect expression of Western attitudes about the impact of aging on cognitive ability. Recently, research has begun looking for more direct linkages between stereotypes and behavior. Support for such a linkage was obtained by Levy and Langer (1994), who found that age differences in memory performance in individuals from the United States and mainland China were related to the degree to which individuals within each of these cultures displayed positive views of aging. Americans held less favorable views toward aging than did the Chinese, and

age differences in memory performance were larger in the former group. In addition, variations in culturally influenced beliefs about aging were found to account for a significant amount of variability in older adults' performance.

Yoon and colleagues (2000) attempted a conceptual replication of this study using Chinese Canadians and Anglophone Canadians and observed similar group differences in attitudes and memory, although the latter were specific to certain types of memory tests. They did not find, however, that positive attitudes about aging mediated the relationship between culture and aging. Despite some differences in findings, an important point of consistency in these two studies was the obtained effects regarding the relationship among culture, age, and memory performance. Both sets of researchers observed smaller age differences in groups with more positive beliefs about aging. The fact that expressed attitudes about aging were not consistent predictors of more general, group-based effects across studies may relate to the fact that explicit and implicit attitudes are not identical and do not always act in concert (e.g., Devine, 1989).

More recently, researchers have explored possible mechanisms underlying the linkages between aging self stereotypes and behavior. Two dominant conceptual frameworks have been used to examine these linkages (see also Wheeler & Petty, 2001).

1. Stereotype Threat

Steele and colleagues (2002) invoked the concept of stereotype threat as a means for explaining the effects of negative stereotypes on performance. They argued that negative stereotypes about a group will have a detrimental impact on the behavior of group members when those individuals are put in the position of potentially confirming that stereotype. Situational cues of which the individual is aware (e.g., participation in a memory experiment) are thought to activate stereotypes (e.g., old people have poor memories), which in turn may negatively impact performance due to a number of factors, including increased anxiety, arousal, and evaluation apprehension, or decreased effort. It has also been hypothesized that threat effects will be greater (a) for individuals who identify with the stereotyped group (b) for those who value the stereotyped ability (c) when the test is perceived as being diagnostic of the stereotyped ability and (d) for those who are aware of the negative implications of the stereotype.

Researchers have begun exploring the possibility that negative stereotypes about aging may result in older adults' experiencing stereotype threat, and several studies have provided results consistent with this possibility. Rahhal, Hasher, and Colcombe (2001) and Hess, Hinson, and Statham (2005) both found that deemphasizing the diagnostic value of a test with respect to the stereotyped ability (i.e., memory) significantly reduced the differences in performance between young and older adults.

In a more focused test of the stereotype threat hypothesis, Hess and co-workers (2003) examined how highlighting negative aging stereotypes influenced memory performance in young and older adults. They found that older adults' performance became progressively worse, and age differences progressively larger, as the negative implications of the aging stereotypes were made more salient. Hess et al. (2003) also found that these apparent threat effects were partially mediated by strategy use. This suggests that threat may have a negative impact on those working memory functions associated with planning and executing a strategy, a finding consistent with other research (e.g., Schmader & Johns, 2003).

Additional findings consistent with a stereotype threat interpretation of the results were that the effects of stereotype salience (a) were only observed for members of the stereotyped group and (b) were strongest for those with the greatest investment in their own memory ability. On the positive side, it is important to note that age differences in performance were essentially eliminated when more optimistic information regarding aging and memory was made salient to participants.

In a somewhat different realm, Auman, Bosworth, and Hess (2005) examined the operation of stereotype threat in medical situations. They found that the activation of negative stereotypes about being a patient resulted in increases in measures of arousal, such as blood pressure and skin conductance. This finding is important given the fact that health problems increase with age, resulting in older adults potentially being more susceptible to multiple stereotype-based influences (e.g., aging and patient status).

Whereas such findings provide support for the potential operation of stereotype threat in later life, some aspects of these studies were not entirely consistent with expectations. For example, Hess and colleagues (2003, 2004) were unsuccessful in obtaining evidence for the mediation of threat-based effects through factors such as anxiety, which are assumed to underlie such effects. The failure to obtain evidence for mediation is not necessarily damning to a stereotype threat explanation, as Steele et al. (2002) suggested that multiple mediators could be operative, with the situation determining the most influential ones. The nonspecificity in the current explication of the framework, however, might also be seen as a bit troubling in terms of establishing the validity of the stereotype threat phenomenon.

Two other studies have provided mixed support for stereotype threat influences on age differences in memory performance. Andreoletti and Lachman (2004) found that varying information regarding the diagnostic value of a memory test for identifying age differences affected not only the memory performance of older adults, but also that of middle-aged and younger adults, but not college students. They also found that these effects were moderated by education. Those with high levels of education benefited from the provision of counterstereotypic information about aging, whereas the performance of those with low levels of education suffered with the presentation of both stereotypic and counterstereotypic information. They concluded that the general susceptibility of their sample to aging stereotypes might be related to their relatively high levels of expressed concerns about their own memory ability.

Chasteen and colleagues (2005) did not find that changing the instructions on a memory task to deemphasize the memory component, thereby reducing its diagnosticity with respect to a stereotyped ability, differentially benefited the recall performance of older adults. They did find, however, that self-reports of stereotype threat (i.e., subjective experience) mediated the effects of age on memory.

Results of these initial studies of stereotype threat and aging are interesting, but somewhat inconsistent. Part of the problem may have to do with the manner in which older adults are recruited and their previous experience in research settings. If older adults believe they are being asked to participate in a study because of their age, threat may have been induced before the participant even arrives in the research setting. This not only complicates investigations of stereotype threat, but it also has important implications for the valid assessment of age differences in performance, with situationally based threat

factors having the potential to exacerbate age effects based in ability (Hess et al., 2003). Clearly, more research is necessary to understand the theoretical and pragmatic implications of stereotype threat.

2. Ideomotor Processes

The stereotype threat framework argues that stereotypes have their primary influence through the conscious experience of threat associated with stereotype activation. This implies that threat effects on performance are mediated by factors reflecting subjective experience, such as anxiety or evaluation apprehension. To this point, attempts at identifying mediators have been relatively unsuccessful. Other research, however, suggests that stereotypes may have a more direct impact on behavior without conscious intervention. This research has its basis in James' (1890) notion of ideomotor action, as elaborated upon by Bargh (1997; Bargh & Ferguson, 2000) and others (e.g., Dijksterhuis, 2001). Within this perspective, a direct link between perception and behavior is assumed, such that the perception of cues associated with specific behaviors results in a relatively automatic tendency to engage in those behaviors. With respect to stereotypes, the assumption is that subtle cues in the environment will activate stereotype-related information, which in turn will activate situation-appropriate behavioral tendencies.

Research with younger adults has demonstrated that a wide variety of behaviors can be affected by the implicit activation of stereotype-related information. Importantly, this research has demonstrated that it is not necessary for the individual to be a member of the group whose stereotype is primed. Thus, young college students can be primed to behave in a manner consistent with a variety of stereotypes, including that of old age. For example, activation of aging stereotypes has resulted in younger adults walking slower (Bargh, Chen, & Burrows, 1996), remembering less (Dijksterhuis et al., 2000), and responding more slowly (Dijksterhuis, Spears, & Lépinasse, 2001) than participants in a control condition. The important factor in these cases appears to be that the individual possesses knowledge relating to the group that can subsequently be activated, with greater knowledge or experience associated with stronger priming effects (e.g., Dijksterhuis et al., 2000). Evidence also shows that stereotype activation effects may be stronger in individuals belonging to the stereotyped group due to a lower threshold of activation associated with such information in group members (e.g. Shih et al., 2002). This suggests that the just-described effects may be even stronger for older adults as out-group stereotypes become in-group stereotypes.

A growing number of studies have examined implicit stereotype activation effects in older adults, with clear evidence of stereotype-based influences on a variety of behaviors. Several studies have examined ideomotor processes with respect to memory. In an initial study in this area, Levy (1996) implicitly primed positive and negative aging stereotypes and then examined changes in performance on a variety of tasks (memory for words, activities paired with photos, and dots placed on a spatial array). A general pattern of improvement following the positive primes and deterioration following negative primes was observed in older adults' performance, although the strength of this effect was somewhat variable across tasks. Consistent with the notion that stereotype threshold activation levels should be higher in nongroup members, these effects were not observed in a sample of young adults. Using a similar procedure, Stein,

Blanchard-Fields, and Hertzog (2002) replicated these results only partially. Hess et al. (2004), however, did replicate Levy's basic findings in two separate experiments using a memory test more typical of those used in studies of cognitive aging (e.g., free recall of a list of words). Hess et al. (2004) hypothesized that stereotype activation effects on performance might be most powerful on tasks with a strong strategic component, perhaps explaining the inconsistency across studies.

Levy and colleagues have demonstrated that implicit priming effects are not constrained to memory. Older adults primed with negative aging stereotypes exhibit greater physiological responses to stress (Levy et al., 2000), reduced walking speed (Hausdorff, Levy, & Wei, 1999), poorer handwriting (Levy, 2000), and greater refusal of life prolonging interventions (Levy, Ashman, & Dror, 1999–2000) when compared to individuals exposed to positive aging-related primes. These findings, along with those relating to memory, demonstrate the potential impact of negative stereotypes in later life as well as the pervasiveness of this impact. They also suggest that stereotypes may have a direct effect on performance through relatively automatic goal structures, with associated activation of beliefs or conscious reactions being unnecessary for performance to be affected. This may, in part, account for some of the previously discussed difficulty in identifying belief–performance relationships.

A limitation of most of the current studies examining the relationship between attitudes and functioning has been that they are cross-sectional in nature and have focused on situation-specific effects. Whereas such findings are informative from both a theoretical and a practical standpoint, it would be important to know what the cumulative effects of negative attitudes across the life span might be. For example, research has demonstrated that activation of negative stereotypes leads to increases in stress-related physiological responses (Auman et al., 2005; Levy et al., 2000), which in turn have been associated with negative consequences on memory and other aspects of functioning (e.g., Lupien et al., 1998; Seeman et al., 1997). Frequent experience with such responses in relationship to negative self-stereotypes over an extended period of time may have negative implications for both physical and cognitive health.

Some evidence for such a relationship can be seen in two studies that found positive attitudes about aging early in life to be predictive of both mortality (Levy et al., 2002) and functional health (Levy, Slade, & Kasl, 2002). Using data from the Ohio Longitudinal Study of Aging and Retirement, these researchers found that those with positive attitudes toward aging at the beginning of the study had higher levels of functional health and lived longer than those with less positive views. In both cases, the effects were obtained while controlling for initial levels of self-reported health, thereby controlling for the possibility that health influenced attitudes. Some caution needs to be exercised in interpreting these findings due to the self-report nature of several measures (e.g., functional health) and to the potential influence of sample attrition over the course of the study. Concern can also be expressed due to the potential overlap among some of the five items on the attitudes questionnaire (e.g., "I have as much pep as I did last year") and physical health. Nonetheless, these provocative findings suggest the potential long-term impact of attitudes on adult development.

In sum, the research reviewed in this section has emphasized how older adults' own attitudes about aging influence their behavior. Integrating these ideas with those from the earlier discussed research (see Section II), it can be seen that the influence of attitudes can be thought of in terms of a reciprocal system in which internal and external influences interact. A variety of cues, including the previously discussed behaviors of others, as well as those associated with threat and ideomotor-related effects, may serve to activate self-related attitudes (see lower portion of Figure 17.1). Depending on the nature of the cue and the associated experience, this activation can then influence an older adult's actual behavior through one or more hypothesized routes, including a relatively direct route reflecting ideomotor processes or mediated routes associated with stereotype threat or self-referent beliefs. The older adult's behavior can then feed back and serve as an additional personal characteristic that influences the probability of stereotype activation in others. This reinforces the reciprocal nature of attitude-based influences. It also provides a means for understanding the long-term and self-perpetuating effects of attitudes on behaviors.

A final point worth mentioning is that activating one's attitudes does not have the inevitable effect of causing the individual to behave in an attitude-consistent manner. Simple awareness that the stereotype has been activated has been associated with attitude suppression or nonconsistent behavior (e.g., Hess et al., 2004; Lepore & Brown, 2002). In addition, individual characteristics, such as the extent to which one values a stereotyped behavior (e.g., Hess et al., 2003) or concerns about one's group being stigmatized (e.g., Brown & Pinel, 2003), can moderate the impact of stereotypes. Such findings are hopeful in identifying means for overcoming the sometimes insidious effects of stereotypes.

IV. Conclusions

This review focused on understanding the nature of attitudes about aging and the mechanisms through which they influence the behavior of older adults. Although this summary of research is by no means exhaustive, several important conclusions can be derived from the representative studies that were discussed. First, negative attitudes about aging are pervasive in our culture and are reflected in affective, cognitive, and behavioral responses of individuals and groups of all ages. In addition, evidence shows that implicit attitudes may be even more strongly negative than explicit ones. Second, evidence also shows that people do not view old age as a homogeneous category. Stereotypes of old age contain several different subtypes of older adults, many of which are negative but also some of which are positive. It has been suggested, however, that even most of the positive subtypes of old age have a subtle, negative evaluative component. Third, individual and situational factors affect the nature of aging attitudes and the probability that they will influence behavior. For example, increasing age and familiarity with older adults are both associated with more complex and positive attitudes toward aging. In addition, stereotypes about aging are most likely to be activated and to influence behavior when individuating information is not available and age-related cues (e.g., physical appearance) are the primary source of information about a person. Fourth, there is clear evidence that the behavior of older adults is affected by the stereotype-influenced responses of others. In many cases, stereotype-consistent behavior is reinforced, further perpetuating negative views of aging.

Research has also clearly demonstrated that older adults' own attitudes about aging can have an effect on their behavior with very little influence from external sources. Evidence shows that self-referent beliefs related to ability are associated with performance and also change with age. In addition, relatively subtle cues in the environment (e.g., being asked one's age, having memory assessed) result in the activation of aging-related attitudes, which in turn can influence performance negatively. Finally, self-related attitudes can have relatively short-term situational effects (e.g., depression of memory performance when stereotype threat is induced), but intriguing evidence suggests that they may have long-term influences as well.

The research reviewed here has tended to focus on negative aging attitudes, which in part reflects the emphasis in the literature. This may also be a reflection of the culture-specific nature of this research. Most of the research reviewed here was conducted in North America and western Europe, and the findings may reflect dominant attitudes and values in these cultures. Such attitudes may not necessarily be representative of other non-Western cultures. Interesting issues for future research concern the extent to which attitudes reflect cultural stereotypes versus personal experiences with older adults and the degree to which cultural differences in attitudes are reflected in different patterns of aging.

In closing, it is important to note that positive messages can be derived from the reviewed literature. First, our attitudes about aging are not all negative, and increased exposure to older adults and education about the aging process have been shown to result in more positive attitudes. Indeed, it has been suggested that increasing understanding of the diversity associated with old age, decreasing our fear of aging, and experience in taking the perspective of older adults might be beneficial for overcoming ageist attitudes in our society. Second, negative attitudes do not always influence our perceptions of older adults. When they are viewed as individuals in terms of their specific personality traits and abilities, others are less likely to use aging-related categories in relating to them. This may require attention to cues other than those associated with a person's age. Even when such cues are present, however, it may take conscious effort to overcome relatively well-ingrained implicit attitudes as well as awareness of the potential influence of such attitudes. Finally, research on implicit attitudes and self-stereotypes has indicated that situationally induced negative influences on a variety of behavioral responses can be overcome by emphasizing positive images of aging and suppressing the activation of negative attitudes.

Acknowledgment

Preparation of this chapter was supported by National Institute on Aging Grants AG05552 and AG20153.

References

Adelman, R. D., Greene, M. G., Charon, R., & Friedman, E. (1990). Issues in the physician-geriatric patient relationship. In H. Giles, N. Coupland, & J. M. Wiemann (Eds.), *Communication, health and the elderly* (pp. 126–134). Glasgow: Manchester University Press.

Andreoletti, C., & Lachman, M. E. (2004). Susceptibility and resilience to memory aging stereotypes: Education matters more than age. *Experimental Aging Research*, 30, 129–148.

Auman, C., Bosworth, H. B., & Hess, T. M. (2005). The effects of health-related stereotypes on physiological responses of hypertensive older adults. *Journal of Gerontology: Psychological Sciences*, 60B, P3–P10.

Avorn, J., & Langer, E. (1982). Induced disability in nursing home patients: A controlled trial. *Journal of American Geriatric Society*, 30, 397–400.

Baltes, M. M., Neuman, E. M., & Zank, S. (1994). Maintenance and rehabilitation of independence in old age: An intervention program for staff. *Psychology and Aging*, 9, 179–188.

Baltes, M. M., & Wahl, H. W. (1992). The dependency-support script in institutions: Generalizations to community settings. *Psychology and Aging*, 7, 409–418.

Baltes, M. M., & Wahl, H. W. (1996). Patterns of communication in old age: The dependence-support script and independence-ignore script. *Health Communication*, 8, 217–231.

Baltes, P.B., & Baltes, M.M. (1990). Psychological perspectives on successful aging: The model of selective optimization with compensation. In M. M. Baltes & P. B. Baltes (Eds.), *Successful aging: Perspectives from the behavioral sciences* (pp. 1–34). New York: Cambridge University Press.

Bandura, A. (1997). *Self-efficacy: The exercise of control*. New York: Freeman.

Bargh, J. A. (1997). The automaticity of everyday life. In R. S. Wyer, Jr. (Ed.), *Advances in social cognition* (Vol. 10, pp. 1–61). Mahwah, NJ: Lawrence Erlbaum.

Bargh, J. A., Chaiken, S., Govender, R., & Pratto, F. (1992). The generality of the automatic attitude activation effect. *Journal of Personality and Social Psychology*, 62, 893–912.

Bargh, J. A., Chen, M., & Burrows, L. (1996). Automaticity of social behavior: Direct effects of trait construct and stereotype activation on action. *Journal of Personality and Social Psychology*, 71, 230–244.

Bargh, J. A., & Ferguson, M. J. (2000). Beyond behaviorism: On the automaticity of higher mental processes. *Psychological Bulletin*, 126, 925–945.

Bargh, J. A., Litt, J., Pratto, F., & Spielman, L. A. (1989). On the preconscious evaluation of social stimuli. In A. F. Bennett & K. M. McConkey (Eds.), *Cognition in individual and social contexts* (pp. 357–370). Amsterdam: North-Holland.

Batson, C. D., Chang, J., Orr, R., & Rowland, J. (2002). Empathy, attitudes, and action: Can feeling for a member of a stigmatized group motivate one to help the group? *Personality and Social Psychology Bulletin*, 28, 1656–1666.

Berry, J. M. (1999). Memory self-efficacy in its social cognitive context. In T. M. Hess & F. Blanchard-Fields (Eds.), *Social cognition and aging* (pp. 70–98). San Diego: Academic Press.

Berry, J. M., West, R. L., & Dennehy, D. M. (1989). Reliability and validity of the memory self-efficacy questionnaire. *Developmental Psychology*, 25, 701–713.

Bieman-Copland, S., & Ryan, E. B. (1998). Age-biased interpretation of memory successes and failures in adulthood. *Journal of Gerontology: Psychological Sciences*, 53B, P105–P11.

Bieman-Copland, S., & Ryan, E. B. (2001). Social perceptions of failures in memory monitoring. *Psychology and Aging*, 16, 357–361.

Biernat, M. (2003). Toward a broader view of social stereotyping. *American Psychologist*, 58, 1019–1027.

Braithwaite, V., Lynd-Stevenson, R., & Pigram, D. (1993). An empirical study of ageism: From polemics to scientific utility. *Australian Psychologist*, 28, 9–15.

Brewer, M. B., Dull, V., & Lui, L. (1981). Perceptions of the elderly: Stereotypes as prototypes. *Journal of Personality and Social Psychology*, 41, 656–670.

Brewer, M. B., & Lui, L. (1984). Categorization of the elderly by the elderly: Effects of perceiver's category membership. *Personality and Social Psychology Bulletin*, 10, 585–595.

Brimacombe, C. A. E., Quinton, N., Nance, N., & Garrioch, L. (1997). Is age irrelevant? Perceptions of young and old adult eye-witnesses. *Law and Human Behavior*, 21, 619–634.

Brown, R. P., & Pinel, E. C. (2003). Stigma on my mind: Individual differences in the experience of stereotype threat. *Journal Experimental Social Psychology*, 39, 626–633.

Camp, C. J., & Pignatiello, M. F. (1988). Beliefs about fact retrieval and inferential reasoning across the adult life span. *Experimental Aging Research*, 14, 89–97.

Caporael, L. R., Lukaszewski, M., & Culbertson, G. (1983). Secondary baby talk: Judgements by institutionalized elderly and their caregivers. *Journal of Personality and Social Psychology*, 44, 746–754.

Capowski, G. (1994). Ageism: The new diversity issue. *Management Review*, 83, 10–15.

Cavanaugh, J. C., Feldman, J. M., & Hertzog, C. (1998). Memory beliefs as social cognition: A reconceptualization of what memory questionnaires assess. *Review of General Psychology*, 2, 48–65.

Cavanaugh, J. C., & Poon, L. W. (1989). Metamemorial predictors of memory performance in young and older adults. *Psychology and Aging*, 4, 365–368.

Chasteen, A. L. (2000). The role of age and age-related attitudes in perceptions of elderly individuals. *Basic and Applied Social Psychology*, 22, 147–156.

Chasteen, A. L. (2005). Seeing eye-to-eye: Do intergroup biases operate similarly for younger and older adults? *International Journal of Aging and Human Development*, 61, 123–139.

Chasteen, A. L., Bhattacharyya, S., Horhota, M., Tam, R., & Hasher, L. (2005). How feelings of stereotype threat influence older adults' memory performance. *Experimental Aging Research*, 31, 235–260.

Chasteen, A. L., Schwarz, N., & Park, D. C. (2002). The activation of aging stereotypes in younger and older adults. *Journal of Gerontology: Psychological Sciences*, 57B, P540–P547.

Cuddy, AJ. C., & Fiske, S. T. (2002). Doddering but dear: Process, content, and function in stereotyping of older persons. In T. D. Nelson (Ed.), *Ageism: Stereotyping and prejudice against older persons* (pp. 3–26). Cambridge, MA: MIT Press.

Devine, P. G. (1989). Stereotypes and prejudice: Their automatic and controlled components. *Journal of Personality and Social Psychology*, 56, 680–690.

Dijksterhuis, A. (2001). Automatic social influence: The perception-behavior links as an explanatory mechanism for behavior matching. K. D. Williams &

J.P Forgas (Eds.), *Social influence: Direct and indirect processes.* (pp. 95–108). Philadelphia: Psychology Press.

Dijksterhuis, A., Aarts, H., Bargh, J. A., & van Knippenberg, A. (2000). On the relation between associative strength and automatic behavior. *Journal of Experimental Social Psychology, 36,* 531–544.

Dijksterhuis, A., Spears, R., & Lépinasse, V. (2001). Reflecting and deflecting stereotypes: Assimilation and contrast in impression formation and automatic behavior. *Journal of Experimental Social Psychology, 37,* 286–299.

Erber, J. T. (1989). Young and older adults' appraisal of memory failures in young and older adult target persons. *Journal of Gerontology: Psychological Sciences, 44,* P170–P175.

Erber, J. T., Etheart, M. E., & Szuchman, L. T. (1992). Age and forgetfulness: Perceivers' impressions of targets' capability. *Psychology and Aging, 7,* 479–483.

Erber, J. T., Prager, I. G., Williams, M., & Caiola, M. A. (1996). Age and forgetfulness: Confidence in ability and attribution for memory failures. *Psychology and Aging, 11,* 310–315.

Erber, J. T., & Rothberg, S. T. (1991). Here's looking at you: The relative effect of age and attractiveness on judgments about memory failure. *Journal of Gerontology: Psychological Sciences, 46,* P116–P123.

Erber, J. T., Szuchman, L. T., & Prager, I. G. (1997). Forgetful but forgiven: How age and lifestyle affect perceptions of memory failure. *Journal of Gerontology: Psychological Sciences, 52B,* P303–P307.

Erber, J. T., Szuchman, L. T., & Rothberg, S. T. (1990). Everyday memory failure: Age differences in appraisal and attribution. *Psychology and Aging, 5,* 236–241.

Finkelstein, L. M., Burke, M. J., & Raju, N. S. (1995). Age discrimination in simulated employment contexts: An integrative analysis. *Journal of Applied Psychology, 80,* 652–663.

Fiske, S. T., Cuddy, A. J. C., Glick, P., & Xu, J. (2002). A model of (often mixed) stereotype content: Competence and warmth respectively follow from perceived status and competition. *Journal of Personality and Social Psychology, 82,* 878–902.

Fiske, S. T., & Neuberg, S. L. (1990). A continuum model of impression formation, from category-based to individuating processes: Influences of information and motivation on attention and interpretation. In M. P. Zanna (Ed.), *Advances in experimental social psychology* (Vol. 23, pp. 1–74). New York: Academic Press.

Fiske, S. T., & Taylor, S. E. (1991). *Social cognition* (2nd edition). New York: McGraw-Hill.

Galinsky, A. D., & Moskowitz, G. B. (2000). Perspective taking: Decreasing stereotype expression, stereotype accessibility, and in-group favoritism. *Journal of Personality and Social Psychology, 78,* 708–724.

Gilewski, M. J., Zelinski, E. M., & Schaie, K. W. (1990). The memory functioning questionnaire for assessments of memory complaints in adulthood and old age. *Psychology and Aging, 5,* 482–490.

Greene, M. G., Adelman, R., Charon, R., & Hoffman, S. (1986). Ageism in the medial encounter: An exploratory study of the doctor-elderly relationship. *Language and Communication, 6,* 113–124.

Greenwald, A. G., Banaji, M. R., Rudman, L. A., Farnham, S. D., Nosek, B. A., & Mellott, D. S.(2002). A unified theory of implicit attitudes, stereotypes, self-esteem, and self-concept. *Psychological Review, 109,* 3–25.

Greenwald, A. G., McGhee, D. E., & Schwartz, J. L. K. (1998). Measuring individual differences in implicit cognition: The Implicit Association Test. *Journal of Personality and Social Psychology, 74,* 1464–1480.

Hale, N. M. (1998). Effects of age and interpersonal contact on stereotyping of the elderly. *Current Psychology: Developmental, Learning, Personality, Social, 17,* 28–47.

Harwood, J., Ryan, E. B., Giles, H. & Tysoski, S. (1997). Evaluations of patronizing speech and three response styles in a non-service-providing setting. *Journal of Applied Communication Research, 25,* 170–184.

Hausdorff, J. M., Levy, B. R., & Wei, J. Y. (1999). The power of ageism on physical function of older persons: Reversibility of age-related gait changes. *Journal of the*

American Geriatrics Society, 47, 1346–1349.

Heckhausen, J., & Baltes, P. B. (1991). Perceived controllability of expected psychological change across adulthood and old age. *Journal of Gerontology: Psychological Sciences, 46,* 165–173.

Heckhausen, J., & Brim, O. G. (1997). Perceived problems for self and others: Self-protection by social downgrading through adulthood. *Psychology and Aging, 12,* 610–619.

Heckhausen, J., Dixon, R. A., & Baltes, P. B. (1989). Gains and losses in development throughout adulthood as perceived by different adult age groups. *Developmental Psychology, 25,* 109–121.

Heckhausen, J., & Krueger, J. (1993). Developmental expectations for the self and most other people: Age grading in three functions of social comparison. *Developmental Psychology, 29,* 539–548.

Hertzog, C., & Hultsch, D. F. (2000). Metacognition in adulthood and old age. In F. I. M. Craik & T. A. Salthouse (Eds.). *The handbook of aging and cognition* (pp. 417–466). Mahwah, NJ: Lawrence Erlbaum.

Hertzog, C., McGuire, C. L., & Lineweaver, T. T. (1998). Aging, attributions, perceived control and strategy use in a free recall task. *Aging, Neuropsychology, and Cognition, 5,* 85–106.

Hess, T. M., Auman, C., Colcombe, S. J., & Rahhal, T. A. (2003). The impact of stereotype threat on age differences in memory performance. *Journal of Gerontology: Psychological Sciences, 58B,* 3–11.

Hess, T. M., Hinson, J. T., & Statham, J. A. (2004). Implicit and explicit stereotype activation effects on memory: Do age and awareness moderate the impact of priming? *Psychology and Aging, 19,* 495–505.

Hultsch, D. F., Hertzog, C., & Dixon, R. A. (1987). Age differences in metamemory: Resolving the inconsistencies. *Canadian Journal of Psychology, 41,* 193–208.

Hummert, M. L. (1990). Multiple stereotypes of elderly and young adults: A comparison of structure and evaluations. *Psychology and Aging, 5,* 182–193.

Hummert, M. L. (1999). A social cognitive perspective on age stereotypes. In T. M. Hess & F. Blanchard-Fields (Eds.), *Social cognition and aging* (pp. 175–196). San Diego: Academic Press.

Hummert, M. L., Garstka, T. A., O'Brien, L. T., Greenwald, A. G., & Mellott, D. S. (2002). Using the implicit association test to measure age differences in implicit social cognitions. *Psychology and Aging, 17,* 482–495.

Hummert, M. L., Garstka, T. A., & Shaner, J. L. (1997). Stereotyping of older adults: The role of target facial cues and perceiver characteristics. *Psychology and Aging, 12,* 107–114.

Hummert, M. L., Garstka, T. A., Shaner, J. L., & Strahm, S. (1994). Stereotypes of the elderly held by young, middle-aged, and elderly adults. *Journal of Gerontology: Psychological Sciences, 49,* P240–P249.

Hummert, M. L. & Ryan, E. B. (1996). Toward understanding variations in patronizing talk addressed to older adults: Psycholinguistic features of care and control. *International Journal of Psycholinguistics, 12,* 149–170.

Ikels, C. (1990). New options for the urban elderly. In D. Davis & E. Vogel (Eds.), *Chinese society on the eve of Tiananmen: The impact of reform* (pp. 215–242). Cambridge, MA: Harvard University Council of East Asian Studies.

James, W. (1890). *Principles of psychology* (Vol. 2). New York: Holt.

Johansson, B, , Allen-Burge, R., & Zarit, S. H. (1997). Self-reports on memory functioning in a longitudinal study of the oldest old: Relation to current, prospective, and retrospective performance. *Journal of Gerontology: Psychological Sciences, 52B,* P139–P146.

Karpinski, A., & Hilton, J. L. (2001). Attitudes and the implicit association test. *Journal of Personality and Social Psychology, 81,* 774–788.

Kemper, S. (1994). "Elderspeak:" Speech accommodation to older adults. *Aging and Cognition, 1,* 17–28.

Kite, M. E., & Johnson, B. T. (1988). Attitudes toward older and younger adults: A meta-analysis. *Psychology and Aging, 3,* 233–244.

Kogan, N. (1979). A study of age categorization. *Journal of Gerontology, 34,* 358–367.

Kwong See. S. T., & Heller, R. B. (2004). Judging older targets' discourse: How do age stereotypes influence evaluations? *Experimental Aging Research, 30*, 63–73.

Kwong See, S. T., Hoffman, H. G., & Wood, T. L. (2001). Perceptions of an old female eyewitness: Is the older eyewitness believable? *Psychology and Aging, 16*, 346–350.

Lachman, M. E. (1986). Locus of control in aging research: A case for multidimensional and domain-specific assessment. *Psychology and Aging, 1*, 34–40.

Lachman, M. E. (2000). Promoting a sense of control over memory aging. In R. D. Hill, L. Bäckman, & A. Stigsdotter-Neely (Eds.), *Cognitive rehabilitation in old age.* New York: Oxford University Press.

Lachman, M. E., Steinberg, E. S., & Trotter, S. D., (1987). Effects of control beliefs and attributions on memory self assessments and performance. *Psychology and Aging, 2*, 266–271.

Lachman, M. E., Weaver, S. L., Bandura, M., Elliott, E., & Lewkowicz, C. J. (1992). Improving memory and control beliefs through cognitive restructuring and self-generated strategies. *Journal of Gerontology: Psychological Sciences, 47*, P293–P299.

Lane, C. J., & Zelinski, E. M. (2003). Longitudinal hierarchical linear models of the memory functioning questionnaire. *Psychology and Aging, 18*, 38–53.

Lepore, L., & Brown, R. (2002). The role of awareness: Divergent automatic stereotype activation and implicit judgment correction. *Social Cognition, 20*, 321–351.

Levy, B. (1996). Improving memory in old age by implicit self-stereotyping. *Journal of Personality and Social Psychology, 71*, 1092–1107.

Levy, B. (2000). Handwriting as a reflection of aging self-stereotypes. *Journal of Geriatric Psychiatry, 33*, 81–94.

Lvey, B. (2003). Mind matters: Cognitive and physical effects of aging stereotypes. *Journal of Gerontology: Psychological Sciences, 58B*, P203–P211.

Levy, B., Ashman, O., & Dror, I. (1999–2000). To be or not to be: The effects of aging stereotypes on the will to live. *Omega: Journal of Death and Dying, 40*, 409–420.

Levy, B., & Langer, E. (1994). Aging free from negative stereotypes: Successful memory in China and among the American deaf. *Journal of Personality and Social Psychology, 66*, 989–997.

Levy, B. R., Hausdorff, J. M., Hencke, R., & Wei, J. Y. (2000). Reducing cardiovascular stress with positive self-stereotypes of aging. *Journal of Gerontology: Psychological Sciences, 55B*, P205–P213.

Levy, B. R., Slade, M. D., Kunkel, S. R., & Kasl, S. V. (2002). Longevity increased by positive self-perceptions of aging. *Journal of Personality and Social Psychology, 83*, 261–270.

Levy, B. R., Slade, M. D., & Kasl, S. V. (2002). Longitudinal benefit of positive self-perceptions of aging on functional health. *Journal of Gerontology: Psychological Sciences, 57B*, P409–P417.

Leyens, J.-P., Yzerbyt, V., & Schadron, G. (1994). *Stereotypes and social cognition.* London: Sage.

Lineweaver, T. T., & Hertzog, C. (1998). Adults' efficacy and control beliefs regarding memory and aging: Separating general from personal beliefs. *Aging, Neuropsychology, and Cognition, 5*, 264–296.

Linville, P. W., Fischer, G. W., & Salovey, P. (1989). Perceived distributions of the characteristics of in-group and out-group members: Empirical evidence and a computer simulation. *Journal of Personality and Social Psychology, 57*, 165–188.

Linville, P. W., Salovey, P., & Fischer, G. W. (1986). Stereotyping and perceived distributions of social characteristics: An application to in-group–outgroup perception. In J. Dovidio & S. L. Gaertner (Eds.), *Prejudice, discrimination, and racism* (pp. 165–208). New York: Academic Press.

Lupien, S., De Leon, M. J., de Santi, S., Convit, A., Tarshish, C., Nair, N. P. V., Thakur, M. McEwen, B. S., Hauger, R. L., & Meaney, M. J. (1998). Cortisol levels during human aging predict atrophy and memory deficits. *Nature Neuroscience, I*, 69–73.

Luszcz, M. A., & Fitzgerald, K. M. (1986). Understanding cohort differences in cross-generational, self, and peer perceptions. *Journal of Gerontology, 41*, 234–240.

Matheson, D. H., Collins, C. L., & Kuehne, V. S. (2000). Older adults' multiple stereotypes of younger adults. *International Journal of Aging and Human Development, 41*, 245–257.

McCann, R., & Giles, H. (2002). Ageism in the workplace: A communication perspective. In T. D. Nelson (Ed.), *Ageism: Stereotyping and prejudice against older persons* (pp. 163–199). Cambridge, MA: MIT Press.

McDonald-Miszczak, L., Hertzog, C., & Hultsch, D. F. (1995). Stability and accuracy in metamemory and aging. *Psychology and Aging, 10*, 553–564.

McFarland, C., Ross, M., & Giltrow, M. (1992). Biased recollections in older adults: The role of implicit theories of aging. *Journal of Personality and Social Psychology, 62*, 837–850.

Miller, L. M. S., & Lachman, M. E. (1999). The sense of control and cognitive aging: Toward a model of mediational processes. *Social cognition and aging* (pp. 17–42). San Diego: Academic Press.

Montepare, J. M., & Zebrowitz-McArthur, L. (1988). Impressions of people created by age related qualities of their gait. *Journal of Personality and Social Psychology, 55*, 547–556.

Mueller, J. H., Wonderlich, S., & Dugan, K. (1986). Self-referent processing of age-specific material. *Psychology and Aging, 1*, 293–299.

Ng, S. H. (2002). Will families support their elders? Answers from across cultures. In T. D. Nelson (Ed.), *Ageism: Stereotyping and prejudice against older persons* (pp. 295–309). Cambridge, MA: MIT Press.

Nosek, B. A., Banaji, M. R., & Greenwald, A. G. (2002). Harvesting implicit group attitudes and beliefs from a demonstration web site. *Group Dynamics: Theory, Research, and Practice, 6*, 101–115.

O'Connor, B. P., & Rigby, H. (1996). Perceptions of baby talk, frequency of receiving baby talk, and self-esteem among community and nursing home residents. *Psychology and Aging, 11*, 147–154.

Parr, W. V., & Siegert, R. (1993). Adults' conceptions of everyday memory failures in others: Factors that mediate the effects of target age. *Psychology and Aging, 8*, 599–605.

Pasupathi, M., & Löckenhoff, C. E. (2002). Ageist behavior. In T. D. Nelson (Ed.), *Ageism: Stereotyping and prejudice against older persons* (pp. 201–246). Cambridge, MA: MIT Press.

Perdue, C. W., & Gurtman, M. B. (1990). Evidence for the automaticity of ageism. *Journal of Experimental Social Psychology, 26*, 199–216.

Petty, R. E., Priester, J. R., & Wegener, D. T. (1994). Cognitive processes in attitude change. In R. S. Wyer, Jr., & T. K. Srull (Eds.), *Handbook of social cognition* (2nd edition, Vol. 2, pp. 69–142). Hillsdale, NJ: Lawrence Erlbaum.

Radecki, S. E., Kane, R. L., Solomon, D. H., & Mendenhall, R. C. (1988). Do physicians spend less time with older patients? *Journal of the American Geriatrics Society, 36*, 713–718.

Rahhal, T. A., Hasher, L., & Colcombe, S. J. (2001). Instructional manipulations and age differences in memory: Now you see them, now you don't. *Psychology and Aging, 16*, 697–706.

Rebok, G. W., & Balcerak, L. J. (1989). Memory self-efficacy and performance differences in young and old adults. The effect of mnemonic training. *Developmental Psychology, 25*, 714–721.

Riggs, K. M., Lachman, M. E., & Wingfield, A. (1997). Taking charge of remembering: Locus of control and older adults' memory for speech. *Experimental Aging Research, 23*, 237–256.

Rodin, J., & Langer, E. J. (1977). Long-term effects of a control-relevant intervention with the institutionalized aged. *Journal of Personality and Social Psychology, 35*, 897–902.

Rosencranz, H. A., & McNevin, T. E. (1969). A factor analysis of attitudes toward the aged. *Gerontologist, 9*, 55–59.

Rubin, K. H., & Brown, I. (1975). A life-span look at person perception and its relationship to communicative interaction. *Journal of Gerontology, 30*, 461–468.

Ryan, E. B. (1992). Beliefs about memory changes across the adult life span. *Journal of Gerontology: Psychological Sciences, 47*, P41–P46.

Ryan, E. B., Giles, H., Bartolucci, G., & Henwood, K. (1986). Psycholinguistic and social psychological components of communication by and with the elderly. *Language and Communication, 6*, 1–24.

Ryan, E. B., & Kwong See, S. (1993). Age-based beliefs about memory changes for self and others across adulthood. *Journal of Gerontology: Psychological Sciences, 48*, P199–P201.

Ryan, E. B., Kwong See, S., Meneer, W. B., & Trovato, D. (1992). Age-based perceptions of language performance among younger and older adults. *Communication Research, 19*, 311–331.

Ryan, E. B., Meredith, S. D., & Shantz, G. D. (1994). Evaluative perceptions of patronizing speech addressed to institutionalized elders in contrasting conversational contexts. *Canadian Journal on Aging, 13*, 236–248.

Schaie, K. W. (1988). Ageism in psychological research. *American Psychologist, 43*, 179–183.

Schaie, K. W. (1993). Ageist language in psychological research. *American Psychologist, 48*, 49–51.

Schmader, T., & Johns, M. (2003). Converging evidence that stereotype threat reduces working memory capacity. *Journal of Personality and Social Psychology, 85*, 440–452.

Schmidt, D. F., & Boland, S. M. (1986). The structure of impressions of older adults: Evidence for multiple stereotypes. *Psychology and Aging, 1*, 255–260.

Seeman, T., McAvay, G., Merrill, S., Albert, M., & Rodin, J. (1996). Self-efficacy beliefs and change in cognitive performance: MacArthur studies of successful aging. *Psychology and Aging, 11*, 538–551.

Seeman, T. E., McEwen, B. S., Singer, B. H., Albert, M. S., & Rowe, J. W., (1997). Increase in urinary cortisol excretion and memory declines: MacArthur studies of successful aging. *Journal of Clinical Endocrinology and Metabolism, 82*, 2458–2465.

Shih, M., Ambady, N., Richeson, J. A., Fujita, K., & Gray, H. M. (2002). Stereotype performance boosts: The impact of self-relevance and the manner of stereotype activation. *Journal of Personality and Social Psychology, 83*, 638–647.

Slotterback, C. S., & Saarino, D. A. (1996). Attitudes toward older adults reported by young adults: Variation based on attitudinal task and attribute categories. *Psychology and Aging, 11*, 563–571.

Steele, C. M., & Aronson, J. (1995). Contending with a stereotype: African-American intellectual test performance and stereotype threat. *Journal of Personality and Social Psychology, 69*, 797–811.

Steele, C. M., Spencer, S. J., & Aronson, J. (2002). Contending with group image: The psychology of stereotype and social identity threat. In M. P. Zanna, (Ed), *Advances in experimental social psychology* (Vol. 34, pp. 379–440). San Diego: Academic Press.

Stein, R., Blanchard-Fields, F., & Hertzog, C. (2002). The effects of age-stereotype priming on memory performance in older adults. *Experimental Aging Research, 28*, 169–181.

Tajfel, H. (1981). *Human groups and social categories: Studies in social psychology.* Cambridge, England: University Press.

Thimm, C., Rademacher, U., & Kruse, L. (1998). Age stereotypes and patronizing messages: Features of age-adapted speech in technical instructions to the elderly. *Journal of Applied Communication Research, 26*, 66–82.

Tuckman, J., & Lorge, I. (1953). The effect of changed directions on the attitudes about old people and the older worker. *Educational and Psychological Measurement, 13*, 607–613.

Warr, P. (1994). Age and employment. In H. C. Triandis, M. D. Dunnette, & L. M. Hough (Eds.), *Handbook of industrial and organizational psychology* (2nd edtion, Vol. 4, pp. 485–550). Palo Alto, CA: Consulting Psychologists Press.

West, R. L., Welch, D. C., & Thorn, R. M. (2001). Effects of goal-setting and feedback on memory performance and beliefs among older adults. *Psychology and Aging, 16*, 240–250.

Wheeler, S. C., & Petty, R. E. (2001). The effects of stereotype activation on behavior: A review of possible mechanisms. *Psychological Bulletin, 127,* 797–826.

Yarmey, D. A., (1984). Accuracy and credibility of the elderly eyewitness. *Canadian Journal on Aging, 3,* 79–90.

Yoon, C., Hasher, L., Feinberg, F., Rahhal, T. A., & Winocur, G. (2000). Cross-cultural differences in memory: The role of culture-based stereotypes about aging. *Psychology and Aging, 15,* 694–704.

Zelinski, E. M., Gilewski, M. J., & Anthony-Bergstone, C. R. (1990). Memory functioning questionnaire: Concurrent validity with memory performance and self-reported memory failures. *Psychology and Aging, 5,* 388–399.

Eighteen

Improving the Mental Health of Older Adults

Bob G. Knight, Brian Kaskie, Gia Robinson Shurgot, and
Jennifer Dave

The aging of the population worldwide suggests that older adults will become a larger part of the client populations for professional psychologists. Also, successive generations of American adults have higher prevalence of mental disorders, suggesting that future cohorts of older adults will have a higher need for psychological services (Koenig, George, & Schneider, 1994). In an analysis of the Americans View Their Mental Health surveys, Swindle and colleagues (2000) report that from 1957 to 1996 the proportion of respondents reporting an "impending nervous breakdown" increased and the use of nonphysician mental health professionals increased. These trends imply that older adults of the future will have both a higher need and a higher demand for psychological services.

In fact, research suggests that the belief that older adults are reluctant to seek mental health services is unfounded. Robb and co-workers (2003) reported similar attitudes between old and young toward mental health service use, with older adults being open to referrals from a wider range of sources (including physicians, clergy, friends, and family). However, older adults reported less experience using mental health services. Rokke and Scogin (1995) reported that older adults had more positive attitudes toward mental health services than younger adults and found that older adults rated psychological treatments as more credible and acceptable than drug therapy for the treatment of depression.

It has often been assumed that therapist ageism was a barrier to older adults receiving appropriate services. The early pessimism regarding working with the elderly was most notably propagated by Freud (1905/1953, p. 264), who wrote that learning ceases after the age of 50. Pessimism continued in decades to come with the loss-deficit model of aging (Berezin, 1963), which holds that depression due to late life losses is an inevitable part of normal aging.

However, the presumed widespread negativity of mental health professionals toward older adults was either exaggerated from the beginning or has changed over time. Scientific studies of attitudes toward the elderly among mental health professionals suggested that they

Handbook of the Psychology of Aging
Copyright © 2006 by Academic Press.

are more positive and more complex than had been assumed (Gatz & Pearson, 1988; Robb, Chen, & Haley, 2002). James and Haley (1995) presented clinical psychologists with vignettes that varied the age and the health status of the client. They reported that bias against clients with physical health problems was stronger than age bias. Lee, Volans, and Gregory (2003) reported that clinical psychology trainees in Britain showed generally positive attitudes toward working with older adults, with many seeing it as challenging and rewarding. Moreover, a survey of psychologists in the United States suggested that most see older adults in the course of their work (Qualls et al., 2002).

This chapter reviews the scientific literature on efforts to improve the mental health of older adults. First, we review psychological interventions with older clients. We then discuss the ethnic diversity of older adults. Rather than attributing low utilization of mental health services by older persons to mutually negative attitudes, we believe that whether older adults receive mental health treatment is largely influenced by public policy, especially as encoded in the Medicare program, and so we review the effects of Medicare policy on access to services among the elderly.

I. Current Research on Psychotherapy with Older Adults

The following sections evaluate interventions that have been used with older adults for specific diagnostic syndromes and for other challenges. In particular, we consider psychological treatments for depression, anxiety, dementia, sleep disorders, alcohol dependence, psychological distress related to physical health problems, and psychological interventions

with family caregivers of frail older adults.

A. Depression

By far, most of the research on interventions with older adults has focused on treating depression. Major depressive disorders appear to affect about 1 to 2% of older adults. Clinically significant symptoms of depression appear in 15% of community resident samples, with higher prevalence in various medical settings, rising to 40% in long-term care (Gatz, 2000).

As outlined by several reviews (Karel & Hinrichsen, 2000; Gatz et al., 1998; Scogin & McElreath, 1994), controlled outcome research in the field suggests that many types of interventions are effective with older adults. Cognitive therapy, which seeks to alter maladaptive cognitions that maintain negative thoughts about oneself and the world (Beck et al., 1979), and behavior therapy, which aims to change a client's activities to modify their mood by teaching skills training, increasing positive events, and decreasing negative events (Lewinsohn, 1974), are the most common psychological interventions studied in depressed older adults.

Pinquart and Sörensen (2001) compiled 122 studies and determined that, overall, psychosocial and psychotherapeutic interventions were effective in decreasing depression scores and improving psychological well-being. Psychosocial interventions (e.g., self-help groups, social activity programs) were not as effective as psychotherapeutic interventions [i.e., cognitive–behavioral therapy (CBT), reminiscence, relaxation] in changing self-rated depression. Particularly effective at improving mental health were cognitive–behavioral therapy and control-enhancing interventions, usually for nursing home residents. They also found that individual psychotherapy interventions were more effective than group ones in reducing clinician-rated depression and self-rated depression.

An analysis of the effectiveness of CBT, desipramine, and a combination of the two showed that all treatments resulted in some decrease in symptoms (Thompson et al., 2001). However, treatment involving CBT resulted in greater therapeutic gains than medication alone. Those with moderate levels of depression showed greater gains than those who were more severely depressed.

In addition to traditional individual psychotherapy, cognitive and behavioral bibliotherapies, in which clients follow a self-help book to decrease depressive symptoms, have been found to be more effective than no treatment, but not significantly different from each other (Scogin, Jamison, & Gochneaur, 1989). At 2-year follow-up, approximately three-quarters of the participants felt less depressed than they had initially and half continued to use the bibliotherapy materials (Scogin, Jamison, & Davis, 1990). In a comparison of bibliotherapy and individual cognitive therapy, both were more effective than the control group and showed decreases in self-reported depression with no differences between the two treatment groups (Floyd et al., 2004).

Less research has been done on interpersonal therapy (IPT), a manualized intervention that focuses on one or two interpersonally relevant problems (Klerman et al., 1984). A review of earlier studies of IPT with older adults found it to be effective (Niederehe, 1994). More recent studies have supported the effectiveness of IPT in treating depression and its recurrence (Miller et al., 2001, 2003; Mossey et al., 1996). Specifically, one study found that clients receiving a combination of nortriptyline and IPT had a lower recurrence rate than those in the drug-alone and IPT-alone groups (Reynolds et al., 1999).

Lynch and colleagues (2003) examined dialectical behavior therapy (DBT) group and telephone coaching as an augmentation to antidepressant medication compared to antidepressant medication treatment alone in the treatment of depressed older adults. DBT group sessions provided education about depression and mindfulness concepts and practices and focused on teaching skills in distress tolerance, emotion regulation, and interpersonal effectiveness. Posttreatment, the combined intervention group experienced reductions in self-rated depression, and both treatment groups had equivalent decreases in interviewer-rated depression scores. The combined treatment group showed more resistance to recurrence of depression. At the 6-month follow-up, 75% of the combined treatment group was in remission, compared to 31% of antidepressant patients.

In conclusion, a number of studies have been performed with older adults demonstrating the effectiveness of psychological interventions for depression. Cognitive–behavioral therapy, and interpersonal therapy have been studied more frequently than other types of therapy and show a greater amount of evidence for efficacy.

B. Anxiety

Although anxiety has been studied frequently in younger adults, research on late-life anxiety is still in its infancy (Stanley & Beck, 2000). The major source of data on the prevalence of anxiety disorders in the elderly comes from the Epidemiological Catchment Area study (ECA) (Regier et al., 1988), which has indicated that approximately 5.5% of older adults suffer from anxiety disorders, although exact numbers vary by specific diagnosis. Anxiety and comorbid disorders in the elderly are often underestimated and overlooked (Lenze et al., 2001).

Medication is often the treatment of first resort for anxiety disorders (Stanley & Beck, 2000). However, empirical evidence of psychological treatment of anxiety disorders has begun to appear in recent years. A majority of these studies have used CBT and/or relaxation training for different anxiety disorders. For example, Mohlman and colleagues (2003) reported that cognitive behavioral treatment for general anxiety disorder (GAD) improved GAD symptoms more than in the wait-list control group. With a second set of participants, they adapted the treatment especially for older adults by including memory aids and frequent review of treatment techniques. These adaptations resulted in a higher percentage of participants who responded to the treatment. Stanley, Beck, and Glassco (1996) found CBT to be effective in reducing negative outcomes (i.e., worry, anxiety, and depression), and treatment gains were maintained even after 6 months.

In their version of CBT, King and Barrowclough (1991) taught anxious clients to construe their anxiety symptoms as nonthreatening, which was effective at decreasing anxiety. Later, Barrowclough et al. (2001) compared CBT and supportive counseling, concluding that CBT was superior at decreasing anxiety and depression scores. At 1-year follow-up, 71% of those in the CBT group showed improvement compared to 39% of those in the counseling group.

Wetherell, Gatz, and Craske (2003) randomly assigned 75 older adults with GAD to a CBT group, a discussion group, or a wait list. Clients in the active conditions met in groups of four to six people for 90 min per week. The CBT condition included relaxation training, cognitive restructuring, and worry exposure. At the end of treatment, 22% of those in the CBT group, 39% in the discussion group, and 86% in the wait-list group were still considered to

have GAD. In the two active groups, worry and anxiety decreased significantly and treatment gains were maintained or increased at 6-month follow-up. Generally, outcomes for the CBT group did not differ significantly from the discussion group.

A study examining the use of relaxation training in older persons with complaints of anxiety led to improvement in self-reported psychiatric symptoms, although trait anxiety remained stable (Scogin et al., 1992). At 1-year follow-up, treatment gains were maintained and trait anxiety decreased, suggesting that with time and practice, techniques may become more effective (Rickard, Scogin, & Keith, 1994).

Generally speaking, a number of cognitive–behavioral treatments are effective for anxiety disorders in older adults.

C. Dementia

Dementias affect about 6 to 8% of persons over 65 and increase with advancing age, doubling in prevalence about every 5 years, so that the prevalence for persons over 85 is about 25% (Gatz, Kasl-Godley, & Karel, 1996; Jorm & Jolley, 1998). Although many types of dementia are not reversible, several psychological treatments have been developed to decrease problem behaviors, improve mood, and slow cognitive decline.

One of the more researched interventions with individuals with dementia is reality orientation (RO). Often implemented in a classroom-style setting and with institutionalized individuals, RO aims to lessen confusion and improve quality of life through the use of orienting tactics and mentally stimulating activities (Taulbee & Folsom, 1966). Spector and co-workers (2000) performed a meta-analysis of six randomized controlled trials of classroom reality orientation. Overall, they found cognitive and behavioral benefits, the long-term effects of which were unclear (due to the lack of follow-up data from many of the studies). In a pilot study by the same research group, those who received RO demonstrated improved cognition and decreased mood symptoms (Spector et al., 2001).

Another often-used treatment for those with dementia is memory training, which can serve to increase cognitive capability. Quayhagen and colleagues (1995) noted that individuals who received a cognitive stimulation program performed better than the control group and placebo group on cognitive and behavioral measures. However, the treatment gains disappeared in under 1 year's time. Moore and co-workers (2001) found that their memory training program served to improve scores of those with dementia on a number of recall and recognition tasks, although no mood measures were taken.

Rapp, Brenes, and Marsh (2002) assessed the effects of a multifaceted group intervention that included education about memory loss, relaxation training, memory skills training, and cognitive restructuring for memory-related beliefs for older adults with mild cognitive impairment. Posttreatment and 6-month follow-up assessments indicated better memory appraisals than controls, however, there were no differences between groups on memory performance.

For more severely demented clients, it is important to enlist the assistance of caregivers to implement behavioral strategies such as increasing pleasant events in order to improve the mood of the client (Teri et al., 1997). These behavioral approaches should be relied on when the client no longer has the capacity to participate directly in therapy.

In sum, results on different treatments for dementia patients are varied. Some evidence shows that interventions to decrease problems behaviors are effective, although adaptations to traditional therapies may need to be made to account for cognitive decline.

D. Sleep Disorders

According to epidemiological reviews, up to 50% of those age 65 and older report frequent sleep disturbances (Foley et al., 1995). Medications are often prescribed for insomnia, although side effects are frequent (Murtaugh & Greenwood, 1995). A meta-analysis by Pallesen, Nordhus, and Kvale (1998) showed that behavioral treatments resulted in significant and long-lasting improvements in the sleep patterns of older insomniacs. Specific behavioral treatments have been reported, including sleep hygiene, which consists of educating those with sleep problems how to engage in healthy sleep habits (e.g., Martin et al., 2000), and sleep restriction, which reduces the amount of time a person is allowed to spend in bed and so avoids the frustration that is believed to perpetuate insomnia (e.g., Morin et al., 1993). CBT models often incorporate the previously listed techniques in combination with cognitive restructuring so that dysfunctional beliefs about sleep are corrected (e.g., Morin et al., 1993). Direct comparisons with medications for sleep are rare; however, Morin and colleagues (1999) found that CBT and pharmacological treatments (combined and alone) improved sleep, although those in the medication-alone group did not maintain their therapeutic gains at 2-year follow up.

Psychological interventions for sleep disorders have generally been found to be effective. They have the potential to provide an alternative treatment without the side effects or long-term negative impact associated with many medications used for sleep.

E. Alcohol Abuse and Dependence

Nonclinical samples show that older adults have lower rates of alcohol abuse and dependence than younger adults. The estimates of alcohol abuse in community samples vary widely from 1 to 15%, with estimates among patients in outpatient primary care running at the high end of the range (11 to 15%; Oslin, 2004). However, alcohol abuse remains a serious problem among the elderly (for a review, see Bucholz, Sheline, & Helzer, 1995). Older adults who abuse alcohol are at risk for physical health problems, as well as psychiatric comorbidity, such as anxiety, depression, and cognitive impairment (Oslin, 2000).

In a review of psychological interventions, Schonfeld and Dupree (1995) reported evidence for the effectiveness of cognitive and behavioral interventions over 12-step and social support models. Carstensen, Rychtarik, and Prue (1985) found that a behavioral treatment program for older males was successful in maintaining treatment gains at a 2-year follow-up.

Greater age seems to function as an access barrier to treatment, likely due to health, mobility, transportation problems, and the effects of cognitive impairment, as Satre et al. (2003, 2004) found in studies of older veterans seeking services in an elder-specific drug and alcohol program. Once treatment is begun, however, evidence shows that older adults have outcomes equal to or better than younger adults, based on short- and long-term studies conducted in a managed care program (Satre et al., 2003).

F. Psychological Distress Related to Health Problems

Most people encounter more health problems as they age; 65% of older adults experience one or more chronic illnesses. Rybarczyk et al. (1992) presented important considerations that should be taken into account when working with those older adults with cooccurring mental illness and physical illnesses. These aim to challenge negative cognitions (i.e., realizing that depression is separate from the illness; challenging the client's feelings of being a burden) and to address practical issues. The effectiveness of CBT in low-income and ethnically varied older primary care patients in a hospital depression clinic was described by Areán and Miranda (1996), who found that depression scores were decreased significantly following 16 weeks of CBT treatment.

Rybarczyk and colleagues (2001) assessed an 8-week mind/body group intervention for older adults with chronic illness. The intervention included education on mind/body relationships, relaxation training, cognitive restructuring, problem solving, communication, and behavioral treatment for insomnia, nutrition, and exercise. At posttreatment, the intervention group showed reductions in self-reported sleep difficulties, pain, anxiety, and depression symptoms compared to the wait list control group. At the 1-year follow-up, the intervention group maintained benefits in sleep and had an increase in health behaviors, but improvements in pain, anxiety, and depression symptoms at posttreatment were not maintained.

Rybarczyk and co-workers (2002) examined the efficacy of an 8-week group cognitive behavioral treatment compared to a 6-week home-based audio-relaxation treatment (HART), and delayed-treatment control for comorbid insomnia and chronic illness in older adults. Compared to the control group, the CBT group had improvements in most self-report measures of sleep at posttreatment and at the 4-month follow-up. There were no improvements in objective measures of sleep such as wrist actigraphy for either treatment condition.

While more research is needed on interventions for psychological distress related to medical problems, these early results are encouraging. Evidence supports a role for psychological interventions in alleviation of depression, anxiety, pain, and other emotional distress among older medical patients.

G. Interventions for Caregivers

This section first considers evaluations of psychological interventions with caregivers of the frail elderly, much of which has used groups as the mode of intervention. One of the more robust findings in the caregiver literature is that those caring for a relative feel burdened and depressed (Schulz & Martire, 2004; Schulz et al., 1995). Several meta-analyses have been published evaluating the effectiveness of caregiver interventions (e.g., Sörensen, Pinquart, & Duberstein, 2002; Brodaty, Green, & Koschera, 2003; Gitlin et al., 2003). These meta-analyses, which overlap considerably in the studies included, show null to small effects for interventions to reduce burden and emotional distress in caregivers. A puzzle in the literature on psychological interventions for older adults is why caregiving interventions appear to be less effective than interventions for clinical depression.

In order to further the understanding of caregiver interventions, the National Institute on Aging sponsored the national multisite REACH study (Resources for Enhancing Alzheimer's Caregivers' Health), in which randomized trials of six types of treatments (psychoeducational, supportive, respite, psychotherapy, interventions to improve care recipient competence, and multicomponent interventions) were compared to control groups and to each other (Gitlin et al., 2003).

In the combined results, there was a statistically significant, although small, effect on burden among the combined interventions. Regarding depression, only one of the interventions (family therapy plus technology) had a significant effect. As indicated by Schulz et al. (2003), the absence of significant clinical effects in interventions with caregivers can be attributed to the fact that many caregivers have subsyndromal levels of psychological distress.

Coon and colleagues (2003) examined depression and anger management group classes based on cognitive behavioral tenets. Coon et al. (2003) found that caregivers in both anger and depression management groups experienced reduced anger and depression and increased self-efficacy at the posttreatment assessment compared to a wait-list control group.

Knight and McCallum (1996) argued that caregiving is a family level problem and that family approaches would be more appropriate, in theory, than individual and group interventions focusing on the primary caregiver alone. The investigation of caregiving interventions in a family context has been limited. Mittelman and colleagues (1995) examined a multicomponent intervention for spouse caregivers of Alzheimer's disease patients that consisted of individual and family counseling sessions over 4 months, followed by weekly support groups and telephone counseling for crises compared to a usual care control group. Eight- and 12-month follow-ups indicated that this intervention was effective in reducing depression among caregivers. These benefits were maintained over a 3-year period (Mittelman et al., 2005).

Overall, psychological interventions for caregivers have tended to have null to small effects. While it would be premature to draw conclusions based on only two studies, the success of the Mittelman group and of the Miami site of

REACH (Eisdorfer et al., 2003; described later in the section on ethnicity) suggests particular promise for family-based approaches.

H. Intervention Section Summary

The effectiveness of psychological interventions for many common problems of older adults have empirical support. In meta-analyses, the effect sizes for psychological interventions for older adults have been similar to those found with younger adults and for medication interventions with older adults. In the few studies in which psychological interventions have been directly compared to psychotropic medications, psychological interventions have been shown to be equally effective and often have lower rates of relapse than medication alone. While it is commonly argued that group psychotherapy is a more cost-effective option, the findings of many (but not all) studies that group interventions result in markedly lower effect sizes suggests a need to rethink this assumption.

Another issue in intervention research is the nearly exclusive focus on white, non-Hispanic populations. The next section discusses ethnic diversity issues and psychological interventions with older clients.

II. Ethnic Diversity and Interventions for Older Adults

In 1990, 13% of American older adults were members of ethnic minority groups. By 2030, the proportion is expected to increase to 25% (AARP, 1996). Considering the projected increase in the diversity of our older adult population in the future, the limited availability of services tailored specifically for ethnic minority older adults, and the limited inclusion of ethnic minorities in psychological interventions, there is a need to continue

to devise culturally tailored interventions and to assess their effectiveness in diverse groups of older adults. Within the older adult literature, much of the focus on diversity has been within the caregiving intervention literature, although some research on psychological interventions with medically ill populations has also made a point to recruit and study ethnic minority samples [e.g., Areán and Miranda (1996) and Rybarczyk et al. (2001), both described in that section in this chapter].

Earlier we discussed general findings from the multi-site REACH studies (Schulz et al., 2003) that examined multicomponent interventions for caregivers of persons with dementia. REACH also incorporated a particular emphasis on including minority populations of caregivers. Gallagher-Thompson and co-workers (2003) assessed a 10-week psychoeducational group that emphasized cognitive and behavioral skills compared to an enhanced support group that focused on guided discussion and empathic listening in a sample of Latino and Anglo female caregivers. Participants in the psychoeducational group showed greater improvement in depressive symptoms and increased use of adaptive coping strategies for both Latina and Anglo caregivers.

Burgio and colleagues (2003) compared group workshops providing basic information about behavior management, problem solving, and cognitive restructuring as part of a multicomponent intervention with African-American and white caregivers to a minimal support condition with brief telephone support and written educational materials. Caregivers in both interventions experienced reduced levels of recipient problem behaviors, burden, and higher satisfaction with leisure activities, but no change in depressive or anxiety symptoms. Interestingly, the skills training intervention was more effective in reducing the burden ratings of African-Americans, whereas the minimal support condition was more effective for white caregivers.

Eisdorfer and colleagues (2003), from the REACH team, assessed a family-based therapy intervention, family therapy augmented by technology, and a minimal support control condition in white American and Cuban American caregivers. The family therapy intervention aimed to restructure interactions within the family and between the family and other systems that could be related to the caregiver's burden. The technology augmentation consisted of a computer–telephone system facilitating linkages with the caregivers' family and supportive resources in the community. At the 18-month follow-up, both Cuban American and white caregivers in the combined family therapy and technology intervention had reductions in depressive symptoms. It is also interesting that family therapy alone reduced depressive symptoms in Cuban American caregivers at the 18-month follow-up, whereas whites showed increases in depressive symptoms. This finding could highlight the promising effectiveness of family therapy with ethnic minority caregivers who tend to endorse higher familism values than white caregivers (Knight et al., 2002).

Overall, these interventions from the REACH program illustrate the importance of exploring ethnic differences in responses to treatment. In some cases, but not all, what is effective with white caregivers was not effective with minority caregivers. Even more neglected is the study of the special mental health needs of lesbian and gay elderly and whether adaptations are needed in mental health treatment with that population (e.g., D'Augelli et al., 2001; Kimmel, Rose, & David, 2005). Clearly, far more research is needed before these differences can be understood and implemented in program and policy changes.

Equally clearly, it is important to make such research a priority.

Despite the known benefits of psychological interventions, older adults' access to mental health services have been restricted, largely due to public policy as encoded in the Medicare program. The next section turns to the consideration of these major federal programs and their influence on mental health service delivery for older adults.

III. Policy Dimensions of Mental Health Services for Older Adults

Despite the development of empirically validated and clinically effective interventions for older adults (Gatz et al., 1998), less than one out of every four older persons with mental illness and substance abuse disorders obtains any type of mental health care (Manderscheid et al., 2001). When older adults with mental illnesses do receive care, they usually rely on nonspecialty providers and rarely receive the most effective forms of treatment. This is a significant public health policy problem. Untreated mental illnesses impair functional ability, limit occupational and leisure opportunities, lower health status, and may be a source of stress to caregivers (Administration on Aging, 2001).

Previous analyses of the intersection between public mental health policies and the growing number of older adults with mental illnesses concluded that the policies implemented through the Medicare insurance program were among most critical to the provision of effective services to older adults with mental illnesses (e.g., Bartels, 2003). The remainder of this section reviews Medicare mental health policies in more detail and considers their application within the usual places of care for older persons with mental illnesses.

A. Medicare

The Medicare health insurance program provides coverage for inpatient psychiatric care, partial hospital care (i.e., day treatment), and outpatient psychiatric services delivered by qualified Medicare providers (Centers for Medicare and Medicaid Services, 2004). Payments for inpatient psychiatric services amounted to $3.2 billion in 2001 (Medicare Payment Advisory Commission, 2004). Day treatment care and outpatient mental health service payments amounted to slightly more than $1.2 billion in 1998 (Office of the Inspector General, 2001a). Still, total allocations for inpatient, day treatment, and outpatient services account for less than 4% of total Medicare spending, and slightly more than 50% of these allocations are provided to cover the service use of disabled beneficiaries who are under the age of 65 and constitute just 14% of the Medicare beneficiary population (Cano et al., 1997).

These figures suggest that Medicare specialty mental health service policies continue to fall short in promoting service use among older beneficiaries. Medicare spends less on mental health services than would be expected relative to private sector spending on mental health and substance abuse services, and relative to the prevalence of mental illness among the older adult population (Knight & Kaskie, 1995). Medicare also continues to allocate a significantly higher amount for inpatient care than day treatment and outpatient services, and thus falls short in providing services in the least restrictive settings possible. These criticisms are not new and go back 30 years and more (e.g., Kahn, 1975).

1. Medicare Part A: Inpatient Services

Under the part A program, Medicare beneficiaries can receive inpatient mental health care provided within a general hospital, qualified freestanding psychiatric hospital (CMS, 2004), or skilled nursing facilities. The deductibles and copayment rates for inpatient psychiatric services equal those for other admitting diagnoses (e.g., physical conditions). However, persons who need long-term care for serious, persistent, or recurring mental illnesses are not provided coverage beyond a lifetime total of 190 days within a dedicated psychiatric inpatient hospital. The provision of inpatient psychiatric care for persons with such long-term needs historically has been left to state, local, and private providers (Sherman, 1996).

Skilled Nursing Facilities (SNF) More than 50% of the 1.6 million older adult nursing home residents have a diagnosable form of mental illness, but only 44,000 of these persons received specialty mental health care from a qualified Medicare provider in 1995 (Cowles, 2004). The provision of specialty care has been curtailed even further since Medicare implemented the nursing home prospective payment system in 1998. The Office of Inspector General (OIG, 2001b) reported that allocations for SNF psychiatric care fell from $211 million to $194 in the very first year after cost containment.

Mental health care provided to nursing home residents is likely to decline even more as the OIG (2001b) argued that as many as 3 out of 10 service claims were "medically unnecessary." The OIG asserted that Medicare allocations for SNF services could be reduced by an additional $30 million and proposed the implementation of a variety of managed behavioral healthcare practices to achieve this outcome.

The OIG perception that many mental health services in nursing homes are medically unnecessary appears to be built upon a mixed bag of evidence.

Some practices are clearly outside the bounds of ethical practice: billing more individual therapy visits than could be accomplished in the time spent in a facility or billing for verbally based therapy with nonverbal demented patients. Some findings of lack of medical necessity were based on inadequate record keeping, which leaves the need for care unknowable. Some findings reflected misunderstandings of quality care codified into bad policy: the determination that no person with a dementia diagnosis could benefit from psychological intervention, the disallowance of interventions provided for the patient's benefit but involving a family member or staff member in the facility, and a decisive preference for medication over psychological interventions.

In response, the American Geriatrics Society and American Association of Geriatric Psychiatry (2003) convened an interdisciplinary panel of experts that defined "best practices" for providing psychiatric care in skilled nursing facilities. These practices focused specifically on managing behavioral symptoms among residents with dementia, a primary concern of the OIG review panel. How the implementation of these best practice guidelines will work under increased cost containment efforts remains to be determined.

2. Medicare Part B: Outpatient Services

Medicare part B covers mental health services provided by a qualified medical doctor, clinical psychologist, clinical social worker, clinical nurse specialist, or physician assistant within an outpatient setting. The types of outpatient services include group and individual psychotherapy, testing and evaluation, family counseling, and psychopharmaceutical management (CMS, 2004).

The most significant expansion of Medicare part B mental health policy occurred between 1987 and 1989. During that time, part B services were extended to include partial hospitalization services for persons who would otherwise require inpatient care. Medicare policies also expanded the array of qualified service providers to include professionals other than medical doctors; community mental health centers were included as qualified service locations; and the annual fiscal limit on outpatient services was removed (in 1987, the annual limit was $500). These policies were designed specifically to increase access and use of outpatient services (Rosenbach & Ammering, 1997). However, Medicare continued to require that beneficiaries assume a 50% copayment for outpatient care, compared to a 20% copay for medical services.

Access and use of outpatient services increased immediately upon implementation of the changes in outpatient reimbursement policies (Rosenbach & Ammering, 1997). Between 1987 and 1992, the use of outpatient mental health services among older persons increased from 14 to slightly more than 25 persons for every 1000 Medicare beneficiaries. Changes in Medicare policy are thus the most effective way to increase access to effective psychological interventions for older adults.

Parity for mental health services with medical services under insurance plans has become an increasingly salient political issue at both state and federal levels over the last decade. The platforms of both major parties endorsed parity in 2004. Medicare and Medicaid are often excluded from proposed federal parity legislation, however. Providers and purchasers claim that the provision of part B services will increase significantly. However, research on the effect of introducing parity in other contexts (e.g., state health insurance programs for persons under the age of 65) showed no deleter-ious effects or significant cost increases (Pacula & Sturm, 2000)

Primary Care Perhaps the most critical issue about the provision of care to persons with mental illnesses concerns the extent to which care is overwhelm-ingly provided by nonspecialist providers in primary care settings. Only 29% of older adults who obtained part B services for a primary psychiatric diagnosis were treated by a specialist (Ettner & Hermann, 1998). The remaining care is obtained from a general practitioner in a primary care setting.

The provision of mental health care within primary care settings can be improved. Integration of a depression screening protocol in primary care settings corresponded with reductions in suicidal ideation and other depressive symptoms (Bruce et al., 2004). Case coordi-nators can also serve to improve the provision of mental health care to older adults in primary care settings (PRISMe; Substance Abuse and Mental Health Services Administration, 2004). However, Bartels (2003) cautioned that current Medicare policies do not provide coverage for the way in which care was provided within these experimental models.

Overall, there have been some promising Medicare policy developments Since the early 1990s. Unfortunately, the prevailing concerns with cost contain-ment and cost cutting in health services tend to undercut efforts to adopt model practices and policies on a nationwide basis. Until mental health services achieve parity with health care services in Medicare, appropriate access nation-wide is likely to be an elusive goal.

IV. Discussion and Conclusions

This chapter considered evidence for the effectiveness of psychological interventions with older adults, the importance of ethnic diversity issues in mental health and aging within the population of dementia caregivers, and the influence of public policies on the accessibility of mental health services for older adults.

The accumulation of evidence for the effectiveness of psychological inter-ventions continues and has grown to encompass a wider array of psychological disorders. Clearly, more needs to be done in this area, especially with regard to substance abuse and the more severe disorders such as dementia and schizo-phrenia. Given that the effectiveness of psychotherapy with older adults has been known for a number of decades, with continuous improvement in the amount and the quality of the empirical research backing this claim (e.g., Gatz et al., 1985; Knight, Gatz, & Kelly, 1992; Smyer, Zarit, & Qualls, 1990), it may be time to shift research strategy from the demon-stration of effectiveness to exploring processes involved in psychological change for older adults and whether there are any observable age differences in those underlying processes.

The growth of minority populations is an important demographic change within the older adult population of the United States and one that psychology needs to address in research, training, and practice. With the small evidence base available, it appears that ethnic differences may well make a difference in the type of services that will prove effective. It is imperative that this becomes a central research priority so that services can develop in an equitable manner for all older adults.

The policy picture has been less con-sistently positive in terms of improve-ment over time. The fairly large expansion in Medicare coverage for outpatient services circa 1987 to 1989 was a positive step, followed by trends toward retrenchment in an era of managed care and cost containment for health services more generally. The historical preference in Medicare policy for inpatient mental health services and for medication over psychological interventions seems likely to continue for the foreseeable future without intentional policy changes toward parity for mental health services under Medicare or toward greater priority for psychological interventions. Despite the current focus on evidence-based care for younger adults, evidence for the effectiveness of psychological interventions with older adults seems not to have had an appreciable effect on mental health policy for older adults.

Maggie Kuhn, social activist and founder of the Grey Panthers, said "Old age is not a disease—it is strength and survivorship, triumph over all kinds of vicissitudes and disappointments, trials and illnesses" (Kuhn, 1979/1996). Knight (2004), in his contextual, cohort-based, maturity, specific challenge model, has argued for a view of psychological interventions for older adults as working with clients who are developmentally more mature, members of earlier-born cohorts, often living in age-specific social contexts and dealing with some of the most challenging problems that people face in the course of the human life span. In this review, we have argued that psychological interventions are shown to be effective in helping older adults overcome a variety of psychological disorders related to these challenges. Much existing mental health policy for older adults ignores this evidence base. However, there has been progress in bringing mental health services for older adults into the public debate on health and mental health services. As noted earlier in this chapter, recent discussions of federal mental health policy by the Surgeon General and by the President's Commission of Mental Health have included older adults' needs and services

for them. The field of psychology is especially well positioned to infuse the public debate with empirical evidence and to expand the options available to older adults facing the specific challenges of later life.

Acknowledgments

Writing of this manuscript by the third author (Gia Robinson Shurgot, Ph.D.) was supported by the Office of Academic Affiliations, VA Special MIRECC Fellowship Program in Advanced Psychiatry and Psychology, Department of Veterans Affairs.

References

Administration on Aging (2001). *Older Adults and Mental Health: Issues and Opportunities*. Washington, DC: Department of Health and Human Services.

Areán, P., & Miranda, J. (1996). The treatment of depression in elderly primary care patients: A naturalistic study. *Journal of Clinical Geropsychology, 2*, 153–160.

Barrowclough, C., King, P., Colville, J., Russell, E., Burns, A., & Tarrier, N. (2001). A randomized trial of the effectiveness of cognitive-behavioral therapy and supportive counseling for anxiety symptoms in older adults. *Journal of Consulting and Clinical Psychology, 69*, 756–762.

Bartels, S. J. (2003). Improving the system of care for older adults with mental illness in the United States: Findings and recommendations for the President's New Freedom Commission on Mental Health. *American Journal of Geriatric Psychiatry, 11*, 486–497.

Beck, A. T., Rush, A. J., Shaw, B. F., & Emery, G. (1979). *Cognitive therapy for depression*. New York: Guilford Press.

Berezin, M. (1963). Some intrapsychic aspects of aging. In N. E. Zinberg & I. Kaufman (Eds.), *Normal psychology of the aging process*. New York: International Universities Press.

Brodaty, H., Green, A., & Koschera, A. (2003). Meta-analysis of psychosocial interventions for caregivers of people with dementia. *Journal of the American Geriatrics Society, 51*, 657–664.

Burgio, L., Stevens, A., Guy, D., Roth, D., & Haley, W. (2003). Impact of two psychosocial interventions on White and African American family caregivers of individuals with dementia. *Gerontologist, 43*, 568–579.

Carstensen, L. L., Rychtarik, R. G., & Prue, D. M. (1985). Behavioral treatment of the geriatric alcohol abuser: A long term follow-up study. *Addictive Behaviors, 10*, 307–311.

Coon, D. W., Thompson, L., Steffen, A., Sorocco, K., & Gallagher-Thompson, D. (2003). Anger and depression management: Psychoeducational skill training interventions for women caregivers of a relative with dementia. *Gerontologist, 43*, 678–689.

D'Augelli, A. R., Grossman, A. H., Hershberger, S. L., & O'Connell, T. S. (2001). Aspects of mental health among older lesbian, gay, and bisexual adults. *Aging & Mental Health, 5*, 149–158.

Eisdorfer, C., Czaja, S. J., Loewenstein, D. A., Rubert, M. P., Argüelles, S., Mitrani, V. B., et al. (2003). The effect of a family therapy and technology-based intervention on caregiver depression. *Gerontologist, 43*, 521–531.

Ettner, S., & Hermann , R. (1998). Inpatient treatment of elderly Medicare beneficiaries. *Psychiatric Services, 49*, 1173–1179.

Floyd, M., Scogin, F., McKendree-Smith, N. L., Floyd, D. L., & Rokke, P. D. (2004). Cognitive therapy for depression: A comparison of individual psychotherapy and bibliotherapy for depressed older adults. *Behavior Modification, 28*, 297–318.

Foley, D. J., Monjan, A. A., Brown, S. L., Simonsick, E. M., Wallace, R. B., & Blazer, D. G. (1995). Sleep complaints among elderly persons: An epidemiologic study of three communities. *Sleep: Journal of Sleep Research & Sleep Medicine, 18*, 425–432.

Freud, S. (1905/1953). On psychotherapy (J. Strachey, trans.). In *The complete psychological works of Sigmund Freud* (Vol. 6). London: Hogarth Press.

Gallagher-Thompson, D., Coon, D. W., Solano, N., Ambler, C., Rabinowitz, Y., &

Thompson, L. W. (2003). Change in indices of distress among Latino and Anglo female caregivers of elderly relatives with dementia: Site-specific results from the REACH national collaborative study. *Gerontologist, 43*, 580–591.

Gatz, M. (2000). Variations on depression in later life. In S. H. Qualls & N. Abeles (Eds.), *Psychology and the aging revolution* (pp. 239–258). Washington, DC: American Psychological Association.

Gatz, M., Fiske, A., Fox, L. S., Kaskie, B., Kasl-Godley, J., McCallum, T., & Wetherell, J. (1998). Empirically-validated psychological treatments for older adults. *Journal of Mental Health and Aging, 4*, 9–46.

Gatz, M., Kasl-Godley, J. E., & Karel, M. J. (1996). Aging and mental disorders. In J. E. Birren & K. W. Schaie (Eds.), *Handbook of the psychology of aging* (4th edition, pp. 365–382). San Diego: Academic Press.

Gatz, M., & Pearson, C. G. (1988). Ageism revisited and the provision of psychological services. *American Psychologist, 43*, 184–188.

Gatz, M., Popkin, S. J., Pino, C. D., & VandenBos, G. R. (1985). Psychological interventions with older adults. In J. E. Birren & K. W. Schaie (Eds.), *Handbook of the psychology of aging* (2nd editon, pp. 755–785). New York: Van Nostrand Reinhold.

Gitlin, L. N., Belle, S. H., Burgio, L. D., Czaja, S. J., Mahoney, D., & Gallagher-Thompson, D., et al. (2003). Effect of multicomponent interventions on caregiver burden and depression: The REACH multisite initiative at 6-month follow-up. *Psychology & Aging, 18*, 361–374.

James, J. W., & Haley, W. E. (1995). Age and health bias in practicing clinical psychologists. *Psychology & Aging, 10*, 610–616.

Jorm, A. F., & Jolley, D. (1998). The incidence of dementia: A meta-analysis. *Neurology, 51*, 728–733.

Kahn, R. (1975). The mental health system and the future aged. *The Gerontologist, 15*, 24–31.

Karel, M. J., & Hinrichsen, G. (2000). Treatment of depression in late life: Psychotherapeutic interventions. *Clinical*

Psychology Review. Special Issue: Assessment and Treatment of older adults, 20, 707–729.

Kimmel, D. C., Rose, T., & David, S. (Eds.) (2005). *Research and Clinical Perspectives on Lesbian, Gay, Bisexual, and Transgender Aging.* New York: Columbia University Press.

King, P., & Barrowclough, C. (1991). A clinical pilot study of cognitive-behavioural therapy for anxiety disorders in the elderly. *Behavioural Psychotherapy, 19,* 337–345.

Klerman, G. L., Weissman, M. M., Rounsaville, B. J., & Chevron, E. S. (1984). *Interpersonal psychotherapy of depression.* New York: Basic Books.

Koenig, H. G., George, L. K., & Schneider, R. (1994). Mental health care for older adults in the year 2020: A dangerous and avoided topic. *Gerontologist, 34,* 674–679.

Knight, B. (2004). *Psychotherapy with older adults* (3rd edition). Thousand Oaks, CA: Sage.

Knight, B., Kelly, M., & Gatz, M. (1992). Psychotherapy with the elderly. In D. K. Freedheim (Ed.), *The history of psychotherapy.* Washington, DC: American Psychological Assn.

Knight, B. G., & Kaskie, B. (1995). Models for mental health service delivery to older adults. In M. Gatz (Ed.), *Emerging Issues in Mental Health and Aging* (pp. 231–255). Washington, DC: American Psychological Association.

Knight, B. G., & McCallum, T. J. (1998). Family therapy with older clients: The contextual, cohort-based, maturity/specific challenge model. In I. H. Nordhus, G. VandenBos, S. Berg, & P. Fromholt (Eds.), *Clinical geropsychology* (pp. 313–328). Washington, DC: American Psychological Association.

Knight, B. G., Robinson, G. S., Flynn Longmire, C., Chun, M., Nakao, K., & Kim, J. H. (2002). Cross cultural issues in caregiving for persons with dementia: Do familism values reduce burden and distress? *Ageing International, 27,* 70–93.

Kuhn, M. (1979/1996). Original quotation from *New Age,* February, 1979. Retrieved from on-line Columbia World of Quotations

(1996) at www.bartleby.com September 24, 2004.

Lee, K. M., Volans, P. J., & Gregory, N. (2003). Attitudes towards psychotherapy with older people among trainee clinical psychologists. *Aging & Mental Health, 7,* 133–141.

Lenze, E. J., Mulsant, B. H., Shear, M. K., Alexopoulos, G. S., Frank, E., Reynolds, C. F., III (2001). Comorbidity of depression and anxiety disorders in later life. *Depression & Anxiety, 14,* 86–93.

Lewinsohn, P. M. (1974). A behavioral approach to depression. In R. J. Friedman & M. M. Katz (Eds.), *The psychology of depression: Contemporary theory and research.* Oxford, England: Wiley.

Lynch, T. R., Morse, J. Q., Mendelson, T., & Robins, C. (2003). Dialectical behavior therapy for depressed older adults: A randomized pilot study. *American Journal of Geriatric Psychiatry, 11,* 33–45.

Manderscheid, R., Atay, J., Hernández-Cartagena, M., Edmond, P., Male, A., Parker, A., & Zhang, H. (2001). Highlights of organized mental health services in 1998 and major national and state trends. In R. Manderscheid & M Henderson (Eds.) *Mental health, United States, 2000,.* Rockville, MD: U. S. Department of Health and Human Services, Center for Mental Health Services.

Martin, J., Shochat, T., & Ancoli-Israel, S. (2000). Assessment and treatment of sleep disturbances in older adults. *Clinical Psychology Review. Special Issue: Assessment and treatment of older adults, 20,* 783–805.

Miller, M. D., Cornes, C., Frank, E., Ehrenpreis, L., Silberman, R., Schlernitzauer, M. A., et al. (2001). Interpersonal psychotherapy for late-life depression: Past, present, and future. *Journal of Psychotherapy Practice & Research, 10,* 231–238.

Miller, M. D., Frank, E., Cornes, C., Houck, P. R., & Reynolds, C. F., III (2003). The value of maintenance interpersonal psychotherapy (IPT) in older adults with different IPT foci. *American Journal of Geriatric Psychiatry, 11,* 97–102.

Mittelman, M. S., Ferris, S. H., Shulman, E., Steinberg, G., Ambinder, A., Mackell, J. A., et al. (1995). A comprehensive support program: Effect on depression in spouse-caregivers of AD patients. *Gerontologist, 35*, 792–802.

Mittelman, M. S., Roth, D., Coon, D., & Haley, W. E. (2004). Sustained benefit of supportive intervention for depressive symptoms in Alzheimer's caregivers. *American Journal of Psychiatry, 161*, 850–856.

Mohlman, J., Gorenstein, E. E., Kleber, M., de Jesus, M., Gorman, J. M., & Papp, L. A. (2003). Standard and enhanced cognitive-behavior therapy for late-life generalized anxiety disorder: Two pilot investigations. *American Journal of Geriatric Psychiatry, 11*, 24–32.

Moore, S., Sandman, C. A., McGrady, K., & Kesslak, J. P. (2001). Memory training improves cognitive ability in patients with dementia. *Neuropsychological Rehabilitation, 11*, 245–261.

Morin, C. M., Stone, J., Trinkle, D., Mercer, J., & Remsberg, S. (1993). Dysfunctional beliefs and attitudes about sleep among older adults with and without insomnia complaints. *Psychology & Aging, 8*, 463–467.

Mossey, J. M., Knott, K. A., Higgins, M., & Talerico, K. (1996). Effectiveness of a psychosocial intervention, interpersonal counseling, for subdysthymic depression in medically ill elderly. *Journals of Gerontology: Series A: Biological Sciences & Medical Sciences, 51A*, M172–M178.

Murtagh, D. R. R., & Greenwood, K. M. (1995). Identifying effective psychological treatments for insomnia: A meta-analysis. *Journal of Consulting & Clinical Psychology, 63*, 79–89.

Niederehe, G. T. (1994). Psychosocial therapies with depressed older adults. In L. S. Schneider, C. F. Reynolds, III, B. D. Lebowitz, & A. Friedhoff (Eds.) *Diagnosis and treatment of depression in late life* (pp. 293–315). Washington, DC: American Psychiatric Association.

Office of Inspector General (2001a). *Medicare part B payments for mental health services*. Washington, DC: Department of Health and Human Services.

Office of Inspector General (2001b). *Mental health services provided in nursing homes*. Washington, DC: Department of Health and Human Services.

Oslin, D. W. (2000). Alcohol use in late life: Disability and comorbidity. *Journal of Geriatric Psychiatry & Neurology, 13*, 134–140.

Oslin, D. W. (2004). Late life alcoholism: Issues relevant to the geriatric psychiatrist. *American Journal of Geriatric Psychiatry, 12*, 571–583.

Pallesen, S., Nordhus, I., & Kvale, G. (1998). Nonpharmacological interventions for insomnia in older adults: A meta-analysis of treatment efficacy. *Psychotherapy, 35*, 472–482.

Pinquart, M., & Sörensen, S. (2001). How effective are psychotherapeutic and other psychosocial interventions with older adults? A meta-analysis. *Journal of Mental Health & Aging, 7*, 207–243.

Qualls, S. H., Segal, D. L., Norman, S., Niederehe, G., & Gallagher-Thompson, D. (2002). Psychologists in practice with older adults: Current patterns, sources of training, and need for continuing education. *Professional Psychology: Research & Practice, 33*, 435–442.

Quayhagen, M. P., Quayhagen, M., Corbeil, R. R., Roth, P. A., & Rodgers J. A. (1995). A dyadic remediation program for care recipients with dementia. *Nursing Research, 44*, 153–159.

Rapp, S., Brenes, G., & Marsh, A. P. (2002). Memory enhancement training for older adults with mild cognitive impairment: A preliminary study. *Aging & Mental Health, 6*, 5–11.

Regier, D. A, Boyd, J. H., Burke, J. D., Rae, D. S., Myers, J. K., Kramer, M., et al. (1988). One-month prevalence of mental disorders in the United States: Based on five epidemiologic catchment area sites. *Archives of General Psychiatry, 45*, 977–986.

Reynolds, C. F., III, Frank, E., Perel, J. M., Imber, S. D., Cornes, C., Miller, M. D., et al. (1999). Nortriptyline and interpersonal psychotherapy as maintenance therapies for recurrent major depression: A randomized controlled trial in patients older than 59 years. *Journal of the American Medical Association, 281*, 39–45.

Rickard, H. C., Scogin, F., & Keith, S. (1994). A one-year follow-up of relaxation training for elders with subjective anxiety. *Gerontologist, 34,* 121–122.

Robb, C., Chen, H., & Haley, W. E. (2002). Ageism in mental health and health care: A critical review. *Journal of Clinical Geropsychology, 8,* 1–12.

Robb, C., Haley, W. E., Becker, M. A., Polivka, L. A., & Chwa, H. J. (2003). Attitudes towards mental health care in younger and older adults: Similarities and differences. *Aging & Mental Health, 7,* 142–152.

Rokke, P. D., & Scogin, F. (1995). Depression treatment preferences in younger and older adults. *Journal of Clinical Geropsychology, 1,* 243–257.

Rosenbach, M. (1997). Trends in Medicare Part B Mental Health Utilization and Expenditures: 1987–1992. *Health Care Financing Review, 18,* 19–42.

Rybarczyk, B., DeMarco, G., DeLaCruz, M., Lapidos, S., & Fortner, B. (2001). A classroom mind/body wellness intervention for older adults with chronic illness: Comparing immediate and 1-year benefits. *Behavioral Medicine, 27,* 15–27.

Rybarczyk, B., Gallagher-Thompson, D., Rodman, J., Zeiss, A., Gantz, F. E., & Yesavage, J. (1992). Applying cognitive-behavioral psychotherapy to the chronically ill elderly: Treatment issues and case illustration. *International Psychogeriatrics, 4,* 127–140.

Rybarczyk, B., Lopez, M., Alsten, C., Benson, R., & Stepanski, E. (2002). Efficacy of two behavioral treatment programs for comorbid geriatric insomnia. *Psychology and Aging, 17,* 288–298.

Satre, D. D., Knight, B. G., Dickson-Fuhrmann, E., & Jarvik, L F. (2003). Predictors of alcohol-treatment seeking in a sample of older veterans in the GET SMART program. *Journal of the American Geriatrics Society, 51,* 380–386.

Satre, D. D., Knight, B. G., Dickson-Fuhrmann, E. & Jarvik, L F. (2004). Substance abuse treatment initiation among older adults in the GET SMART program: Effects of depression and cognitive status. *Aging & Mental Health, 8,* 346–354.

Satre, D. D., Mertens, J., Areán, P. A., & Weisner, C. (2003). Contrasting outcomes of older versus middle-aged and younger adult chemical dependency patients in a managed care program. *Quarterly Journal of Studies on Alcohol, 64,* 520–530.

Schonfeld, L., & Dupree, L. W. (1995). Treatment approaches for older problem drinkers. *International Journal of the Addictions, 30,* 1819–1842.

Schulz, R., Burgio, L, Burns, R., Eisdorfer, C., Gallagher-Thompson, D., Gitlin, L., & Mahoney, D. (2003). Resources for enhancing Alzheimer's caregiver health (REACH): Overview, site- specific outcomes, and future directions. *Gerontologist, 43,* 514–520.

Schulz, R., & Martire, L. M. (2004). Family caregiving of persons with dementia: Prevalence, health effects, and support strategies. *American Journal of Geriatric Psychiatry, 12,* 240–249.

Schulz, R., O'Brien, A. T., Bookwala, J., & Fleissner, K. (1995). Psychiatric and physical morbidity effects of dementia caregiving: Prevalence, correlates, and causes. *Gerontologist, 35,* 771–791.

Scogin, F., Jamison, C., & Davis, N. (1990). Two-year follow-up of bibliotherapy for depression in older adults. *Journal of Consulting & Clinical Psychology, 58,* 665–667.

Scogin, F., Jamison, C., & Gochneaur, K. (1989). Comparative efficacy of cognitive and behavioral bibliotherapy for mildly and moderately depressed older adults. *Journal of Consulting & Clinical Psychology, 57,* 403–407.

Scogin, F., & McElreath, L. (1994). Efficacy of psychosocial treatments for geriatric depression: A quantitative review. *Journal of Consulting and Clinical Psychology, 62,* 69–74.

Scogin, F., Rickard, H. C., Keith, S., Wilson, J., & McElreath, L. (1992). Progressive and imaginal relaxation training for elderly persons with subjective anxiety. *Psychology & Aging, 7,* 419–424.

Sherman, J. J. (1996). Medicare's mental health benefits: Coverage, use, and expenditures. *Journal of Aging & Health, 8,* 54–71.

Smyer, M. A., Zarit, S. H., & Qualls, S. H. (1990). Psychological intervention with the aging individual. In J. E. Birren & K. W. Schaie (Eds.), *Handbook of the psychology of aging* (3rd edition, pp. 375–403). San Diego: Academic Press.

Sörensen, S., Pinquart, M., & Duberstein, P. (2002). How effective are interventions with caregivers? An updated meta-analysis. *Gerontologist, 42,* 356–372.

Spector, A., Davies, S., Woods, B., & Orrell, M. (2000). Reality orientation for dementia: A systematic review of the evidence of effectiveness from randomized controlled trials. *Gerontologist, 40,* 206–212.

Spector, A., Orrell, M., Davies, S., & Woods, B. (2001). Can reality orientation be rehabilitated? Development and piloting of an evidence-based programme of cognition-based therapies for people with dementia. *Neuropsychological Rehabilitation, 11,* 377–397.

Stanley, M. A., & Beck, J. G. (2000). Anxiety disorders. *Clinical Psychology Review. Special Issue: Assessment and Treatment of Older Adults, 20,* 731–754.

Stanley, M. A., Beck, J. G., & Glassco, J. D. (1996). Treatment of generalized anxiety in older adults: A preliminary comparison of cognitive-behavioral and supportive approaches. *Behavior Therapy, 27,* 565–581.

Swindle, R., Heller, K., Pescosolido, B., & Kikuzawa, S. (2000). Responses to nervous breakdowns in America over a 40-year period: Mental health policy implications. *American Psychologist, 55,* 740–749.

Taulbee L. R., & Folsom J. C. (1966). Reality orientation for geriatric patients. *Hospital and Community Psychiatry, 17,*133–135.

Teri, L., Logsdon, R. G., Uomoto, J., & McCurry, S. M. (1997). Behavioral treatment of depression in dementia patients: A controlled clinical trial. *Journals of Gerontology: Series B: Psychological Sciences & Social Sciences, 52B,* P159–P166.

Thompson, L. W., Coon, D. W., Gallagher-Thompson, D., Sommer, B. R., & Koin, D. (2001). Comparison of desipramine and cognitive/behavioral therapy in the treatment of elderly outpatients with mild-to-moderate depression. *American Journal of Geriatric Psychiatry, 9,* 225–240.

Wetherell, J. L., Gatz, M., & Craske, M. G. (2003). Treatment of generalized anxiety disorder in older adults. *Journal of Consulting & Clinical Psychology, 71,* 31–40.

Nineteen

Adaptive Technology

Charles T. Scialfa and Geoff R. Fernie

Technology can be used either to adapt the environment so that it is more accommodating for people with physical, cognitive, or sensory impairments or to equip individuals with means to compensate for their impairments. This adaptive (assistive) technology has the potential to increase the quality of life and independence as well as reducing health care costs (Agree & Freedman, 2000; Mann, 2001). Two movements have had a great impact on the use of adaptive technology to increase environmental accessibility. One is the introduction of accessibility legislation prompted by people with disabilities insisting on built environments and services that do not discriminate against them. The second is the universal design philosophy, under which the goal is to create products and environments that are accessed and used more easily by a wider public (Story, 1998). Although both approaches help large proportions of the public, it is important to recognize their limitations. Some people have needs that can only be met by specialized and often customized devices. Also, a universally designed product or environment is likely to be less costly and carry less stigma,

but it is of no value if the user cannot actually perform the desired function.

While technological development is a given in the history of humankind, elders generally lag behind their younger counterparts in its use, at least in technologies developed for the general population (e.g., the Internet). Thus, today's cohort of young adults will likely be quite comfortable in their later years with technologies saturating the market today (e.g., cell phones) but emerging or unforeseen technologies will be foreign to them.

In addition to this lag effect, access to and use of technology by older people is by no means universal. Socioeconomic status, health, education, race, ethnicity, and work status are but some of the factors that predict who will use technology and with what regularity they will use it. This is more true for those who have stopped working or who are living without younger people in the home (Willis, 2004). Certainly one of the challenges for society will be to minimize access gaps so that inequalities in services and opportunities do not become more problematic.

This chapter covers many major life domains for the older person and includes

Handbook of the Psychology of Aging

relatively low-level functions such as dressing and hygiene, but also treats more demanding activities such as driving and human–computer interaction. In addition, because functional ability in the aged ranges from those who are multiply disabled to individuals who are more robust than many of their juniors, we will summarize an extremely diverse set of adaptive technologies. This emphasis on inclusiveness implies that some areas must be omitted and others covered with less depth than might otherwise be the case. To mitigate these acknowledged deficiencies, we will point the reader, in advance, to domain-specific references that will paint with a much finer stroke.

General references on gerontechnology include edited volumes by Charness and Schaie (2003), Fisk and Rogers (2001), Kwon and Burdick (2004), and a recent work entitled, "Technology for Adaptive Aging" (Pew & van Hemel, 2004). For those interested in driving, the National Academy of Sciences and Transportation Research Board has a recent release (National Academies of Science, 2004) that covers many pertinent issues, including driver capabilities, roadway design, training, and alternative means of mobility. Medical issues are covered in works edited by Rogers and Fisk (2001) and Park, Morrell, and Shifren (1999).

I. Eating

Difficulties with eating are extremely common among older people and may present in the form of physiological impairments in the swallowing process, physical impairments that interfere with the ability to effectively transport food from the table to the mouth, and/or behavioral conditions that interfere with the safe intake of sufficient nutrients. Swallowing disorders (dysphagia) are common among people who have had strokes (Murry et al., 1999); clinical signs of swallowing difficulty have been observed in as many as 70% of institutionalized older people (Steele et al., 1997). People with dysphagia are at risk for choking, aspiration (entry of material into the airway), and inadequate nutritional intake; airway obstruction, aspiration pneumonia, and malnutrition are serious consequences. Direct therapy for swallowing impairment usually involves exercises and maneuvers designed to enhance the function of specific muscles or organs in the mouth and pharynx (Huckabee & Cannito, 1999). Texture modification (i.e., thickening liquids and mincing or pureeing solid foods) is the most frequently used intervention for dysphagia in hospitals and long-term care facilities (Robbins et al., 2002).

The simplest assistive devices include some utensils and cooking knives with handgrips that are universally designed to make them easier to manipulate. Alternatively, occupational therapists will sometimes make use of thermally deformable plastics to change the shape of handles of utensils to match the needs of individuals. Devices have been developed for automating the process of lifting a spoon full of food to the mouth.

Conventional orthotic solutions to providing upper limb function have included systems where the weight of the user's arm is supported on a pivoting mechanical arm so that the user only has to provide sufficient force to initiate the movement and balance the load. Motorized upper limb orthotics have also been attempted. One exciting recent advance is the effort to rehabilitate the function of upper limbs following a stroke using functional electrical stimulation (Popovic et al., 2005).

II. Hygiene

Independent function in the bathroom is of critical importance. Loss of the ability to function in this room frequently precipitates admission to an institutional environment. Most of the assistive technology in this bathroom is focused on providing access to the toilet and either a bathtub or a shower.

Getting on and off a toilet is made more difficult for many people by the fact that toilet seats in North America tend to be lower to the ground than most other seating. Ways of increasing the height of existing toilets are to add a raised seat or to mount the toilet on a raised pedestal. Grab bars can be beneficial; however, it is also important to remember that people who transfer from a wheelchair need to have an unobstructed path to make that transfer. The optimum layout in a multiuser setting is to have the toilet placed with space on either side for wheelchair access and to equip it with hinged grab bars on both sides.

The most accessible solution to bathing is a roll-in shower stall with a built-in seat and grab bars. Some people still prefer to use a tub and a variety of designs have been produced to make this possible. Added features might include a wider side that acts as a seat for transferring. Another common and successful way of adapting an ordinary tub for access is to install a lift platform on the inside.

Attention has also been focused on technologies to assist people with cognitive impairments in their use of the bathroom. The idea that computer vision (e.g., digital imaging and pattern recognition) and artificial intelligence could enable the environment to monitor the actions of a user and to intervene intelligently with verbal prompts when needed has been demonstrated to have potential even with people with moderate to severe dementias (Mihailidis, Barbenel, & Fernie, 2004). Even if practical routine application of the technology is eventually limited to milder levels of cognitive impairment, the combination of enhanced privacy and independence for

the individual and a reduction in burden for the caregiver might have important effects on the ability to avoid premature admission to an institution. Mihailidis and Fernie (2002) described the use of artificial intelligence in the broader context of design.

III. Health

Issues related to health, disability, and disease are confronted on an everyday basis by most older adults. Older people are more likely than others to see doctors, require hospitalization, suffer from multiple chronic conditions, be disabled, take medications, reside in institutions, make use of home health care, and visit health professionals. The economic consequences are of concern and likely to become even more so as "baby-boomers" move in larger numbers into that part of the life span where the most expensive health care is required. Ironically, technology has been a major factor in the increased costs in health care, but it can also reduce the price tag by allowing greater numbers of people to "age in place" and by delivering medical services and products more efficiently.

Willis (2004) pointed out that technology is being used by many people to gain knowledge about health. Almost two-thirds of Internet users in the United States (73 million people) have gone online in search of health information. This means that more adults go online for medical advice on any given day than actually visit health professionals. The information they find is used to self-diagnose, confer with health care professionals, make critical health decisions, and facilitate caregiving (Fox & Rainie, 2000). However, the Internet is not a one-way street. Currently, data gathered from home medical devices, "on the body" and "in the body" biosensors can be stored and transmitted automatically to others

(Mynatt et al., 2001) who are involved in the health care of an older person. In a more reciprocal vein, currently a variety of synchronous, multipoint, desktop communication suites exist that allow for shared data, audio and video streaming, group workspaces, and archiving. The applications to telehealth are obvious (Hanson & Clark, 2000).

One area in which technology has been used, albeit at a relatively low level, is in fostering adherance to prescription drug use. Aldults younger than 70 or so are quite diligent in taking their medications (Morrell et al., 1997; Park et al., 1999), but adherance among very old people can be improved with memory aids and organizational charts (Park et al., 1992). More effective instructional design of prescription information may facilitate comprehension and adherance (Morrow et al., 1998; Morrow & Leirer, 1999). However, these methods do not work for everyone and those who are having difficulties with comprehension and prospective memory are particularly vulnerable to errors. One can imagine that, with little difficulty, currently available technologies could be put to good use here. For example, the same bar code readers that Morrell and Leirer (1998) have used to study medication adherance could be used in the home, integrated with personal computers or personal data assistants (PDAs), to store data on medications, check for harmful interactions, present multimedia instruction on loading drug organizers and, perhaps, monitor adherance. An alternative has been presented by Pollack and colleagues (Pineau et al, 2003; Pollack et al., 2003), who have used a personal robot to remind older people living in an institution of the medications they must take.

Technological benefits presuppose a well-informed and capable consumer of health care who is willing and able to use the resources available and here is where a good deal of work needs doing.

Although the reliability of health information, including that on the Internet, is relatively high (Eysenbach et al., 2002), there are no widely accepted means of certification and consumers are consulted rarely in design. There is a persistent mismatch between the complexity of health information provided to elders and their ability to comprehend it. In part, this is due to low health literacy (Baker et al., 2000; Echt & Morrell, 2005), but, despite "plain language" regulations in many countries, it is also attributable to materials that are written at too high a reading level using unnecessarily complicated syntax and cognitively inefficient organization (Morrow et al., 1998). On the consumer side of the issue, older adults are not inclined to engage in rigorous searches for quality health care information (Fox & Rainie, 2000), have difficulty searching and navigating Web sites (Grahame et al., 2004; Laberge & Scialfa, 2005; Sit, 1998), and are less able to generate strategies in solving health-related problems (Berg et al., 1999). Additionally, health care devices such as home glucometers that are promoted as easy to use are, in fact, quite complex and prone to human error (Rogers et al., 2001). In addition, there are issues of access, privacy, and cost, issues that are only partially amenable to technological solutions.

Lest the reader depart this topic with a pessimistic outlook, there are several successful applications of adaptive technology in health care for older adults. One, described by Echt and Morrell (2005) is the U.S. National Institute of Health Senior Health Project. In this effort to bring age-related health information to the World Wide Web, cognitive ergonomics principles were used to migrate conventional text to the new environment, evaluate the material vis-à-vis the older user's ability to understand it, and engage elders in participatory design so as to enhance usabilty.

Another positive example can be found in multimedia training tools for health products and services (Mykityshyn et al., 2002).

IV. Communications

Many aspects of technology treated elsewhere in this chapter deal directly or indirectly with communication. Thus, for example, navigation aids in the car or effective prescription labeling are intended to communicate information that is critical for the person to whom it is directed. The following section discusses communication more directly. The focus is on hearing aids, hand-held devices (e.g., cell phones), and the Internet.

A. Hearing Aids

Hearing loss is common among older adults and can be seen in deficits with pure-tone sensitivity, temporal processing, localization, and speech perception, particularly in noise-filled environments (for a review, see Schneider & Pichora-Fuller, 2000). Although newer assistive listening devices such as phone and television amplifiers and loop systems for conferencing are receiving greater use, many older people attempt to redress their hearing loss with a hearing aid. This is a wise choice. Treated hearing loss is associated with higher levels of social support, less depression, and less paranoia (Seniors Research Group, 1999) and hearing loss is correlated with declines in cognitive function (Lindenberger & Baltes, 1997). Still, many people who have hearing loss do not have a hearing aid and even those who purchase hearing aids often do not use them. Research indicates that many users are dissatisfied with the performance of their hearing aids because they amplify noise as well as signal and may

be difficult to adjust and maintain (Meister & van Wedel, 2003). It may also be the case that older people do not receive after-purchase counseling that is sufficient to use the devices properly (Kochkin, 2002).

Developments in signal processing and the use of directional microphones will undoubtedly lead to more intelligent hearing aids for the future. However, these improvements do not help all listeners in the same way. For example, Lunner (2003) reported that elders with the better working memory derived the most benefit from a hearing aid that adjusted amplification and compression constants to increase dynamic range when speech was detected. Importantly, as hearing aid technology becomes more complex, it will require greater presale testing to ensure the best match between the device and the client's needs, as well as greater training to teach the user how to optimize performance of the device across a range of listening environments.

There are other ways in which technology may facilitate the efficient use of hearing aids. Virtual listening environments that more closely resemble natural settings could be used in both assessment and counseling stages. As well, the Internet provides a vehicle for social support and education among the hearing impaired. Kochkin (2002) reported that many older adults want online hearing assessments and counseling regarding their hearing aids. Cummings et al. (2002) found that an online support group for the hearing impaired benefited users in the development of social support. In fact, it was those who had the less well-developed social support offline who derived the most benefit from the group. This is a wonderful example of how technology can provide access to crucial interactions for those most at risk.

B. Computing on the Move

Tasks that once were available only on desktop PCs are being performed on smaller and hand-held devices, including cellular telephones, personal digital assistants (PDAs), and vehicular intelligent transportation systems (ITS). Just a few years ago, it was estimated that about 46–50% of households in Canada and the United States have a cellular phone and, in some European and Asian nations, the numbers approach 80–90%. PDAs are less common, but their potential equals that of laptop computing (Ipsos-Reid, 2001). These devices may help older adults to continue productive and independent lifestyles but they must be designed adequately to meet the perceptual and cognitive changes of old age.

Many hand-held and vehicular devices rely primarily on a visual user interface to present information. However, because these systems are often portable and used in diverse environments, they present new problems in designing for older adults. Most notable is the reduced screen size and resolution. A typical cell phone, for example, has a resolution of 96×65 pixels, and a typical PDA displays information at 240×320 pixels (Kärkkäinen & Laarni, 2002). Because of these limitations, designers often compact large amounts of information by miniaturizing and crowding text and graphics, thus requiring users to have relatively good acuity. Omori et al. (2002) reported that by increasing font size of mobile phones, both older and younger adults increased their reading speed and made significantly fewer errors. However, because screen "real estate" is limited, increasing the size of text and objects comes at a cost. Users will either be forced to scroll or go through multiple menus to find needed information or developers will need to consider eliminating options and functions.

The portable nature of hand-held devices means that they will be used in varying and degraded lighting conditions that will impact older users who have declines in contrast sensitivity and glare recovery (Scialfa et al., 2004). Although most hand-held devices have luminance and contrast controls, they can be buried deep in menus in the interface, making them difficult to access. Some hand-held devices take advantage of reversing polarity to aid low-luminance viewing, however, this reduces legibility on devices that rely on a monochrome screen (Muter, 1996). A final way that hand-held devices and ITS displays overcome low luminance conditions is by providing backlighting for their controls. Most cellular phones have this capability, but many of the "hard buttons" on PDAs do not.

Although a great deal of information is presented visually, for some devices, such as cellular phones and music players, the transmission of sound is the primary method of communication. PDAs, home health products, and ITS applications use auditory alerts to notify users of an upcoming event or unsafe conditions. Sounds are also used in more subtle ways to provide feedback that an action has occurred. In more advanced systems, voice recognition software interprets human voice commands and digitized speech is used to respond. Given that many older adults have hearing impairments (see Schneider & Pichora-Fuller, 2000), devices that utilize auditory output need to consider their limitations. Unfortunately, there is a paucity of research examining auditory factors and usability, especially in older adults.

Signal compression of analog and digital cellular phones will likely have a greater impact on older people, particularly if there is a reduction in the higher frequencies normally affected by *presbycusis*. Ambient noise is also a concern because the listening environments (e.g., a car or public space) are often more complex and less suited to auditory communication than a private home. Computer-generated speech may be more problematic for older adults, not only because of environmental noise, but also because it lacks the prosody and inflections that aid speech comprehension (Kiss & Ennis, 2001). Voice recognition systems also have more difficulty with older adult speech, perhaps because of its greater variability.

A final concern with small devices is the difficulty older adults may have manipulating their controls. Most of these devices, due to their smaller size, require fine motor movements to tap onto very small targets (e.g., the keys of a virtual keyboard), to press small buttons, or to write with a stylus. The controls give little tactile feedback to indicate that they have been used. Such features, designed for maximum function and minimum size, will present substantial usability problems for older people, in whom motor control shows systematic decline (Ketchem & Stelmach, 2004).

V. The Internet and World Wide Web

During the past decade, the Internet has become one of the most important computer applications for older adults. In the year 2000, adults over the age of 60 represented the fastest growing group of Internet users (Silver, 2001) and almost one-half of elder users access the Internet daily. Communication is facilitated via the Internet because electronic mail allows greater flexibility in developing and maintaining personal relationships and because information can be acquired via the World Wide Web (Fox, 2001). There is certainly great potential, realized in notable cases such as SeniorNet (Ito et al., 2001), for the Internet to build

social support and, while the impact on psychological well-being is an unresolved issue (Chen & Persson, 2002; Wright et al., 2000), many elders report that usage lets them transcend physical and economic limitations to mobility and increases cognitive activity (McMellon & Schiffman, 2002). As well, the future will undoubtedly involve a substantial role of the Internet for learning, job related or avocational, among older people (see Willis, 2004).

Although many older adults take to these affordances with zeal, in order to use the Internet efficiently, they must overcome a number of personal, hardware, and software obstacles. Numerous age-related changes in vision, hearing, and touch will make it more difficult to process computer-generated text, images, and sound (Scialfa et al., 2004). In part, these can be overcome by intelligent, user-centered design, as has been espoused repeatedly but with only limited success (Mead et al., 2002; National Institute on Aging, 2004; Strong, Walker, & Rogers, 2001). Appropriate choice and design (e.g., Worden et al., 1997) of input devices are critical because older adults have difficulty with mouse control, small keyboards, and other data entry tools requiring fine motor control (Chaparro et al., 1999; Charness et al., 2005; Wright et al., 2000).

Even in the absence of disability or disease, the cognitive demands of Internet use are imposing. Both verbal and spatial working memory are taxed because browsing and searching can lead down navigation routes that are difficult to retrace under divided-attention conditions. Attention is also an issue when designers use devices, such as pop-up windows, that are explicitly intended to draw the user from her or his primary task. Prospective memory failures are embarrassing at best, as when we forget to attach a file before mailing it. While semantic memory might transfer from past experience to some processes (e.g., cutting and pasting) and structures (e.g., an hierarchically organized file system) in the "e-world," without appropriate training the potential for transfer is often an unknown to the elder neophyte. Other procedural and declarative knowledge must be acquired. Familiarity and understanding of graphical tools are by no means assured.

These are not merely theoretical sources of performance problems for older Internet users (Laberge & Scialfa, 2005). Older adults have difficulty using data fields, key words, or Boolean operators when carrying out online searches (Mead et al., 2000). They also exhibit greater navigational and search problems when Web pages have a large number of links, are poorly organized, or present information in unexpected areas (Lin, 2001; Grahame et al., 2004).

Many of these problems can be mitigated through appropriate design and others may be dealt with via enlightened training. At least for some applications, older adults learn to use technologies better through the use of advanced organizers such as outlines, preparatory notes, and flowcharts (Zandi & Charness, 1989), incremental, part-task instruction (Rogers et al., 1996), randomized compared to blocked training (Jamieson & Rogers, 2000), action-oriented compared to conceptual training (Mead & Fisk, 1998), worked examples (van Gerven et al., 2002), and multimedia presentations that allow for easier imitation (Mykityshin et al., 2002). Whether these approaches generalize across tasks, people, and domains is an important issue for the future.

VI. Mobility

Let us begin with the manually propelled chair. The ideal situation for such chairs

is with the large propulsion wheels placed as closely to the center of gravity as possible so that the user is almost balanced on them and turning is optimized. This configuration also results in very little weight being applied to the smaller, front castors, resulting in reduced drag. However, wheelchairs with wheels close to the center of gravity have not been traditionally prescribed for seniors and nonathletic users because of the risk of tipping over backward. Simple but effective antitipping devices and recognition of the importance of wheelchair skills training have changed this (Kirby et al., 2001).

Appreciation of the significance of wheel configuration and placement has also come to the field of powered wheelchairs — scooters and power bases. The simplest scooters change direction by changing the direction of the front wheel. The power base changes direction by controlling the direction of rotation and relative speed of the two drive wheels. The lowest cost scooters generally have a motor attached to the swiveling front wheel. This is suitable for travel on level indoor surfaces, but is much less adequate for outside driving where a better solution is to drive the rear wheels, as these are supporting most of the weight. Most scooters are three-wheeled. Much greater stability is afforded by four-wheeled designs. However, there is a trade-off with maneuverability, as four-wheel designs have a particularly large turning radius. Scooters, in general, have much larger turning circles than power-based wheelchairs and are not very useful in confined indoor spaces. The steering column also obstructs coming up close to a table, which is offset in many designs by being able to swivel the user's seat so that he/she sits facing sideways to the vehicle when at the table.

Powered wheelchairs come in three general configurations. The most common configuration prior to the last decade was to place the drive wheels at the rear and castor wheels at the front. Such rear wheel drive chairs have good traction, especially going up slopes, but need to be driven backward in order to access confined spaces, rather like parallel parking a car between two other vehicles. Front wheel drive chairs are easier to maneuver but tend to present more problems in the control of their steering at speed and have a greater tendency to tip forward when braking, especially on a downhill slope. Midwheel drive chairs have become much more popular in recent years, but are not without difficulties either.

Two alternative configurations are noteworthy. Fernie et al. (2001) developed a chair where the drive wheels are mounted close to the center of the chair and are forced downward by a spring so that all wheels are always in contact with the ground. This chair also has the advantage that the drive wheels can be rotated about the center axis to provide the option of sideways movement. The other notable variation on design is the IBOT, which is capable of rising from a four-wheeled configuration to balance on two wheels. Balancing is achieved by a gyroscopic control system. Cooper et al. (2003) found that the IBOT was most useful outdoors where there is sufficient space for it to operate in the two-wheel balancing mode.

Rolling walkers provide less mobility assistance than wheelchairs but are much more numerous. These are folding walking aids that have four wheels, a seat, and a storage basket. The walkers help with balance by providing tactile feedback. They provide a means of resting, as most of them have a seat. Pippin and Fernie (1997) also found that walkers exhibited a social function by causing others to assist the users by opening doors and reaching for objects placed too high or low on shop shelves. They found that walkers were also valued because they encouraged social interaction by providing a topic of conversation. However, studies by Bateni and associates (2004) identified potential risks of increased falls because the frame obstructs compensatory stepping when people experience a lateral disturbing perturbation. The forward/backward safety is also an issue, particularly when transferring into and out of the seat because walkers have a tendency to slide even with the brakes applied (Finkel, Fernie, & Cleghorn, 1997). A notable recent attempt has been made to overcome these limitations by providing a heavier, more stable base that is powered (Slevin, 2001).

Various other configurations of walkers exist. So-called stable walkers (sometimes known as walking frames) have no wheels so that there is no possibility of rolling and causing a loss of balance when weight is applied. However, they must be picked up and repositioned with almost every step that is taken. These actions require sufficient strength and present some risks. The most common compromise is to use a walker with two wheels on the front legs and no wheels on the rear legs so that the user lifts the rear legs and rolls the walker forward. This avoids the need to lift the walker but ensures that it has a reduced tendency to roll away when weight is applied to it.

The most commonly used assistive mobility device is the cane. Research by Bateni et al. (2004) demonstrated that canes can inhibit important compensatory-grasping maneuvers. These studies have also shown that users are reluctant to release their grasp of a cane at a time when balance is lost. This can inhibit reactions involving grasping other stable objects in the environment such as a stair rail, which might provide more effective assistance in recovery from a balance perturbation.

In fact, laboratory studies show that users attempt to grasp the stair rail or other objects while still holding the cane. The message to take from this research is that people who use a cane should be trained to use stair rails and to transfer the cane to the opposite hand if necessary so that the hand closest to the rail can grasp it effectively.

VII. Driving

The automobile is a primary means of maintaining mobility and social connectedness. Easy access to a car improves elder mobility, enhances functional independence, and allows for the maintenance of social support in a world characterized by urban sprawl. At the same time, it is generally admitted that, when equated for exposure (e.g., miles driven per annum), older adults are involved in a larger number of automobile accidents than all save the very young (Hakamies-Blomqvist, 2004). Clearly then, at least for the foreseeable future, technologies that allow older people to drive safely will have an impact on a significant segment of the population.

Adaptive processes are seen readily, both today and throughout automotive history, in older drivers, the vehicles, and the roadways along which they travel. As Smiley (2004) summarized, older people, particularly those experiencing perceptual and cognitive decline, change their driving habits so that they have less exposure to risk, especially at night, during hours of heavy traffic flow, along high-speed motorways, and in inclement weather (Ball et al., 1998; Hakamies-Blomqvist & Walstrom, 1998). The automotive industry, motivated by a variable admixture of profit and government prodding, has improved their product continuously so as to reduce the risk of accident and improve the crashworthiness of the automobile should an

accident occur. Examples include anti-glare and antireflective coatings on the windshield, variable speed window wipers, and day-time running lights. As well, roadway engineers regularly introduce technological changes (e.g., super-reflective signage and rumble strips to warn against driving on the shoulder) to make roadways safer. Computing and the car are now combining to produce adaptive technologies far more ambitious than those seen heretofore.

Three trends are important in discussing adaptive technology and older drivers. First, the automobile will be the primary mode of transportation for some time to come and, with demographic trends pointing to a continued "graying" of the population, this implies that increasing numbers of elder drivers will be on the road, even though in some cases they do not possess the capacity to drive safely. Second, as mentioned earlier, both the automobile and the roadway environments are continually being reinvented with technologies that reduce risk. Third, technology is bringing to drivers activities not related to driving but which engage them while on the road (e.g., cell phone use, Internet).

Before moving to the car and highway, let us consider the older driver. Schieber's (2003) review of age-related deficits in sensory and cognitive function documents many of the changes that can influence an older person's decision to drive selectively or avoid driving altogether. However, there are many people who continue to drive when they should not. Given the rarity with which physician's offer advice against continuing behind the wheel (Hakamies-Blomqvist & Walstrom, 1998), there will likely be increased public interest in developing remediation for those who can be trained to correct unsafe behavior and an increased need to restrict or prohibit driving among those who cannot. However, individualized, face-to-face training is expensive and comprehensive screening tests that assess both sensory and cognitive function are not being used today.

Several research groups (Owsley et al., 1998; Lundberg et al., 2003) have presented evidence that functions such as memory, attention, and vision can discriminate elders who have driving accidents from those who do not. They have also shown that one's ability to process peripheral information can be improved with training, and because peripheral processing is critical to some of the driving conditions that pose special difficulty for older people (e.g., negotiating intersections), this type of work provides a model for delivering remediation via personal computer and for testing older drivers with economies not realized currently. At a more technologically sophisticated level, Porter and Whitton (2002) integrated a global positioning system with video cameras in a vehicle to monitor driving behavior and showed that while older adults generally drove more safely than their younger counterparts, they had greater difficulties with turning, signaling, and inattention. Such an implementation could be used not only to monitor at-risk drivers for extended periods of time, but might also allow for performance feedback that can modify risky driving habits such as maintaining unsafe headways (Ben-Yaacov et al., 2002).

Driving performance is being made safer, at least in theory, by a variety of intelligent transportation systems (ITS) that assist the driver with way finding, adjusting speed and headway in response to hazards, warning of impending collisions, and enhancing vision under degraded conditions such as fog and darkness. Caird (2004) reviewed the small but growing body of studies examining how older adults accept and use these systems. Firm conclusions on their benefits are difficult to make at present,

but several issues arise frequently enough to bear mention. Older adults are likely to use an ITS system if they perceive that it promotes their safety or reduces driving demands. They tend to look for longer durations at visual displays in the vehicle (McKnight & McKnight, 1993), which will put them at greater risk. Perhaps this is one reason they prefer and perform best with auditory compared to visual aids (Liu, 2001). There is the largely unexplored area of trust and complacency with automation that is invariably fallible. If the older people believe that they can do a more reliable job on their own, they will not use an ITS system, even if it reduces risk objectively. Finally, it is an irony of this domain that improvements to the characteristics of the automobile or environment may actually increase risky behavior and mask deficits that would otherwise serve as evidence that driving should be restricted or discontinued.

Moving to the area of in-vehicle technology that is unrelated to driving, the most notable example today is the cellular phone. As with any emerging technology, older adults use cell phones while driving less than younger people. This will change in the next decade because cell phone use among those in their forties is large and growing. Data on cell phone use and driving are clear: Whether assessed in a simulator or on the road, whether measured behaviorally or epidemiologically, driving performance deteriorates while using a cell phone, which is true for both hand-held and hands-free units (Horrey & Wickens, 2004). Some data indicate that older people are affected disproportionately when talking while driving, but even if the effect of cell phones and age are additive, their generally slower responses will put them at great risk, particularly under time-limited conditions.

VIII. The Future

In a field as rapidly developing as adaptive technology, it is risky to predict far into the future. Still, there are some trends, illustrated earlier, that have enough momentum to persist for the intermediate term. One of them is the increasing presence of increasingly complex computers in everyday life. This "ubiquitous" computing influences health, communications, mobility, learning, and growing older "in place," allowing for greater independence but also presenting challenges of information integration, privacy, and trust. A second trend is that demographically influenced market forces will compel various industries (e.g., transportation and housing) to design for both healthy and less well-off older adults in order to maximize financial strength. A third pattern is that both public and private-sector funding agencies are placing greater priority on supporting interdisciplinary teams that can take adaptive technology from the drawing board to the consumer. Finally, there is the growing sophistication of the older adult population that will make it easier for them to accept adaptive technology but will also increase their expectations of what technology can accomplish.

There is a persistent issue of the "disconnect" between those developing technologies and those who work with elders or, for that matter, the older people themselves. Integrative, interdisciplinary applications of technology to older adults will only come about when academics are trained better in technology itself. Also, developers must be more willing to draw from gerontologists and elders as they develop, test, refine, and market their products. This is a demanding and daunting necessity, requiring that each group of experts develop new languages, procedures, and perspectives in order to optimize the process.

One way in which this symbiosis will be felt is in methodology. Most of the the authors and readers of this *Handbook* are unaccustomed to relinquishing the experimental control that augments internal validity but is time-consuming, expensive, and often does not generalize. This is also similar for development engineers, whose focus has been on whether the technology "works" in the mechanical and not the human sense. As Hertzog and Light (2004) pointed out, nontraditional tools such as focus groups, usability analysis, participatory design, small-n longitudinal studies, and the analysis of covariance structures can provide invaluable weapons to the gerontechnologist's armamentarium. While many would nod approval of this view, to embrace it carries significant implications for how we evaluate and fund research proposals, develop editorial policies for peer-review journals, allocate raises and promotions, and communicate with the public.

References

Agree, E., & Freedman, V. (2000). Incorporating assistive devices into community-based long-term care. *Journal of Aging and Health, 12,* 426–450.

Baker, D., Gazmararina, J., Sudano, J., & Patterson, M. (2000). The association between age and health literacy among elderly persons. *Journal of Gerontology: Social Sciences, 55B,* S368–S374.

Ball, K., Owsley, C. Stalvey, B., Roenker, D., Sloane, M., & Graves, M. (1998). Driving avoidance and functional impairment in older drivers. *Accident Analysis & Prevention, 30,* 313–322.

Bateni, H., Heung, E., Zettl, J., & McIlroy, W., & Maki B. (2004). Can use of walkers or canes impede lateral compensatory stepping movements? *Gait and Posture, 20,* 74–83.

Bateni, H., Zecevic, A., McIlroy W., & Maki, B. (2004). Resolving conflicts in task demands during balance recovery: Does holding an object inhibit compensatory grasping? *Experimental Brain Research, 157,* 49–58.

Ben-Yaacov, A., Maltz, M., & Shinar, D. (2002). Effects of an in-vehicle collision avoidance warning system on short- and long-term driving performance. *Human Factors, 44,* 335–342.

Berg, C., Meegan, S., & Klaczynski, P. (1999). Age and experiential differences in strategy generation and information requests for solving everyday problems. *International Journal of Behavioral Development, 23,* 615–639.

Caird, J. (2004). In-vehicle intelligent transportation systems (ITS) and older drivers' safety and mobility. In *Transportation in an Aging Society: A Decade of Experience.* Washington, DC: National Academy of Sciences, Transportation Research Board.

Chaparro, A., Bohan, M., Fernandez, J., Choi, S., & Kattel, B. (1999). The impact of age on computer input device use: Psychophysical and physiological measures. *International Journal of Industrial Ergonomics, 23,* 503–513.

Charness, N., Holley, P., Feddon, J., & Jastrzembski, T. (2005). Light pen use and practice minimize age and hand performance differences in pointing tasks.

Charness, N., & Schaie, K. W. (Eds.) (2003). *Impact of technology on successful aging.* New York: Springer.

Chen, Y., & Persson, A. (2002). Internet use among young and older adults: Relation to psychological well-being. *Educational Gerontology, 28,* 731–744.

Cooper, R., Boninger, M., Cooper, R., Dobson, A., Kessler, J., Schmeler, M., & Fitzgerald, S. (2003). Use of the Independence 3000 IBOT Transporter at home and in the community. *Journal of Spinal Cord Medicine, 26,* 79–85.

Cummings, J., Sproul, L., & Keisler, S. (2002). Beyond hearing: Where real-world and online support meet. *Group Dynamics: Theory, Research and Practice, 6,* 78–88.

Czaja, S. J., & Lee, C. C. (2001). The Internet and older adults: Design challenges and opportunities. In N. Charness, D. C. Park, & B. A. Sabel (Eds.), *Communication, technology, and aging: Opportunities and challenges for the future* (pp. 60–78). New York: Springer.

Echt, K., & Morrell, R. (2005) Promoting health literacy in older adults: An overview of the promise of interactive technology.

Eysenbach, G., Powell, J., Kuss, O., & Sa, E.-R. (2002). Empirical studies assessing the quality of health information for consumers on the World Wide Web: A systematic review. *Journal of the American Medical Association, 287,* 2691–2700.

Fernie, G., Griggs, G., Holliday, P., Pacitto, M., & Wilcox P. (2001) Function and performance of the Rocket multi-directional powered wheelchair. *Proceedings of the Seventeenth International Seating Symposium,* February 22–24, 2001, Orlando, FL; Pittsburgh, PA: University of Pittsburgh.

Finkel J., Fernie, G., & Cleghorn, W. (1997) A guideline for the design of a four-wheeled walker. *Assistive Technology, 9,* 116–129.

Fisk, A., & Rogers, W. (Eds.) (2001). *Handbook of human factors and the older adult.* San Diego: Academic Press.

Fox, S. (2001). *Wired seniors: A fervent few, inspired by family ties.* Pew Internet and American Life Project. http://www.pewinternet.org.

Fox, S., & Rainie, L. (2000). *The online health care revolution: How the Web helps Americans take better care of themselves.* Pew Internet and American Life Project. http://www.pewinternet.org.

Grahame, M., Laberge, J., & Scialfa, C. (2004). Age differences in search of web pages: The effects of link size, link number and clutter. *Human Factors.*

Hakamies-Blomqvist, L. (2004). Safety of older persons in traffic. In *Transportation in an aging society: A decade of experience.* Washington, DC: National Academy of Sciences, Transportation Research Board.

Hakamies-Blomqvist, L., & Wahlstrom, B. (1998). Why do older drivers give up driving? *Accident Analysis and Prevention, 30,* 305–315.

Hanson, E., & Clarke, A. (2000). Role of telematics in assisting family carers and frail older people at home. *Health and Social Care in the Community, 8,* 129–137.

Hertzog, C., & Light, L. (2004). Methodological issues in the assessment of technology use for older adults. In R. Pew & S. van Hemel (Eds.), *Technology for adaptive aging*. Washington, DC: National Academy of Sciences.

Horrey, W., & Wickens, C. (2004). Cell phones and driving performance: A meta-analysis. *Proceedings of the Human Factors and Ergonomics Society 48th Annual Meeting*, San Diego, CA.

Huckabee, M., & Cannito, M. (1999). Outcomes of swallowing rehabilitation in chronic brainstem dysphagia: a retrospective evaluation. *Dysphagia, 14*, 93–109.

Ipsos-Reid (2001). On the run with technology. *World Monitor, 2*, 26–34.

Irvine, A., Ary, D., & Burgeois, M. (2003). An interactive multimedia program to train professional caregivers. *The Journal of Applied Gerontology, 22*, 269–288.

Ito, M., O'Day, V., Adler, A., Linde, C., & Mynatt, E. (2001). Making a place for seniors on the net: SeniorNet, senior identity and the digital divide. *Computers in Society*, September, 15–21.

Jamieson, B., & Rogers, W. (2000). Age-related effects of blocked and random practice schedules on learning a new technology. *Journal of Gerontology: Psychological Sciences, 55B*, P343–P353.

Kärkkäinen, L., & Laarni, J. (2002). Designing for small display screens. *Proceedings of the Second Nordic Conference on Human-Computer Interaction* (pp. 227–230). Aarhus, Denmark.

Ketchem, C., & Stelmach, G. (2004). Movement control in the older adult. In R. Pew, & S. van Hemel (Eds.) (2004). *Technology for adaptive aging*. Washington, DC: National Academy of Sciences.

Kirby, R., Lugar, J., & Breckenridge, C. (2001). New wheelie aid for wheelchairs: Controlled trial of safety and efficacy. *Archives of Physical Medicine and Rehabilitation, 82*, 380–390.

Kiss, I., & Ennis, T. (2001). Age-related decline in perception of prosodic affect. *Applied Neuropsychology, 8*, 251–254.

Kochkin, S. (2002). Factors impacting consumer choice of dispenser and hearing aid brand; use of ALDs and computers. *The Hearing Review*, December, 2002.

Kwon, S., & Burkick. D. (Eds.) (2004). *Gerontechnology; research and practice in technology and aging: A textbook and reference for multiple disciplines*. New York: Springer.

Laberge, J., & Scialfa, C. (2005). Predictors of web navigation performance in a lifespan sample of adults. *Human Factors*.

Lin, D.-Y. M. (2001). Age differences in the performance of hypertext perusal. *Proceedings of the Human Factors and Ergonomics Society 45th Annual Meeting*, 211–215.

Lindenberger, U., & Baltes, P. (1997). Intellectual functioning in old and very old age: Cross-sectional results from the Berlin aging study. *Psychology and Aging, 12*, 410–432.

Liu, Y.-C. (2001). Comparative study of the effects of auditory, visual and multimodality displays on drivers' performance in advanced traveler information systems. *Ergonomics, 44*, 425–442.

Lundberg, C., Hakamies-Blomqvist, L., Almqvist, O., & Johannson, K., (2003). Licence suspension revisited: A 3-year follow-up study of older drivers. *Journal of Applied Gerontology, 22*, 427–444.

Lunner, T. (2003). Cognitive function in relation to hearing aid use. *International Journal of Audiology, 42*, S49–S58.

Mann, W. (2001). The potential of technology to ease the care provider's burden. *Generations, 25*, 44–48.

McKnight, J.A., & McKnight, S.A. (1993). The effect of cellular phone use upon driver safety. *Accident Analysis and Prevention, 25*, 259–265.

McMellon, C., & Schiffman, L. (2002). Cybersenior empowerment: How some older individuals are taking control of their lives. *The Journal of Applied Gerontology, 21*, 157–175.

Mead, S., & Fisk, A. (1998). Measuring skill acquisition and retention with an ATM simulator: The need for age-specific training. *Mi*, 516–523.

Mead, S., Lamson, N., & Rogers, W. (2002). Human factors guidelines for Web site usability: Health-oriented Web sites for older adults. In R. Morrell (Ed.),

Older adults, health information and the World Wide Web. Mahwah, NJ: Lawrence Erlbaum.

Mead, S., Sit, R., Rogers, W., Jamieson, B., & Rousseau, G. (2000). Influence of general computer experience and age on library database search performance. *Behavior and Information Technology, 19,* 107–123.

Meister, H., & van Wedel, H. (2003). Demands on hearing aid features: Special signal processing for elderly users? *International Journal of Audiology, 42, Supplement 2,* S58–S62.

Mihailidis, A., Barbenel, J., & Fernie, G. (2004). The efficacy of an intelligent orthosis to facilitate handwashing by persons with moderate-to-severe dementia. *Neuropsychological Rehabilitation, 14,* 135–171.

Mihailidis, A., & Fernie, G. (2002). The importance of using "context-aware" design principles when developing cognitive assistive devices for older adults. *Gerontechnology, 2,* 173–188.

Morrell, R., Park, D., Kidder, D., & Martin, M. (1997). Adherence to antihypertensive medications across the lifespan. *Gerontologist, 37,* 609–619.

Morrow, D., Hier, C., Menard, W., & Leirer, V. (1998). Icons improve older and younger adults' comprehension of medication information. *Journals of Gerontology Series B Psychological Sciences & Social Sciences, 53B,* P240–P254.

Morrow, D., & Leirer, V. (1999). Designing medication instructions for older adults. In D. Park, R. Morrell, W. Roger, & K. Shefrin (Eds.), *Processing of medical information in aging patients: Cognitive and human factors perspectives* (pp. 249–265).

Morrow, D., Leirer, V., Andrassy, J., Hier, C., & Menard, W. (1998). The influence of list format and category headers on age differences in understanding medication instructions. *Experimental Aging Research, 24,* 231–256.

Murry T, Carrau R, & Eibling D. (1999). Epidemiology of swallowing disorders. In R. Carrau & T. Murry (Eds.), *Comprehensive management of swallowing disorders,* (pp. 3–9). San Diego: Singular.

Muter, P. (1996). Interface design and optimization of reading of continuous text.

In H. van Oostendorp & S. de Mul (Eds.), *Cognitive aspects of electronic text processing* (pp. 161–180). Norwood, NJ: Ablex.

Mykityshyn, A., Fisk, A., & Rogers, W. (2002). Learning to use a home medical device: Mediating age-related differences with training. *Human Factors, 44,* 354–364.

Mynatt, E., Melenhorst, A.-S., Fisk, A., & Rogers, W. (2001). Aware technologies for aging in place: Understanding user needs and attitudes. *Pervasive Computing, April–June,* 36–41.

National Academies of Science (2004). *Transportation in an aging society: A decade of experience.* Washington, DC: National Academy of Sciences, Transportation Research Board.

National Institute on Aging (2004). *Making your Web site senior friendly.* Washington, DC: NIA.

Omori, M., Watanabe, T., Takai, J., Takada, H., & Miyao, M. (2002). Visibility and characteristics of the mobile phone for elderly people. *Behaviour and Information Technology, 21,* 313–316.

Owsley, C., Ball, K., McGwin, G., Sloane, M., Roenker, D., White, M., & Overley, T. (1998). Visual processing impairment and risk of motor vehicle crash among older adults. *Journal of the American Medical Association, 279,* 1083–1088.

Park, D., Hertzog, C., Leventhal, H., Morrell, R., Leventhal, E., Birchmore, D., Martin, M., & Bennett, J. (1999). Medication adherence in rheumatoid arthritis patients: Older is wiser. *Journal of the American Geriatrics Society, 47,* 172–183.

Park, D., Morrell, R., Frieske, D., & Kincaid, D. (1992). Medication adherence behaviors in older adults: Effects of external cognitive supporters, *Psychology and Aging, 7,* 252–256.

Park, D., Morrell, R., & Shifren, K. (Eds.) (1999). *Processing of medical information in aging patients: Cognitive and human factors perspectives.* Mahwah, NJ: Lawrence Erlbaum.

Pew, R., & van Hemel, S. (Eds.) (2004). *Technology for adaptive aging.* Washington, DC: National Academy of Sciences.

Pineau, J., Montemerlo, M., Pollack, M, Roy, N., & Thrun, S. (2003). Towards robotic assistants in nursing homes: Challenges and results. *Robotics and Autonomous Systems, 42,* 271–281.

Pippin, K., & Fernie, G. (1997). Designing devices that are acceptable to frail elderly: A new understanding based upon how older people perceive a walker. *Technology and Disability, 7,* 93–102.

Pollack, M., Brown, L., Colbry, D., McCarthy, C., Orosz, C, Peintner, B., Ramakrishnan, S., & Tsamardinos, I. (2003). Autominder: An intelligent cognitive orthotic system for people with memory impairment. *Robotics and Autonomous Systems, 44,* 273–282.

Popovic, M., Thrasher, T., Zivanovic. V., Takaki, J., & Hajek, V. (2005). Neuroprosthesis for restoring reaching and grasping functions in severe hemiplegic patients.

Porter, M., & Whitton, J. (2002). Assessment of driving with the global positioning system and video technology in young, middle-aged and older drivers. *Journal of Gerontology: Medical Sciences, 57A,* M578–M582.

Robbins, J., Nicosia, M., Hind, J., Gill, G., Blanco, R., & Logemann, J. (2002). Defining physical properties of fluids for dysphagia evaluation and treatment. *Perspectives on Swallowing and Swallowing Disorders (Dysphagia). American Speech-Language Hearing Association Special Interest Division 13 Newsletter, 11,* 16–19.

Rogers W., & Fisk, D. (Ed.) (2001). *Human factors interventions for the health care of older adults.* Mahwah, NJ:Lawrence Erlbaum.

Rogers, W., Mykityshyn, A., Campbell, R., & Fisk, A. (2001). Only three easy steps? User-centered analysis of a "simple" medical device. *Ergonomics in Design, 9,* 6–14.

Rogers, W. A., Fisk, A. D., Mead, S. E., Walker, N. & Cabrera, E. F. (1996). Training older adults to use automatic teller machines. *Human Factors, 38,* 425–433.

Schieber, F. (2003). Human factors and aging: Identifying and compensating for age-related deficits in sensory and cognitive function. In N. Charness & K.W. Schaie (Eds.),

Impact of technology on successful aging. (pp. 42–84) New York: Springer.

Schneider, B., & Pichora-Fuller, M. (2000). Implications of perceptual deterioration for cognitive aging research. In F. Craik & T. Salthouse (Eds.), *The handbook of aging and cognition* (2nd edition, pp. 155–219). Mahwah, NJ: Lawrence Erlbaum.

Scialfa, C., Ho, G., & Laberge, J. (2004). Perceptual aspects of gerontechnology. In S. Kwon & D. Burdick (Eds.), *Gerotechnology: Research and practice in technology and aging.* New York: Springer.

Seniors Research Group (1999). *The consequences of untreated hearing loss in older persons.* Washington, DC: The National Council on the Aging.

Silver, C. (2001). Internet use among older Canadians (Statistics Canada Catalogue No. 56F0004MIE, No. 4). Retrieved June 6, 2002 from http://www.statcan.ca/english/IPS/Data/56F0004MIE2001004.htm.

Sit, R. (1998). On-line library catalog seach performance by older adult users. *Library and Information Science Research, 20,* 115–131.

Slevin F. (2001). A smart walker. *Gerontechnology, 1,* 130.

Smiley, A. (2004). Adaptive strategies of older drivers. In *Transportation in an aging society: A decade of experience.* Washington, DC: National Academy of Sciences, Transportation Research Board.

Steele, C., Greenwood, C., Ens, I., Robertson, C., & Seidman-Carlson, R. (1997). Mealtime difficulties in a home for the aged: Not just dysphagia. *Dysphagia, 12,* 43–50.

Story, M. (1998). Maximizing usability: The principles of universal design. *Assistive Technology, 10,* 4–12.

Strong, A., Walker, N., & Rogers, W. (2001). Searching the World Wide Web: Can older adults get what they need? In W. Rogers & A. Fisk (Eds.), *Human factors interventions for the health care of older adults.* Mahwah, NJ: Lawrence Erlbaum.

van Gerven, P., Paas, F, Van Merrienboer, J., & Schmidt, H. (2002). Cognitive load theory and aging: effects of worked examples on training efficiency. *Learning and Instruction, 12,* 87–105.

Willis, S. (2004). E-learning in current and future elder cohorts. In R. Pew & S. van Hemel (Eds.), *Technology for adaptive aging.* Washington, DC: National Academy of Sciences.

Worden, A., Walker, N., Bharat, K., & Hudson, S. (1997). Making computers easier for older adults to use: Area cursors and sticky icons. *Proceedings of CHI '97* (pp. 266–271). New York: ACM.

Wright, P., Bartram, C., Rogers, N., Emslie, H., Evans, J., Wilson, B., & Belt, S. (2000). Text entry on handheld computers by older users. *Ergonomics, 43,* 702–716.

Zandi, E., & Charness, N. (1989). Training older and younger adults to use software. *Educational Gerontology, 15,* 615–631.

Part Four

Complex Behavioral Concepts and Processes in Aging

Twenty

Wisdom and Aging

Gerard M. Brugman

I. Introduction

Sometime between 2870 and 2675 B.C., Ptah Hotep, Vizir to Pharaoh Issi, wrote books on worldly wisdom. The books — dedicated to his son — contained instructions pertaining to proper behavior and were probably used for philosophy in schools (Erman, 1995). These wisdom books are supposed to have been the source of the Hebrew wisdom literature (Assmann, 1997; Bryce, 1979). Almost five millenia later, psychologists have started to study wisdom.

The study of wisdom as an independent subject in (psycho-)gerontology has indeed a remarkable short history. Even when we disregard those five millenia, it is still rather late when we take into considerion the strong tie with aging present in common sense notions of wisdom and in early scientific theorizing on wisdom. Possible explanations for this late start can be found in the dominance of the deficit paradigm in early gerontology and difficulties in the assessment of wisdom being an elusive construct. At the end of the 1980s, wisdom research actually started. Before that time wisdom was only part of broader theories, such as

Erikson's theory of psychosocial development. Wisdom was considered to be the result of the successful outcome of the last psychosocial conflict, or ego-integrity (Erikson, 1959, 1976). Kohlberg's theory of moral reasoning also incorporated wisdom, albeit implicitly, notably in his theoretical notions on moral development and aging. The last stage of the development of moral reasoning was hypothesized to be a stage of existential scepsis (Kohlberg, 1973). Furthermore, some scattered publications on wisdom could be found (see Clayton, 1975). The actual first steps were made in the form of a historical analysis of the concept (Clayton & Birren, 1980), whereas the first empirical studies on wisdom were directed to implicit theories (Clayton & Birren, 1980; Holliday & Chandler, 1986; Sternberg, 1985). The general goal in this first period around 1980 was a conceptual exploration of the concept (for an overview of studies on implicit theories of wisdom, see Sternberg & Lubart, 2001).

This chapter builds on earlier contributions. It is organized as follows: As the history of wisdom in philosophy is almost as old as human civilization itself, this chapter, albeit briefly, examines the philosophical roots of psychological theories

Handbook of the Psychology of Aging
Copyright © 2006 by Academic Press.

on wisdom. Next, we discuss recent developments in theorizing on wisdom; empirical results with respect to wisdom and its correlates are also presented. Furthermore, attention is paid to development and age-related differences, culture, and the stimulation of wisdom. Finally, we will offer some suggestions for future research and theorizing.

A. Wisdom in the Five Preceding Editions of the Handbook

In the second edition of this handbook (Birren & Schaie, 1985), Labouvie-Vief cleared the way for the study of wisdom as an independent object for psychological theorizing and research, although the term "wisdom" as such was not used and could not be found in the subject index. However, her chapter turned out to be a prelude for the wisdom agenda in the following two decennia. Starting from a neo-Piagetian framework, Labouvie-Vief tried to integrate wisdom-related concepts in the framework of postformal thinking. Later notions of Sternberg (e.g., adaptive function of intelligence) and Baltes (e.g., pragmatics of life, the selective optimization with compensation model in relation to wisdom) rely heavily on this notion of postformal intelligence. In discussing one of the functions of wisdom, or passing information to next generations, she paved the way for evolutionary approaches (Csikszentmihalyi & Rathunde, 1990; Schloss, 2000). Furthermore, Labouvie-Vief argued that there is no guarantee for certainty. Everyone must accept responsibility for his or her own thought and "this can create an obsession for finding safe techniques to secure truth" (Birren & Schaie, 1985, p.522). This element is present in the meta-criteria of Baltes (management of uncertainty) and obviously in epistemic approaches of wisdom (Brugman, 2000;

Kitchener, 1983; Meacham, 1990) in which wisdom is conceived of as an epistemic stance: Wisdom as a midway between certainty and doubt respectively as expertise in uncertainty. Finally, when discussing intersystemic thinking she pointed at the capacity to integrate different perspectives, and as such her theory is the precursor to the reflective judgment theory (Kitchener, 1983). With respect to the relationship between aging and postformal thinking, she stressed that not every adult will attain this level of adaptive intelligence.

In the third edition of this handbook (Birren & Schaie, 1990), Simonton explored the relationship between creativity and wisdom. He argued that the swansong phenomenon, a term derived from Adorno's notion *Spätstil*, denoting the exceptional high-level creative activity in old age, is a manifestation of the coinciding of wisdom and creativity in old age (see also Beckerman, 1990; Dittmann-Kohli, 1993). He argued, like Labouvie-Vief (1985) did earlier, that the acquisition of wisdom is by no means guaranteed among the elderly.

With respect to the possible relationship between wisdom and creativity, Simonton cleared the land for the contribution of Sternberg and Lubart in the fifth edition (Birren & Schaie, 2001). The balance theory of wisdom was presented in which Sternberg and Lubart tried to integrate wisdom, creativity, and intelligence: Wisdom is thought to be the synthesis between creativity and intelligence. This balance theory of wisdom is discussed later in this chapter.

II. Philosophical Roots of Psychological Conceptualizations of Wisdom

Psychological theorizing about wisdom owes much to philosophy. A good overview of the philosophical roots of wisdom can be found in one of the first publications in psychology on wisdom by Clayton and Birren (1980). A quarter of a century later, several psychological theories on wisdom have been developed, empirical research has been conducted, and in that sense it is useful to see to what degree several elements of philosophical systems have been incorporated in contemporary theorizing in psychology. Before presenting new developments in psychological theorizing on wisdom, we will linger for a moment on its philosophical roots.

Taking an overview of the history of philosophy, a global trend in conceptualizations of wisdom can be discerned (Brugman, 2000). The conceptualization of wisdom develops from "knowing rules of conduct" via "living a virtuous life" and having "faith in god" to a more sceptical variant, stressing the idleness of everything, and managing the uncertainties of life (Nietzsche, 1972; Schopenhauer, 1976). As a matter of fact, almost every element is present simultaneously throughout history as well as in contemporary Western conceptualizations, perhaps, with respect to the latter, with the exception of "faith in god" which element can only be discerned in the more "spiritual variants" outside the mainstream.

The next section distinguishes two main approaches of wisdom in psychology: the pragmatic approach (the Berlin wisdom paradigm, the balance theory), focusing on knowledge about the pragmatics of life in service of the self and the common good; and the epistemic approach (theory on the midway between certainty and doubt, the epistemic theory and the theory of reflective judgment), focusing on an attitude toward knowledge.

A preliminary inspection of those two main approaches with respect to their "philosophical roots" reveals that almost all central philosophical notions about wisdom have been incorporated in psychological theories. The Berlin wisdom paradigm (Baltes & Staudinger, 2000), with emphasis on (expert) knowledge about the fundamental pragmatics of life, can be traced back to Ptah Hotep (Egypt, middle period, c.2675 B.C.), author of the first wisdom books, in which wisdom was seen as knowledge about the rules for conduct (Erman, 1995). With respect to the moral loading of the concept of wisdom within this paradigm, the Berlin wisdom paradigm pays a tribute to Plato as well as to Aristotle and the Stoa for whom a virtuous life was the heart of wisdom.

The same holds for the balance theory (Sternberg, 2003): Central to this theory is the notion of "the common good," a notion derived directly from Aristotle's ethics (1970). For Aristotle, however, the good of the community is a more perfect good than the good for the individual. This theory is also tributary to Augustinus of Hippo (354–430 A.D.), who put a strong emphasis on moral perfection (Curley, 1996). The epistemic approaches pay a tribute to Socrates (Plato, 1997), Pyrrhon (Bett, 2000), Sextus Empiricus (1987, 1993), the Hellenistic sceptics such as Carneades (Long, 1986), Hume (1965, 1978, 1985), and Montaigne (1991), and to philosophers of the 19th century such as Schopenhauer (vanity of the world) (1976) and Nietzsche (a way of dealing with knowledge) (Sloterdijk, 1983).

Not all aspects of wisdom in philosophical descriptions can be found in contemporary psychological theories. Several elements are lacking. Among these are faith in god, self-sufficiency, humility, living according to nature, bravery, and duty. However, there is certainly a strong common element in philosophical and psychological notions: Both emphasize knowing how to live, the good life or eudaimonia, which implies assumptions about the meaning of life,

Table 20.1
Four Types of Sages[a]

Polonius	Paternal wisdom: experience, admonition and advice; pragmatic knowledge, proverbial wisdom, traditional; akin to *phronèsis* or practical wisdom (Long, 1986)
Prospero	Magic wisdom: magic, alchemy; mystery, based on esoteric knowledge of the cosmic world
Solomon	Judicial and political wisdom: judgment, decision, prediction; outstanding feature is the sharpness of unbiased judgment based on knowledge of the social world
Jacques	Sceptic wisdom: a nonnormative wisdom characterized by distance, melancholy, irony and doubt; shift from problem solving to problem-finding orientation; frame of orientation is the nonlogical, contradictory, impermanent nature of the universe; it challenges the very idea of wisdom as virtue

[a]After Assmann (1994, 1997)

virtue, and acknowledgment of human limitations.

III. The Concept of Wisdom: Theories

Several theories, hypotheses, and definitions of wisdom have been developed (see Simonton, 1990; Sternberg & Lubart, 2001; Sternberg, 1990) in which two main approaches can be discerned: a pragmatic and an epistemic approach, representing two opposing world views in Western culture, both of which have a long tradition. In terms of Frye's mythopoetic structures (Frye, 1957; Murray, 1985), one might describe the pragmatic approach as romantic/comedic, characterized by achievement and control, and the epistemic approach as ironic/tragic, characterized by a failure to achieve and the absence of control.

Pragmatic theories lay emphasis on the know how of living in an ethical perspective: wisdom is the instrument to be used for living a good life, with respect to oneself and to others, whereas epistemic theories highlight the limitations of human endeavors, especially with respect to knowing reality. They put emphasis on our powerlessness and on restrictions in our capacity to act on reality, if not on "...die unmittelbare, aufrichtige, und feste Überzeugung von der Eitelkeit aller

Dinge..." (Schopenhauer, 1976, p.251) or "the direct, sincere, and firm conviction of the vanity of everything in this world."

It goes without saying that there are more theories (see Sternberg & Lubart, 2001). However, the two approaches mentioned do cover most of the domain of the study of wisdom in Western psychology (for cultural differences, see Takahshi, 2000a,b, 2002; Yang, 2001).

Assmann (1991, 1994) has differentiated among four manifestations of wisdom, which shed some additional light on the differences between these two main approaches of wisdom in psychology (see Table 20.1).

Jacques the sceptic represents the epistemic approach, whereas Polonius, the fatherly wisdom, represents the pragmatic approach. The wisdom of Solomon is grossly neglected in psychological theories, whereas the wisdom of Prospero is abundantly present, however, outside mainstream psychology.

The theories within these approaches differ with respect to the amount of empirical evidence supporting the theory. The pragmatic approach of the group around Baltes, i.e., the Berlin wisdom paradigm, in an empirical sense, is the most robust one, with an increasing body of empirical evidence (Baltes & Freund, 2003a,b; Baltes, Glück, & Kunzmann, 2002; Baltes & Kunzmann, 2003a,b; Pasupathi & Staudinger, 2001;

Pasupathi, Staudinger, & Baltes, 2001; Paul & Baltes, 2003; Staudinger, 1999; Staudinger & Pasupathi, 2003; Staudinger & Leipold, 2003).

The second pragmatic theory, Sternberg's balance theory, is an extension of a more general theory of intelligence: the wisdom, intelligence, and creativity synthesized theory (WISC). Sternberg (2003) conceives of wisdom as a form of practical intelligence. Empirical evidence is still lacking, although Sternberg anounced a large-scale wisdom project aimed at stimulation of wisdom in an educational setting. The theoretical construction is outlined, and research to furnish the necessary empirical support is in progress.

Empirical evidence for the epistemic approach is meager. The reflective judgment theory has yielded some interesting studies, however, which are, because of their sequential design, unique in this research domain (Kitchener, et al., 1989, 1993). The theory of Meacham (1983, 1990) is, thus far, not empirically tested, while there is only limited evidence supporting the epistemic theory (Brugman, 2000).

A. Pragmatic Theories

1. The Berlin Wisdom Paradigm

The Berlin wisdom paradigm as described in earlier volumes of this handbook (Simonton, 1990; Sternberg & Lubard, 2001) actually started in the beginnings of the 1990s, built on theoretical notions on adult intelligence developed in the 1980s by Baltes and Dittmann-Kohli (Baltes, Dittmann-Kohli, & Dixon, 1984; Dittmann-Kohli, 1984). What is its status fifteen years later? As from the start, wisdom is seen as a body of expert knowledge about the meaning and conduct of life. A new element was introduced by Baltes & Staudinger (2000) in which wisdom was expanded with

"the orchestration of human development towards excellence" while attending conjointly to personal and collective well-being. Relying on, among many others, Plato (1997), Zeno of Citium (Kristeller, 1991), Augustinus of Hippo (Curley, 1996), Montaigne (1991), Pierre Charron (1971), and Kant (Honderich, 1995), virtue entered the stage in psychology. The two ways of conceptualizing wisdom as distinguished by Kramer (2000) are present in the Berlin wisdom paradigm: (1) a rare, highly exercised and developed form of cognitive expertise about the domain of human affairs that allows for multiple conduits and (2) a constellation of personal attributes reflecting a high degree of cognitive, affective, and behavioral maturity that allows for an unusual degree of sensitivity, broad-mindedness, and concern for humanity.

Noteworthy is that age, notably being old, disappeared from the model as a fostering experiental context, as empirical research did not support this part of the model: in most empirical studies thus far no age differences have been found (Ardelt, 1997; Baltes & Smith, 1990; Baltes et al., 1995; Brugman, 2000; Maercker & Smith, 1991; Roth et al., 1990; Staudinger, 1999; Staudinger et al., 1998; but see Happé, Winner, & Brownell, 1998; Kitchener et al., 1989). Research is conducted with respect to adolescence as a period in which possibly the "seeds of wisdom" can be found (Pasupathi, Staudinger, & Baltes, 2001; Staudinger & Pasupathi, 2003).

Wisdom is now defined as a cognitive and motivational metaheuristic (pragmatic) that organizes and orchestrates knowledge toward human excellence in mind and virtue, both individually and collectively (Baltes & Staudinger, 2000) (see Figure 20.1).

Although wisdom involves cognitive, emotional, and motivational characteristics, it is neither a variant of intelligence

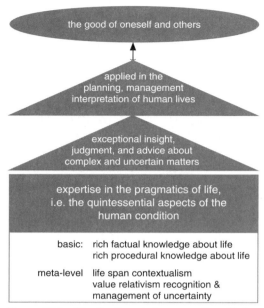

the good of oneself and others

applied in the
planning, management
interpretation of human lives

exceptional insight,
judgment, and advice about
complex and uncertain matters

expertise in the pragmatics of life,
i.e. the quintessential aspects of the
human condition

basic: rich factual knowledge about life
              rich procedural knowledge about life

meta-level   life span contextualism
              value relativism recognition &
              management of uncertainty

Figure 20.1 The Berlin wisdom paradigm (Baltes & Kunzmann, 2003).

nor of personality dimensions that can be assessed by psychometric tests (Baltes & Kunzmann, 2003). In this sense the Berlin wisdom paradigm departs from Sternberg's balance theory (2003) in which wisdom is defined as a form of practical intelligence.

As the management of human lives is part of the model, study of the relationship between wisdom and selective optimization with compensation (SOC) (Baltes, Dittmann-Kohli, & Dixon, 1984) marks possibly a new direction in the research (Baltes & Freund, 2003). Wisdom is conceived of as the theoretical knowledge about the good and right life, SOC as its practical implication.

Although the Berlin wisdom paradigm figures largely in the field of wisdom research, some questions remain open in this theory (see also Ardelt, 2004). First, thus far the nature of the investigations has been cross-sectional, whereas with respect to wisdom, period and cohort effects cannot be ruled out. Second, correlations among the five criteria range

between .55 and .83, which is quite high (consistency coefficients range between .59 and .94) (Baltes et al., 1995). In their analyses, criteria are used as equivalent and compensating indicators: Estimates of wisdom level are based on summation of the scores across the criteria.

This raises two questions. First, as the five criteria do have much common variance, it is not quite clear why the separate rating of the criteria is maintained, in any case with respect to the basic and the meta-level criteria. Second, wisdom nominees score higher on meta-criteria (management of uncertainty, life span contextualism, and value relativism) compared with community samples. This might imply that meta-criteria are not equivalent with the basic, or the wisdom-related knowledge, criteria. As wisdom nominees perform better, this might imply that meta-level criteria are more essential. Some support for this possibility was reported in an earlier investigation (Baltes et al., 1995). Clinical psychologists outstripped old professionals on the wisdom tasks. Clinical psychologists have a large body of knowledge concerning "the pragmatics of life", it is their job. If asked to suggest solutions to an existential problem of a client, they can easily serve up numerous alternatives. It is, however, disputable if clinical psychologists as such are or have grown more "wise" than other individuals. Differential item functioning analyses might shed some light on possible differential meanings of the items for different groups.

Finally, the nature of the existential problems used in the research conducted by the Berlin group is somewhat restricted to "white middle class" problems. It would be interesting to see if a relationship exists between performance on the existential dilemmas thus far used, i.e., triggering Polonius' wisdom (paternal), and tasks consisting of political dilemmas, i.e., triggering

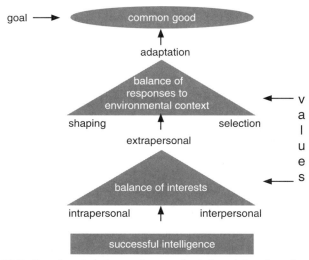

Figure 20.2 Sternberg's balance theory of wisdom (after Sternberg, 2003).

Solomon's wisdom (judicial, political) (Assmann, 1994). Moreover, it is needless to say that knowledge about wisdom in the political realms is badly needed.

2. Balance Theory

A recently developed theory on wisdom is Sternberg's (1998, 2003) balance theory. Wisdom is embedded in a broader framework of cognition and is part of the wisdom, intelligence, and creativity synthesized theory (WICS): Wisdom is the *practical* aspect of intelligence, combined with conventional intelligence — the academic aspect of intelligence — and creativity. Sternberg (1998, 2000b, 2001a, 2003; Sternberg & Lubart, 2001) has been working on a theoretical framework regarding intelligence for a long time. Sternberg (1985) was among the first to investigate implicit theories about wisdom, creativity, and intelligence and had affirmed that people can differentiate between those concepts.

In his WICS, Sternberg combines the academic, creative, and practical aspects of intelligence. Whereas intelligence and creativity are, respectively,

the thesis and the antithesis, wisdom is the synthesis (Sternberg & Lubart, 2001).

Sternberg defines wisdom as "...the application of successful intelligence and creativity as mediated by values towards the achievement of a common good through a balance among (a) intrapersonal, (b) interpersonal, and (c) extrapersonal interests, over (a) short and (b) long terms, in order to achieve a balance among (a) adaptation of existing environments (Sternberg, 2003, p.152) (see Figure 20.2).

Although Erasmus wrote his *Praise of Folly* almost 500 years ago (Erasmus, 2004) and despite the existence of the Russian *yurodivy*, or holy fool, Sternberg considers foolishness as the absence of wisdom. Foolish people are susceptible to four fallacies of thinking: egocentrism, omniscience, omnipotence, and invulnerability. Wise people are supposed to be free of these forms of bias.

The core concept in the balance theory is *tacit knowledge* (Sternberg, 2001). Formal knowledge can be relevant to wise judgments, but the stuff of tacit knowledge is "when to apply this knowledge, where to apply it, how to apply it, to whom to apply it, even why to apply it" (Sternberg, 2003, p.155).

Finally, being based on successful intelligence, Sternberg (2000) considers wisdom as a form of giftedness. In other words, wisdom is a rare phenomenon. This fits nicely into the final sentence of one of the first publications on wisdom in psychology by Clayton: "... where are the wise men? Have they ever existed?" (1975, p.128). Several elements in this definition deserve attention. *First*, like the Berlin wisdom paradigm, it has an explicit *moral* loading, notably striving for the common good, comparable to Kohlberg's fifth stage of moral reasoning and to the notion that wisdom is used for the good of oneself and others (Pasupathi, Staudinger, & Baltes, 2001). This moral loading may, however, pose a problem for assessment, as different people may have different perceptions about what can be considered as "common good." Sternberg (2003) argues that a terrorist can be everything but wise. However, one might assume that a terrorist considers his suicidal attack to be an action serving his own version of the common good. Moreover, his or, for that matter, her sacrifice might exemplify a balance between interests in the realms Sternberg mentions. What the terrorist considers as good is, however, considered as evil in other cultures and vice versa. Actually, this follows directly from Baltes' meta-criterium of value relativism: The wise person acknowledges that values can vary over time and cultures. As a result, the prototypical terrorist Sternberg mentions is perhaps not wise, but for another reason. What renders the terrorist unwise from an epistemic perspective is that he is acting on the basis of some absolute truth. Therefore, he is neither a good manager of uncertainties nor does he exhibit the necessary value relativism. A doubtful terrorist is a contradiction in terms. Too much emphasis on your own

"truth," be it with respect to religion or political systems, does not take into account the possibility of other "truths."

Second, a core element in the definition is the *balance* between several realms of interests, thereby deviating from Aristotle's (1970) notion of the primacy of the common good over the good for the individual. Here too, an assessment problem may arise: A balance of interests can only be assessed by looking for consensus among judges about the degree in which a decision is balanced. It forms a threat for the reliability, as well as for the validity of wisdom assessment. The same problem hampers the epistemic theory of Meacham (see the next paragraph) in which the concept of balance is also vital. Results of the project based on the balance theory will perhaps give a decisive answer.

B. Epistemic Theories: Wisdom as Expertise in Uncertainty

Although notions such as management of uncertainty are part of the wisdom theories discussed earlier, as is the case for the Berlin wisdom paradigm (Baltes & Smith, 1990), uncertainty constitutes the very center of the approach of wisdom found in epistemic theories.

1. Meacham

Meacham was among the first psychologists to focus on one's attitude toward knowledge as the pivotal element in wisdom (1983, 1990; see also Sternberg & Lubart, 2001; Simonton, 1990). His point of departure is the assumption that in individuals there is a specific ratio between what one knows and what one knows, one does not know. The position on these two dimensions can change and when they change unevenly, this affects the ratio between the two. A child knows relatively less than an adult, but when the child is sufficiently aware of the fact that much more is to be known, the ratio [knowing/knowing what one does not know] can be smaller than that of the adult who is convinced that what he knows is almost everything that can be known. When a child grows older and acquires more knowledge and is convinced that what is still to be known grows disproportionally, the ratio will get even smaller. Montaigne's *Que sçay-je* (1580/1991) is a good reflection of such a small ratio.

For Meacham, wisdom consists of finding a balance between certainty and doubt or finding the hypothetical midway between the two. Too much doubt or certainty is incompatible with wisdom. With respect to old age, Meacham argues that, because of an impressive accumulation of knowledge gathered throughout life, this may result in an increase of confidence in one's knowledge or one's certainty; in other words, loss of wisdom. However, negative life events may lead to a decrease in confidence, i.e., to an increase of doubt, which also implies loss of wisdom.

His wisdom model consists of two dimensions: the age-independent core of wisdom, or the balance between certainty and doubt, and an age-dependent dimension, labeled quality, or the profoundness of wisdom (more or less akin to the basic criteria from the Berlin wisdom paradigm and to the tacit knowledge from Sternberg's balance theory). In this view, people are born wise and most of them lose it with time. Although the theory is quite daring, it has not, thus far, resulted in empirical investigations, likely because concepts such as *midway* or *balance* are difficult to operationalize. Yet, one of his — notably for that early period of wisdom research — daring hypotheses — wisdom is unrelated to age — has been strongly supported by research conducted in the framework of theories with competing assumptions.

2. Kitchener: Reflective Judgment Theory

An early theory on a wisdom-related field, the reflective judgment theory, was developed by Kitchener (1983). Although the theory is not about wisdom per se (Kitchener & Brenner, 1990), it fits well into the epistemic paradigm in which wisdom is defined as an attitude toward knowledge (Meacham, 1990).

The reflective judgment theory is a stage theory on the development of one's epistemic stance. In seven stages the individual develops from just accepting knowledge with no inclination to justify it to the final stage in which knowledge is constructed via a process of reasonable inquiry into generalizable conjectures about the problem, while the justification of knowledge is probabilistic and proceeds via evidence and argument using generalizable criteria (see Table 20.2). This last stage is akin to the scepticism of the third Academy of Carneades (214–219 B.C.). Carneades is described by Philo of Larissa as a modest sceptic with a fallibilist philosophy (Brittain, 2001; Hankinson, 1995; Long, 1986).

We discuss later her perspective regarding the development and stimulation of reflective judgment. Meanwhile, it can be concluded that her theory and research are ahead of the dominant Berlin wisdom paradigm, which, after assuming that old age constitutes a fostering experiental context (Baltes & Smith, 1990), focused only recently (Pasupathi, Staudinger, & Baltes, 2001) on adolescence as the period in which the "seeds of wisdom" are to be found.

Table 20.2
Kitchener's Stages of Reflective Judgment (1983)

View on knowledge	Concept of justification
1. Knowledge simply exists	No justification needed
2. Knowledge is absolutely certain	Beliefs are unjustified or justified by authority
3. Knowledge is absolutely certain or temporarily uncertain	Justification by authority; when this is not possible, then intuition will do
4. Knowledge is idiosyncratic	Justification by idiosyncratic reasons
5. Knowledge is contextual and subjective	Justification in particular context via rules of inquiry for that context
6. Knowledge is personally constructed via evaluations of evidence, opinions of others, etc.	Justification by comparing evidence on different sides of an issue and across contexts and then constructing solutions evaluated by personal criteria
7. Knowledge is constructed via a process of reasonable inquiry into generalizable conjectures about the problem	Probabilistic justification via evidence and argument using generalizable criteria

3. Epistemic Wisdom Theory

This theory originates in the sceptic tradition in the Hellenistic philosophy (Hankinson, 1995), but later developments in the sceptic tradition have also been incorporated in the theory, notably the writings of David Hume (1974, 1978, 1985). The epistemic wisdom theory (Brugman, 2000) departs from Hellenistic scepticism, grounded by Pyrrhon of Elis (Bett, 2000; Burnyeat & Frede, 1997; Floridi, 2002; Hankinson, 1995; Sextus Empiricus, 1993). The core of this Hellenistic sceptism, as passed down by Sextus Empiricus in the second century, six centuries after the original form of the theory was devised by Pyrrhon of Elis (365–275 B.C.), consists of *suspending judgment*, or "epochè". For the Pyrrhonian sceptics the only way leading to eudaimonia, or the good life, was to be found in a specific epistemological stance, mirrored in the sceptical sequence: Given an argument, sceptics were always looking for counter arguments (opposition), without being able to decide which of the two was the better (isosthenia), leading to suspending judgment (epochè). This would lead to "ataraxia," or tranquility of mind, finally resulting in "adoxastos," or living without beliefs. "Adoxastos" was considered to be the ultimate source of eudaimonia, or the good life.

Characteristic for the skeptics was (a) their passionate quest for truth, (b) their acknowledgment of the obstacles lying on the road to truth, and (c) their attempt to relate their epistemological stance to fundamental questions of conduct in life and, for that matter, eudaimonia, or the good life (Burnyeat & Frede, 1997; Hankinson, 1995). All the steps in this sequence can be connected with psychological prerequisites. *Investigation* requires openness to new experiences and a minimal level of intelligence, whereas for *opposition*, dialectical thinking is appropriate.

Departing from this skeptical sequence, a model is developed in which three components can be discerned: meta-cognition, personality/affect, and behavior (see Figure 20.3).

The core of wisdom is *acknowledging uncertainty*, which fosters a more flexible attitude toward information. This renders the individual invulnerable to clinging to fixed ideas, which are often the cause of conflicts within the person, and between persons, nations, or ethnic

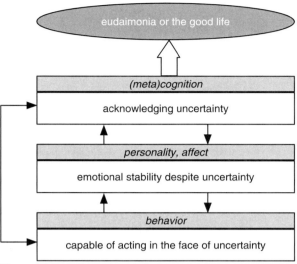

Figure 20.3 Epistemic wisdom model (Brugman, 2000).

groups. Furthermore, it enables a more effective approach to the complexities of life by not putting it in a mental straitjacket. However, acknowledgment of uncertainty is not sufficient. Two other components, the personality/affect component and the behavioral component, must be considered as necessary conditions as well.

Similar to the Berlin wisdom paradigm, personality factors and affect are vital for wisdom. As mentioned earlier, according to Labouvie-Vief (1985) people tend to cling to fixed ideas in the search for certainty out of fear of the unknown, and of uncertainty because this implies the impossibility to predict outcomes, thereby implying loss of control. As a result, emotional stability is necessary for the individual to cope effectively with uncertainties and to be resigned to unpredictability or the loss of control (Brugman, 2000; Paul & Baltes, 2003; Staudinger et al., 1998).

Furthermore, openness to new experiences is needed. Fixed notions, clinging to certainties, precludes looking for (often) contradictory information. Moreover, openness to new experiences goes with tolerance for ambiguity (Brugman, 1996), a characteristic that is an important element in the notion of dialectical thinking (Riegel, 1973). Empirical evidence supports the notion that wisdom and openness are moderately associated in young and older adults (Kramer, 2000). Brugman (2000) reported significant correlations between .27 and .41, with Staudinger and colleagues (1998) reporting a correlation of .25.

The third component is behavioral in nature (agògè), notably being capable of acting in the face of uncertainty. One of the arguments against scepticism has always been that it implies inertia (Weintraub, 1997). What is the use of acting if one is not certain about one's knowledge about reality. A nice illustration of Cratylus (c.400 B.C.) is given by Ayer (1971). Cratylus decided never to make a statement whose truth he could not be certain. In the end he was reduced to wagging his finger. According to Bertrand Russell the task of philosophy is teaching "how to live without certainty, and yet without being paralysed by hesitation..." (1994, p. 14). Several solutions for this problem have been suggested (DeRose & Warfield, 1999; Hankinson, 1995; Mates, 1996; Norton, 1993; Sextus Empiricus, 1993; Unger, 1975, 1984; Vogt, 1998; Williams, 1996). The Hellenistic sceptics offered a simple solution: Act according to *appearances* (azètètos), without making any definite statements about the nature of reality, living a life without commitments. David Hume (1740/1978) did find his way out by means of *biperspectivalism*: As philosophical reflection and common sense are irreconcilable, we have no other choice than to oscillate between them. When we act, we have to detach ourselves from philosophical reflection (see also Williams, 1996). Finally, Vaihinger (1927/1986) argued that the only possibility to escape inertia is to make use of deliberate *fictions*: in other words, we have to act *as if*.

Only partial empirical support for the epistemic wisdom theory is available. A questionnaire (see Table 20.3), devised to assess epistemic wisdom, correlated significantly with well-being and with openness to new experience in samples of young and old subjects, albeit the relationship with emotional stability did not reach significance (Brugman, 2000).

C. Preliminary Conclusion about Epistemic Theories

In sum, the Berlin wisdom paradigm defines wisdom as expertise in the pragmatics of life serving the good of oneself and others. The balance theory assumes that high-level practical intelligence serves to balance different types of interests in order to reach a common good. The epistemic theories, finally, conceive of wisdom as an epistemical, notably sceptical attitude toward knowledge, serving eudaimonia or the good life, by leading to tranquility of mind, to cautiousness in judgments, and carefully balancing the pros and cons of different perspectives.

The main differences between pragmatic and epistemic approaches are the status of (1) knowledge and (2) virtue. For the pragmatic theories, (expert-) knowledge or tacit knowlegde about the pragmatics of life is vital to wisdom. The epistemic theories, however, emphasize the attitude toward knowledge. Virtue, finally, is the core of the pragmatic theories and is absent in the epistemic theories.

Although descriptions of wisdom differ in many respects, several common elements can be distracted.

1. In the realm of cognition, the concept of *uncertainty* is ubiquitous in the numerous theories, except in the balance theory. It is explicitly present in the epistemic wisdom theories and in the Berlin wisdom paradigm, as one of the wisdom criteria is "management of uncertainty." It is also implicitly present in the Berlin wisdom paradigm, as wisdom refers to dealing with important life problems, and those problems are inherently ill-defined problems (see also Dittmann-Kohli, 1984).

2. Almost all wisdom theories imply *personal well-being* as a result of wisdom, notwithstanding Brecht's sigh that 'Beneidenswert, wer frei davon!' (Those who are free from wisdom are to be envied) (Brecht, 1981, p.1119) and a lamentation in the bible: 'If my fate is the same as that of a fool, what was my wisdom for. And in this way, I had to conclude that wisdom is idle too' (Ecclesiastes, 2–15).

3. The relationship with personality, notably with openness to new experience, is emphasized in the epistemic theory and in the Berlin wisdom paradigm.

Table 20.3

Overview of Instruments for the Assessment of Wisdom

Assessment type	Author(s)	Description	a/interrater reliability	Validity, relationship with other constructs
Scoring responses on vignettes for wisdom-related criteria	Baltes (Pasupathi, Staudinger, & Baltes, 2001)	Wisdom-related dilemmas (e.g., how to respond to call from friend who says he wants to commit suicide)	Interrater reliability: 0.59/0.94a = 0.51/0.56	Higher performance by wisdom nominees compared with non nominees (Baltes et al., 1995; Mearcker, Böhmig, & Staudinger, 1998)
	Sternberg (2003);	24 vignettes (// BWP)	In progress	In progress
	Kitchener et al. (1989, 1993)	Reflective judgment interview: seven questions about four ill-structured social/physical science problems	Interrater reliability: 0.78 test–retest reliability (over a 3-month interval): 0.71/0.83 ?a = 0.62/0.96	
Questionnaires	Brugman (2000)	Epistemic cognition questionnaire: 15-item scale of three components: meta-cognitive, personality, and behavior	a = 0.67	Associated with well-being and openness to experience
	Webster (2003)	Self-assessed wisdom scale: 30 items assessing five interrelated dimensions of wisdom	a = 0.78	Associated with generative and ego-integrity measures
	Jason et al. (2001)	Foundational value scale: 5 components: harmony, warmth, intelligence, nature, and spiritual	Adequate internal and test/retest reliability	
	Perry et al. (2002)	Adolescent wisdom scale: self-rating of 23 attributes associated with wisdom	High internal consistency	Associated with less involvement with alcohol use, cigarette use, and violent behaviors
Indirect measures	Happé, Winner, & Brownell (1998);	Theory of mind tasks (versus control tasks and jumbled text fragments)	no data	
	Ardelt (1997)	Haan's ego ratings/California 100 item Q-sort deck	Interrater reliability 0.51/0.62	

4. Most theories hypothesize that the seeds of wisdom are to be found in adolescence and early adulthood.

IV. Empirical Research

Since the last edition of this handbook (Birren & Schaie, 2001) there has been a steady stream of empirical publications, especially by the Berlin wisdom paradigm group (Aspinwall & Staudinger, 2003; Baltes & Freund, 2003a,b; Baltes, Glück, & Kunzmann, 2002; Baltes & Kunzmann, 2003; Kunzmann & Baltes, 2003a,b; Pasupathi, Staudinger, & Baltes, 2001; Paul & Baltes, 2003; Staudinger & Leipold, 2003; Staudinger & Pasupathi, 2003) and theoretical publications around the balance theory (Halpern, 2001; Kuhn & Udell, 2001; Paris, 2001; Sternberg, 2000a,b, 2001a,b,c, 2003). There are some empirical and theoretical contributions stemming from the epistemic theories.

Before discussing research with respect to correlates of wisdom, developmental aspects, education for wisdom, and culture, we first discuss some of the instruments used thus far to measure wisdom and wisdom-related variables, categorized according to their theoretical rationale (for an overview, see Table 20.3).

A. Assessment

1. Pragmatic Approach

In the *Berlin wisdom paradigm* (Baltes & Smith, 1990), subjects are requested to comment on hypothetical existential problems. An example of such a wisdom-related dilemma is: "In thinking over his or her life, a person realizes that he or she has not achieved all he or she once imagined. What could one or the person do and think in such a situation?" (Pasupathi, Staudinger, & Baltes, 2001, p. 354).

Comments given by the subject are scored by trained raters on five wisdom criteria, two basic criteria: (1) rich factual knowledge, (2) rich procedural knowledge and three meta-level ones, (3) relativity, (4) uncertainty management, and (5) life span contextualism.

Sternberg reported (2003) that with respect to instruments to assess wisdom in the framework of the *balance theory*, work is in progress. The instrument consists of 26 life problems. Based on an example provided, these problems are very much like those used by the Berlin wisdom paradigm: Moral dilemmas of the Prospero or garden-variety type, e.g., making a choice between love and career. No indications are given, thus far, about scoring of the protocols, e.g., with respect to the *balance* among intra-, inter-, and extrapersonal interests.

2. The Epistemic Approach

In the *reflective judgement interview* (Kitchener, 1983; Kitchener et al., 1989, 1993), subjects have to respond to a standard set of seven questions about four ill-structured problems from the social and physical sciences, e.g., problems about the safety of chemical additives to food or the building of the pyramids.

The responses are scored, i.e., estimating the stage that appears in the response (see Table 20.2), by certified raters, using scoring rules developed by Kitchener and King (1985).

The *epistemic cognition questionnaire* (ECQ15) (Brugman, 2000) is an instrument devised to assess wisdom, conceived as expertise in uncertainty. By means of PCA, three basic epistemic elements of wisdom could be extracted: (1) acknowledgment of ungraspability of reality, (2) adoxastos or tranquility of mind, and (3) being able to act despite uncertainty.

3. Miscellaneous

Other instruments have been developed outside the two approaches outlined earlier. Departing from Clayton and Birren's (1980) notion of wisdom as the integration of cognitive, reflective, and affective qualities, Ardelt (1998) argued that too much emphasis has been given to cognitive aspects of wisdom. She therefore used instruments assessing affect: *Haan's ego ratings/California 100 item Q-sort deck*.

Happé, Winner, and Brownell (1998) developed *theory of mind tasks* akin to the *means-end problem-solving procedure* by Heidrich and Denney (1994) (see also Platt & Spivack, 1975). Wisdom is defined as superior social insight. The subjects are told short stories and have to answer questions from memory in which they must infer personal motives of the protagonists of these stories.

Webster (2003) devised the *self-assessed wisdom scale* (SAWS), which is a 30-item questionnaire. Wisdom is seen as a multidimensional construct encompassing five dimensions: experience, emotions, reminiscence, openness, and humor. The SAWS correlated significantly with the wisdom-related Eriksonian constructs generativity and ego integrity.

Jason and colleagues (2001) developed the *foundational value scale*. Factor analysis revealed five components: harmony, warmth, intelligence, nature, and spirituality.

The *adolescent wisdom scale* by Perry and associates (2002) is a self-rating questionnaire, consisting of 23 attributes associated with wisdom and is validated in a sample of 2027 high school seniors. The development of the scale was part of an alcohol-use prevention program.

Table 20.3 presents an overview of the instruments, including data, if available, about reliability and validity.

B. Correlates of Wisdom

As age is believed not to be a predictor of wisdom during adulthood and old age (Staudinger, 1999), it is useful to look at other correlates or predictors of wisdom, such as intelligence, creativity, moral reasoning, and personality. Some of these correlates have received attention by researchers from the very beginning of wisdom research, notably personality traits, educational status, and gender (see Staudinger et al., 1998). With age ceasing to be a predictor in adulthood, studies into these correlates take on more significance.

1. Intelligence and Creativity

Lemaire (Day, Gordon, & Williamson, 1998) discerned six aspects of the wisdom of Solomon (Kings, 3–11). Wisdom is (1) a special gift from Yahweh, (2) superior, even divine, (3) associated with the exercise of justice, (4) political wisdom, (5) technical wisdom, and (6) intelligence and knowledge. So, already in the Bible, intelligence is one of the aspects of wisdom.

More recently, as seen in the discussion of the balance theory, Sternberg (2003) pursued the relationship further. He hypothesized a Hegelian relationship among intelligence, creativity, and wisdom. Intelligence is the thesis, creativity the antithesis, and wisdom the synthesis. Sternberg expected an increasing interest in research on creativity and wisdom, as the first is needed to adapt to and shape our rapid changing society, whereas the second is needed more and more to make sense of it. Nevertheless, wisdom, creativity, intelligence are part of the same intellectual system (the WICS). Baltes and Kunzmann (2003) took an opposite position in that they argue that wisdom is not to be conceived as a variant of intelligence.

Table 20.4
Intellectual versus Wisdom-Related Knowledge (Ardelt, 2000a)

	Intellectual knowlege	Wisdom-related knowledge
Goals	Quantitative, discovery of new truths	Qualitative, rediscovery of significance of old truths
Approach	Scientific, logos	Spiritual, mythos
Range	Time bound, particularistic	Timeless, universal
Acquisition	By detached experience	By combination of cognition and self-reflection
Effects on the knower	Belief knowledge, if scientifically arrived, is limitless	Acceptance of limits of knowledge
Relation to aging	Reversed U-shaped pattern	Potentially positive

Simonton (1990) discussed the implication of theories of creative production: an antithetical longitudinal relationship should exist between creativity and wisdom. However, as mentioned earlier, he argued that the phenomenon of the *swan song* might be the manifestation of mature wisdom.

Horn and Masunaga (2000) argued that wisdom involves some aspects of mature human intelligence. Such mature intelligence includes expert knowledge, a vital element of wisdom according to them. Crystallized intelligence and long-term working memory abilities increase with age throughout adulthood. According to Horn and Masunaga (2000) wisdom is a form of reasoning relying heavily on a large body of expert knowledge, built up through learning over a long period of time. This implies a positive relationship between wisdom and age in adulthood, a relationship for which there is no empirical support (see, e.g., Staudinger, 1999).

Earlier research by Staudinger et al. (1998) revealed that intelligence alone accounted for only 1% of the wisdom variance, just like the interaction of intelligence and personality. An interesting finding with respect to the development of wisdom was reported by Staudinger and Pasupathi (2003). In an adolescent sample (14–20 years), intelligence and personality were the strongest unique predictors of wisdom, whereas in an adult sample (35–75 years), the interaction between intelligence and personality turned out to be the strongest predictor. In terms of adaptive intelligence, some findings suggest that wisdom and optimal adaptation, in the form of selective optimization with compensation, go together (Baltes & Freund, 2003a,b).

Finally, Ardelt (2000) discussed two forms of knowledge in relation to aging: intellectual and wisdom related (see Table 20.4). She argued that wisdom-related knowledge rather than intellectual knowledge is crucial for successful aging, as wisdom-related knowledge would help older individuals prepare for their own physical and social decline, if not for their own death. This does, however, not exclude the necessity to pay attention to what she labels as survival skills, notably intellectual knowledge, enabling elderly people to keep up with technological changes in society. In this respect, it has to be kept in mind that the relationship of future generations of elderly with societal, notably technological, change will be different from that relationship in the present population of elderly.

2. *Moral Reasoning and Moral Values*

There is a kind of moral revival going on in wisdom research. Virtue, values, concern for humanity, and the common good, elements that were implicit in earlier theories on wisdom (see Baltes & Smith, 1990), have become explicit in the more recent versions of the same theories (Baltes & Staudinger, 2000) and in newly developed ones (Sternberg, 2003). The future will tell if this extension of the construct wisdom further into the ethical domain will bear fruit or if it turns out to be a moral Trojan horse that is dragged into the empirical stronghold of wisdom. Kunzmann and Baltes (2003) presented some empirical data on values: A value orientation that focuses conjointly on other enhancing values is present in individuals scoring high on their measures of wisdom.

Not only (prosocial) values are at stake. Wisdom also becomes associated with high levels of moral reasoning. A study by Pasupathi and Staudinger (2001) revealed a positive relationship between wisdom — as assessed by the Berlin vignets — and moral reasoning in an adult sample (20–87 years). In individuals with a high level of moral reasoning, wisdom was age related, which suggests that a threshold of moral reasoning should be reached for wisdom to develop. This finding makes for a complex relationship between moral reasoning and wisdom, keeping in mind the following findings. There is empirical evidence, longitudinal and cross-sectional, for (1) a positive relationship between reflective thinking and age in adolescence (Kitchener et al., 1989); (2) a positive relationship between wisdom-related knowledge (but not for the meta-criteria) and age in adolescence (Pasupathi, Staudinger, & Baltes, 2001); (3) a positive relationship between age and moral reasoning in childhood, adolescence, and early adulthood (Damon, 2000; Kohlberg, 1973); (4) elderly performing worse on moral reasoning dilemmas than adults (Armon, 1984; Kohlberg, 1973; Power, Power, & Snarey, 1988; Walker, 1986); and (5) the absence of a relationship between age and wisdom in adulthood and old age (Staudinger, 1999).

It will take some more research and theorizing before these findings can be integrated into a comprehensive model.

3. *Personality, Affect, and Motivation*

Personality factors are among the first ones studied in relation to wisdom. Openness to experience is the most frequently reported predictor of wisdom (Kramer, 2000). The same finding is reported by Brugman (2000) with respect to openness, although the expected relationship with emotional stability (see Figure 20.3) was not found. The other three personality factors of the big five (extraversion, agreeableness, and conscientiousness) did not correlate with wisdom either.

In the study of Staudinger and colleagues (1998), personality factors accounted for 2% of the variance, whereas the interaction of intelligence and personality accounted for an additional 1%. Kunzmann and Baltes (2003) reported higher affective involvement in individuals scoring higher on wisdom-related knowledge. Finally, they reported a joint motivational commitment to developing the potential of oneself and that of others. The general tenet of their research, thus far, is that wisdom involves emotional and motivational characteristics, although it does not coincide with them.

4. Eudaimonia, Quality of Narratives, and Reminiscence

In general, wisdom has been associated with the good life. In Greek and Hellenistic philosophy, acquiring wisdom, even the striving for it, was not a guarantee for happiness to be sure, but at least the road to happiness (Algra et al., 1999; Hossenfelder, 1996; Long & Sedley, 1992; Onfray, 1990).

Ardelt (1997, 2000b) reported that in a sample of elderly women wisdom was a strong predictor of life satisfaction, independent of objective circumstances, such as financial situation, physical environment, and socioeconomic status.

In the context of a so-called positive psychology, Baltes, Glück, and Kunzman (2002) discussed the role wisdom plays in successful life span development: It is the aim of positive psychology to catalyze change in academic psychology from a preoccupation with the production of knowledge for repairing the worst things in life to building the best qualities in life, and wisdom is supposed to be an important instrument in this sense. Some research has been conducted that might shed some light on the topic. Kramer (2000) reported that wise people show less despair and less dissatisfaction by grappling with existential issues and finding purpose and meaning in adverse experiences. Kunzmann and Baltes (2003) found a relationship among wisdom-related knowledge and lower negative and pleasant feelings, a stronger focus on personal growth, and a lower tendency toward values revolving around a pleasurable life (see also Baltes & Kunzmann, 2003).

Research has also been conducted on the relationship among wisdom, reminiscence and life narratives (see e.g., Glück, Bluck, Baron & McAdams, 2005). Life review was already part of the Berlin wisdom paradigm from the start (Baltes & Smith, 1990), and the relationship with wisdom is obvious as life narratives and reminiscence have to do with giving meaning to the life lived thus far. In a study by Brugman (2000), wisdom was a predictor of narrative coherence and well-being in a sample of Russian elderly. Further analyses of the same data (Brugman & Ter Laak, 2004) in a subsample of convinced communist party members showed that wisdom is associated with more effective dealing with existential problems: Reconstructing the life story when radical ruptures in the life story, caused by the fall of the U.S.S.R., make such a reconstruction inevitable (see also Randall & Kenyon, 2002).

We conclude that there is some empirical support for the notion that wisdom and the good life go together.

C. Developmental Change, Age-Related Differences, and the Role of Experience

Since the publication of the fifth volume of this handbook (Birren & Schaie, 2001), there has been an increasing interest in developmental aspects of wisdom (Ardelt, 2000a; Daiule, Buleau, & Rawlins, 2001; Damon, 2000; Olejnik, 2002; Perry et al., 2002; Staudinger & Pasaputhi, 2003; Schloss, 2000; Takahashi & Overton, 2003), in spite of strong empirical support for the notion that wisdom, as assessed by a wide range of instruments, is an age-independent variable, in any case during adulthood and old age (Brugman, 2000; Pasupathi, Staudinger, & Baltes, 2001; Staudinger, 1999). It must, however, be kept in mind that almost all the evidence is based on cross-sectional studies [but see Kitchener et al. (1993) for a study with a sequential design on the development of a wisdom-related concept, i.e., reflective judgment, in adolescents and young adults]. It is not unlikely that this conclusion is biased by period and cohort effects. Wisdom is defined in terms of tacit knowledge by the leading theorists in the field (Paul & Baltes, 2002; Sternberg, 2003) and with respect to knowledge that it is not too daring to argue that radical changes in the availability of information have taken place and that there are considerable differences between cohorts with respect to their access to information. This is not to say that the sheer availability of information is supportive for the development of wisdom, but the availability of information implies an increase of the chance that there is contradictory information. This confrontation with contradictions might lead to an increase, and perhaps a better management, of uncertainty and it might lead to an increase in value relativism. However, the same informational changes might lead to the opposite effect: In order to manage the sometimes overwhelming amount of available information, one might be inclined to simplify it and to seclude oneself from contradictory information (see also Meacham, 1983, 1990).

The absence of empirical support for a positive age–wisdom relationship in adulthood and old age poses a possible threat for theories based on concepts such as expertise (e.g., the Berlin wisdom paradigm, Baltes et al., 1995), stage-like development (e.g., Erikson, see Hoare, 2002), and the role of specific experiences (see Kinnier et al., 2001). These theories are confronted with the problem that a positive age–wisdom relationship is implied by their approach: With time, one develops expertise, wisdom is usually seen as a characteristic of last stages of development, and acquiring experience is a function of time too.

Several hypotheses are suggested to solve this problem, a problem that in part, can be reduced to differences between a *developmental* versus an *individual difference* approach. Horn and Masunaga (2000) argue that wisdom is only a potential in old age, as does

Ardelt (2000a,b). She argues that the relationship between wisdom and aging is *potentially* positive. It is potentially age related in the sense that wisdom, being timeless and universal knowledge (as opposed to intellectual knowledge (see Table 20.4)), enables elderly people to prepare for the physical and social decline of old age. She puts a strong emphasis on reminiscence and life review and on the pursuit of spiritual realization, although she does not specify what is meant by that last pursuit. Youth and adulthood, however, are reserved for the pursuit of intellectual knowledge, whereas old age is reserved for wisdom-related knowledge.

Another solution for the age paradox is offered by Erikson (Hoare, 2002). Erikson overturned in the end his lifelong belief that integrity and wisdom are products of the last stage of life. He replaced wisdom with faith as the final form of achievable, existential hope.

The same position is taken by Pascual-Leone (2000), who argued that higher, wisdom-related stages are an expectable but often missed outcome of adult development. An elegant way out can be found in an old publication of Riegel (1973). First, he hypothesized that there is a postformal dialectical stage. This stage of dialectical operations has characteristics that are strongly related to wisdom (see also Kramer, 2000). Moreover, he argued that each preceding stage, i.e., the standard Piagetian stages of cognitive development, can have — albeit not necessarily — a dialectical conclusion. As a result, wisdom-related characteristics can be present at all levels, be it stage bound.

Meacham (1983, 1990) suggested another solution. Defining wisdom as an equilibrium between certainty and doubt, he first defined the core of wisdom, which is a specific ratio between what one actually knows and what can be potentially known. This core characteristic has no relationship with age. The second characteristic of wisdom is labeled "the quality of wisdom," or its profoundness. This feature may change as a function of age. This notion of a differential developmental process, with some aspects appearing earlier in the course and others later, can also be found in publications from the Berlin wisdom paradigm (see Pasupathi, Staudinger, & Baltes, 2001). A hypothesis for which some empirical evidence is provided (Staudinger & Pasupathi, 2003) is that there is a specific order in which their five wisdom criteria appear. They suggest the following order: (1) rich factual knowledge, (2) rich procedural knowledge, (3) life span contextualism, (4) value relativism, and (5) recognition and management of uncertainty. In sum, first the basic criteria and then meta-level ones develop. Moreover, because this wisdom-related content appears to be age specific, adolescents are better at solving dilemmas associated with adolescence, e.g., dilemmas about sexual experiences or grades. An interesting finding in this respect is that community samples usually perform better according to basic criteria than to meta-level criteria. This is not true for the wise nominees. This might be interpreted as support for the position, taken by Meacham, that meta-level criteria, notably uncertainty management, are the age-independent core of wisdom. His age-dependent "quality of wisdom" can be seen as "wisdom-related knowledge," a basic-level criterium in the Berlin wisdom paradigm.

As indicated at the start of this section, there is a increasing flow of publications on developmental aspects of wisdom. The focus of attention is adolescence. Because there is no relationship between wisdom and age in adulthood and old age, one might find a relationship, or "the seeds of wisdom,"

at an earlier stage of development; witness the following citation:

I was alone in the apartment and it was bliss. I said to myself: 'There are two solutions: One is to somehow change my life, but that's impossible; the other is to end my life, but that's impossible, too. So there's only one thing to do.' And I laughed at the unwitting absurdity of the alternative: 'The only thing to do is to go on living, without changing anything. But that's impossible too. Here we have three impossibilities, of which the last is the most possible impossibility.' (Lugovskaya, 2003, p.77).

This is the diary entry of the 7th of January 1934 by the 14-year-old Nina Lugovskaya, a girl living in Moscow and victim of the Great Terror. Early evidence for the hypothesis that adolescence is the cradle of wisdom can be found within the context of the reflective judgment theory (Kitchener, 1983; Kitchener et al., 1989, 1993). In this theory, the period from adolescence to early adulthood is characterized by a transition from a stage in which knowledge is seen as absolutely certain (stage 3), via one in which knowledge is seen as idiosyncratic (stage 4), one in which knowledge is conceived as contextual (stage 5). In early adulthood, the final stage, knowledge is personally constructed via evaluation of evidence (see Table 20.2). The period studied by means of a sequential design coincides with the age groups compared (cross-sectional design) by Pasupathi, Staudinger, and Baltes (2001) (16 resp. 14 to 34 resp. 37 years) in their study on wisdom in adolescence and early adulthood. Findings of both studies point in the same direction, which is the more significant, considering the fact that different measures and designs are used.

The study of Pasupathi, Staudinger, and Baltes (2001) provided more information that might shed some light on what is happening during adolescence. First, they observed in the group of adolescents more between and within variability than was the case in the group of young adults.

Furthermore, they reported only a partial age-match effect: Adolescents performed at the same level on adolescent tasks as on adult tasks, whereas young adults did better on adult tasks. The authors suggested that adults may lose their expert knowledge for problems more specific for adolescents. What remains unclear is whether this (partial) age match plays a differential role for basic and meta-level criteria.

There was a gender effect in adolescents, with girls outperforming boys. No such effect was found in adults. Maybe adolescent girls are more involved in the kind of problems presented in the vignettes.

Adolescents, like adults, perform better on basic criteria than on meta-level criteria, but the discrepancy between meta-level and basic criteria in adolescents was greater than in adults.

Finally, life span contextualism, or considering the temporal contexts in which circumstances are embedded, yielded the best results compared with the other two meta-level criteria, notably value relativism and recognition of uncertainty. In sum, the results provided partial support for the hypothesis that the cradle of wisdom is found in adolescence.

Outside the Berlin wisdom paradigm and the reflective judgment theory, some research has been focusing on adolescents. Damon (2000) also assumed that the roots of wisdom are found in adolescence. He considered the ability to understand oneself in terms of moral purposes that guide one's critical life choices an essential precursor of wisdom. Fry (1998) argued in the same vein that both personal meaning and wisdom have their origins predominantly in interpersonal relations and social transactions. More specifically, he stresses the role of tutors and mentors, the role of reference groups, and the need for hardiness training.

However, there is conflicting evidence too. Comparing different age groups (15–20, 25–35, 40–50, 60–70), Olejnik (2002) reported the absence of age differences in dialectical/relativistic and procedural knowledge dimensions of wisdom (Berlin wisdom paradigma criteria). We have to wait for more longitudinal, if not sequential, studies for more firm conclusions.

1. Specific Experiences as a Determinant in the Development of Wisdom

The role of experience in the development of wisdom has always been stressed in psychological as well as in implicit theories. However, the nature of this role has remained obscure. As experience accumulates with age, theories stressing the role of experience in the development of wisdom have to explain the absence of an age–wisdom relationship (Kinnier et al., 2001; Kramer, 2000). Statistically the chance of being confronted with a critical event increases with age, making the chance of becoming wise according to these theories more probable. The solution suggested here is that it is not experience as such that is important, but the specific nature of the events encountered in life.

Kramer (2000) stressed the role of unusual if not radical life experiences in the emergence of wisdom. Such experiences foster introspection, reflection on the human condition, and counseling others. However, the question remains unanswered what is first. One might argue that individuals differ to the degree in which events prompt them to reflect on the human condition. In other words the effects of the same events may be quite different for different individuals. Actually, every event, however unremarkable, can be a trigger for introspection and reflection.

Lu (2001) reported a differential effect of specific life experiences on the five wisdom criteria. The criterium "procedural knowledge" correlated with spending more time reading newspapers. Furthermore, scores on "factual knowledge" were higher in subjects with experience in managerial positions, whereas scores on uncertainty, life span contextualism, and value relativism, being meta-criteria, were higher for persons who had participated in community activities.

Linley (2003) discussed the role of wisdom in adaptation to psychological trauma. Departing from the Berlin wisdom paradigm and the basic philosophical tenets of Hegel, he argued that wisdom is both a process and an (possible) outcome of the process of adaptation to trauma. He conceptualizes wisdom, borrowing from the Berlin wisdom paradigm, as the recognition and management of uncertainty, the integration of affect and cognition, and the recognition and acceptance of human limitation (Meacham, 1983, 1990; Taranto, 1989). The Hegelian conceptualization is proposed as life (thesis), trauma (antithesis), and wisdom (synthesis).

With respect to the nature of experience considered to enhance wisdom, Kinnier and co-workers (2001) interviewed adults that had been confronted with life-threatening situations and discovered that these individuals advocated, among others, less materialism and a more caring attitude toward others. These characteristics are akin to those mentioned in relation to wisdom (Kunzmann & Baltes, 2003).

The conclusion drawn by Pasupathi, Staudinger, and Baltes, (2001) on this topic is that wisdom develops idiosyncratically and nonnormatively in adulthood. However, there is good reason to expect age-related *normative* increases in wisdom-related performance during adolescence, which increase might be considered as a developmental task during this life stage (Heymans, 1994).

Given (a) substantial (cross-sectional) evidence pointing in the direction of the absence of age differences in adulthood and old age and (b) scarce evidence for age-related change in adolescence and early adulthood (Kitchener et al., 1993; Pasupathi & Staudinger, 2001), more longitudinal and sequential empirical research in adolescence and research on determinants of idiosyncratic development of wisdom in adulthood are advisable to arrive at more firm conclusions.

D. Education

The Old Testament discerns three pathways to wisdom: Through parental advice, faith, and *formal training* (Day, Gordon, & Williamson, 1998). Again, psychologists lag a bit behind. Something akin can be found in the 7th century with Virgilius Maro Grammaticus (Law, 1995). In his grammaires dramatisées, he described *sapientia* as the ultimate goal of all human striving. He paid special attention to obstacles in the attainment of wisdom, notably avarice. A much used concise summary said: "Industrious reading, assiduous questioning, scorn for the riches, and *honouring your teacher* are the four keys to wisdom" (Law, 1995, p.42). However, negative ideas about the role of formal education in the development of wisdom can also be found. In the 15th century, Nicolai de Cusa (1988) strongly argued for wisdom as derived directly from experience as opposed to wisdom extracted from books by learned men. In his *Idiotia de Sapientia*, a learned man sighs, "If the food of wisdom is not in the books of the sages, where might it be found elsewhere" (1988, pp. 4–5). Montaigne (1580, 1991) can be mentioned as well: "I have seen in my time hundreds of craftsmen and ploughmen wiser and happier than University

Rectors — and whom I would rather be like" (p. 542).

These ideas fit very well in the balance theory of Sternberg (2003) in which the role of tacit knowledge is emphasized as well, although one of the procedures Sternberg suggests in presenting his educational ideas is just "reading classic works of literature and philosophy to learn and reflect on the wisdom of the sages" (p.165), which does not fit very well in the writings of Nicolai de Cusa.

Pascual-Leone (2000) made a distinction between two pathways to accelerate access to wisdom: (1) the natural life-experience path and (2) the meditation path. In both of them, maturational organismic factors and mental attentional mechanisms are supposed to play a role.

With respect to education, there has been a discussion initiated by Sternberg about the possibility to "teach" wisdom. He argues that intelligence-related skills are a necessary but not a sufficient basis for education. Sternberg has actually started a project, attempting to measure and infuse wisdom-related skills in a sample of 600 middle school students, before, during, and after a curriculum of 12 weeks.

Sternberg repeats several reasons why wisdom should be part of the curriculum. First, he argues that knowledge as such is insufficient for wisdom. It is no guarantee for satisfaction and happiness. Second, wisdom provides a mindful and considered way to enter deliberative values into important judgments. Finally, wisdom may lead to a better and more harmonious world (Sternberg, 2003, p.163). One might add that we have indeed a long way to go.

With respect to developing wisdom in the classroom, he devised 16 principles of wisdom derived from his balance theory, varying from "demonstrating how wisdom is critical for a satisfying life," "teaching role-model wisdom, because what you do is more important than what you say," "helping students to balance their own interests," to "teaching students to search for and then try to reach the common good — a good where everyone wins" (p.165). Furthermore, he tries to give some concrete procedures to follow in teaching wisdom in which he emphasizes the role of dialectical thinking. As yet no results of the project are available. His plans have, in any case, resulted in a critical discussion in the educational psychologist (Halpern, 2001; Kuhn & Udell, 2001; Paris, 2001; Perkins, 2001; Stanovich, 2001; Sternberg, 2001a,b).

There is, however, a study in which empirical results about the stimulation of wisdom-related thinking are presented (see Figure 20.4). Kitchener and colleagues (1993) reported practice effects for the reflective judgment interview, although the amount of practice was minimal. It consisted of a highly supportive condition of the original reflective judgment interview.

The simple conclusion is that reflective judgment can be stimulated, but the results of this rather isolated investigation do not warrant a general conclusion.

V. Final Remarks

Some general trends are visible in wisdom research and theorizing after the last edition. The Berlin wisdom paradigm has consolidated its prominent place in wisdom research and theorizing. The balance theory of wisdom has been elaborated in which wisdom is placed in a broader framework of intelligence, an educational program based on this theory is on its way, but the theory still lacks empirical support. Research stemming from the epistemic approach is still scarce.

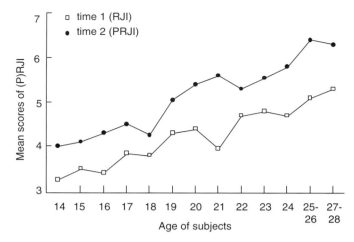

Figure 20.4 Mean reflective interview (RJI) time 1 and mean prototypic reflective judgment interview (PRJI) time 2 scores (after Kitchener et al., 1993). Mean scores correspond with the stages of reflective judgment (see Table 20.2).

With respect to the concept itself, some extensions have taken place. First, the concept now has an explicit moral loading. There might be a danger in introducing elements such as value and virtue in the description of wisdom, which are hard to assess. Moreover, the wise person may become a politically correct new saint. The wise person described in psychological theories might meet the same fate as the sage, once described by the Stoa as one who

... never errs, never fails to grasp things with complete security. His knowledge is logically equivalent to truth, since it is based upon the causal nexus which controls cosmic events. Unlike the ordinary man who utters some true statements which he cannot prove against every attempt to overturn them, the wise man's judgments are infallible, since he knows why each of them must be true (Long, 1986, p.130).

Such a sage is pure fiction, if not nonhuman. This argument is akin to the 19th century discussion on the moral qualities of artists, a discussion raised by the German art-historian Winckelmann (1977): An artist, reaching for beauty and truth, cannot be anything else than morally perfect. In other words, esthetics and ethics coincide,

beauty and truth coincide: The brush of the artist should be dunked in wisdom (p.39). Such artists and sages just do not exist. Second, the concept of wisdom is widened in the sense that its adaptive value is increasingly emphasized. The balance theory defines wisdom as high level practical intelligence, and recent investigations in research of the Berlin wisdom paradigm focus on the relationship between selective optimization with compensation (SOC) and wisdom. Due to the lack of support for the initial hypothesis of the age relatedness of wisdom, two trends are discernible. First, there is increasing research activity in the realm of adolescent development. Second, the search for other determinants of wisdom has intensified. As a result, there is an increase in theorizing and research about correlates and precursors of wisdom, and research into the relationship of wisdom with variables such as the good life and moral reasoning is intensified.

Finally, there is some attention for the construction of new instruments to assess wisdom and the first steps are taken with respect to the stimulation of wisdom. Building upon the trends described earlier, some suggestions for future wisdom research and theorizing will be presented.

With respect to adulthood and old age, more attention should be paid to determinants of interindividual differences and intraindividual change in wisdom, focusing on the role of experience. This might interact with personality traits. One might hypothesize that openness to experience or emotional stability interacts with experience, rendering it fruitful or not. Furthermore, additional research is needed into the nature of experience and the interaction between age and experience. Therefore, longitudinal or sequential studies are needed. Cross-sectional designs leave too many questions unanswered.

Research into adolescence as the possible cradle of wisdom has just started and it has to be continued, with special attention to *differential* developmental processes. Although some first promising steps have been taken, more research has to be devoted to the question of which aspects of wisdom develop first, which later, or, even, which aspects do not develop at all.

Although enlarging the concept of wisdom with a moral component might not be wise, a promising domain seems to be research into the *relationship* between wisdom and moral reasoning.

Vital for the future of wisdom research is the quality of the instruments for the assessment of the wisdom construct. With respect to the most frequently used instrument, the Berlin vignettes, one might suggest some broadening of the content of the vignettes from personal to more extrapersonal topics. It would be interesting to see if scores on vignettes about political or ecological affairs differ from scores on vignettes concerning private moral dilemmas. More information is also needed about the relationship between basic and meta-level criteria, especially to answer the question if

simple summation of scores of the different criteria as an estimate of wisdom is allowed.

Given an increasing number of different instruments to assess wisdom, validity studies might be very useful: Do the different instruments measure the same construct and do they do so in different populations differing in culture or age?

With respect to culture it may be useful to expand research into wisdom in other cultures than Western countries. Studies so far have restricted themselves mainly to Western countries and Western-oriented cultures such as Japan or Taiwan. One might think of studies focusing on islamic or African cultures.

Finally, as many characteristics of our Western society, relevant for the development of wisdom, e.g., information technology and the resulting changes in the availability of information and globalization, are changing rapidly, research has to focus on changes in wisdom and conceptions of wisdom and its manifestations within our culture over time. As in studies on the development of wisdom, sequential studies are indispensable to answer questions about cohort differences and historical change with respect to wisdom.

Acknowledgments

This chapter has profited substantially from the comments of Paulien Kintz and my colleagues Dr. Jan ter Laak and Professor Dr. Peter Heymans.

References

Algra, K., Barnes, J., Mansfeld, J., & Schofield, M. (Eds.) (1999). *The Cambridge history of Hellenistic philosophy.* Cambridge: Cambridge University Press.

Ardelt, M. (1997). Wisdom and life satisfaction in old age. *Journal of Gerontology, 52B,* pp. 15–27.

Ardelt, M. (2000a). Intellectual versus wisdom-related knowledge: The case for a different kind of learning in later years of life. *Educational Gerontology, 26,* 1–15.

Ardelt, M. (2000b). Antecedents and effects of wisdom in old age: A longitudinal perspective on aging well. *Research on Aging, 22,* 360–394.

Ardelt, M. (2004). Wisdom as Expert Knowledge System: A critical review of a contemporary operationalization of an ancient concept. *Human Development, 47,* 257–285.

Aristotle (1970). *Ethics.* Harmondsworth: Penguin.

Arlin, P. K. (1975). Cognitive development: A fifth stage? *Developmental Psychology, 2,* 602–606.

Armon, C. (1984). Ideals of the good life and moral judgment: Ethical reasoning across the life span. In M. L. Commons, F. A. Richards, & C. Armon (Eds.), *Beyond formal operations* (pp. 357–380). New York: Praeger.

Aspinwall, L. G., & Staudinger, U. M. (Eds.) (2003). *A psychology of human strengths: Fundamental questions and future directions for a positive psychology.* Washington, DC: APA.

Assmann, A. (Ed.) (1991). *Weisheit; Archäologie der literarischen Kommunikation 3.* München: Wilhelm Fink Verlag.

Assmann, A. (1994). Wholesome knowledge: Concepts of wisdom in a historical and cross-cultural perspective. In D. L. Featherman, R. M. Lerner, & M. Perlmutter (Eds.), *Life-span development and behavior* (Vol. 12, pp. 188–224). Hillsdale, NJ: Lawrence Erlbaum.

Ayer A. J. (1971). *The problem of knowledge.* Harmondsworth: Penguin.

Baltes, P. B., & Dittmann-Kohli, F. (1982). Einige einführende Überlegungen zur Intelligenz im Erwachsenenalter. *Neue Sammlung, 22,* 261–278.

Baltes, P. B., Dittmann-Kohli, F., & Dixon, R. A. (1984). New perspectives on the development of intelligence in adulthood: Towards a dual-process conception and a model of selective optimization with compensation. In P. B. Baltes & O. G. Brim (Eds.), *Life-span development and behavior* (Vol. 6, pp. 33–76). New York: Academic Press.

Baltes, P. B., & Freund, A. M. (2003a). The intermarriage of wisdom and selective optimization with compensation: Two meta-heuristics guiding the conduct of life. In C. Keyes & J. Haidt (Eds.), *Flourishing: Positive psychology and the life well-lived* (pp. 249–273). Washington, DC: APA.

Baltes, P. B., & Freund, A. M. (2003b). Human strengths as the orchestration of wisdom and selective optimization with compensation. In L. G. Aspinwall & U. M. Staudinger (Eds.), *A psychology of human strengths: Fundamental questions and future directions for a positive psychology* (pp. 23–35). Washington, DC: APA.

Baltes, P. B., Glück, J., & Kunzmann, U. (2002). Wisdom: Its structure and function in regulating successful life span development. In C. R. Snyder & S. J. Lopez (Eds.), *Handbook of positive psychology* (pp. 327–347). London: Oxford University Press.

Baltes, P. B., & Kunzmann, U. (2003). Wisdom. *Psychologist, 16,* 131–133.

Baltes, P. B., & Smith, J. (1990). Weisheit und Weisheitsentwicklung: Prolegomena zu einer psychologische Weistheitstheorie. *Zeitschrift für Entwicklungspsychologie und Pädagogische Psychologie, 22,* 95–135.

Baltes, P. B., & Staudinger, U. M. (2000). Wisdom: A metaheuristic (pragmatic) to orchestrate mind and virtue towards excellence. *American Psychologist, 55,* 122–136.

Baltes, P. B., Staudinger, U., Maercker, A., & Smith, J. (1995). People nominated as wise: A comparative study of wisdom-related knowledge. *Psychology & Aging, 10,* 155–166.

Beckerman, M. (1990). Leos Janácek and 'The Late Style' in music. *The Gerontologist, 30,* 632–635.

Bett, R. (2000). *Pyrrhon, his antecedents, and its legacy.* Oxford: Oxford University Press.

Birren, J. E. (Ed.) (1959). *Handbook of aging and the individual.* Chicago: University of Chicago Press.

Birren, J. E., & Fisher, L. M. (1990). The elements of wisdom: Overview and integration. In R. J. Sternberg (Ed.), *Wisdom, its nature, origins, and development* (pp. 317–332), Cambridge: Cambridge University Press.

Birren, J. E., & Schaie, K. W. (Eds.) (1985). *Handbook of the psychology of aging* (2nd edition). New York: Van Nostrand Reinhold.

Birren, J. E., & Schaie, K. W. (Eds.) (1990). *Handbook of the psychology of aging.* (3rd edition). San Diego: Academic Press.

Birren , J. E., & Schaie, K. W. (Eds.) (2001). *Handbook of the psychology of aging* (5th edition). San Diego: Academic Press.

Birren, J. E., & Schroots, J. F. (1996). Concepts, theory, and methods in the psychology of aging. In J. E. Birren & K. W. Schaie (Eds.), *Handbook of the psychology of aging* (4th edition, pp. 3–23). San Diego: Academic Press.

Brecht, B. (1981). *Die Gedichte von Bertolt Brecht in einem Band.* Frankfurt am Main Suhrkamp.

Brice, G. E. (1979). *A legacy of wisdom: The Egyptian contribution to the wisdom of Israel.* Cranbury, NJ: Associated University Press.

Brittain, C. (2001). *Philo of Larissa. The last of the Academic Sceptics.* Oxford: Oxford University Press.

Brown, W. S. (Ed.) (2000). Understanding wisdom: Sources, science and society (Vol. 3, pp. 361–391). Philadelphia, PA: Templeton Foundation Press.

Brugman, G. M. (1994a). Wisdom as high level epistemic cognition & aging: A developmental task analysis. In J. ter Laak, A. Podolskii & P. G. Heymans (Eds.), *Developmental tasks: Towards a cultural analysis of human development* (pp. 259–273). Dordrecht/Boston: Kluwer.

Brugman, G. M. (1996). Problem finding: Discovering and formulating problems. In A. J. Cropley & D. Dehn (Eds.), *Fostering the growth of high ability: European perspectives* (pp. 139–156). Norwood, NJ: Ablex.

Brugman, G. M. (1997). Wisdom as moderate scepsis: Changes over the life-span. *Revista de Psicologia, 15,* 3–53.

Brugman, G. M. (2000). *Wisdom: Source of narrative coherence and eudaimonia.* Delft, The Netherlands: Eburon.

Brugman, G. M., & Ter Laak, J. J. F. (2004). Narrative change. *Journal of Developmental Psychology, 25,* 42–56.

Bryce, G. E. (1979). *A legacy of wisdom. The Egyptian contribution to the wisdom of Israel.* Lewisburg, PA: Bucknell University Press.

Burnyeat, M. & Frede, M. (Eds.) (1997). *The original sceptics: A controversy.* Indianapolis/Cambridge: Hackett.

Charron, P. (1601, 1971). *Of wisdom* (De la sagesse). New York: Da Capo Press.

Cicero (1994). *Academica I & II* (Transl. H.Rackham). London: Loeb.

Clayton, V. (1975). Erikson's theory of human development as it applies to the aged: A contradictive cognition. *Human Development, 18,* 119–128.

Clayton, V., & Birren, J. E. (1980). The development of wisdom across the lifespan: A reexamination of an ancient topic. In P. B. Baltes & O. G. Brim (Eds.), *Lifespan development and behavior* (Vol. 3, pp. 103–135). New York: Academic Press.

Csikszentmihalyi, M., & Rathunde, K. (1990). The psychology of wisdom: An evolutionary interpretation. In R. J. Sternberg (Ed.), *Wisdom; its nature, origin, and development* (pp. 25–51). Cambridge: Cambridge University Press.

Curley, A. J. (1996). *Augustine's critique of skepticism. A study of contra academicus.* New York: Peter Lang.

Cusa, Nicolaus de (1450, 1988). *Idiotia de sapientia.* Hamburg: Felix Meiner Verlag GmbH.

Daiute, C., Buteau, E., & Rawlins, C. (2001). Social-relational wisdom: Developmental diversity in children's written narratives about social conflict. *Narrative Inquiry, 11,* 277–306.

Damon, W. (2000). Setting the stage for the development of wisdom: Self-understanding and moral identity during adolescence. *Laws of life symposia series* (Vol. 3, pp. 339–360). Philadelphia, PA: Templeton Foundation Press.

Day, J., Gordon, R. P., & Williamson, H. G. M. (Eds.) (1998). *Wisdom in ancient Israel.* Cambridge: Cambridge University Press.

DeRose, K., & Warfield, T. A. (1999). *Skepticism.* Oxford: Oxford University Press.

Dittmann-Kohli, F. (1984). Weisheit als mögliches Ergebnis der Intelligenzentwicklung im Erwachsenenalter. *Sprache & Kognition*, 2, 112–133.

Dittmann-Kohli, F. (1993). Produktivität und Kreativität im Alter: Eine psychologische Perspektive. In U.Weisner (Ed.), *Picasso – letzte Bilder. Werke 1966–1972* (pp. 172–178). Bielefeld: Kunsthalle Bielefeld.

Erasmus, D. (1994). *Lof en blaam* (including Praise of Folly). Amsterdam: Atheneum/ Polak & Van Gennep.

Erikson, E. H. (1959). *Identity and the life cycle*. New York: International University Press.

Erikson, E. H. (1976). *Aging, death and the completion of being*. Philadelphia, PA: University of Pennsylvania Press.

Erman, A. (1995). *Ancient Egyptian poetry and prose*. New York: Dover Publications, Inc.

Floridi, L. (2002). *Sextus Empiricus. The transmission and recovery of Pyrrhonnism*. Oxford: Oxford University Press.

Fry, P. S. (1998). The development of personal meaning and wisdom in adolescence: A reexamination of moderating and consolidating factors and influences. In P. T. Wong & P. S. Fry (Eds.), *The human quest for meaning: A handbook of psychological research and clinical applications* (pp. 91–110). Mahwah, NJ: Lawrence Erlbaum.

Frye, N. (1957). *Anatomy of criticism; four essays*. Princeton: Princeton University Press.

Furrow, J. L., & Wagener, L. M. (2000). Lessons learned: The role of religion in the development of wisdom in adolescence. In W. S. Brown (Ed.), *Understanding wisdom: Sources, science and society. Laws of life symposia series* (Vol. 3, pp. 361–391). Philadelphia, PA: Templeton Foundation Press.

Gent, (1966). Der Begriff der Weisen. *Zeitschrift für Philosophische Forschung*, 20, 77.

Glück, J., Bluck, S., Baron, J., & McAdams, D. (2005). The wisdom of experience: Autobiographical narratives across adulthood. *International Journal of Behavioral Development*, 29, 197–208.

Halpern, D. F. (2001). Why wisdom? *Educational Psychologist*, 36, 253–256.

Hankinson, R. J. (1995). *The sceptics*. London/ New York: Routledge.

Happé, F. F. E., Winner, E., & Brownell, H. (1998). The getting of wisdom: Theory of mind in old age. *Developmental Psychology*, 34, 358–362.

Heidrich, S. M., & Denney, N. W. (1994). Does social problem differ from other types of problem solving during the adult years? *Experimental Aging Research*, 20, 105–126.

Heymans, P. G. (1994). Developmental tasks: A cultural analysis of human development. In J. ter Laak, P. G. Heymans & A. I. Podol'skij (Eds.), *Developmental tasks: Toward a cultural analysis of human development* (pp. 3–34). Dordrecht: Kluwer Academic Press.

Hoare, C. H. (2002). *Erikson: On development in adulthood*. Oxford: Oxford University Press.

Holliday, S. G., & Chandler, M. J. (1986). *Wisdom: Explorations in adult competence*. Basel: Karger.

Honderich, T. (1995). *The Oxford companion to philosophy*. Oxford: Oxford University Press.

Horn, J., & Masunaga, H. (2000). On the emergence of wisdom: Expertise development. In W. S. Brown (Ed.), *Understanding wisdom: Sources, science and society. Laws of life symposia series*, (Vol. 3, pp. 245–276). Philadelphia, PA: Templeton Foundation Press.

Hossenfelder, M. (1996). *Antike Glückslehre*. Stuttgart: Kröner.

Hume, D. (1740, 1965). In J. M. Keynes & P. Sraffa (Eds.), *An abstract of a Treatise of human nature 1740: A Pamphlet hitherto unknown by David Hume*. Conn.: Hamden.

Hume, D. (1740, 1978). In L. A. Selby-Bigge & P. H. Nidditch (Eds.), *A treatise of human nature*. Oxford: Oxford University Press.

Hume, D. (1741, 1985). In E. F. Miller (Ed.), *Essays: Moral, political, and literary*. Indiannapolis: Liberty Fund.

Hume, D. (1777, 1974). In P. H. Nidditch (Ed.), *Enquiries concerning human understanding and concerning the principles of morals*. Oxford: Clarendon Press.

Jason, L., Reichler, A., King, C., Madsen, D., Camacho, J., & Marchese, W. (2001).

The measurement of wisdom: A preliminary effort. *Journal of Community Psychology, 29*, 585–598.

Kinnier, R. T., Tribbensee, N. E., Rose, C. A., & Vaughan, S. M. (2001). In the final analysis: More wisdom from people who have faced death. *Journal of Counseling and Development, 79*, 171–177.

Kitchener, K. S. (1983). Cognition, metacognition, and epistemic cognition. *Human Development, 26*, 222–232.

Kitchener, K. S., & Brenner, H. G. (1990). Wisdom and reflective judgment: Knowing in the face of uncertainty. In R. J. Sternberg (Ed.), *Wisdom; its nature, origin, and development* (pp. 212–229). Cambridge: Cambridge University Press.

Kitchener, K. S., & King, P. M. (1985). *Reflective judgment scoring rules* (available from K. S. Kitchener, School of Education, University of Denver, 2450S, Vine Street, Denver, Colorado 80208).

Kitchener, K. S., King, P. M., Wood, P. K., & Davison, M. L. (1989). Sequentiality and consistency in the development of reflective judgment: A six-year longitudinal study. *Journal of Applied Developmental Psychology, 10*, 73–95.

Kitchener, K. S., Lynch, C. L., Fischer, W., & Wood, P. K. (1993). Developmental range of reflective judgment: The effect of contextual support and practice on developmental stage. *Developmental Psychology, 29*, 893–906.

Knight, A., & Parr, W. (1999). Age as a factor in judgments of wisdom and creativity. *New Zealand Journal of Psychology, 28*, 37–47.

Kohlberg, L. (1973). Stages and aging in moral development: Some speculations. *The Gerontologist, 13*, 497–502.

Kramer, D. (2000). Wisdom as a classical source of human strength: Conceptualization and empirical inquiry. *Journal of Social and Clinical Psychology, 19*, 83–101.

Kristeller, P. A. (1991). *Greek philosophers of the Hellenistic age*. New York: Columbia University Press.

Kuhn, D., & Udell, W. (2001). The path to wisdom. *Educational Psychologist, 36*, 261–264.

Kunzmann, U., & Baltes, P. B. (2003a). Wisdom-related knowledge: Affective, motivational, and interpersonal correlates. *Personality & Social Psychology Bulletin, 29*, 1104–1119.

Kunzmann, U., & Baltes, P. B. (2003b). Beyond the traditional scope of intelligence: Wisdom in action. In R. J. Sternberg & J. Lautrey (Eds.), *Models of intelligence: International perspectives* (pp. 329–343). Washington, DC: APA.

Labouvie-Vief, G. (1985). Intelligence and cognition. In J. E. Birren & K. W. Schaie (Eds.), *Handbook of the psychology of aging* (2nd edition, pp. 500–530). New York: Van Nostrand Reinhold.

Law, V. (1995). *Wisdom, authority and grammar in the seventh century: Decoding Virgilius Maro Grammaticus*. Cambridge: Cambridge University Press.

Linley, P. A. (2003). Positive adaptation to trauma: Wisdom as both process and outcome. *Journal of Traumatic Stress, 16*, 601–610.

Long, A. A. (1986). *Hellenistic philosophy; stoics, epicureans, sceptics*. Avon: Bath Press.

Long, A. A. (1996). *Stoic Studies*. Cambridge: Cambridge University Press.

Long, A. A., & Sedley, D. N. (1992). *The Hellenistic philosophers*. Cambridge: Cambridge University Press.

Lopez, S., & Snyder, C. R. (Eds.) (2003). *Positive psychological assessment: A handbook of models and measures*. Washington, DC: APA.

Lu, I. H. (2001). Older adults' wisdom on a "life-planning task": Characteristics and relations to life experiences. *Japanese Journal of Educational Psychology, 49*, 198–208.

Lugovskaya, N. (2003). *The diary of a Soviet schoolgirl*. Moscow: Glas/Chicago: Northwestern Univerity Press.

Mates, B. (1996). *The sceptic way: Sextus Empiricus's outlines of Pyrrhonism*. New York: Oxford University Press.

Maercker, A., Böhmig-Krumhaar, S., & Staudinger, U. (1998). Existentielle Konfrontation als Zugang zu weisheitsbezogenem Wissen und Urteilen: Eine Untersuchung von Weisheitsnominierten.

Zeitschrift für Entwicklungspsychologie und Pädagogische Psychologie, 30, 2–12.

Maercker, A., & Smith, J. (1991). *Weisheit am Beispiel menschlicher Grenzsituationen.* Poster 10. Tagung für Entwicklungspsychologie. Köln, 23–25 Sept. 1991.

Meacham, J. A. (1983). Wisdom and the context of knowledge: Knowing that one does not know. *Contributions to Human Development, 8,* 111–134.

Meacham, J. A. (1990). The loss of wisdom. In R. J. Sternberg (Ed.), *Wisdom, its nature, origins, and development* (pp. 181–211), Cambridge: Cambridge University Press.

Montaigne, M. de (1580, 1991). In M. A. Screech (Ed.), *The complete essays.* Harmondsworth: Penguin Books.

Murray, K. (1985). Life as fiction. *Journal for the Theory of Social Behaviour, 15,* 173–188.

Nietzsche, F. (1972). Wissenschaft und Weisheit im Kampfe. *F.Nietzsche Werke* Bd.III (pp. 1041–1056). Frankfurt/M: Verlag Ullstein GmbH.

Norton, D. F. (1993). *The Cambridge companion to Hume.* Cambridge: Cambridge University Press.

Olejnik, M. (2002). Wisdom as the meaning of life construction. The case of the biological evaluation. *Polish Psychological Bulletin, 33,* 23–30.

Onfray, M. (1990). *Cynisms: Portrait du philosophe en chien.* Paris: Bernard Grasset.

Paris, S. G. (2001). Wisdom, snake oil, and the educational marketplace. *Educational Psychologist, 36,* 257–260.

Pascual-Leone, J. (2000). Mental attention, consciousness, and the progressive emergence of wisdom. *Journal of Adult Development, 7,* 241–254.

Pasupathi, M., & Staudinger, U. M. (2001). Do advanced moral reasoners also show wisdom? Linking moral reasoning and wisdom-related knowledge and judgment. *International Journal of Behavioral Development, 25,* 401–415.

Pasupathi, M., Staudinger, U. M., & Baltes, P. B. (2001). Seeds of wisdom: Adolescents' knowledge and judgments about difficult life problems. *Developmental Psychology, 37,* 351–361.

Paul, U. K., & Baltes, P. B. (2003). Wisdom-related knowledge: Affective, motivational, and interpersonal correlates. *Personality and Social Psychology Bulletin, 29,* 1104–1119.

Pennebaker, J. W., & Stone, L. D. (2003). Words of wisdom: Language use over the life span. *Journal of Personality & Social Psychology, 85,* 291–301.

Perkins, D. N. (2001). Wisdom in the wild. *Eductional Psychologist, 36,* 265–368.

Perry, C. L., Komro, K. A., Jones, R. M., Munson, K, Williams, C. L., & Jason, L. (2002). The measurement of wisdom and its relationship to adolescence substance use and problem behaviors. *Journal of Child and Adolescent Substance Abuse, 12,* 45–63.

Plato (1997). *Complete works.* Ed. J. M. Hooper. Indiapolis/Cambridge: Hackett.

Platt, J., & Spivak, G. (1975). The MEPS procedure manual. Philadelphia: Community Mental Health/Mental Retardation.

Power, F. C., Power, A. R., & Snarey, J. (1988). Integrity and aging: Ethical, religious, and psychosocial perspectives. In D. K. Lapsley & F. C. Power (Eds.), *Self, ego, and identity* (pp. 131–150). New York: Springer Verlag.

Randall, W., & Kenyon, G. M. (2002). Reminiscence as reading our lives: Towards a wisdom environment. In J. D. Webster & B. K. Haight (Eds.), *Critical advances in reminiscence work: From theory to application* (pp. 233–253). New York: Springer.

Riegel, K. F. (1973). Dialectic operations: The final period of cognitive development. *Human Development, 16,* 346–370.

Roth, D., Pratt, M., Humsberger, B., & Pancer, M. (1990). *Wisdom: Everyday judgments and formal ratings of reasoning.* Paper presented at the Canadian Psychological Meetings, Ottawa, Canada, June 1990.

Russell, B. (1994). *History of Western philosophy.* London: Routledge.

Schloss, J. P. (2000). Wisdom traditions as mechanisms for organismal integration: Evolutionary perspectives on homeostatic "laws of life." In W. S. Brown (Ed.), *Understanding wisdom: Sources, science and society.* (Vol. 3, pp. 153–191).

Philadelphia, PA: Templeton Foundation Press.

Schopenhauer, A. (1851, 1976). *Aphorismen zur Lebensweisheit.* Frankfurt am Main: Insel Verlag.

Schopenhauer, A. (Ed.) (1851, 1996). *Über die Universitäts-Philosophie. Parerga und Paralipomena I* (pp. 171–242). Sämtliche Werke, Band IV. Stuttgart/Frankfurt am Main: Suhrkamp Taschenbuch Verlag.

Sextus Empiricus (1987). *Against the physicists/Against the ethicists.* Transl. R. G. Bury. London: Loeb.

Sextus Empiricus (1993). *Outlines of Scepticism.* Transl. R. G. Bury. London: Loeb.

Simonton, D. K. (1990). Creativity and wisdom in aging. In J. E. Birren & K. W. Schaie (Eds.), *Handbook of the psychology of aging* (3rd edition, pp. 320–329). San Diego: Academic Press.

Sloterdijk, P. (1983). *Kritik der zynischen Vernunft.* Frankfurt am Main: Suhrkamp Verlag.

Stanovich, K. E. (2001). The rationality of educating for wisdom. *Educational Psychologist, 36,* 247–251.

Staudinger, U. M. (1999). Older and wiser? Integrating results on the relationship between age and wisdom-related performance. *International Journal of Behavioral Development, 23,* 641–664.

Staudinger, U., & Leipold, B. (2003). The assessment of wisdom-related performance. In S. Lopez & C. R. Snyder (Eds.), *Positive psychological assessment: A handbook of models and measures* (pp. 171–184). Washington, DC: APA.

Staudinger, U. M., Maciel, A. G., Smith, J., & Baltes, P. B. (1998). What predicts wisdom-related performance? A first look at personality, intelligence, and facilitative experiental contexts. *European Journal of Personality, 12,* 1–17.

Staudinger, U. M., & Pasupathi, M. (2003). Correlates of wisdom-related performance in adolescence and adulthood: Age-graded differences in 'paths' towards desirable development. *Journal of Research on Adolescence, 13,* 239–268.

Sternberg, R. J. (1985). Implicit theories of intelligence, creativity, and wisdom. *Journal of Personality and Social Psychology, 49,* 607–627.

Sternberg, R. J. (Ed.) (1990). *Wisdom; its nature, origin, and development.* Cambridge: Cambridge University Press.

Sternberg, R. J. (1998). A balance theory of wisdom. *Review of General Psychology, 2,* 347–365.

Sternberg, R. J. (2000a). Wisdom as a form of giftedness. *Gifted Child Quarterly, 44,* 252–260.

Sternberg, R. J. (2000b). Intelligence and wisdom. In R. J. Sternberg (Ed.), *Handbook of intelligence* (pp. 631–649). Cambridge: Cambridge University Press.

Sternberg, R. J. (2001a). What is the common thread of creativity? Its dialectical relation to intelligence and wisdom. *American Psychologist, 56,* 360–362.

Sternberg, R. J. (2001b). Why schools should teach for wisdom: The balance theory of wisdom in educational settings. *Educational Psychologist, 36,* 227–245.

Sternberg, R. J. (2001c). How wise is it to teach wisdom? A reply to five critiques. *Educational Psychologist, 36,* 269–272.

Sternberg, R. J. (2003). *Wisdom, intelligence, and creativity synthesized.* Cambridge: Cambridge University Press.

Sternberg, R. J., & Lubart, T. I. (2001). Wisdom and creativity. In J. E. Birren & K. W. Schaie (Eds.), *Handbook of the psychology of aging* (5th edition, pp. 500–522). San Diego: Academic Press.

Takahashi, M. (2000a). Towards a culturally inclusive understanding of wisdom: Historical roots in the East and West. *International Journal of Aging and Human Development, 51,* 271–230.

Takahashi, M. (2000b). The concept of wisdom: A cross-cultural comparison. *International Journal of Psychology, 35,* 1–9.

Takahashi, M., & Overton, W. F. (2003). Wisdom: A culturally inclusive developmental perspective. *International Journal of Behavioral Development, 26,* 269–277.

Taranto, M. A. (1989). Facets of wisdom: A theoretical synthesis. *International Journal of Aging and Human Development, 29,* 1–21.

Thomson, D. (2001). The getting and losing wisdom. *Journal of Religious Gerontology*, *12*, 77–88.

Unger, P. (1975). *Ignorance: A case for Scepticism.* Oxford: Oxford University Press.

Unger, P. (1984). *Philosophical relativity.* Minnesota: University of Minnesota Press.

Vaihinger, H. (1927, 1986). *Die Philosophie des Als Ob. System der theoretischen, praktischen und religiösen Fiktionen der Menschheit auf Grund eines idealistischen Positivismus.* Aalen: Scientia Verlag.

Vogt, K. M. (1998). *Skepsis und Lebenspraxis. Das pyrrhonische Leben ohne Meinungen.* München/Freiburg: Verlag Karl Alber.

Walker, L. J. (1986). Experiental and cognitive sources of moral development in adulthood. *Human Development, 29,* 113–124.

Webster, J. D. (2003). An exploratory analysis of a self-assessed wisdom scale. *Journal of Adult Development, 10,* 13–22.

Weintraub, R. (1997). *The sceptical challenge.* London/New York: Routledge.

Williams, M. (1996). *Unnatural doubts. Epistemological realism and the basis of scepticism.* Princeton, NJ: Princeton University Press.

Wink, P., & Helson, R. (1997). Practical and transcendent wisdom: Their nature and some longitudinal findings. *Journal of Adult Development, 4,* 1–15.

Winckelmann, J. (1825). *Sämtliche Werke.* Donauöschingen: Verlag Deutscher Classiker.

Winckelmann, J. (1977). *Gedanken über der Nachahmung der griechischen Werke in der Malerei und Bildhauerkunst.* Stuttgart: Ph.Reclam Verlag.

Yang, S. (2001). Conceptions of wisdom among Taiwanese Chinese. *Journal of Cross-Cultural Psychology, 32,* 662–680.

Twenty-One

Autobiographical Memory and the Narrative Self over the Life Span

James E. Birren and Johannes J. F. Schroots

I. Introduction

The purpose of this chapter is to explore the narrative self of the individual in relation to the dynamics of autobiographical memory across the life span. This chapter defines autobiographical memory as a type of episodic memory for information related to the self, in the form of both memories (retrospective memory) and expectations (prospective memory). "If retrospective memory relates to the retrieval of memories, experiences, or past events in the present, then prospective autobiographical memory is concerned with the retrieval of expectations, anticipations, or future events, which likewise are based on present memory functioning" (Schroots, van Dijkum, & Assink, 2004, p. 70).

Recognition of the complexity of aging has resulted from the increasing number of longitudinal studies in which genetics, health, the physical and social environments of individuals, and their behavior are found to interact over the course of life (Schroots & Birren, 1993; Schaie, 2005). Slowest to emerge have been explorations of the roles in aging related to "top down" concepts of the control of human behavior, such as purpose, intentionality, wisdom, religious beliefs, and value-determined choices (Birren & Schroots, 2001). In a broad view, there are emerging issues of the extent to which one's interpretation of life and beliefs of control and values influence longevity and quality of life.

A new approach to exploring aging from a psychological perspective derives from the individual's interpretation of causality in life. Such information can only be obtained from individuals themselves, a combination of autobiographical memories, and a personal synthesizing organization of them, called the "self."

There is a growing agreement among researchers that there is an important and strong relationship between self and autobiographical memory. Conway and Pleydell-Pearce (2000, p. 261) argue that autobiographical memory is part of the self and of fundamental significance for emotions and the experience of personhood, i.e., for the experience of enduring as an individual, in a culture, over time.

Who am I? What am I? The source of the information lies in autobiography. An autobiography is the story of an individual's life told or written by himself or herself that is based on the recall of memories, events, experiences, and relationships with other persons. The narrative self reflects the awareness of the individual's particular being or identity as distinguished from that of other persons.

Although autobiographical memories and autobiographical narratives are closely related to each other, memory researchers and narrative researchers have gone their separate ways, using different concepts, theories, and methods within their own traditions (Robinson & Taylor, 1998). Studies of autobiographical memory follow mostly the experimental tradition of "bottom up" research at the event level of individual lives. Studies of life stories and narratives, however, follow a more existential–phenomenological "top down" approach.

This chapter attempts to bring together two areas of contemporary interests in psychology: autobiographical memory and the emergence of the narrative self. It is another window through which we can gain an understanding of the complexities and the course of human life. This chapter begins with studies of autobiographical memory at the event level of analysis, as life events are the building blocks of life stories (Bluck & Habermas, 2001).

II. Autobiographical Memory

A. History

The psychological study of memory started more than a century ago and can be characterized by two different traditions (Baddeley, 1999). The first tradition relates to experimental research on learning and memory, initiated by the German psychologist Ebbinghaus in 1885 with the publication of his epoch-making book on higher mental processes of memory (*Ueber das Gedächtnis*). Ebbinghaus adapted Fechner's experimental, psychophysical methods to the study of memory as a pure function of learning, independent of meaning and content. To this end, he studied the structure, organization, and accuracy of memory under controlled laboratory conditions using nonsense syllables as stimuli. Ebbinghaus was the first to publish the experimental results of measuring forgetting as a function of time, represented in the famous "forgetting curve" (Boring, 1950).

The second tradition in memory research was started by the British psychologist Francis Galton. In 1879 he conducted what is now often considered to be the first empirical study of autobiographical memory. Galton displayed a word to himself and then allowed the word to elicit some type of association, the so-called "prompt word" technique. As psychology developed as a natural science, the experimental laboratory tradition of Ebbinghaus was followed during the next 100 years and Galton's approach passed into oblivion with the exception of Sir Frederic Bartlett's (1932) work, which criticized the experimental study of memory for its use of meaningless stimulus material. Bartlett advocated a different approach in which subjects learn and recall meaningful material under naturalistic conditions. Presumably, the past experimental research excluded many important variables influencing the functions of memory and their organization.

Since the 1970s there has been an upsurge in the interest of "everyday memory." Crovitz and Schiffman (1974) modified Galton's "prompt word" technique by presenting subjects with a word and then asking them to think of a specific memory they associated with that word. Later researchers extended this cued-memory technique by sampling autobiographical memory without restrictions on time of occurrence or kind of experience (Rubin, 1986).

B. Definitions

In the past decades, the concept of autobiographical memory was under discussion among memory researchers, who at first studied the psychological function of memory in general, but later made a distinction between long- and short term memory (Broadbent, 1958). Short-term or working memory refers to the temporary storage of material necessary for performing a range of complex tasks such as comprehension, reasoning, and long-term learning. Long-term memory refers to more durable encoding and storage systems. This division puts autobiographical memory in the long-term memory category.

In 1972 Tulving divided long-term memory into episodic and semantic memory, the first referring to personally experienced events and the last to general facts, e.g., knowing how to read and write. According to this finer distinction, autobiographical memory should be conceived as a form of episodic memory. Tulving (2002) developed the concept of episodic memory in more detail, pointing out three important elements: (1) a sense of subjective time, which enables one to travel back in time in one's own mind; (2) the ability to be aware of subjective time, which is called "autonoetic awareness"; and (3) a "self" that can travel in subjective time. Tulving does not use the term "autobiographical memory" and the as yet unsolved question is whether episodic memory and autobiographical memory are different terms for the same memory system. Rubin (1995, p. 1) had a pragmatic answer to this academic question when he stated that "definitions should not be set a priori, but should reflect the natural cleavages that researchers found in nature." Bluck and Habermas (2001) described research on "autobiographical memory" generally, "as any sort of research in which individuals recall episodes from their own past; the focus in most research is on the recall of specific, individual memories of particular events" (p. 135).

Definitions of autobiographical memory refer invariably to the individual's past, i.e., retrospective memory. Recently, however, some experimental researchers have shown interest in prospective memory, which can be defined "... as remembering at some point in the future that something has to be done, without any prompting in the form of explicit instructions to recall" (Maylor et al., 2002, p. 236). This definition, which emphasizes the memory function of "remembering to remember," covers only partly prospective *auto*biographical memory functioning. As Tulving argues, episodic memory enables the *autos* or "self" (from Greek) to travel in subjective time, not only back in time, but also forward into the future. Human beings are living their lives in time and are aware both of what has been and what may come.

C. Patterns of Events

Life stories, narratives, and similar autobiographical reports are composed of personal memories, experiences, expectations, and anticipations, which are usually labeled with the generic term of life events. Life events are the building blocks of life stories or, to put it differently, the story of a life is given substance, size, and shape by the events it embodies (Bluck, 2001; deVries & Watt, 1996). The sampling of autobiographical memory in terms of life events without restrictions on time of occurrence or type of event produces some remarkable patterns, which are described by

Conway and Pleydell-Pearce (2000) as follows: (a) *Forgetting* or retention curve in the form of a mathematical power function. The pattern of this curve shows a steep drop in the beginning of the retention period (so-called recency effect) and a slower decline as retention time increases (cf. Ebbinghaus, 1885). (b) *The childhood amnesia* pattern reflects the reduction or absence of memories coming from the first years of life. (c) *The autobiographical memory bump* pattern is only found for people over the age of 40. The distribution of memories departs from a simple forgetting function and turns into a roughly bimodal distribution of memories with a concentration of memories between 10 and 30 years of age, called the "bump," and another from the recent past (recency effect).

Many interpretations have been proposed regarding this complex, bimodal pattern, for which Rubin, Rahhal, and Poon (1998) have produced conclusive evidence: "... for older adults the period from 10 to 30 years of age produces recall of the most autobiographical memories, the most vivid memories, and the most important memories. It is the period in which are developed peoples' favorite films, music, and books, and the period from which they judge the most important world events to have originated" (p. 3). Conway and co-workers (2005) confirmed the universality of the bump pattern in a cross-cultural investigation of autobiographical memory, i.e., similar retrieval curves were observed in which the periods of childhood amnesia and the bump were the same across five cultural groups from Japan, China, Bangladesh, England, and the United States. In explaining the bump pattern, Rubin and colleagues (1998) proposed four possible theoretical accounts from four different areas of psychology. The following summary, which has been liberally composed of their comprehensive

literature review, provides an outline of the four arguments.

1. Cognitive Account

Events from early adulthood are remembered best because they occur in a period of transitions from rapid change to stability. In times of rapid change many novel events are encountered, which benefit recall as follows. First, when a novel event is encountered at the end of a period of change, there is more effort after meaning, which increases the event's memorability. Second, there may be a lack of proactive interference, which is an important cause of forgetting because the novel event is different from what has preceded it. Third, the first time that an event occurs it should be more distinctive both because of its novelty and because more attention is paid to details that the individual will learn to ignore in later occurrences. Such distinctiveness is an aid to later memory. Rubin and colleagues also noted the benefits of stability on later recall, i.e., events from stable periods are more likely to serve as prototypes or models for future occurrences and thus may be retrieved and rehearsed more as new events are retrospectively compared to them. Further, once a stable cognitive structure has been established, this structure will serve as a stable organization to cue events.

2. Cognitive Abilities/Neural Substrate Account

If cognitive abilities were to rise and fall as a function of age with the same time course as that for the bump, this rise and fall would account for enhanced memory in early adulthood if one assumes that people learn in proportion to their ability. In contrast, if there was a rapid, major increase in abilities followed by a period of relative stability, or slow decline, then a more complex explanation would be needed. The latter pattern is the case, both for cognitive processing speed and memory test data as for fluid intelligence. At the neural level, both patterns could exist, i.e., an aspect of neural development could either follow a course similar to the pattern of cognitive abilities, with a rapid rise and slow decline, or it could peak sharply in early adulthood.

3. Narrative/Identity Account

A sense of identity develops in late adolescence. If identity is viewed as a narrative of the important aspects of one's life and if much of identity is formed in early adulthood, there will be more events in that narrative that come from early adulthood than would be expected from a monotonic forgetting function. In addition, events from this period will be more likely to be organized and incorporated into an overall story or view of the self and thus benefit mnemonically from all the advantages of such a schematic organization as well as from increased spaced rehearsal.

4. Genetic Fitness Account

Early adulthood could be special because it is the time of the greatest potential to reproduce. That is, the increase in memory during the bump could serve the cognitive functions needed in selecting the best mate. In addition, it might not have been as common for our ancestors to live as long as we now do, so there might have been less selection pressure for a high level of functioning beyond a certain age.

All four accounts derive their interpretative power mainly from descriptive evidence, but fail to give an explanation for the emergence of the autobiographical memory bump over the life span. Schroots (2003) and colleagues suggested a *dynamic* explanation in terms of a "dual process theory of ontogenesis," stating that two synchronic life span forces of growth and senescing, respectively, generate the bump via relatively more intensive encoding of information between 10 and 30 years of age. Support for this theory was obtained by the construction, computer simulation and empirical validation of a mathematical model, called Janus after the Roman god with two faces—one face looking into the future and one into the past. Essentially, the Janus model describes the synchronic course of two limited growth and decline curves from birth to death and their impact on neurobehavioral functioning of autobiographical memory, as demonstrated empirically for autobiographical data collected with the life-line interview method for three age groups, young, middle-aged, and older adults (Schroots & van Dijkum, 2004).

With regard to prospective autobiographical memory, we want to note that Schroots, van Dijkum, and Assink (2004) observed forgetting curves, including proximity patterns or recency for all three age groups, but that a similar pattern as the bump for past events did not occur in the future curve of middle-aged and older adults.

D. Affective Valence of Life Events

While the bump pattern of the recall of autobiographical memories of events is a well-established, universal phenomenon, little is known about the life span distribution of events in terms of affect or emotion. Although the terms "affect" and "emotion" have different meanings, in practice they are used more or less interchangeably (Strongman, 1996). Many studies of life events have focused predominantly on the negative aspects and consequences of important life events for individual health and well-being (Zautra, Affleck, & Tennen, 1994).

The question arises whether the one-sided emphasis on so-called critical, stressful, or negative life events does justice to the whole range of memories and expectations over the life span.

Using a time line, deVries and Watt (1996), reported that the majority of life events were rated as positive for both past and future of the individual. However, older respondents reported less positive events for the future than middle-aged and younger people. Martin and Smyer (1990) asked participants to report about life events that had occurred at different times in their life span and found that the ratio of positive and negative events was 1.6, which means that for each 10 negative events there were 16 positive events. In a study where depressed and nondepressed participants were asked to retrieve 30 memories, all participants recalled more positive than negative memories (Yang & Rehm, 1993). Using a diary self-report memory method, Thompson (1998) found a small effect of pleasantness such that positive events were remembered slightly better than negative events. Robinson and Taylor (1998) simply asked women to tell about their lives resulting in more pleasant than unpleasant memories. In general, most research suggests that people remember more positive events than negative events.

In contrast, Assink and Schroots (2002) reported that in a study of 98 persons with the life-line interview method as many positive events as negative events were found for both past and future of the individual. In addition they reported that the distribution of positive and negative events over past and future is dependent on age, i.e., the older people are, the more positive they are about the past and the less positive about the future, whereas the younger people are, the more positive they are about the future and less positive about the past. Based on the affective ratings of both past and

future events (total life), an interaction effect of age and gender was observed on the mean affect for life in general, with young women being more positive about life than young men, whereas middle-aged and older men were more positive about life than middle-aged and older women. Finally, Assink and Schroots (2002) demonstrated a "positive affect bump" for middle-aged and older adults who remember more positive events for the period of about 10 to 40 years of age than for other periods of life. These findings are fairly consistent with the study results of Berntsen and Rubin (2002) and Rubin and Berntsen (2003), who also reported a clear bump for positive events, but a monotonically decreasing retention function for negative events. Briefly summarized, there is increasing evidence that pleasant and unpleasant memories follow a differential retention function in middle-aged and older adults.

Walker, Skowronski, and Thompson (2003) mentioned the well-known phenomenon that in surveys of subjective well-being, people generally report that they are happy with their lives. In an attempt to explain this phenomenon, Walker and colleagues (2003) referred to studies of autobiographical memory. From a temporal perspective, there is some similarity between autobiographical memory and subjective well-being, i.e., both concepts refer to the past and future of the individual as constructed in the present. Subjective well-being refers not only to the evaluation of the present life situation, but also to appraisal of the past and expectations for future well-being. It is not surprising then that in various life span studies of subjective well-being, similar affect patterns are demonstrated as for autobiographical memory. Generally, young adults rate their past well-being lower and future well-being higher than present subjective well-being; middle-aged adults believe that they will function at about the same level of well-being in the future as they do in the present, and older adults rate their past well-being higher and their future well-being lower than their present well-being (Keyes & Ryff, 1999; Staudinger, Bluck, & Herzberg, 2003). The question arises as to what extent life events are related to individual levels of subjective well-being.

To our knowledge there are only two studies directly concerned with the relationship between subjective well-being and autobiographical memory. Suh, Diener, and Fujita (1996) explored the effect of past events on subjective well-being in a 2-year longitudinal study and found that only life events during the previous 3 months influenced life satisfaction and positive and negative affect. These findings are partly in accordance with the results of the time-line study of deVries and co-workers (2001), who asked young, middle-aged, and older participants to identify in units of time (e.g., days, months, years) what was or will be the best and worst time of their lives as an indication for subjective well-being: "With minor exception, the best of times appear to be the times of the present, including the period immediately preceding and following. In relative contrast to the best times, the identification of worst times was not clearly related to age and is much more variable" (pp. 146–147). The results of the time-line study differentiate the findings of Suh and colleagues (1994) in that results show that only recent events have an impact on subjective well-being in the sense that distant negative events may also influence the individual's level of well-being.

Summarizing, it can be concluded that (a) most people remember more positive events than negative events, in particular for the autobiographical memory bump period, and (b) primarily recent or proximate events affect individual well-being.

E. Content of Lives

So far we have discussed the view that life stories and similar autobiographical data are composed of elementary pieces or memories of life events, which may form particular patterns with certain affective qualities. The question now arises what type of events people of different ages remember from their past or expect for the future. In order to answer this question, the content of life events has to be analyzed, which is usually a problematic task as quantitative and qualitative approaches in science and the humanities merge into one another almost imperceptibly (Denzin & Lincoln, 2000). From a methodological perspective, the minimal ambition should be to categorize the (unstructured) autobiographical data in such a way that they can be analyzed statistically (Schroots & Birren, 2002). A quick glance, however, at the research literature in the field of life stories, narratives, life review, and reminiscing is not very encouraging, i.e., many different lists and schemes of categories are proposed, as well as many different ways of analyzing and reporting data (Haight & Webster, 1995).

After a partial successful attempt to compare the life stories of the life-line interview method (LIM) and time line (TL) in terms of type of events, Schroots and Assink (2004) concluded that there is a real need for the standardization of the content analysis of autobiographical material, particularly for standard coding lists. In order to fill this need, Schroots and Assink (2004) developed a coding list for the categorization of life events and classified the events into nine categories (relations, school, work, health, growth, home, birth, death, and other) representing the most important themes and domains of life and borrowed wholly or partly from Birren and Hedlund (1987), Sugarman (1986), deVries and Watt (1996), and Zautra, Affleck, and Tennen (1994). These nine categories were subdivided systematically into 40 subcategories in all so as to produce a more detailed classification of events. Finally, a coding list has been compiled with typical examples of LIM life events, which run, for example, as follows: "I married my sweetheart from high school after graduation at age 17" and "I lost my father when I was four years old."

Despite lacking standards for the content analysis of autobiographical data, a global review of different studies shows some similarity in type of reported life events between men and women of different ages. For instance, Baum and Stewart (1990), as well as deVries and Watt (1996), found that women generally are more focused on school issues, romance, and childbirth, whereas work-related events are more important for men. Younger adults mention more school-related events, friendship, and sexuality; middle-aged adults mention more childbirth and growth activities; and older respondents mention war, retirement, and health as being more important. Changes over the life span in the interactions of cognition, motivation, and emotion have been studied by Carstensen and colleagues (2003). Chapter 15 discusses the relationships of these components of behavior in relation to aging.

Elnick et al. (1999) studied the content of life events reported in the bump period by individuals aged 40 year and older and found that the predominant category in this period relates to "family/relation" type of events. Rönka, Oravala, and Pulkkinen (2003) asked 283 men and women at age 36 to report important turning points in their life; most turning points involved family life (e.g., marriage, divorce, birth of a child), followed by turning points relating to education, work, and social transitions. They also found differences between men and women, i.e., women mention more often events related to family building and to changes in the health of people close to them, whereas men are more focused on the work sphere. These findings are not much of a surprise, nor is the conclusion that positive turning points are usually related to the birth of a child, marriage, and success in realizing one's own goals, whereas negative turning points are related to losses and include, for example, interpersonal problems and failures in regard to one's own goals (Rönka et al., 2003).

The capacity to recall events with age should be differentiated from the evaluation of events on an emotional basis. Thus one may recall a strict disciplinarian teacher who was disliked but later in life may be regarded as "doing a good job, and I now realize how much good she did for me." The emotional valence may change with age, but the recall of the details of the classroom scenes may remain stable.

In this context, it should be emphasized that gender, age of respondent, and age at occurrence of a certain event have an effect on the affective rating of events as the same event can be experienced in quite different ways depending on personality, life stage, earlier experiences, and experiences in the lives of others to whom the individual is related (Settersten, 1999). For example, Neugarten (1977) claimed that the timing of salient events is very important. Unanticipated, off-time events, e.g., death of a child, require greater adjustment than anticipated on-time events (death of parent at old age) and consequently will be accompanied by a stronger affect and presumably influence the readiness for later recall.

In a LIM study of 47 men and 51 women, almost equally divided over a younger (18–30), a middle-aged (31–55) and an older (56–84) age group,

Schroots and Assink (2005) analyzed the content of 98 life stories at the event level. The first pattern of events that emerged from the data confirmed the general findings of the aforementioned studies that men are more oriented toward work and that women are more concerned with health and birth. Middle-aged men, for instance, have few ideas how life will look after retirement, whereas middle-aged women have a much broader perspective and mention events from various domains such as work, health, growth, and death. These findings, stereotypic as they may seem, are consistent with recent life span models of male adult development with work at the center of the model, whereas models of women's development are more varied (Sterns & Huyck, 2001).

A more surprising pattern emerging from Schroots and Assink's content analytic study is that in adolescence — contrary to stereotypic expectations — young men report relational events, such as falling in love, more often than young women. With regard to the future of young adults, it was observed that young women expect almost no events in the period of 41 to 50 years of age; obviously they have difficulties forming an idea of this period. Schroots and Assink also noted that young men — contrary to young women — expect the death of their parents.

In middle age, adolescence is generally remembered as a positive period, but — contrary to young adults — middle-aged women report more memories concerning relationships from adolescence than middle-aged men. Some of these men had recently experienced the death of one of their parents, which had a great impact, as anticipated when they were younger (see earlier discussion).

As is the case with younger and middle-aged men, older men report the death of a parent, in contrast to women. For older women, life looks less rosy after the age of forty, as somehow anticipated when they were younger (see earlier discussion). They are confronted with problems in various domains of life such as relational problems, illness of parents and partner, and problems with their own health. With regard to the future of older men, Schroots and Assink observed another remarkable pattern, i.e., older men expect their partners to die earlier than themselves. This is a paradoxical finding, not only because married women or female partners are generally younger than their husband or partner, but also because women have a longer life expectancy. Whatever the case may be, the content analysis of Schroots and Assink's data suggests that the death of parents or partner is a much bigger issue for men than for women.

In closing this section we would like to mention the type and affect of life events as recalled from the bump period. Generally speaking, the bump period is dominated by memories of school (tens) and relations (twenties); also, more positive than negative events are recalled from this period (Schroots & Assink, 2005). The latter is in accordance with the findings of Berntsen and Rubin (2002) that older respondents show a clear bump in their twenties for the most important and happiest memories.

Summarizing, it should be noted that content analysis of autobiographical material at the microlevel of life events follows out of necessity a more inductive (i.e., hypotheses generating) than deductive (i.e., hypotheses testing) procedure. However, the obvious disadvantages of this approach in terms of testing hypotheses are outweighed by the advantages of the inductive enterprise in terms of theory formation and analytic transparency. The emerging patterns of events in the lives of individuals are, in retrospect, the final evidence that inductive procedures are sound scientific practice.

F. Life in the Middle: An Illustration

In 1995 Birren stated that "the study of aging has become a field of knowledge that is data rich and theory poor, a vast collection of un-integrated pieces of information" (p. 1). The study of life stories from the perspective of autobiographical memory runs the same risk of fragmentation and incoherence, as life stories are deconstructed at the event level by age, gender, affect, content, time perspective (past, future), and so on, resulting in a plethora of stratified data patterns. To produce order out of chaos and to illustrate the emerging patterns of life, Schroots and Assink (2005) made an attempt to reconstruct life stories for three age groups of men and women by compressing the LIM event data set in such a way that the most important patterns of life events were left. By way of illustration, the "average" life story of middle-aged adults is sketched in the form of a so-called "Portrait of Life."

Past. Recall of childhood by middle-aged women is mainly dominated by events concerning education and relocation, in contrast to men who have merely negative memories of their elementary school period. Adolescence is remembered as a positive period by both men and women. Young men seem to be more occupied with relationships in adolescence than young women; for the middle-aged group, however, it is the other way around, middle-aged women report more memories concerning relationships from adolescence than middle-aged men, who for their part report memories from the domains school and work. Middle-aged women have experienced adolescence as a period of personal growth. When they are in their twenties, women get married, but for some of them the relationship ends in a divorce. Middle-aged men also start a family life in this period, but when they are in their thirties, work issues are emerging (problems in the work situation, getting another job). Some of these middle-aged men have recently experienced the death of one of their parents which had a great impact, as anticipated when they were younger.

Future. Thinking about their future, middle-aged men report mainly work-related events (getting another job, retirement). In the near future both middle-aged men and women expect a change in the work domain. Some men expect to get divorced in this period, which is about 10 years after women mention this event. Middle-aged men do not have any idea yet about how life will look after retirement. Women have a broader perspective and mention events in different domains (work, health, growth, death). Their future time perspective extends that of men and they are afraid to lose their partner.

It should be noted that the aforementioned "average" life story of people living in the middle consists of two parts, past and future, which correspond with the way respondents are asked to report about their lives: first the events from their past and then the events they expect for the future. In this context it is illuminating that Berntsen and Rubin (2002) made a conceptual distinction between life narrative and life script.

Life script is generic (it deals with cultural norms and expectations to the content and order of a typical life course), whereas a life narrative is concrete (it deals with the individual life as actually lived, reconstructed, and narrated by a concrete individual). Life script deals with cultural expectations, whereas life narrative deals with personal memories" (p. 640).

Findings of the Schroots and Assink (2004) study show that when young, middle-aged, and older people are asked to tell about their past and future life, their past life story consists of personal memories, whereas their future life story is more general and prototypical.

G. Memory and the Self

Many psychologists agree about the importance of the "self" in organizing and regulating mental life. They conceive of the self as a richly interconnected knowledge structure — the sum total of stored information about personal attributes and experiences. The self plays a preeminent role in the encoding of life events and the retrieval of memories. "Numerous experiments have shown that when we encode new information by relating it to the self, subsequent memory for that information improves compared to other types of encoding (Schacter, 2001, p. 150).

Conway and Pleydell-Pearce (2000, p. 261) elaborated on the relationship between autobiographical memory and the self as follows: "Autobiographical memory is of fundamental significance for the self, for emotions, and for the experience of personhood, that is, for the experience of enduring as an individual, in a culture, over time." Starting from this perspective, Conway and Pleydell-Pearce (2000) developed an integrative, hierarchical model of a so-called "self-memory system" that links an autobiographical knowledge base with information at three different hierarchical levels of specificity (i.e., lifetime periods, general events, and event-specific knowledge) to personal goals. These goals function as control processes in the self-memory system and modulate the construction of memories. Autobiographical memories are encoded and later retrieved in ways that serve the self's goal agendas. As such, current goals influence how autobiographical information is absorbed and organized in the first place, and goals generate retrieval models to guide the search process later. The autobiographical knowledge base also helps ground the self's goals. People formulate goals for the future that are reasonably in line with the information encoded as lifetime periods, general events, and event-specific knowledge. Bluck and Habermas (2001) extended Conway and Pleydell-Pearce's cognitive-oriented self-memory system by introducing their "life story schema" of four types of coherences (temporal, biographical, causal, and thematic coherence), i.e., a skeletal mental representation of life's major components and links, which frames the interaction between self and memory such that the individual engages not only in goal-pursuit to reduce self-discrepancies but also in meaning making, both to understand the past and to predict the future (McAdams, 2003).

III. The Narrative Self

A. History and Definition

The present purpose is to characterize the status of research and scholarship about the narrative self in relation to autobiographical memory and its role in the organization of behavior. Personal experiences lead to the formation of autobiographical memories and evolve into development of a narrative self, the self we tell our selves we are and also tell others.

The self is an important determinant of decisions we make so that our behavior is congruent with our views of our selves. It is not surprising that the self is viewed differently in the many scholarly fields: Philosophy, religion, psychology, sociology, neuroscience, and literature. They have different emphases about the self being formed from within and without, from sins and good works, from experiences, and from self-determination and free will.

In its history, psychology did not encourage the study of the narrative self as it was soft, subjective, and difficult to relate it to more elemental psychological processes. More recently, studies of the "inside" or personal views of life are becoming more frequent. Views of the narrative self have been encouraged by a wide range of reminiscence methods, professional orientations, different settings, and populations (see Bornat, 1994; Reker & Chamberlain, 2000). Purposes range from serving scholarly interests to serving populations at need, e.g., depressed or demented persons. A window was opened on the subject matter by Butler's 1963 article on life review indicating that there was motivation in late life to engage in a review of the contents of one's life.

The broad range of literature that has emerged since Butler's article appeared has provided a richness to the subject matter, but it is difficult at the present time to integrate the information into a coherent picture. The sources of information range from the study of elemental processes of memory (bottom up study) to the life stories gathered by psychologists, sociologists, and anthropologists (top down study) and the life stories and views of the self of patients treated by social workers, nurses, and other clinicians.

The narrative self or our identity is built upon our vast store of autobiographical memories of the events of our lives. What we recall and how we interpret our memories comprise the stories of our lives. Heikkinen pointed out that "The identity of the self is constructed in and through the story, the narrative that runs from beginning to end, from birth to the death of the self" (1996, p. 187). McAdams (1996) added that "...identity is a quality of the mature Me, a way of telling the Me in adolescence and adulthood so that the Me appears (to the self and others) to be unified and purposeful" (p. 134). Others have called the organization of the narrative self as "coherence." Although there is a common drive for coherence, our narrative selves can embrace contradictions and myths as autobiographical memories are recalled, omitted, or reinterpreted, according to a present view of the self. The narrative self is a product of self making that provides us with meaningfulness and uniqueness that come from "... distinguishing ourselves from others, which we do by comparing our self-told accounts of ourselves with the accounts that others give us of themselves, which add further ambiguity. For we are forever mindful of the difference between what we tell ourselves about ourselves and what we reveal to others" (Bruner, 2003, p. 211).

In a hierarchical view of the organization of human behavior, the narrative self and its construction can be viewed as lying close to wisdom, as it deals with uncertainty and how "...the elements of the story must be interpreted, and the links between them be established" (Brugman, 2000, p. 4). Thus the development of wisdom and display of wise behavior is viewed as depending on a knowledge of the self. In summary, the narrative self is the product of a dynamic process involving memory, cognition, emotion, and motivation that equips an individual to take a top down view of himself or herself and make choices that are consistent with evolving values and goals.

B. The Emerging Self

Studies have been done on the development of the self in childhood and adolescence (Fivush & Haden, 2003) and are also reported on middle age and older adults (Birren et al., 1996). This gives rise to the expectation that the narrative self will come to be viewed as a lifelong dynamic process and the subject matter will find a place in developmental and general psychology.

Studies of the emergence of the self in children from the postnatal period to age 7 have shown that development of the self follows a pattern as the children develop the capacity "... to make increasingly distinct *contrasts* between the self and other aspects of the world of experience" (Nelson, 2003, p. 4). Six successive levels of understanding have been described that develop and culminate at ages five to seven years in "Cultural Self Understanding." Further, "...a narrative and cultural self emerges from the social, cognitive, and representational self established in the years two to six" (Nelson, p. 24).

Reinforcing the image of the self that the child develops is the reminiscing that the parents, particularly the mother, do (Reese & Farrant, 2003). The shared reminiscence between parents and children is heavily influenced by culture and leads to secure or avoidant attachment and the memories that are carried forward into adult life. The complexity of the subjective experience of an event is illustrated in an example provided by Reese and Farrant (2003).

For example, the event of feeding ducks at the park appears at the outset to be a positive event, at least when compared to a negative event such as attending a funeral. However, the event may have consisted of the mother refusing to give the child any bread because he was noisy on the drive over, and scolding him for getting dirty. These negative aspects of the event could actually be reinforced in later discussions of the past event if the mother focused exclusively on the child's misbehavior (p. 44).

Here we have a condensed picture of the complexity of the interrelationships between memories of scenes and what is later recalled in adulthood. The context of events may have differing influences on the recall of sibling memories and formation of the narrative self depending on subjective experiences of events and the manner in which parents and family may later reminisce about an event. In addition to pointing out the relationship between reminiscence and culture, Reese and Farrant (2003) also pointed out that attachments, secure and insecure, are influenced by culture. They concluded, "The implications for autobiographical memory and self would then depend on the valued forms of reminiscing in the culture. If it is psychologically adaptive in that culture for children to adopt a less elaborative manner of reminiscing and a sense of self that is interdependent with others, then a secure rather than insecure attachment should lead to that outcome" (p. 45).

Haden (2003, p. 66) concluded that the styles of parent–child interactions and cultural influences on family patterns of reminiscing "…can be critical to the construction of a self-narrative or life history that will at least in part reflect variation in the way communities socially share understanding and experience." Cultural differences and their influences on different views of the self have been compared across Korea, China, India, and the United States by Leichtman, Wang, and Pillemer (2003, pp. 73–97). They also pointed out that "The production and maintenance of autobiographical memories over the life course is a complex process that takes place within biological, psychological, and environmental contexts" and added "…we recognize that memory is a product of multiple levels of contextual influence (p. 94)."

In addition, gender also influences how individual's autobiographical memories are described in culturally appropriate ways (Hayne & MacDonald, 2003; Fivush & Buckner, 2003). What these studies have shown is that the self and autobiographical memories emerge early in life and, as the self is established, it becomes a selective factor in what is recalled.

McAdams (2003) pointed out that there is a lifelong process of defining the self while individuals lead active lives that also have future goals. Thus all of the researchers and scholars emphasize the dynamic process of individuals developing a sense of self from a tremendous range of life experiences and being confronted with the need to select autobiographical memories to construct a narrative self and tell a life story to oneself and others.

To this view, Bruner added that "Self-making is a narrative art, and although it is more constrained by memory than fictions, it is uneasily constrained…" (Bruner, 2003, p. 210). He pointed out that the making of the narrative self comprises a mixture of inside and outside information or experiences. He defines "inside" as consisting of memories, feelings, ideas, beliefs, and subjectivity. This "inside" interacts with the "outside," which consists of cultural influences that tell us how to interpret and communicate our views to ourselves and others. This leads to the issue for future research to determine the extent to which the narrative self is an arbitrary construction or one based on lifelong experience.

C. The Self and Existential Meaning

Reker and Chamberlain (2000) discussed the dynamics of the interpretation of life in terms of meaningfulness, the motivation to "... understand how events in life fit into a larger context. It involved the process of creating and discovering meaning, which is facilitated by a sense of coherence (order, reason for existence) and a sense of purpose (mission in life, direction)" (p. 1). They distinguished this type of existential meaning from "implicit or definitional meaning," which refers to the "attachment of personal significance to objects or events in life" (p. 1).

"From a life span perspective, the will to meaning is a continuous process, triggered by changing circumstances, shifting value orientations, and renewed aspirations. While themes and the course of meaning may change throughout the life span, the central features of the will to meaning in preserving one's identity and promoting one's sense of coherence remain unchanged" (Reker & Chamberlain, 2000, p. 2). They further pointed out the advantage of looking at existential meaning at different stages of the life span and transitions for understanding life span human development.

Existential meaning implies that individuals find unity in their lives, that the selves they tell themselves they are are integrated. Hermans (2000) pointed out that the self can have several voices that are not reducible to a single one. Kenyon (2000) explored the background of the interpretations of the self in philosophy. His view supports the idea that the self can be viewed in different ways, with different voices or in contradictory ways, "...existential meaning manifests itself in the paradox of living an inner life or *inside* story, while we simultaneously live with other persons in a culture and a society" (p. 7). He also supports the view that the self continues to develop over the life span. "In narrative terms, the experience of existential meaning, again paradoxically, involves the loss of letting go of an old story, as part of our becoming a new story, or experiencing new meaning" (Kenyon, 2000, p. 8). Here a bridge needs to be provided between empirical science and modern philosophy. This bridge needs to be crossed if we are to gain understanding of the contribution to the narrative self derived from institutional memberships and religion (see McFadden, 2000).

It seems useful to point out the differences in scholars' interests in the narrative self who might be identified as either constructionists or empiricists. The constructionists emphasize the subjectivity and arbitrariness of the life story and its plot. In contrast, the empiricists are interested in the objectivity and veracity of the life story and the memories upon which it is based. Interpreting a life story from a constructionist position focuses on the subjective usefulness of the life story and autobiographical memories. In contrast, the empiricists wish to link the life story with other data leading to verification of inferences. For example, a constructionist may claim in his/her life story that he/she is a channelist to persons in a next world. The empiricist would seek evidence of other world communication, in addition to the usefulness of the belief by the individual that he or she is a channelist.

The dynamics of the developing self and the important implications for behavior were characterized by Holstein and Gubrium (2000), "Nearly everything we attempt or accomplish today is done in relation to what kind of selves we are" (p. 10). Further, "...individual identity is the basis for all manner of choices and decision-making that affect our lives. Cradle to grave, we perennially refer to our selves to make sense of our conduct and experience, and to guide related actions. The self, in other words, is not only something we are, but an object we *actively* construct and live by."

D. Components of the Self

The narrative self appears to have several components. Reedy and Birren (1980) contrasted three aspect of the self: the ideal self, the real self, and the social image self. The ideal self is the person we would like to be, reflecting our aspirations and goals. The real self is the person we believe ourselves to be, our capacities, strengths, and weaknesses. The social image self is what we believe to be the views of other persons toward us. An important feature of the three selves is the distance among them. That is, an adolescent may have high ideals of what to achieve in life but does not believe he or she is near that actual ideal state.

Furthermore, the social image can be quite different because of the comments of parents and peers and feedback from school reports. The basic hypothesis is that from our autobiographical memories there emerges with age a trend toward adjusting our self views. Our expectations related to the ideal self are modified in the light of experience with work, relationships, family, sports, and other activities such as art or music. At the same time, the real self is brought more in line with the ideal as experiences of living reveal strengths (or weaknesses) not realized in youth. The social image self moves closer to the ideal and real selves as more feedback is provided by the years of engagement in life's activities with other persons. In brief, the basic hypothesis is that the distances among the components of the self move closer together with age and presumably result in less internal tension and more contentment with life (Figure 21.1).

The idea that the components of the self are dynamic and can be changed was further studied by Birren and Reedy (1980). Pre- and postparticipation measurements were made on a group of 45 subjects in a 10-session guided autobiography program. The three components of the self were found to move more closely together. Also, generalized views of the participants of other persons

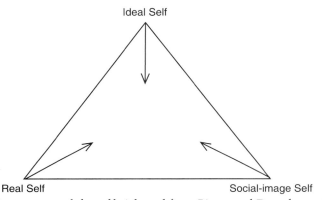

Figure 21.1 Components of the self. Adapted from Birren and Deutchman (1991, p. 11).

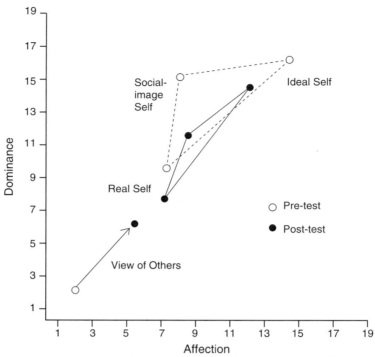

Figure 21.2 Mean scores before and after the autobiography class for real, ideal, and social-image selves and for the view of others, as measured by the Leary interpersonal checklist. Adapted from Reedy and Birren (1980).

moved more closely to their own views of self. This suggests that group participation facilitates reducing the distance among the three components of self and also reduced the distance between the self and others (Figure 21.2).

Research on the narrative self and reminiscence has touched upon therapeutic and coaching applications of recalling life memories. In a sense this involves the renegotiating of the narrative self, i.e., adapting views of the self to current challenges. In Erikson's view of developmental psychology, individuals go through stages of adapting to new challenges or demands (Hoare, 2002). Adaptations to natural events, such as deaths and home destruction from fire or floods, and social events, such as divorce and retirement, can initiate changes or renegotiations in the way the self is viewed by men and women (Barnes & Parry, 2004).

Such changes in the self can invoke selective changes in memories, e.g., those that fit a view of the self as being strong or weak.

A growing interest in the ambiguities of growing older in contemporary societies has prompted research on the influence of the narrative self on adaptations that individuals make. A study was conducted on 423 community residents 70 years and older. The researchers, Windle and Woods (2004), concluded that "The results add to the evidence from an increasing number of studies that demonstrates how psychological resources underlie the processes of adaptation to the changing situations that accompany increasing age and prevent negative outcomes" (p. 583). In this study the narrative self is regarded as a psychological resource. Presumably the narrative self as a psychological resource can have positive and negative outcomes on lives.

E. Future Perspectives

It is important to know the extent to which our subjective or internal views of our selves are influenced over time, our health, disabilities, activity level, and productivity, as they are measured objectively. Also, the way we view ourselves may, over time, influence our network of relationships that are important to the maintenance of well-being in the later years (Burnside & Schmidt, 1994).

Narrative selves are thought to be a dynamic product of autobiographical memories of experienced events. As discussed earlier, they also have a relationship to the futures individuals may project or want in their lives. The part of the self that embraces aspirations and goals is increasingly recognized as being influenced by religion and spiritual beliefs (McFadden, 1996). Like the narrative self, religious beliefs change over the life span (Coleman, Ivani-Chalian, & Robinson, 1998) and presumably influence the evolving narrative self, although not much research has been conducted on the relationship.

Manifestations of the self are observed in many ways, such as in the clothes we wear and the language style we use. We might hear a woman trying on a dress and saying, "This dress doesn't look right on me." Implicit is some comparison of the image projected by wearing the dress and the ideal self and the actual self of the person. Choice of clothing obviously reflects contemporary styles and culture but also expresses the narrative self, i.e., how the individual wants to project his or her image in relation to the mode of the period. Also word choice reflects the kind of image a person wants to project. Use of humor, flattery, sarcasm, ridicule, and verbal aggression reflects the culture of the individual but

also reflects the self that is being expressed (Berekmoes & Vingerhoets, 2004).

Presumably "Who I am" and "Who I want to be" affect our choices of purchases and complex behaviors. There is also the issue to be explored of the extent to which the individuals scan their autobiographical memories to guide their choices and answer implicit questions of "Does this look like me?" or "Does this sound like me?" Further research questions can be raised about comparing ones image with that of parents and other persons. To answer such questions, the linkage among autobiographical memories, the narratives, and behavior choice has to be explored through further research. Behind this complex picture is the view that the narrative self influences behavior choice and is an important area of study.

The narrative self is thought to be important in the choices individuals make and the outcomes of their lives, e.g., as scholars, artists, missionaries, martyrs, and terrorists. Further research is needed to identify the views of the self that contemporary martyrs and violent activists develop from their autobiographical memories that lead to or justify their actions. A tradition in the Japanese culture has been a ritual suicide, "hara-kiri," when face or honor was lost. This was an honorable form of suicide presumably based on a individual's view of himself and was necessary to recover an acceptable view of the social self. In this example, we suspect that the individual views himself in comparison with the memories of models of behavior passed on within families and the broader culture. The individual is viewing extreme choices of behavior and tries to balance the influence of cognitive, motivational, and emotional influences in his views of himself.

At a more abstract level, future research should be encouraged on how individuals project causality in their narrative selves. What are the consequences of individuals viewing themselves as products of predestiny or as products of life as lived? It seems plausible that the outcomes of individuals' lives are influenced greatly by their narrative selves and the generalizations they have made about causality.

One of the unresolved issues is the relationship between the narrative self and other functions of the central nervous system. Some psychologists give emphasis to the role of cognition in the formation of self and identity and minimize the roles of emotion, motivation, and intention (Kahsima, Foddy, & Platow, 2002). Clearly the self is complex and it evolves as one grows up, grows old, and is exposed to different social and physical circumstances. Yet the self does not appear to be a linear product of experiences and related memories. The self does not appear to be only the product of passive experience but rather a result of the individual's developing intentions interacting with memory.

Expansion of research with brain scanning methods is also expected to contribute to our knowledge about the organization of the narrative self. In fact, the abstract concept of the self is already being explored in brain imaging studies (Heatherton, Macrae, & Kelley, 2004; Mitchell, Heatherton, & Macrae, 2002; Macrae et al., 2004; Craik et al., 1999). Such research will help reveal how individuals' concepts of themselves influence their choices of behavior and decisions, i.e., top down regulation of behavior.

Exploring the inside of life, our personal views of ourselves, supplements what we have learned about the organization of behavior in more traditional designed research. One may expect from the growth of interest in autobiographical memory and the narrative self that future large-scale longitudinal studies will include the gathering of information from individuals about their "inside" views of themselves. Such studies can provide answers to questions about growing up and growing old and the outcomes of particular self views.

IV. Summary

This chapter brings together two areas of growing contemporary interest in the psychology of aging: autobiographical memory and the narrative self. The recall of autobiographical memories over the life span is a dynamic process. Research has shown that older people remember relatively more memories from adolescence and early adulthood, the "bump" period, than from other periods of life. In general, people also remember more positive events than negative events over the life span, and over the bump period in particular. The affect of past and future perspective changes with age, i.e., young adults recall relatively more negative events from their past than they expect from the future, whereas older people recall their past more positively and view their future more negatively. Evidence has further shown that memories recalled by men are more oriented toward work and women's memories toward health and family. Obviously the recall of autobiographical memory is a dynamic process related to age and gender.

Autobiographical memories also enter a dynamic relationship with developing selves. The self emerges from the events of a lifetime, their interpretation, and weaving into a life story. The narrative self is the self that individuals tell themselves and others that they are. The narrative self is regarded as important in the choices and decisions individuals make. For this reason it is anticipated that future longitudinal studies will include interpretations of life from the inside views of subjects, including how they project causality in their lives. The influence of the narrative self upon life outcomes of health, quality of life, productivity, and contentment largely remains to be explored.

References

Assink, M. H. J., & Schroots, J. J. F. (2002). The distribution of affect over the life span. *Hallym International Journal of Aging, 4*, 99–117.

Baddeley, A. D. (1999). *Essentials of human memory*. East Sussex: Psychology Press.

Barnes & Parry (2004). Renegotiation of identity and relationships: Men and women's adjustment to retirement. *Ageing & Society, 24*, 213–233.

Bartlett, F. (1932). *Remembering*. Cambridge: Cambridge University Press.

Baum, S. K., & Stewart, R. B. (1990). Sources of meaning through the lifespan. *Psychological Report, 67*, 3–14.

Berekmoes, C., & Vingerhoets, G. (2004). Neural foundations of emotional speech processing. *Current Directions in Psychological Science, 13*, 182–185.

Berntsen, D., & Rubin, D. C. (2002). Emotionally charged autobiographical memories across the life span: The recall of happy, sad, traumatic, and involuntary memories. *Psychology and Aging, 17*, 636–652.

Birren, J. E. (1995). Editorial: New models of aging: Comment on need and creative efforts. *Canadian Journal on Aging, 14*, 1–3.

Birren, J. E., & Deutchman, D. E. (1991). *Guiding autobiography groups for older adults*. Baltimore, MD: Johns Hopkins University Press.

Birren, J. E., & Hedlund, B. (1987). Contribution of autobiography to developmental psychology. In N. Eisenberg (Ed.), *Contemporary topics in developmental psychology* (pp. 394–415). New York: Wiley.

Birren, J. E., Kenyon, G. M., Ruth, J. E., Schroots, J. J. F., & Svensson, T. (Eds.) (1996). *Aging and biography: Explorations in adult development*. New York: Springer.

Birren, J. E., & Schroots, J. J. F. (2001). The history of geropsychology. In J. E. Birren &

K. W. Schaie (Eds.), *Handbook of the psychology of aging* (5th edition, pp. 3–28). San Diego: Academic Press.

Bluck, S., & Habermas, T. (2001). Extending the study of autobiographical memory: Thinking back about life across the life span. *Review of General Psychology, 5*, 135–147.

Boring, E. G. (1950). *A history of experimental psychology* (2nd edition). New York: Appleton-Century Crofts.

Bornat, J. (Ed.) (1994). *Reminiscence reviewed*. Philadelphia, PA: Open University Press.

Broadbent, D. E. (1958). *Perception and communication*. New York: Pergamon Press.

Brugman, G. (2000). *Wisdom: Source of narrative coherence & eudaimonia*. Delft, The Netherlands: Eburon.

Bruner, J. (2003). Self making narratives. In R. Fivush & C. A. Haden (Eds.), *Autobiographical memory and the construction of a narrative self* (pp. 209–225). Mahwah, NJ: Lawrence Erlbaum.

Burnside, I., & Schmidt, M. G. (Eds.) (1994). *Working with older adults*. Boston, MA: Jones & Bartlett.

Butler, R. N. (1963). The life review: An interpretation of reminiscence in the aged. *Psychiatry, 26*, 63–76.

Carstensen, L. L. Fung, H. H. & Charles, S. T. (2003). Socioemotional selectivity theory and the regulation of emotion in the second half of life. *Motivation & Emotion, 27*, 103–123.

Coleman, P. G. (1986). *Ageing and reminiscence processes*. New York: Wiley.

Coleman, P. G., Ivani-Chalian, C., & Robinson, M. (1998). The story continues: Persistence on life themes in old age. *Ageing & Society, 18*, 389–419.

Conway, M. A., & Pleydell-Pearce, C. W. (2000). The construction of autobiographical memories in the self-memory system. *Psychological Review, 107*, 261–288.

Conway, M. A., Wang, Q., Hanyu, K., & Haque, S. (2005). A cross-cultural investigation of autobiographical memory: On the universality and cultural variation of the reminiscence bump. *Journal of Cross-Cultural Psychology, 36*, 1–11.

Craik, F. I. M., Moroz, T. M., Moscovitch, M., Stuss, D. T., Wincour, G., Tulving, E., & Kapur, S. (1999). In search of the self: A positron emission tomography study. *Psychological Science, 10,* 26–34.

Crovitz, H. F., & Schiffman, H. (1974). Frequency of episodic memories as a function of their age. *Bulletin of the Psychonomic Society, 4,* 517–518.

Denzin, N. K., & Lincoln, Y. S. (Eds.) (2000). *Handbook of qualitative research* (2nd edition). Thousand Oaks, CA: Sage.

deVries, B., Blando, J., Southard, P., & Bubeck, C. (2001). The times of our lives. In G. Kenyon, P., Clark, & B. deVries (Eds.), *Narrative gerontology: Theory, research and practice* (pp. 137–158). New York: Springer.

deVries, B., & Watt, D. (1996). A lifetime of events: Age and gender variations in the life story. *International Journal of Aging and Human Development, 42,* 81–102.

Ebbinghaus, H. (1885/1964). *Memory: A contribution to experimental psychology.* New York: Dover.

Elnick, A. B., Margrett, J. A., Fitzgerald, J. M., & Labouvie-Vief, G. (1999). Benchmark memories in adulthood: Central domains and predictors of their frequency. *Journal of Adult Development, 6,* 45–59.

Fivush, R., & Buckner, J. P. (2003). Creating gender and identity through autobiography narratives. In R. Fivush & C. A. Haden (Eds.), *Autobiographical memory and the constructions of a narrative self.* (pp. 149–167). NAWAH, NJ: Lawrence Erlbaum.

Fivush, R., & Haden, C. A. (Eds.) (2003). *Autobiographical memory and the construction of a narrative self: Developmental and cultural perspectives.* Nahwah, NJ: Lawrence Erlbaum

Galton, F. (1879). Psychometric experiments. *Brain, 2,* 149–162.

Haden, C. A. (2003). Joint encoding and joint reminiscing: Implications for young children's understanding and remembering. In R. Fivush & C. A. Haden (Eds.), *Autobiographical memory and the construction of a narrative self: Developmental and cultural perspectives* (pp. 49–69). Nahwah, NJ: Lawrence Erlbaum.

Haight, B. K., & Webster, J. D. (Eds.) (1995). *The art and science of reminiscing: Theory, methods, and applications.* Washington, DC: Taylor & Francis.

Hayne, H., & MacDonald, S. (2003). The socialization of autobiographical memory in children and adults: The roles of culture and gender. In R. Fivush & C. A. Haden (Eds.), *Autobiographical memory and the construction of a narrative self: Developmental and cultural perspectives* (pp. 99–120). Nahwah, NJ: Lawrence Erlbaum.

Heatherton, T. F., Macrae, G. N., & Kelley, W. M. (2004). What the social brain sciences can tell us about the self. *Current Directions in Psychological Science, 13,* 190–193.

Heikkinen, R. L. (1996). Experienced aging as elucidated by narrative. In J. E. Birren, G. M. Kenyon, J. R. Ruth, J. J. F. Schroots, & T. Svensson (Eds.), *Aging and biography: Explorations in adult development* (pp. 187–204). New York: Springer.

Hermans, H. J. M. (2000). Meaning as movement. In G. T. Reker & K. Chamberlain (Eds.), *Exploring existential meaning* (pp. 23–38). Thousand Oaks, CA: Sage.

Hoare, C. H. (2002). *Erikson on development in adulthood.* New York: Oxford University Press.

Holstein, J. A., & Gubrium, J. F. (2000). *The self we live by: Narrative identity in a postmodern world.* New York: Oxford University Press.

Kahsima, Y., Foddy, M., & Platow, M. (Eds.) (2002). *Self and identity: Personal, social, and symbolic.* Nahwah, NJ: Lawrence Erlbaum.

Kenyon, G. M. (2000). Philosophical foundations of existential meaning. In G. T. Reker & K. Chamberlain (Eds.), *Exploring existential meaning* (pp. 7–22). Thousand Oaks, CA: Sage.

Kenyon, G. M., & Randall, W. L. (1997). *Restorying our lives.* Westport, CT: Praeger.

Keyes, C. L., & Ryff, C. D. (1999). Psychological well-being in midlife. In S. L. Willis & J. D. Reid (Eds.), *Life in the middle: Psychological and social development in middle age* (pp. 161–180). San Diego: Academic Press.

Koenig, H. G., McCullough, M. E., & Larson, D. B. (Eds.) (2001). *Handbook of religion and health.* Oxford: Oxford University Press.

Leichtman, M. D., Wang, Q., & Pillemer, D. P. (2003). Cultural variations in interdependence and autobiographical memory: Lessons from Korea, China, India, and the United States. In R. Fivush & C. A. Haden (Eds.), *Autobiographical memory and the construction of a narrative self: Developmental and cultural perspectives* (pp. 73–98). Nahwah, NJ: Lawrence Erlbaum.

Macrae, C. N., Moran, J. M., Heatherton, T. F., Banfield, J. F., & Kelley, W. M. (2004). Medial prefrontal activity predicts memory for self. *Cerebral Cortex, 14,* 647–654.

Martin, P., & Smyer, M. A. (1990). The experience of micro- and macroevents: A life-span analysis. *Research on Aging, 12,* 294–310.

Maylor, E. A., Darby, R. J., Logie, R. H., Della Sala, S., & Smith, G. (2002). Prospective memory across the lifespan. In P. Graf & N. Ohta (Eds.), *Lifespan development of human memory* (pp. 235–256). Cambridge: The MIT Press.

McAdams, D. P. (1996). Narrating the self. In J. E. Birren, G. M. Kenyon, J. E. Ruth, J. J. F. Schroots, & T. Svensson (Eds.), *Aging and biography: Explorations in adult development* (pp.131–148). New York: Springer.

McAdams, D. P. (2003). Identity and the life story. In R. Fivush & C. A. Haden (Eds.), *Autobiographical memory and the construction of a narrative self* (pp. 187–207). Nahwah, NJ: Lawrence Erlbaum.

McFadden, S. H. (1996). Religion, spirituality, and aging. In J. E. Birren & K. W. Schaie (Eds.), *Handbook of the psychology of aging.* 4th ed., (pp. 162–177). San Diego, CA: Academic Press.

McFadden, S. H. (2000). Religion and meaning in life. In G. T. Reker & K. Chamberlain (Eds.), *Exploring existential meaning in late life* (pp. 171–183). Thousand Oaks, CA: Sage.

McFadden, S. H., Brennan, M., & Patrick, J. H. (Eds.) (2003). *New directions in the study of late life religiousness and spirituality.* New York: Springer.

Mitchell, J. P., Heatherton, T. F., & Macrae, C. N. (2002). Distinct neural systems subserve person and object knowledge.

Proceedings of the National Academy of Sciences, US, 99, 15238–15243.

Nelson, K. (2003). Narrative and self, myth and memory: Emergence of the cultural self. In R. Fivush & C. A. Haden (Eds.), *Autobiographical memory: Theoretical and applied perspectives* (pp. 3–28). Nahwah, NJ: Lawrence Erlbaum.

Neugarten, B. L. (1977). Personality and aging. In J. E. Birren & K. W. Schaie (Eds.), *Handbook of the psychology of aging* (pp. 626–649). New York: Van Nostrand-Reinhold.

Reedy, M. N., & Birren, J. E. (1980). *Life review through autobiography.* Poster session, Annual Meeting of the American Psychological Association, Montreal, Canada.

Reese, E., & Farrant, K. (2003). Social origins of reminiscing. In R. Fivush & C. A. Haden, (Eds.), Autobiographical memory: Theoretical and applied perspectives (pp. 29–48). Nahwah, NJ: Lawrence Erlbaum.

Reker, G. T., & Chamberlain, K. (Eds.) (2000). *Exploring existential meaning*: Thousand Oaks, CA.: Sage.

Robinson, J. A., & Taylor, L. R. (1998). Autobiographical memories and self-narratives: A tale of two stories. In C. P. Thompson, D. G. Herrmann, D. Bruce, J. Don Read, D. G. Payne, & M. P. Toglia (Eds.), *Autobiographical memory: Theoretical and applied perspectives* (pp. 125–143). London: Lawrence Erlbaum.

Rönkä, A., Oravala, S., & Pulkkinen, L. (2003). Conceiving the past and future. *Personality and Social Psychology Bulletin, 7,* 807–818.

Rubin, D. C. (Ed.) (1986). *Autobiographical memory.* Cambridge: Cambridge University Press.

Rubin, D. C. (Ed.) (1995). Remembering our past. Cambridge: Cambridge University Press.

Rubin, D. C., & Berntsen, D. (2003). Life scripts help to maintain autobiographical memories of highly positive, but not highly negative events. *Memory & Cognition, 31,* 1–14.

Rubin, D. C., Rahhal, T. A., & Poon, L. W. (1998). Things learned in early adulthood are remembered best. *Memory & Cognition, 26,* 3–19.

Schacter, D. (2001). *The seven sins of memory.* Boston: Houghton Mifflin.

Schaie, K. W. (2005). *Developmental influences on adult intelligence.* New York: Oxford University Press.

Schroots, J. J. F. (2003). Life-course dynamics: A research program in progress from The Netherlands. *European Psychologist, 8,* 192–199.

Schroots, J. J. F., & Assink, M. H. J. (2004). LIM/life story: A comparative content analysis. *Tijdschrift voor Ontwikkelingspsychologie, 25,* 3–40.

Schroots, J. J. F., & Assink, M. H. J. (2005). Portraits of life: Patterns of events over the lifespan. *Journal of Adult Development, 12,* 183–198.

Schroots, J. J. F., & Birren, J. E. (1993). Theoretical issues and basic questions in the planning of longitudinal studies of health and aging. In J. J. F. Schroots (Ed.), *Aging, health and competence: The next generation of longitudinal research* (pp. 3–34). Amsterdam: Elsevier Science.

Schroots, J. J. F., & Birren, J. E. (2002). The study of lives in progress: Approaches to research on life stories. In G. D. Rowles & N. E. Schoenberg (Eds.), *Qualitative gerontology: A comparative perspective* (2nd edition, pp. 51–65). New York: Springer.

Schroots, J. J. F., & van Dijkum, C. (2004). Autobiographical memory bump: A dynamic lifespan model. *Dynamical Psychology,* http://www.goertzel.org/dynapsyc/2004/autobio.htm.

Schroots, J. J. F., van Dijkum, C., & Assink, M. H. J. (2004). Autobiographical memory from a lifespan perspective. *International Journal of Aging and Human Development, 58,* 91–115.

Settersten, R. A. (1999). *Lives in time and place: The problems and promises of developmental science.* New York: Baywood.

Sherman, E. (1991). *Reminiscence and the self in old age.* New York: Springer.

Staudinger, U. M. (1989). *The study of life review.* Berlin: Max-Planck Institute.

Staudinger, U. M., Bluck, S., & Yorck Herzberg, P. (2003). Looking back and looking ahead: Adult age differences in consistency of diachronous ratings of subjective well-being. *Psychology and Aging, 18,* 13–24.

Sterns, H. L., & Huyck, M. H. (2001). The role of work in midlife. In M. E. Lachman (Ed.), *Handbook of midlife development* (pp. 447–486). New York: Wiley.

Strongman, K. T. (1996). Emotion and memory. In C. Magai & S. H. McFadden (Eds.), *Handbook of emotion, adult development and aging* (pp. 133–147). San Diego: Academic Press.

Sugarman, L. (1986). *Life-span development: Concepts, theories and interpretations.* London: Methuen & Co.

Suh, E., Diener, E., & Fujita, F. (1996). Events and subjective well-being: Only recent events matter. *Journal of Personality and Social Psychology, 70,* 1091–1102.

Thompson, C. P. (1998). The bounty of everyday memory. In C. P. Thompson, D. J. Herrmann, D. Bruce, J. Don Read, D. G. Payne, & M. P. Toglia (Eds.), *Autobiographical memory: Theoretical and applied perspectives* (pp. 29–44). London: Lawrence Erlbaum.

Tulving, E. (1972). Episodic and semantic memory. In E. Tulving & W. Donaldson (Eds.), *Organization of memory* (pp. 381–403). New York: Academic Press.

Tulving, E. (2002). Episodic memory: From mind to brain. *Annual Review of Psychology, 53,* 1–25.

Walker, W. R., Skowronski, J. J., & Thompson, C. P. (2003). Life is pleasant – and memory helps to keep it that way! *Review of General Psychology, 7,* 203–210.

Webster. J. D., & Haight, B. K. (Eds.) (2002). *Critical advances in reminiscence work: From theory to application.* New York: Springer.

Windle, G., & Woods, R. T. (2004). Variations in subjective well-being: The mediating role of a psychological resource. *Ageing & Society, 24,* 583–602.

Yang, J. A., & Rehm, L. P. (1993). A study of autobiographical memories in depressed and non-depressed elderly individuals. *International Journal of Aging and Human Development, 36,* 39–55.

Zautra, A. J., Affleck, G., & Tennen, H. (1994). Assessing life events among older adults. In M. P. Lawton & J. A. Teresi (Eds.), *Annual review of gerontology and geriatrics* (Vol. 14, pp. 324–352). New York: Springer.

Twenty-Two

Religion and Health in Late Life

Neal Krause

Psychologists have been studying religion for over 100 years (e.g., James, 1902/1997). Recently, however, there has been a dramatic resurgence of interest in religion fueled primarily by empirical research on religion and health. As a mounting number of studies suggest, older people who are more deeply involved in religion tend to enjoy better physical and mental health than older adults who are not religious (Koenig, McCullough, & Larson, 2001). It should be emphasized that a good deal of this research has taken place within gerontology. In fact, as Levin (2004) points out, this is one place where gerontology has made its influence and contributions especially well known.

However, work on religion is far from complete because we still do not know precisely how the potentially salubrious effects of religion on health arise. This task is not easy because religion is a complex phenomenon that consists of a number of different dimensions. Evidence of this may be found, for example, in research by Fetzer Institute/National Institute on Aging Working Group (1999). These investigators identified 12 different facets or dimensions of religion.

Research on religion and health is also hampered by challenges that are not often encountered elsewhere. More specifically, this research is marred by a good deal of controversy, most of which involves methodological issues (Sloan, Bagiella, & Powell, 1999). For example, Sloan et al. (1999) argued that many researchers fail to control for confounding measures and often fail to adjust data for the fact that multiple comparisons (i.e., multiple tests of significance) have been performed. Unfortunately, this controversy is more emotionally charged than many other academic debates. One way to resolve these problems is to derive more compelling theories and to present more persuasive empirical findings.

It would be difficult to examine all 12 dimensions of religion identified by the Fetzer Institute/National Institute on Aging Working Group (1999) in this chapter. Consequently, the discussion that follows focuses on six dimensions of religion that appear to have the greatest potential for illuminating the nature of the relationship between religion and health in late life. The six dimensions examined are church attendance, prayer, religious coping responses, forgiveness, church-based social support, and religious meaning. In the process of exploring these dimensions of religion, an emphasis is placed on two issues that should add to our understanding of the field. First, an effort is made to highlight the changes in each dimension that might occur across the life course and how these changes may influence health and well-being. Pursuing these issues should help ensure that the study of religion and health gets an even stronger geronto-logical voice. Second, an effort is made to look for logical connections among the different dimensions of religion. Each facet of religion does not operate in isolation from the others, even though some studies make it appear as if this were so. It is time to move beyond the identification of potentially important dimensions of religion to the business of building causal models. Although it is too early to devise definitive models, reflecting on how dimensions of religion might be interrelated is a neces-sary first step.

After reviewing the different dimen-sions of religion, the discussion provided closes with an examination of broader life course issues in the study of religion. Here, an emphasis is placed on approach-ing the study of age-related change in religion in new ways that are capable of accommodating the diverse ways in which religiousness is manifest over the life course.

I. Church Attendance

A. Church Attendance, Health, and Well-Being

Initially, a good deal of the empirical work on religion and health focused solely on the relationship between the frequency of church attendance and health. Especially compelling find-ings have emerged from studies on the frequency of church attendance and

mortality. This work reveals that people who attend worship services more often are less likely to die over the course of a study than individuals who do not go to church as frequently (Hummer et al., 1999). Researchers soon realized, however, that it was difficult to explain these findings because attending religious services is a complex form of behavior that exposes a person to a wide range of religious influences. For example, attend-ing worship services involves engaging in rituals (e.g., communion), prayer, listen-ing to sermons, listening to or partici-pating in religious music, and interacting with fellow church members. As a result, it is difficult to know which factor (or factors) influences health.

Given this lack of conceptual clarity in measures of church attendance, research-ers began to explore a wide range of more focused aspects of religion (e.g., prayer; see Poloma & Gallup, 1991). As a result, church attendance is presently used in one of two ways in empirical research. First, it is included in some analyses as a control variable. Here, investigators try to show how other facets of religion, such as church-based social support, contribute to health and well-being above and beyond the influ-ence of church attendance. Second, other researchers try to document how church attendance affects health by developing causal models. In this instance, church attendance is used as an exogenous variable, and an effort is made to show that it affects health indirectly through other dimensions of religion. For example, there is some evidence that more frequent church attendance is associated with receiving more support from fellow church members and that church-based support is, in turn, associated with less psycholo-gical distress (Nooney & Woodrum, 2002). The second use of church atten-dance is the more rewarding of the two. Instead of trying to pit one dimension of religion against another in a misguided effort to see which has the greatest direct effect on health, causal models show how various facets of religion work together as part of a larger process that may ultimately influence the health of older people.

B. Change in Church Attendance over the Life Course

There is some evidence that rates of church attendance change over the life course. For example, some studies indicate that church attendance is relatively high early in life, tapers off in young adulthood, but then subsequently increases throughout the rest of life (Bahr, 1970). However, there are two reasons why this research falls short. First, a good deal of this work is based on cross-sectional data. As discussed in Section VII, a number of serious shortcomings arise when researchers try to study age-related change with data that have been gathered at a single point in time. Second, this work fails to do justice to the complex patterns that are present because significant variation in church attendance may arise solely within late life. More specifically, research indicates that rates of church attendance are relatively high among the young-old. However, as the inevitable decline of physical and mental functioning sets in, the frequency of church attendance begins to decline among the old-old, especially the oldest-old (Koenig et al., 2001).

However, rather than signaling a disengagement from religion, older adults may simply rely on other ways to practice their faith. For example, some may continue to follow worship services on television and the radio. In addition, a number of congregations have outreach services for home-bound elders. This involves having members of the congregation go out to the homes of elderly shut-ins to provide them with tapes of services or to help them celebrate communion. Finally, there is consistent evidence that some private religious practices, such as prayer, may not decline with advancing age (Barna, 2002).

II. Prayer

A. Prayer, Health, and Well-Being

William James claimed that prayer is "...the very soul and essence of religion" (James, 1902/1997, p. 486). Describing prayer as "...religion in action...," James believed that prayer is the arena in which the work of religion is done (p. 486). Similar views were expressed by Martin Luther, who argued that religion is "...prayer and nothing but prayer" (as reported by Heiler, 1932, p. xiii). Research on the frequency of prayer is consistent with these views because this work indicates that prayer may be the most common form of religious practice. More specifically, Gallup and Lindsay (1999) reported that over 90% of adult Americans pray and 74% indicate they pray at least once a day. Given the central role of prayer in religious life, it is not surprising to find it has been the subject of considerable research (e.g., Poloma & Gallup, 1991).

Even though a good deal of research has examined the relationship between prayer and health, most studies focus solely on how often people pray (e.g., Levin, Taylor, & Chatters, 1994). Although this research is important, it says nothing about the purpose, content, experiences, or expectations of the person who prays. As a result, it is difficult to pinpoint the precise mechanisms that may link prayer with health in late life. Fortunately, some progress has been made in this respect. For example, some investigators have focused on the content of prayer (i.e., they study what people pray for specifically and how they go about praying). This research suggests that meditative or contemplative prayer exerts a more beneficial effect on well-being than other types of prayer (e.g., petitionary prayer) (Poloma & Gallup, 1991). Other investigators report that prayer is an important coping resource that helps people deal more effectively with the noxious effects of stress (Pargament, 1997).

Two recent studies help extend research on prayer and health in new directions. The first study focuses on praying for other people. Based on data from a nationwide survey, the author found that praying for others provides health-related benefits to the person offering the prayer (Krause, 2003a). In order to see why this may be so, it is important to reflect on what praying for others may actually entail. Praying for others involves asking God to help someone else. If a person feels their prayers have been answered, and significant others got what they needed, then praying for others may be construed as a form of social support. This is important because research in secular settings reveals that helping others often provides health-related benefits for support providers as well as support recipients (Reissman, 1965).

The second study has to do with beliefs about how prayer operates. The author's research reveals that feelings of self-esteem are higher among older people who believe that only God knows when it is best to answer a prayer and only He knows the best way to answer it (Krause, 2004a). In contrast, self-esteem tends to be lower among elderly people who believe prayers are answered right away and they get exactly what they ask for.

Another possible explanation for the relationship between religion and health may be found in the work of Benson (1996). His research revealed that engaging in religious rituals, such as prayer, elicits the relaxation response. The relaxation response involves a series of physiological changes in the body, including decreased metabolism, lower blood pressure, and a decline in heart rate. These physiological changes are important because they are associated with better health.

Other potential mechanisms have been identified by Levin (2004). He argues that congregational prayer makes people feel that they are more closely connected to others, thereby eradicating feelings of loneliness and social isolation. This is important because a considerable number of studies link social isolation with poor health (Cohen, 2004). In addition, Levin (2004) further proposes that prayer provides a deep sense of meaning in life and that deriving a sense of meaning is associated with better health.

B. Change in Prayer over the Life Course

Research by Gallup and Lindsay (1999) indicated that older people pray more often than younger adults. However, as the discussion provided earlier reveals, this is an overly simplistic way of assessing prayer. Perhaps one of the most comprehensive studies of age differences in prayer was conduced by Peacock and Poloma (1999). Their research examined age differences in different types of prayer (e.g., meditative, petitionary, ritualistic). Their findings reveal that people aged 65 and over are more likely than younger adults to offer each type of prayer. The work of Peacock and Palmoa (1999) further revealed that positive prayer experiences (e.g., feeling divinely inspired during prayer or receiving deeper religious insight during prayer) tend to be encountered more often by older than by younger adults. Unfortunately, this study is based on cross-sectional data, making it difficult to distinguish among age, period, and cohort effects.

Although there is some evidence that prayer changes with age, it is difficult to determine why this is so. Fortunately, some insights may be found by extending Schulz and Heckhausen's (1996) life course theory of control. Their theory was developed to explain how older adults adjust to the inevitable decline of resources in late life. The distinction between primary and secondary control figures prominently in this perspective. Viewed in general terms, primary control refers to efforts aimed at changing the external environment, whereas secondary control is concerned with changing internal cognitions (e.g., attitudes, attributions, and perceptions) rather than altering the external world. Following the theory of selection, optimization, and compensation (Baltes, 1991), Schulz and Heckhausen (1996) argued that as people age, and their resources dwindle, they gradually relinquish primary control in some areas of life so available resources can be devoted to maintaining primary control in other domains.

Although Schulz and Heckhausen (1996) did not discuss the use of religion in the process they described, it is possible to extend their work to show how religion (and especially prayer) might be involved. Some older people cope with diminishing age-related resources by relying on God-mediated control (Berrenberg, 1987). Although it is hard to find a good definition of God-mediated control, this construct is based on the notion that problems in life can be overcome by turning things over to God. However, it is important to reflect on how this is accomplished. This is where prayer comes in. Some researchers argue that Hallesby's (1994) book on prayer is one of the definitive works in the field (Faber, 2002). Hallesby maintains that

"Helplessness is the real secret and the impelling power of prayer" (1994, p. 23). He goes on to argue that, when praying, "...all that is necessary is to be reconciled with one's helplessness and let our holy and almighty God care for us" (p. 26). Viewed within the context of the present discussion, Hallesby's (1994) work reveals that prayer is one of the primary mechanisms for turning control of life over to God. If this extension of the work of Schulz and Heckhausen (1996) is valid, then turning control of life over to God through prayer may be a form of secondary control and may help explain why prayer increases with advancing age.

III. Religious Coping Responses

A. Religious Coping, Health, and Well-Being

One of the major functions of religion is to help people deal with adversity. Although this may happen in a number of ways, extensive research by Pargament (1997) suggested that religion helps by providing people with time-honored coping responses. These coping mechanisms involve specific cognitive and behavioral responses that people may initiate in an effort to either ward off or diminish the impact of undesirable stressful events. This means, for example, that people may deal with a stressor by turning to God for guidance and strength.

Pargament's (1997) research indicated that people who engage in positive religious coping responses are less likely to suffer from the health-related effects of stress than individuals who do not rely on positive religious coping responses. However, his work further showed that people may also respond to stress by turning to negative religious coping responses. For example, some individuals may believe they are facing adversity because God is punishing them for something they did in the past. Others may feel abandoned by God when especially noxious events are encountered. In essence, this type of coping response aims to reduce distress by attributing responsibility for a life event to someone other than the self (i.e., God). Pargament's (1997) research suggested that people who turn to negative religious coping responses tend to experience more psychological stress. Moreover, his work showed that the magnitude of the impact of negative coping response on well-being is greater than the corresponding effect of positive coping responses. Research on negative coping responses is important because it shows that religion may have an adverse, as well as a beneficial, effect on health and well-being.

B. Change in Religious Coping over the Life Course

Unfortunately, most of the research on religious coping responses has been done with younger adults. As a result, we know little about change in the use of religious coping responses with advancing age. Some evidence shows that older people are more likely to rely on positive religious coping responses than younger individuals (Pargament, 1997), but it is not clear why this may be so. On the one hand, the positive relationship between age and religious coping may simply be due to the fact that people become more involved in religion generally as they grow older. Alternatively, one might argue that the greater use of religious coping responses is a function of age-related change in the nature of the stressors that people face. More specifically, problems such as declining cognitive functioning and the death of a loved one become more

frequent with age. Unfortunately, these problems are very difficult to eradicate or change. As Gottlieb (1997) pointed out, religion may, therefore, be especially useful for coping with this type of difficulty.

Neither of these explanations is very satisfying. Instead, we need a better rationale that is more firmly grounded in a fully articulated theory of development in late life. Unfortunately, there do not appear to be any theoretical discussions of the developmental mechanisms that drive age-related change in the use of religious coping responses. Developing the necessary theoretical groundwork should be a high priority for those working in this field.

IV. Forgiveness

A. Forgiveness, Health, and Well-Being

Research reveals that virtually every major religion in the world places a significant emphasis on the importance of forgiving others (Rye et al., 2000). This is especially true with respect to the Christian faith. As a result, it is not surprising to find there has been a good deal of work in the field. However, as this research has evolved, it has become evident that there are a number of ways in which forgiveness can be practiced (McCullough, Pargament, & Thoresen, 2000). More specifically, there is forgiveness of others, forgiveness of self by God, forgiveness of self by others, and self-forgiveness. So far, most research has focused on forgiving others. A good deal of this work has been done outside the context of religion (Enright & North, 1998). Even so, research in secular settings is relevant for two reasons. First, the findings from these studies indicate that people who forgive other individuals tend to have better mental health than individuals who are less willing to forgive other people for the things they have done (Thoresen, Harris, & Luskin, 2000). Unfortunately, less research has been done on forgiving others and physical health status. Second, some evidence shows that people who are more involved in religion are more likely to forgive others than individuals who are less religious (Bono & McCullough, 2004).

Krause & Ellison, (2003) found evidence that the process of forgiving others may be more complicated than it seems. More specifically, the study indicates that how an older person goes about forgiving others may be important. Based on earlier qualitative research, it was found that some older adults tend to forgive others right away (Krause & Ingersoll-Dayton, 2001). In contrast, other elderly people require transgressors to perform acts of contrition before they are willing to forgive them. These acts of contrition involve making an apology, promising not to commit the transgression again, and making restitution whenever possible. Quantitative findings indicate that forgiving others right away tends to exert a positive effect on a wide range of mental health outcomes, whereas requiring others to perform acts of contrition has a negative effect on well-being (Krause & Ellison, 2003). An effort was also made to determine why some older people are willing to forgive right away, whereas others are not. Research revealed that those who forgive right away do so because they believe God has forgiven them right away for their own transgressions. This finding is important because it shows that the different modes of forgiveness may be interrelated.

Clearly, a good deal of work remains to be done on forgiveness. For example, researchers have yet to resolve thorny issues involving the difference between forgiveness and reconciliation.

This problem arises because people may say they have forgiven others, but find it is difficult to truly put the transgression behind them and restore a damaged relationship to where it was before the problem arose.

We also need to know much more about self-forgiveness. Enright and colleagues defined self-forgiveness as "...a willingness to abandon self-resentment in the face of one's own acknowledged objective wrong while fostering compassion, generosity, and love toward oneself" (Enright & the Human Development Group, 1996, p. 116). Research by Maltby, Macaskill, and Day (2001) indicated that failure to forgive one's self is associated with greater psychological distress among younger people. Similarly, Toussaint and co-workers (2001) reported that self-forgiveness is associated with fewer symptoms of depression among people of all ages, including the elderly.

Finally, we need to know more about why forgiveness may be related to health. One potentially important mechanism has been identified by Bono and McCullough (2004). Research reviewed by these investigators suggests that forgiveness is associated with lower levels of anger and hostility. This is important because a vast literature links anger and hostility with an increased risk of cardiovascular disease (for a review of this research, see Bono & McCullough, 2004). Similarly, Worthington (2004) provided evidence indicating that people who forgive more readily tend to experience fewer negative emotions, and individuals who experience fewer negative emotions tend to have more effective immune functioning.

B. Change in Forgiveness over the Life Course

Some investigators suggest that an important facet of forgiveness — vengefulness

— is a trait (McCullough et al., 2001). To the extent this is true, forgiveness should remain fairly stable over the life course. However, research by a number of investigators suggests this may not be so. For example, Mullet and colleagues conducted several studies on the relationship between age and forgiving others (e.g., Girard & Mullet, 1997). This research revealed that there is a steady increase in the propensity to forgive others from adolescence through old age. Unfortunately, this work suffers from two limitations. First, data are cross-sectional. In addition, it is not entirely clear why these age-related changes arise.

Some insight into the relationship between age and forgiving others may be found in Butler's research on the life review (Butler & Lewis, 1982). These investigators maintained that as people enter late life, they invest a significant amount of time reviewing the experiences they have had with an eye toward weaving the story of their lives into a more coherent whole. Themes of forgiveness figure prominently in this process. More specifically, Butler and Lewis (1982) argued that one of the key developmental tasks in the life review process is the "...expiation of guilt, the resolution of intrapsychic conflicts, and the reconciliation of family relationships" (p. 326).

Research on forgiveness is important because it provides one way of showing how the work we do can be used to improve the quality of life of our aging population. If forgiveness becomes more important with age and if we can learn more about the best way to forgive others, then we should have a solid foundation for clinical intervention. In fact, significant inroads have already been made in this respect. A number of investigators have devised clinical interventions aimed at fostering forgiveness through secular

(Hargrave & Andersen, 1992) as well as religious means (Worthington, 1993).

V. Church-Based Social Support

A. Church-Based Social Support, Health, and Well-Being

Josiah Royce was a leading philosopher of his day and a close friend of William James. In 1911, Royce (1912/2000) delivered a series of lectures that were designed to confront what he felt were serious oversights in the work of James (1902/1997). Chief among these oversights was the emphasis placed by James (1902/1997) on the role of unconscious processes in the generation of religious feelings and religious insights. Royce (1912/2000) argued that instead of arising from within the individual, the impetus for religious experiences and sentiments was decidedly social in nature. More specifically, he maintained that "...our social experience is our principle source of religious insight. And the salvation that this insight brings to our knowledge is salvation through the fostering of human brotherhood" (1912/2000, p. 58). In essence, Royce was arguing that social relationships form the foundation of religion. These observations are important because a vast literature conducted in secular settings reveals that social relationships have a profound effect on physical and mental health (Cohen, 2004). As a result, any discussion of the relationship between religion and health cannot afford to overlook the potentially important role played by social relationships in the church.

However, the task of examining social ties in the church is challenging because, as research reveals (Krause, 2002a), there are at least 12 different dimensions or components of church-based social relationships. A good deal of this involves church-based social support, which has to do with assistance exchanged among people who worship in the same congregation.

This is not the place to conduct an in-depth review of social relationships in the church. Such an undertaking would require a separate chapter. Instead, one way to approach this vast domain is to selectively review how church-based social support may influence health and whether there is anything about this type of assistance that is unique to religious settings.

People at church may help each other in a number of ways. For example, as research suggests (Krause, 2002a), individuals who worship together may exchange emotional and tangible assistance. This is important because a considerable number of studies conducted in secular settings indicate that emotional and tangible support tend to bolster the health and well-being of older people (Cohen, 2004). There are a number of ways in which this can happen. For example, as research in secular settings reveals, tangible and (especially) emotional support may affect health by helping older people cope more effectively with the deleterious effects of stress. In addition, these secular studies indicate that the beneficial effects of support arise because informal others help replenish key psychological resources that have been eroded by stressful events (i.e., self-esteem and feelings of personal control; for a detailed discussion of this research, see Krause, 2005). If emotional and tangible support outside the church function in this manner, then it is reasonable to assume that emotional support and tangible help provided by fellow church members may operate in much the same way. However, it is surprising to find that relatively little research has been done on these issues with older adults.

Fellow church members may also help each other in ways that are largely unique to religious institutions and that typically do not arise in the secular world. One unique function of social ties in the church may be found in research on spiritual support (Krause, 2002b). Spiritual support is assistance that is intended to explicitly enhance the religious beliefs, religious behavior, and religious experiences of the recipient, e.g., a fellow church member may help an older person find solutions to their problems in the Bible or they may help them get to know God better.

There are at least two reasons why spiritual support is important. First, as research indicates, spiritual support is associated with a greater use of positive religious coping responses (Krause et al., 2001). This is important because, as noted earlier, the use of positive religious coping responses is associated with better physical and mental health (Pargament, 1997). Second, there is some evidence that spiritual support makes older people feel closer to God, and those who feel closer to God are likely to be more optimistic (Krause, 2002b). This is noteworthy because this study shows that greater optimism is, in turn, associated with better health.

Although we are beginning to better understand how church-based social support may influence health, a number of potentially important mechanisms have not been evaluated empirically. One that is based on secular research in social psychology appears to be especially promising. Building on long-standing principles in the field, Trice and Wallace (2003) maintain that a sense of self arises from the reflected appraisals of significant others. However, they go on to point out that this process is more complex than it seems initially. Social psychologists argue that the self is a multifaceted entity that is composed of a number of different components.

One is the ideal self. This represents how people would like to see themselves and what they aspire to become. Trice and Wallace (2003) reviewed research showing that a focal person will readily internalize reflected appraisals provided by others when these appraisals are consistent with and bolster the ideal self. Moreover, the focal person will be more likely to behave in a manner that is consistent with the ideal self when it is reinforced by feedback from significant others. Simply put, this research reveals that close others tend to call out the best in us. And when they do, we are more likely to act in accordance with these positive ideals.

What is missing from the discussion provided by Trice and Wallace (2003) is a sense of what the ideal self encompasses and who people actually aspire to become. It is precisely at this point that religion may make a significant contribution. More specifically, religion provides a number of goals and ideals that people are encouraged to pursue. Cast within the context of the work reviewed by Trice and Wallace (2003), this means that religion may play a significant role in shaping the ideal self. Because all facets of the self arise only from interaction with others, it follows that an important function of church-based social support is to encourage the development and adoption of an ideal self that is based on religious principles and teachings. In fact, this may well be one of the most important functions of spiritual support. Viewed in this way, religion may be construed as the search for, and effort to attain, a specific type of ideal self.

B. Change in Church-Based Social Support over the Life Course

There does not appear to be any research in the literature on age-related change in church-based social support. Even so,

it is possible to speculate on this issue by turning to secular theoretical perspectives on aging and social relationships.

Carstensen's (1991) theory of socioemotional selectivity is helpful in this regard. She maintains that as people grow older, they tend to place greater value on relationships that are emotionally close. As a result, the number of ties maintained with others declines, but the emotional closeness of those that remain intensifies. Virtually every religion extols the virtues of loving one another and taking care of those in need. In addition, as discussed earlier, all major religious traditions encourage the forgiveness of others. This suggests that social ties in the church may be deeper, and more emotionally focused, than social relationships in secular settings. If this is true, then socioeomotional selectivity theory would predict that church-based emotional support should become increasingly important as people grow older.

A similar view on age-related change in social relationships is provided by Tornstam's (1997) theory of gerotranscendence. He argued that as people get older, they experience a profound shift in the way they view the world. Part of this shift involves the way social relationships are formed. Tornstam (1997) maintained that with advancing age, people become more selective in the relationships they form and they prefer deeper relationships with a few individuals instead of a larger number of more superficial ties. If social relationships in the church tend to have a deeper, more emotional focus, then Tornstam's (1997) theory would predict that they should become especially important as people go through late life.

Although there is a reasonable basis for expecting church-based social ties to become increasingly important with age, there is little empirical research on this issue. However, some indirect evidence may be found (Krause & Wulff, 2005). This study revealed that, after the frequency of church attendance is controlled statistically, there are no age differences in the proportion of friends found in church. We need to know a good deal more about age-related change in church-based social support.

VI. Religious Meaning in Life

A. Religious Meaning, Health, and Well-Being

Another of the primary functions of religion is to provide people with a sense of meaning in life. Evidence of this may be found in the classic work of Clark (1958), who argued that "...religion more than any other human function satisfies the need for meaning in life" (p. 419). Reker (1997) defined meaning as "...having a sense of direction, a sense of order, and a reason for existence, a clear sense of personal identity, and a greater social consciousness" (p. 710). Religious meaning is simply a sense of meaning that arises specifically from the beliefs, teachings, and practices of a given faith.

The author has conducted two studies that link religious meaning with psychological well-being in late life. The first study indicates that older adults who derive a sense of meaning in life from religion tend to have higher levels of life satisfaction, self-esteem, and optimism than elderly people who do not find meaning in life through religion (Krause, 2003b).

The second study extends these insights in two ways (Krause, 2004b). First, it shows that finding meaning in life through religion is also associated with fewer symptoms of depression. More importantly, however, this study suggests that religious meaning arises from a complex process that involves several other facets of religion. More specifically, data indicate that older people who go to church more often tend to get more emotional and spiritual support from the people who worship there. The findings further reveal that more emotional and spiritual support from fellow church members is, in turn, associated with a greater sense of religion-based meaning in life. These results serve to underscore a theme that runs throughout this chapter — different dimensions of religion work synergistically to bolster health and well-being in late life. Moreover, by demonstrating that religious meaning arises from interaction with fellow church members, this study shows why Royce (1912/2000) may have been right: Social relationships may indeed form the essence of religion.

Although researchers are beginning to make inroads in the study of religious meaning in life, they must grapple with problems that have plagued the study of meaning in the secular literature for decades. As Baumeister (1991) pointed out, conceptualizing and measuring secular meaning in life is a difficult task. This is complicated by the fact that research on secular meaning in life reveals that this construct encompasses a number of different factors or dimensions (Debats, 1998). Researchers who focus on religious meaning have yet to confront these issues, but they will have to if they hope to move the field forward.

The theoretical underpinnings of research on religious meaning, health, and well-being are not well developed. Consequently, insight into how religious meaning may affect health and well-being must be gleaned from secular research on meaning in life. This work reveals there are at least four ways in which the beneficial effects of religious meaning may arise.

The first may be found in the work of Frankl (1984). According to his view, having a sense of meaning in life is a vitally important resource for dealing with stressful life events. More specifically, he argues that "There is nothing in the world, I venture to say, that would so effectively help one survive even the worst conditions as the knowledge that there is meaning in one's life" (Frankl, 1984, p. 126). However, it is still not clear why meaning should be such an effective coping resource. Fortunately, Frankl (1984) provided further insight into this issue. He maintained that having a sense of meaning in life helps people grow in the face of adversity. This is important because a small but fascinating literature reveals that highly challenging events may sometimes foster positive change and personal growth and that people who are able to reap these benefits tend to enjoy better physical and mental health (Tedeschi & Calhoun, 2004).

In order to understand the second way that religious meaning may influence health and well-being, it is necessary to return to issues in conceptualization and measurement of meaning. Based on research conducted in secular settings, some investigators conclude that having goals to strive for is one important component of meaning in life (Debats, 1998). Goals are targets for the future. Goals help organize current activities and provide a conduit for channeling energies, efforts, and ambitions. However, even though goals are oriented toward the future, they also provide more immediate rewards by promoting a sense of hope and optimism. The essence of this perspective was captured some time ago in Cooley's (1927) discussion of plans, which are closely akin to goals. He maintained that "Able men plan and strive not as being discontented now, but because they need to continue in the hope and sense of achievement they already have. They bring the future into the scene to animate the present.... Our plans are our working hopes and our chief

treasures" (Cooley, 1927, p. 205). It is important to have goals because the sense of optimism and hope they promote may have significant health-protective effects (Peterson, Seligman, & Vaillant, 1988).

The insights provided by Cooley (1927) are helpful because they can be used to illuminate the nature and impact of a sense of religiously based meaning in life as well. Providing people with a set of goals is one of the many important functions of religion. For example, some researchers maintain that one goal of leading a religious life is to develop a deeper more mature faith and greater devotion to God (Koenig, 1994). Although this goal is difficult to attain and is often a lifelong process, endorsing and pursuing this goal may, nevertheless, provide the sense of hope and optimism described by Cooley (1927).

The third way in which religious meaning may influence health is found in secular research reviewed by Ryff and Singer (1998). These investigators pointed out that people with a greater sense of meaning in life tend to enjoy better health because meaning has direct physiological effects on the body. In particular, the positive emotions associated with having a sense of meaning in life may improve health by enhancing immune functioning.

The final way that a sense of religious meaning in life may influence health may be found by turning to problems that have plagued the field for some time. A number of researchers argue that values and beliefs are an integral component of religion (Fetzer Institute/National Institute on Aging Working Group, 1999). However, this is a difficult area to study because the number of religious values and beliefs that people hold are virtually limitless. This poses significant challenges for those interested in studying the relationship among religious values, religious beliefs, and health.

There are two ways to approach this problem. The first involves comparing and contrasting the effects of particular religious values and beliefs on health. However, the scope of this task makes it virtually impossible to complete. Moreover, the prospects of trying to show that some religious beliefs and values are more important than others raises a host of ethical issues. The second approach to getting a handle on religious values and beliefs involves looking beyond their content to the functions they perform. It is precisely at this point that research on the meaning in life can be helpful. As Baumeister (1991) persuasively argued, values and beliefs are important primarily because they give rise to a sense of meaning in life. In a world where the utility and worthiness of specific thoughts and actions are often unclear, values provide the basis for selecting among different options by giving the assurance that personal choices are, in the words of Baumeister (1991), right, good, and justifiable. If values are an important component of meaning, and if they provide a sense of direction, purpose, and legitimacy in daily life, then it is not hard to see how they can enhance feelings of psychological well-being among older people.

B. Change in Religious Meaning over the Life Course

Although there does not appear to be any empirical research in the literature, it is possible to use existing theoretical work to argue that the sense of meaning in life provided by religion may become increasingly important as people grow older. Evidence of this may be found in Erikson's (1959) widely cited theory on development across the life course. He maintained that the life span is divided into eight stages and that each

stage poses unique developmental challenges. The final stage, which arises in late life, is characterized by the crisis of integrity versus despair. This is a time of deep introspection when older individuals try to accept the kind of person they have become over the years. This is accomplished by trying to reconcile what one set out to do in life with what has actually been accomplished. If this crisis is resolved successfully, elderly people develop a deeper sense of meaning in life. However, if it is not resolved successfully, they slip into despair. Viewed more broadly, this theoretical perspective suggests that as people get older, they carefully reevaluate the past in an effort to make sense of the things that have happened to them. Ultimately, the goal of this process is to imbue life with a deeper sense of meaning.

If aging involves a search for a deeper sense of meaning in life and religion provides one way of finding it, then it follows that as people grow older, they may be especially inclined to turn to religion for this purpose. It appears that Erikson was well aware of the relationship between religion and a sense of meaning in life. As Hoare (2002) reported, by the time he reached 80 years of age, Erikson had replaced the word "integrity" with the word "faith" (p. 90).

VII. Issues in Assessing Life Course Changes in Religion

As the discussion provided up to this point consistently reveals, involvement in many dimensions of religion may change with age. In particular, people appear to become more involved in religion as they grow older. However, this does not necessarily mean that the same individual becomes more deeply involved in all facets of religion. Instead, it is more likely that people become more involved in only some dimensions of religion with advancing age. For example, one person may rely more on church-based social support, whereas another individual may utilize religious coping responses more often. The fact that religion speaks to a range of different age-related needs highlights one reason why it has persisted for centuries. The essence of this perspective was captured by James (1902/1997), who maintained that "The divine can mean no single quality, it must mean a group of qualities, by being champions of which in alternation, different men may all find worthy missions" (p. 509). If religion helps different people in different ways, then we must find a way to comes to grips with this diversity as we study change in religion over the life course. In order to see how this might be accomplished, it is necessary to review briefly how researchers approach the study of age-related change in religion. Typically they have taken one of three ways to address this issue.

First, the wide majority of investigators conduct cross-sectional surveys of older and younger adults. Then, they simply compare the responses of older and younger people to questions that cover a number of different facets of religion. For example, some researchers report that those who are presently older pray more than those who are currently younger (Levin, Taylor, & Chatters, 1994). Unfortunately, problems arise with this strategy because data have been gathered at a single point in time. As discussed earlier, it is not possible to distinguish among age, period, and cohort effects.

The second approach to studying age differences in religion improves upon the first because it relies on data that have been gathered from the same individuals over fairly long periods of time. This second approach is exemplified by the work of Wink and Dillon (2001). These investigators studied change in the importance of religion over time using data provided by the same respondents over a 40-year period. Their findings revealed that religion was initially quite important early in life, but then declined around age thirty or forty. However, their data further indicate that the importance of religion then increased significantly around age fifty or sixty.

Although findings from long-term studies are important, there is a potentially serious shortcoming in this approach. More specifically, focusing on aggregate age-related change in religion creates the impression that all people follow a single trajectory of religious involvement over the life course. However, if the insights of James (1902/1997) are accurate, this is not likely to be the case. The limitations associated with searching for a single pattern of change in religion over the life course are illustrated by investigators who take a third approach to research in this field. These researchers gather data on change in religion retrospectively by asking study participants a series of questions about their involvement in religion at specific times in their lives. This means, for example, that older respondents are asked to think back to when they were 20 years of age and report how often they went to church or how often they prayed. These questions are then repeated for different points in the life course (e.g., age forty, age fifty, and age sixty).

The main contribution of this strategy arises from the way in which data are analyzed. Rather than searching for a single trajectory of religious involvement over the life course, researchers who follow this strategy look for multiple patterns of change in religiousness as people grow older. This research reveals, for example, that some individuals remain deeply religious throughout life, others are never involved in religion at any time, and yet others follow a nonlinear pattern of change similar to the one reported by Wink and Dillon (2001) (see George et al., 2004; Ingersoll-Dayton, Krause, & Morgan, 2002). This more complex view of religion and life course is consistent with the basic tenets of Nelson and Dannifer's (1992) aged heterogeneity hypothesis. These investigators maintain that regardless of the conceptual domain under study, there is a general tendency toward greater differentiation among people with advancing age.

Although the insights provided by studies on multiple patterns of change in religion are intriguing, there are limitations in the work that has been done so far. In particular, the fact that data are gathered retrospectively raises the possibility that the findings may be biased by faulty recall as well as inaccurate reporting. Even so, results emerging from this work set an exciting agenda for the future. First, researchers need to identify the different ways in which differing dimensions of religion change as people grow older. Recent advances in the estimation of individual growth curves should be especially helpful for achieving this goal (Raudenbush & Bryk, 2002). This can obviously also be done with longitudinal data mentioned in the second approach discussed earlier. Then, researchers can identify the social and psychological factors that set an individual on one path instead of another. Following this strategy should enable us to move the classic insights of James (1902/1997) beyond the realm of abstract theory to the development of multiple, empirically grounded trajectories of change in religiousness over the life course.

VIII. Conclusions

As the discussion provided throughout this chapter reveals, a good deal of research has been done on the relationship between religion and health in late life. This work provides mounting evidence that religion may indeed have a beneficial effect on the physical and mental health of older people. Although the accelerating pace of this research is encouraging, there is still a great deal we do not know. A number of unresolved issues and unexamined questions were identified earlier, but, this hardly exhausts all the issues that need to be addressed.

With the exception of Pargament's (1997) research on negative religious coping responses, the discussion provided in this chapter has been solely concerned with the potentially beneficial effects of religion. However, as Pargament's (1997) work reveals, there may be a dark underside to religion as well. We need to know more about this because it is important to provide a more balanced view of the bad as well as the good effects of religion. Fortunately, some progress has been made in this respect. More specifically, there are two other ways that religion may erode health and well-being. First, as research reveals, negative interaction may arise in the church and, if it does, people may experience more symptoms of depression (Krause, Ellison, & Wulff, 1998). Second, research suggests that people who have doubts about their faith tend to experience more symptoms of psychological distress (Krause, 2003c). We need to know if there are other negative aspects of being involved in religion. For example, the research that has been done so far on negative interaction in the church focuses primarily on conflict that arises within a congregation (i.e., within-group conflict). However, it would be interesting to see if conflict involving people outside the church (e.g., between-group conflict arising from intolerance of other religions) is associated with more physical or mental health problems as well. In the process, research is needed to directly compare and contrast the relative impact of positive and negative facets of religion on health and well-being in late life.

The discussion provided earlier was cast solely in terms of age-related change in religion. However, this ignores the possibility that there may be cohort differences in religion as well. This issue has rarely been discussed in the literature on religion and health, but it should be. We need basic historical research that probes the differences and similarities in religious involvement across different cohorts of older people. Some thought-provoking evidence of cohort differences is provided by Meredith and Schewe (2002). Their research revealed that levels of religious commitment tend to be higher in the World War II cohort (i.e., those born between 1922 and 1927) than in the cohorts born before and after them. In the process of doing this kind of research, however, it is important to emphasize that the goal is not to see whether age or cohort effects are more important. Instead, it is likely that both operate at the same time. As a result, research is needed to evaluate the relative contributions of both life course factors.

Six dimensions of religion were discussed earlier, but this hardly covers the full content domain of this construct. Research has been conducted in a number of other areas, and it appears that some of them may influence health and well-being in late life. For example, research reveals that older people who feel they have developed a deep personal relationship with God tend to rate their health more favorably than older adults who do not feel close to God (Krause, 2002b). Although a good deal of ground has been covered, researchers

have yet to fully grasp the depth and breadth of religion. As a result, continued effort is needed to flesh out the content domain of religion in late life.

There is extensive evidence of pervasive race differences in levels of religious involvement, as well as marked race differences in the relationship between religion and health. For example, as research reviewed by Taylor, Chatters, and Levin (2004) reveals, older African–Americans tend to be more deeply involved in religion than older whites. Moreover, this research indicates that various dimensions of religion tend to exert a more beneficial effect on the health and well-being of older blacks than older whites. We need to know whether religion also exerts protective effects on older adults in other racial and ethnic groups. For example, more studies are needed that compare and contrast religion and health among older Hispanics and older whites.

However, race represents only one way of exploring the heterogeneity of our aging population. Another important factor is gender. Fairly extensive evidence now shows that older women are more deeply involved in religion than older men (Levin et al., 1994). Even so, it is surprising to find that less is known about the differential impact of religion on health and well-being between older men and older women. More research is needed on this issue. In the process, researchers must remember that gender is nested within race, and as a result, we need to know more about how race and gender intersect to influence health and well-being in late life.

In addition to looking at variations by race and gender, it would also be important to consider cross-national variations in the relationship between religion and health. Some work has already been done in this area (e.g., Lalive d'Epinay & Spini, 2004), but this research has been concerned primarily with the frequency of church attendance and health. Clearly, studies are needed on cross-national differences in other facets of religion. In addition, we need to know more about the relationship between religion in Asian nations and health in late life. Research in non-Western settings may yield especially valuable insights. For example, when individuals go to Shinto shrines in Japan, they are more likely to engage in private devotionals than group worship activities (Nelson, 2000). As a result, social relationships with fellow worshipers may be weaker in Japan than in the United States. It was argued earlier, that the relationship between church attendance and health may be explained, at least in part, by the social relationships that arise with fellow church members. If relationships with fellow worshipers in Japan are not as closely knit, then it follows that the relationship between worshiping in religious shrines in Japan and health may not be as strong as the corresponding relationship between church attendance and health in the West.

Finally, the religious and secular worlds do not constitute highly segregated or compartmentalized domains of life. Instead, older people constantly shift from one world to the other. We need to know more about the interface between religious and secular life. For example, research is needed to see if social relationships in the church influence the way older people interact with individuals in the secular world.

Religion is one of the oldest institutions in human society. The very fact that it has persisted for thousands of years suggests it must be performing some important social function and that it must be meeting some basic psychological needs. Significant inroads have been made in identifying these functions, but at the same time, it should be evident that the field is wide open. The findings that have emerged so far are tantalizing, but the gaps in our knowledge are great. A necessary first step in moving the field forward involves developing an appreciation for the work that has been done and the possibilities that exist. Viewed in this way, the research reviewed in this chapter reveals we are on our way, and the work that lies ahead holds out the promise of illuminating some of the most enduring questions about the purpose and meaning of growing old.

References

Bahr, H. M. (1970). Aging and religious disaffiliation. *Social Forces, 49*, 59–71.

Baltes, P. B. (1991). The many faces of aging: Toward a psychology of old age. *Psychological Medicine, 21*, 837–854.

Barna, G. (2002). *The state of the church – 2002*. Ventura, CA: Issachar Resources.

Baumeister, R. F. (1991). *Meanings of life.* New York: Guilford.

Benson, H. (1996). *Timeless healing: The power and biology of belief*. New York: Scribner.

Berrenberg, J. L. (1987). The belief in personal control scale: A measure of God-mediated and exaggerated control. *Journal of Personality Assessment, 51*, 194–206.

Bono, G., & McCullough, M. E. (2004). Religion, forgiveness, and adjustment in older adulthood. In K. W. Schaie, N. Krause, & A. Booth (Eds.), *Religious influences on health and well-being in the elderly* (pp. 163–186). New York: Springer.

Butler, R. N., & Lewis, M. I. (1982). *Aging and mental health.* St. Louis: Mosby.

Carstensen, L. L. (1991). Selectivity theory: Social activity in life span context. *Annual Review of Gerontology and Geriatrics, 11*, 195–217.

Clark, W. H. (1958). *The psychology of religion.* New York: Macmillan.

Cohen, S. (2004). Social relationships and health. *American Psychologist, 59*, 676–684.

Cooley, C. H. (1927). *Life and the student: Roadside notes on human nature, society, and letters.* New York: Knopf.

DeBats, D. L. (1998). Measurement of personal meaning: The psychometric properties of the life regard index. In P. T. P. Wong & P. S. Fry (Eds.), *The human quest for meaning* (pp. 237–259). Mahwah, NJ: Lawrence Erlbaum.

Enright, R. D. and the Human Development Study Group (1996). Counseling within the forgiveness triad: On forgiving, receiving forgiveness, and self-forgiveness. *Counseling and Values, 40*, 107–126.

Enright, R. D., & North, J. (1998). *Exploring forgiveness.* Madison, WI: University of Wisconsin Press.

Erikson, E. (1959). *Identity and the life cycle.* New York: International University Press.

Faber, M. D. (2002). *The magic of prayer: An introduction to the psychology of faith.* Westport, CT: Praeger.

Fetzer Institute/National Institute on Aging Working Group (1999). *Multidimensional measurement of religiousness/spirituality for use in health research.* Kalamazoo, MI: Fetzer Institute.

Frankl, V. (1984). *Man's search for meaning.* New York: Simon & Schuster.

Gallup, G., & Lindsay, D. M. (1999). *Surveying the religious landscape: Trends in U.S. beliefs.* Harrisburg, PA: Morehouse.

George, L. K., Hayes, J. C., Flint, E. P., & Meador, K. G. (2004). Religion and health in life course perspective. In K. W. Schaie, N. Krause, & A. Booth (Eds.), *Religious influences on health and well-being in the elderly* (pp. 246–282). New York: Springer.

Girard, M., & Mullet, E. (1997). Forgiveness in adolescents, young, middle-aged, and older adults. *Journal of Adult Development, 4*, 209–220.

Gottlieb, B. H. (1997). Conceptual and methodological issues in the study of coping with chronic stress. In B. H. Gottlieb (Ed.), *Coping with chronic stress* (pp. 3–40). New York: Plenum.

Hallesby, O. (1994). *Prayer.* Minneapolis: Augsburg.

Hargrave, T. D., & Andersen, W. T. (1992). *Finishing well: Aging and reparation in the intergenerational family.* New York: Brunner/Mazel.

Heiler, F. (1932). *Prayer: A study of the history and psychology of religion.* New York: Oxford University Press.

Hoare, C. H. (2002). *Erikson on development in adulthood.* New York: Oxford University Press.

Hummer, R., Rogers, R., Nam, C., & Ellison, C. G. (1999). Religious involvement and US adult mortality. *Demography, 36*, 273–285.

Ingersoll-Dayton, B., Krause, N., & Morgan, D. L. (2002). Religious trajectories and transitions over the life course. *International Journal of Aging and Human Development, 55*, 51–70.

James, W. (1902/1997). *William James: Selected writings.* New York: Book-of-the-Month Club.

Koenig, H. G. (1994). *Aging and God.* New York: Haworth Pastoral Press.

Koenig, H. G., McCullough, M. E., & Larson, D. B. (2001). *Handbook of religion and health.* New York: Oxford University Press.

Krause, N. (2002a). Exploring race differences in a comprehensive battery of church-based social support measures. *Review of Religious Research, 44*, 126–149.

Krause, N. (2002b). Church-based social support and health in old age: Exploring variations by race. *Journal of Gerontology: Social Sciences, 57B*, S332–S347.

Krause, N. (2003a). Praying for others, financial strain, and physical health status in late life. *Journal for the Scientific Study of Religion, 42*, 377–391.

Krause, N. (2003b). Religious meaning and subjective well-being in late life. *Journal of Gerontology: Social Sciences, 58B*, S160–S170.

Krause, N. (2003c). A preliminary assessment of race differences in the relationship between religious doubt and depressive symptoms. *Review of Religious Research, 45*, 93–115.

Krause, N. (2004a). Assessing the relationships among prayer expectancies, race, and self-esteem in late life. *Journal for the Scientific Study of Religion, 43*, 395–408.

Krause, N. (2004b). Religion and mental health. In R. Hummer & C. G. Ellison (Eds.), *Religion, family, and health.* Oxford University Press.

Krause, N. (2005). Social relationships in late life. In R. H. Binstock & L. K. George (Eds.), *Handbook of aging and the social sciences,* (6th edition). San Diego: Academic Press.

Krause, N., & Ellison, C. E. (2003). Forgiveness by God, forgiveness of others, and psychological well-being in late life. *Journal for the Scientific Study of Religion, 42,* 77–93.

Krause, N., Ellison, C. E., & Wulff, K. M. (1998). Church-based emotional support, negative interaction, and psychological well-being: Findings from a national sample of Presbyterians. *Journal for the Scientific Study of Religion, 37,* 725–741.

Krause, N., Ellison, C. G., Shaw, B. A., Marcum, J. P., & Boardman, J. (2001). Church-based social support and religious coping. *Journal for the Scientific Study of Religion, 40,* 637–656.

Krause, N., & Ingersoll-Dayton, B. (2001). Religion and the process of forgiveness in late life. *Review of Religious Research, 42,* 252–276.

Krause, N., & Wulff, K. M. (2005). Friendship ties in the church and depressive symptoms: Exploring variations by age. *Review of Religious Research, 46:* 325–340.

Lalive d'Epinay, C. J., & Spini, D. (2004). Commentary: Religion and health: A European perspective. In K. W. Schaie, N. Krause, & A. Booth (Eds.), *Religious influences on health and well-being in the elderly* (pp. 44–58). New York: Springer.

Levin, J. S. (2004). Prayer, love, and transcendence: An epidemiologic perspective. In K. W. Schaie, N. Krause, & A. Booth (Eds.), *Religious influences on health and well-being in the elderly* (pp. 69–95). New York: Springer.

Levin, J. S., Taylor, R. J., & Chatters, L. M. (1994). Race and gender differences in religiosity among older adults: Findings from four national surveys. *Journal of Gerontology: Social Sciences, 49,* S137–S145.

Maltby, J., Macaskill, A., & Day, L. (2001). Failure to forgive self and others: A replication and extension of the relationship between forgiveness, personality, and social desirability and general health. *Personality and Individual Differences, 30,* 881–885.

McCullough, M. E., Pargament, K. I., & Thoresen, C. E. (2000). *Forgiveness: Theory, research, and practice.* New York: Guilford.

McCullough, M. E., Bellah, C. G., Kilpatrick, S. D., & Johnson, J. L. (2001). Vengefulness: Relationships with forgiveness, rumination, well-being, and the Big Five. *Personality and Social Psychology Bulletin, 27,* 610–610.

Meredith, G. E., & Schewe, C. D. (2002). *Defining markets defining moments.* New York: Hungry Minds.

Nelson, E. A., & Dannifer, D. (1992). Aged heterogeneity: Fact or fiction? The fate and diversity in gerontological research. *The Gerontologist, 32,* 17–23.

Nelson, J. K. (2000). *Enduring identities: The guise of Shinto in contemporary Japan.* Honolulu: University of Hawaii Press.

Nooney, J., & Woodrum, E. (2002). Religious coping and church-based social support as predictors of mental health outcomes: Testing a conceptual model. *Journal for the Scientific Study of Religion, 41,* 359–368.

Pargament, K. I. (1997). *The psychology of religion and coping: Theory, research, and practice.* New York: Guilford.

Peacock, J. R., & Poloma, M. M. (1999). Religiosity and life satisfaction across the life course. *Social Indicators Research, 48,* 321–345.

Peterson, C., Seligman, M., & Vaillant, G. (1988). Pessimistic explanatory style is a risk factor for physical illness: A thirty-five year longitudinal study. *Journal of Personality and Social Psychology, 55,* 23–27.

Poloma, M. M., & Gallup, G. H. (1991). *Varieties of prayer: A survey report.* Philadelphia: Trinity Press International.

Raudenbush, S. W., & Bryk, A. S. (2002). *Hierarchical linear models: Applications and data analysis methods.* Thousand Oaks, CA: Sage.

Reissman, F. (1965). The "helper" therapy principle. *Social Work, 10,* 27–32.

Reker, G. T. (1997). Personal meaning, optimism, and choice: Existential predictors of depression in community and institutional elderly. *The Gerontologist, 37,* 709–716.

Royce, J. (1912/2000). *The sources of religious insight.* Washington, DC: The Catholic University of America Press.

Rye, M. S., Pargament, K. I., Ali, A., Beck, G. L., Dorff, E. N., Hallisey, C., Narayanan, V., &

Williams, J. G. (2000). Religious perspectives on forgiveness. In M. E. McCullough, K. I. Pargament, & C. E. Thoresen (Eds.), *Forgiveness: Theory, research, and practice* (pp. 17–40). New York: Guilford.

Ryff, C. D., & Singer, B. (1998). The contours of positive human health. *Psychological Inquiry, 9,* 1–28.

Schulz, R., & Heckhausen, J. (1996). A life span model of successful aging. *American Psychologist, 51,* 702–714.

Sloan, R. P., Bagiella, E., & Powell, T. (1999). Religion, spirituality, and medicine. *Lancet, 353,* 664–667.

Taylor, R. J., Chatters, L. M., & Levin, J. S. (2004). *Religion in the lives of African Americans: Social, psychological, and health perspectives.* Thousand Oaks, CA: Sage.

Tedeschi, R. G., & Calhoun, L. G. (2004). Posttraumatic growth: Conceptual foundations and empirical evidence. *Psychological Inquiry, 15,* 1–18.

Thoresen, C. E., Harris, A. H., & Luskin, F. (2000). Forgiveness and health: An unanswered question. In M. E. McCullough, K. I. Pargament, & C. E. Thoresen (Eds.), *Forgiveness: Theory, research and practice* (pp. 254–280). New York: Guilford.

Tornstam, L. (1997). Gerotranscendence: The contemplative dimension of aging. *Journal of Aging Studies, 11,* 143–154.

Toussaint, L. L., Williams, D. R., Musick, M. A., & Everson, S. A. (2001). Forgiveness and health: Age differences in a U. S. probability sample. *Journal of Adult Development, 8,* 249–257.

Trice, D. M., & Wallace, H. M. (2003). The reflected self: Creating yourself as (you think) others see you. In M. R. Leary & J. P. Tangney (Eds.), *Handbook of self and identity* (pp. 91–105). New York: Guilford.

Wink, P., & Dillon, M. (2001). Religious involvement and health outcomes in late adulthood: Findings from a longitudinal study of women and men. In T. G. Plante & A. C. Sherman (Eds.), *Faith and health: Psychological perspectives* (pp. 75–106). New York: Guilford.

Worthington, E. L. (1993). *Psychotherapy and religious values.* Grand Rapids, MI: Baker Book House.

Worthington, E. L. (2004). Commentary: Unforgiveness, forgiveness, religion and health during aging. In K. W. Schaie, N. Krause, & A. Booth (Eds.), *Religious influences on health and well-being among the elderly* (pp. 187–201). New York: Springer.

Author Index

Subject Index